Reader's Digest

EAT BETTER, LIVE BETTER

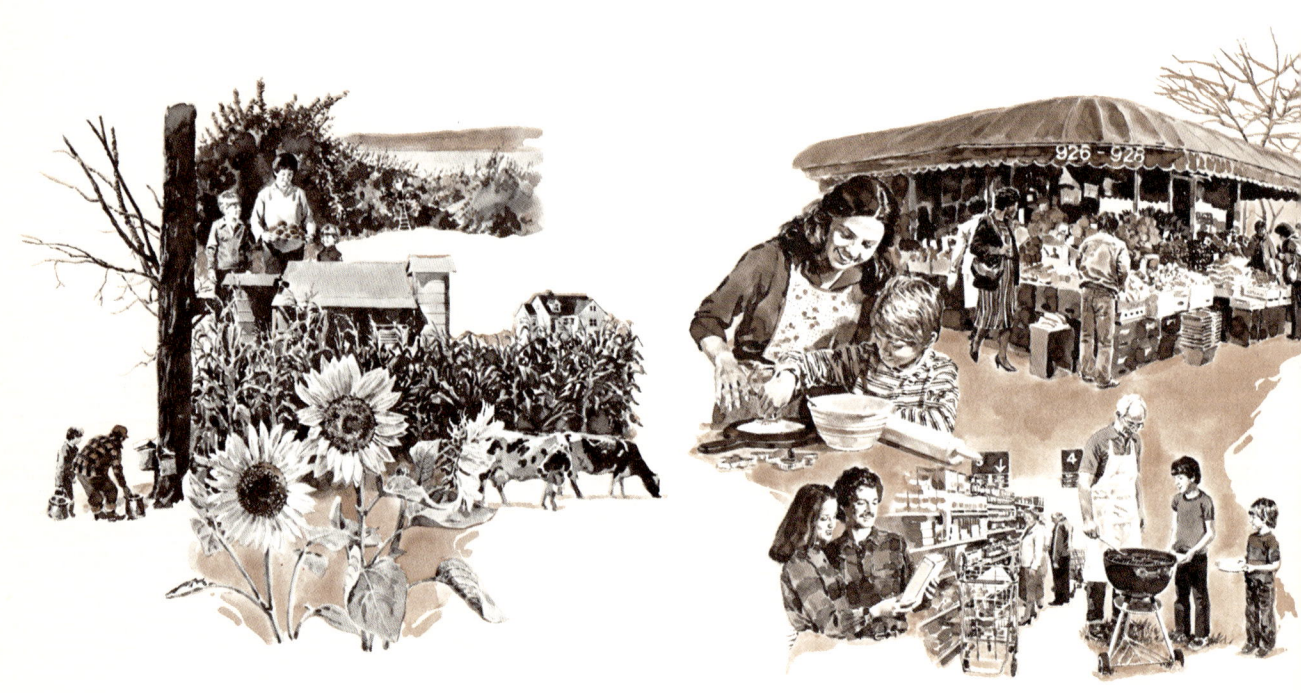

Reader's Digest

EAT BETTER, LIVE BETTER

A Commonsense Guide to Nutrition and Good Health

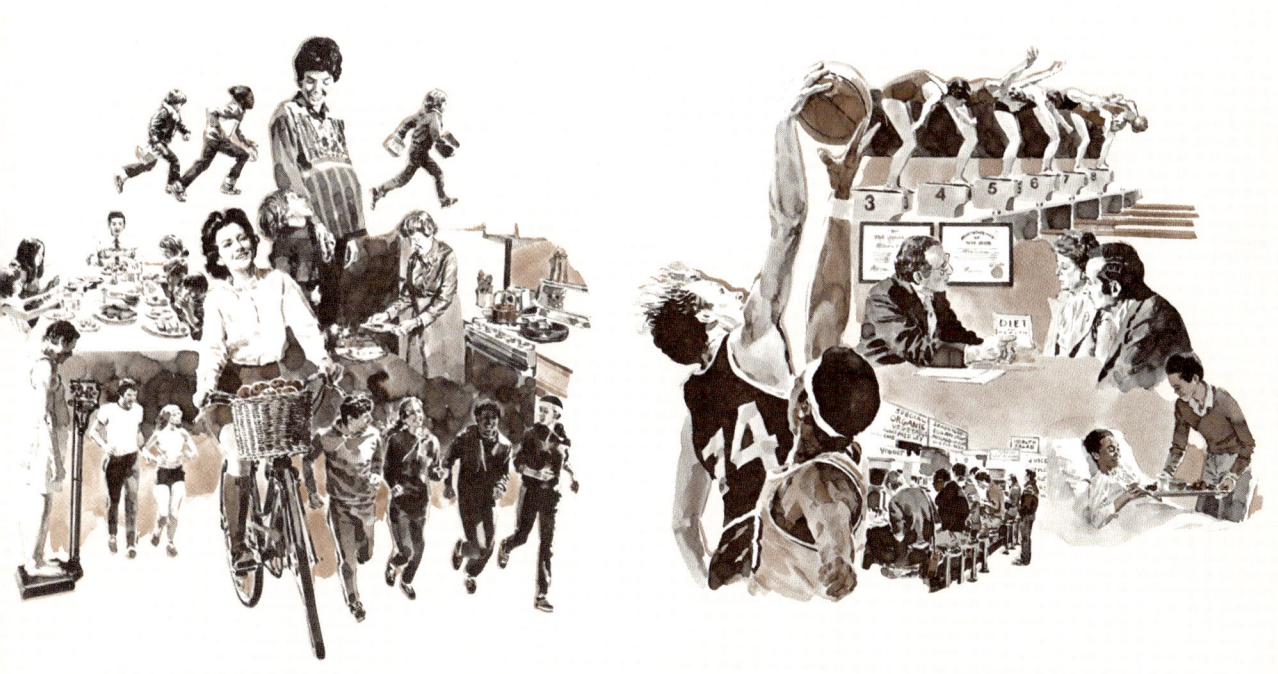

The Reader's Digest Association, Inc.

Pleasantville, New York/Montreal

Eat Better, Live Better

Editor: Joseph L. Gardner
Art Editor: Robert Grant
Associate Editor: Kaari Ward

Research Editors: Muriel Clarke, Mary Jane Hodges
Associate Editors: Ben Etheridge, Sally French,
Therese Hoehlein-Cerbie, Sharon Fass Yates
Copy Editor: Elaine Andrews
Art Assistant: Marlene Rimsky
Editorial Assistant: Ann Purdy
Index: Georgea Atkinson Pace
Food Charts Typist: Grace Del Bagno

Contributing Writers: Robert Bahr, Rebecca Davenport,
Martha Fay, Sara Stein, Karen Theroux

Recipe Consultant: Michèle Urvater

The editors are grateful for the assistance of the Board
of Consultants who reviewed selected portions of the text.
Other consultants are acknowledged on page 399.

BOARD OF CONSULTANTS

Johanna Dwyer, D.Sc.
Chairperson, Francis Stern
   Nutrition Center
Tufts New England Medical Center
Boston

Victor Herbert, M.D., J.D.
Chief, Hematology and Nutrition
   Laboratory
Bronx VA Medical Center
New York

Jerome L. Knittle, M.D.
Professor and Director, Division of
   Nutrition and Metabolism
Mount Sinai School of Medicine
New York

In preparing this volume for publication, the editors have used
reliable and current information. However, there
may be some inconsistencies because of the nutrient
variation in foods and differences among the various sources
consulted. Nothing contained herein is to be construed as a diet
recommended or endorsed by The Reader's Digest Association, Inc.
Individuals should not attempt to gain or lose weight or treat
ailments through diet without consulting a physician.

The acknowledgments and credits that appear on pages 399 - 401
are hereby made a part of this copyright page.
Copyright © 1982 The Reader's Digest Association, Inc.
Copyright © 1982 The Reader's Digest Association (Canada) Ltd.
Copyright © 1982 Reader's Digest Association Far East Ltd.
Philippine Copyright 1982 Reader's Digest Association Far East Ltd.
Reproduction in any manner, in whole or in part, except as
authorized by the Copyright Act, is prohibited.
All rights reserved.
Library of Congress Catalog Card Number 82-60100
ISBN 0-89577-141-1

Printed in the United States of America

Foreword

"The simple fact is that our diets have changed radically within the last 50 years, with great and often very harmful effects on our health. These dietary changes represent as great a threat to public health as smoking. Too much fat, too much sugar or salt, can be and are linked directly to heart disease, cancer, obesity and stroke.... In all, six of the ten leading causes of death in the United States have been linked to our diet."

With these sobering words, Senator George McGovern introduced a landmark U.S. Senate report to the press and public in January 1977. Its premise was that overeating, improper food choices, and alcohol were the main causes of the nation's high rate of obesity and the high incidence of the so-called killer diseases. At least 20 percent of American adults—some estimates put the figure as high as 40 percent—are overweight. Close to one million Americans die each year of heart and artery diseases, more than cancer, stroke, and accidents combined. By setting Dietary Goals for the United States, the Senate report was intended to have a profound effect on the eating patterns of the nation.

The Select Committee on Nutrition and Human Needs of the U.S. Senate was formed in 1968. Originally, it concentrated on programs to eliminate hunger by pulling together information and research from the agriculture and food industries. But as time passed, it became evident that there was a greater problem: an affluent nation stuffing itself with the wrong kinds of food.

Before publication of the Dietary Goals, federal involvement in nutrition had focused on human needs for vitamins, minerals, and protein, as for example in the Recommended Dietary Allowances (see pages 32-33). Now, for the first time, a government body was making recommendations to guide public policy with respect to all the nutrients—carbohydrates and fats as well as protein. The Dietary Goals, in brief, were:

1. Avoid overweight;
2. Increase complex carbohydrates;
3. Eat less sugar;
4. Cut down on fats;
5. Reduce consumption of saturated fats;
6. Reduce cholesterol consumption;
7. Limit salt intake.

In terms of the food Americans put on their dining tables, the Dietary Goals emphasized eating more fruits and vegetables, whole-grain cereals and breads, fish, lean meats such as chicken and turkey, and eating less of fatty meats, butterfat, eggs, and highly salted or sugared foods.

"Nutrition and health education are offered at the same time as barrages of commercials for soft drinks, sugary snacks, high-fat foods, cigarettes, and alcohol," Dr. Beverly Winikoff of the Rockefeller Foundation pointed out at the McGovern press conference. "We put candy machines in our schools, serve high-fat lunches to our children, and place cigarette machines in our work places. The American marketplace provides easy access to sweet soft drinks, high-sugar cereals, candies, cakes, and high-fat beef, and more difficult access to foods likely to improve national nutritional health." The recommendations outlined in the Dietary Goals, she maintained, could reverse the trend.

Dissenting Voices

Predictably, the Dietary Goals report proved controversial. "The McGovern Committee proposes to mount a campaign that will persuade consumers to fill their shopping carts mainly with whole wheat bread, spaghetti and potatoes," said Thomas H. Jukes, a research biochemist at the University of California, Berkeley. "It is a dreary prospect." Representatives of the food industry protested, as did some members of the committee, who suggested a warning: "... science cannot at this time insure that an altered diet will provide improved protection from certain killer diseases."

Of course, there is truth in some of the dissents. An improved diet by itself is no guarantee against contracting a disease or of recovering from one. But it can lower the likelihood of disease or lessen the severity, especially if accompanied by the elimination or reduction of other risk factors in one's lifestyle such as physical inativity, smoking, and alcohol or drug abuse. And in February 1980 the Departments of Agriculture and Health and Human Services issued a set of Dietary Guidelines for Americans that simplified and modified the Dietary Goals (see pages 96-97). This continues to be the basis of government nutrition information and programs.

Even before the Dietary Goals were published, Americans had begun to change their attitudes about food. In the decade 1970-1980, consumption of fresh fruit and vegetables, chicken, fish, margarine, and skim milk was up; eggs, butter, sugar, coffee, and whole milk was down. With or without the endorsement of Washington, nutrition had become a subject of widespread interest. Yet, at the same time, Americans were spending $5 billion annually (total food expenditure: $302.9 billion) on vitamin supplements that most nutrition scientists say are unnecessary for those on a balanced diet. And overweight people were going on crash diets and spending more than $200 million annually on dietary aids that don't and can't work. It was plain that a concerned nation needed more accurate information about food and health. EAT BETTER, LIVE BETTER presents the current facts about nutrition and how it affects our health in one easy-to-read volume.

Four Books in One

The volume is divided into four distinct parts (see Contents opposite). "ABC's of Nutrition" is a primer on the necessary nutrients that fuel your body: carbohydrates, fats, proteins, vitamins, minerals, and water. It concludes with 42 pages of charts giving the nutritive value of foods commonly found in the American diet.

"Family Food Guide" offers a detailed manual on buying foods and beverages with nutrition as the most important consideration, market-basket tips for the shopper, and the latest information on how to store foods safely so as to preserve quality. Following practical suggestions for food preparation is a special section: "Cooking the Nutritious Way," 200 delicious recipes selected for their economy and ease of preparation and to help introduce variety into your menus.

"Eating for Good Health," the third part of EAT BETTER, LIVE BETTER, confronts the American concern with overweight by reviewing reducing diets, spas, and support groups. It tells you how to change your habits and learn to eat sensibly—with diet suggestions for each member of your family, from baby to grandmother. Proper nutrition is only part of the story, and thus Part 3 concludes with another special section: "Fitness Through Exercise." Here you will learn why it is important to add physical activity to your daily routine. The illustrated pages will help you pick an activity, sport, or exercise routine to trim your shape, firm up your muscles, and increase your cardiorespiratory efficiency.

Concluding the volume is "Special Diets for Special Needs." Here are diet tips for dealing with such common ailments as cold, fever, sore throat, diarrhea, or constipation and facts you need to know if you or someone in your family is put on a sodium-, sugar-, or fat-controlled diet or one that calls for increased fiber. There is also a review of elimination diets to detect food allergies and suggestions for coping with lactose or gluten intolerance. Finally, if you have a picky eater, a vegetarian, or an athlete in the family, you can learn what special dietary needs he or she may have.

"People don't eat nutrition—they eat food," the late anthropologist Dr. Margaret Mead once said. Nonetheless, the exhaustive introduction to the subject contained in this commonsense guide to nutrition and good health can help you and every member of your family become more aware of food *as* nutrition. The decision to be healthy and fit is within your grasp. Take the sensible, down-to-earth approach to eating outlined in this book; forget the fads, gimmicks, and quick-weight-loss schemes. Change your life-style—and add happy, healthy years to your life.

THE EDITORS

Contents

1. ABC's of Nutrition   9
Necessary Nutrients: Carbohydrates, Fats,
   Proteins, Vitamins, Minerals, Water
Nutritive Value of Foods

2. Family Food Guide   95
The Basic Four Food Groups
Buying Guide: Vegetables, Fruits, Fish, Meat,
   Poultry, Eggs, Cheese, Legumes, Grains,
   Herbs and Spices
Gathering Foods from the Wild
Beverages: What's Good for You
Market Basket
Keeping Foods Fresh
Preparation Techniques

Special Section: Cooking the Nutritious Way   218

3. Eating for Good Health   281
Dealing with Overweight
Eating Sensibly

Special Section: Fitness Through Exercise   320

4. Special Diets for Special Needs   353
Food and Health/Nutrition Obstacles
Dealing with Common Ailments: Liquid, Soft,
   and Bland Diets; High-Fiber Diets
Detecting Food Allergies: Elimination Diets
Food Intolerance: Lactose- and
   Gluten-Restricted Diets
Coping with Dietary Limitations: Sodium-,
   Sugar-, and Fat-Controlled Diets
Self-imposed Food Restrictions: Picky Eaters,
   Vegetarian Diets, The Athlete's Diet

Bibliography, Acknowledgments and Credits,
   Index   398

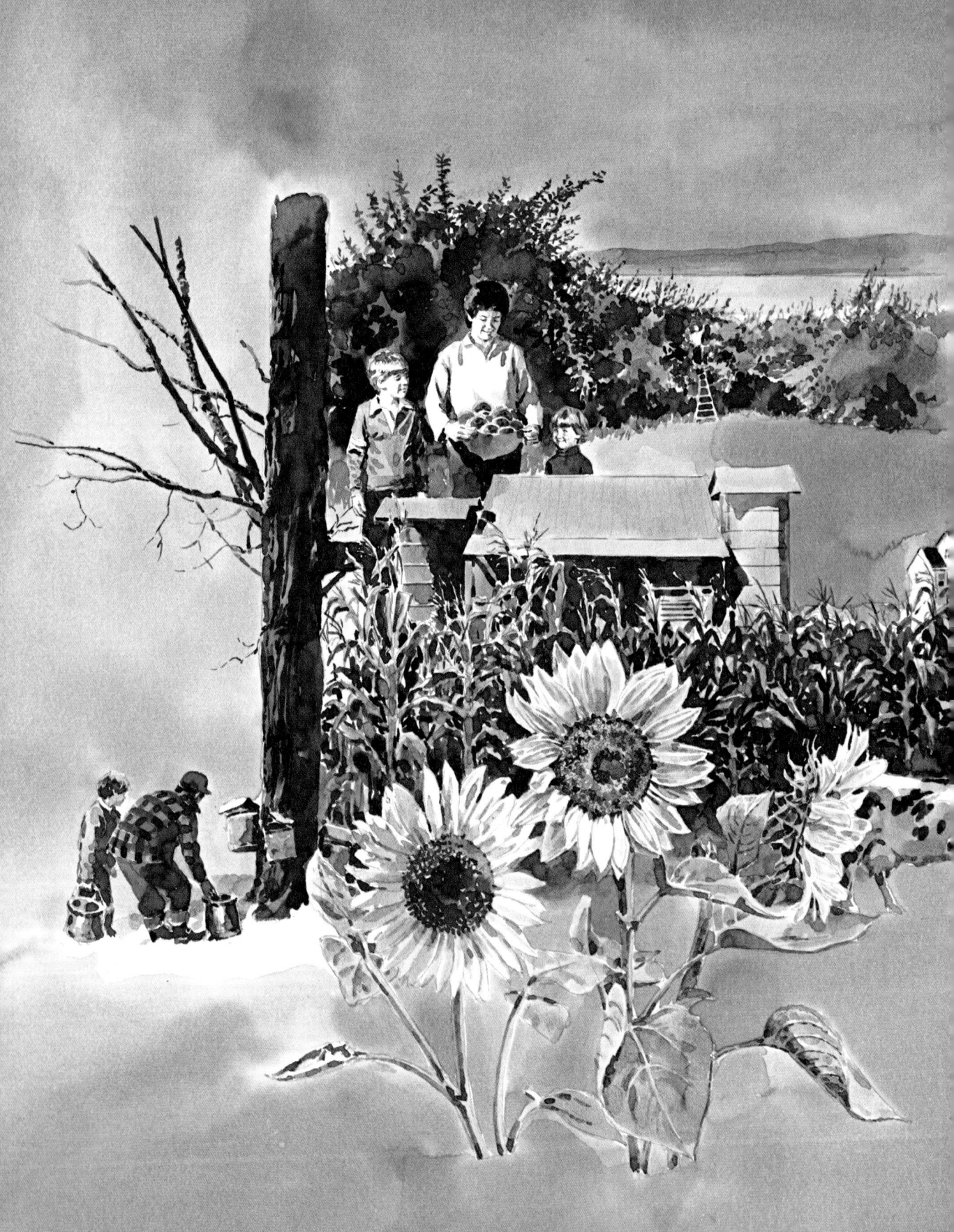

1. ABC'S OF NUTRITION

A concise introduction to the essential nutrients needed for human life and growth —and how much of these you require to maintain good health. Plus detailed charts showing the nutrient content and calorie counts of common foods that make up the American diet: Nutritive Value of Foods.

Necessary Nutrients
   Food and Your Body 10
      The Digestive System 11
      Calories Equal Energy 12
   The Underrated
      Carbohydrates 13
      Complex Carbohydrates . . 15
   The American Sweet
      Tooth 16
      Facts About Fiber 18
   The Unavoidable Fats 20
      Cutting Down on Fats . . . 21
      Cholesterol 22
   The Powerful Proteins 24
      The Remarkable Soybean 25
      Amino Acid Patterns 26
      Protein Myths 29

What You Should Know
      About Vitamins 30
      A Nutrition Glossary 31
   Recommended Dietary
      Allowances 32
      Guide to Vitamins 36
   Food and Drug
      Interactions 38
   Vitamin C Questions
      and Answers 41
   Over-the-Counter
      Vitamins 42
   Minerals Your Body Needs . 44
      Guide to Minerals 46
      Sodium in Your Diet 48
   The Importance of Water . . . 50
Nutritive Value of Foods 51

Necessary Nutrients/Food and Your Body

A nutrient is a substance found in food and needed by the body for life and health. Nutrition scientists today have identified about 40 essential nutrients, which are classified as vitamins, minerals, amino acids (building blocks of proteins), essential fatty acids (in fats), and water. "Essential" means we must obtain these nutrients from our diets either because we cannot make them at all in our bodies or we cannot make enough of them. In addition, we need carbohydrates, fats, and proteins as fuel for energy; an ideal fuel mix is probably about 12 percent calories from proteins, 30 to 35 percent from fats, and the rest from carbohydrates.

Although individual nutritional requirements vary, all of us have a continual need for nutrients from each group—for energy, growth, replacement, and maintenance of body tissue, and for regulation of vital physiological processes. Understanding the roles nutrients play enables us to appreciate their value and to determine optimum individual needs, avoiding excesses that may be wasted or may build up in the body in potentially harmful amounts, or deficiencies that will prevent the body from operating at its peak.

All the nutrients needed for a healthy human body are obtained from food or are manufactured by the body. The food we eat, however, must undergo dramatic physical and chemical changes in order for the essential nutrients it contains to be used to fuel the body. These changes are carried out in the digestive system.

How Digestion Works

The purpose of digestion is to free nutrients by breaking down the large molecules in which most are found into simpler forms small enough (and soluble enough) to pass from the digestive system into the cells where they are needed. However, these nutrients are worthless if digestion is impaired.

Digestion incorporates a wide variety of mechanical and chemical steps that are suited to breaking down particular types of nutrients. Hormonal processes come into play before, during, and after digestion since the secretions and muscular movements of the digestive tract can be triggered by hormonal secretions or inhibited in part by psychological factors outside the body. The mechanical processes take place throughout the entire cycle of digestion. The chemical processes act, by means of acids, enzymes, and alkalis, primarily on proteins, fats, and carbohydrates, since vitamins and minerals are able to be absorbed for the most part by the body in their original form, once they are split off from the foods that bind them.

Water is a vital medium in the entire digestive process, aiding secretions in softening, diluting, and dissolving nutrients and in transporting them to the cells. In the mouth, food begins to be broken down both mechanically and chemically. It is masticated, or chewed, and reduced to small particles that are more accessible to digestive chemicals. The chewed food mixes with saliva and becomes softer and easier to swallow, while ptyalin, an enzyme in the saliva, begins to chop up starches in the food into their constituent molecules of simpler sugars.

While the food remains in the mouth, its pleasant taste creates a stimulus for continued eating and for secretion of more saliva. The food is then pushed farther into the digestive system by swallowing, a reflex contraction caused by the presence of food on the back of the tongue. Wavelike muscular motions (called peristalsis) propel the food through the esophagus (in about five seconds) then through the cardiac sphincter, a circular band of muscle that guards the entrance to the stomach and prevents food from returning to the esophagus.

The stomach, somewhat like a rotating cement mixer on a truck, acts on food mechanically and chemically, and also serves as a reservoir. The stomach is an elastic organ, divided into three sections: the cardiac, or the upper, portion; the fundus, or the large, rounded, central portion; and the pylorus, or the lower outlet.

As food first enters the stomach, it spreads toward the outer edge; food swallowed later moves toward the center. This enables the mass of food to maintain the proper alkaline or neutral pH that allows the salivary digestion that started in the mouth to continue. Meanwhile, the outer layers are being digested by acid gastric juices. Here and elsewhere in the digestive system, the pH (acid or alkaline quality) of the food's surroundings works to facilitate certain digestive processes and retard others. Without this important control, digestion would not be possible.

The stomach moves in rhythmic, muscular contractions and eventually combines all of the food with the gastric juices, forming a semisolid mixture known as chyme. The gastric juice contains hydrochloric acid, which creates an acidic medium to aid in the splitting of proteins and to destroy microorganisms and protect the body from food-borne infection; mucin, which acts as a lubricant to help move food through the digestive tract, and protects the tract itself; and the enzymes pepsin and gastric lipase, which help to split protein and fat molecules, respectively. The amount of gastric juice present in the stomach will be increased by smelling, tasting, or simply thinking about food, but secretions will be inhibited by emotions such as anger or fear or by repulsive sights or odors.

On the average, foods remain in the stomach for about 4 hours. The actual transit time, however, depends on the type of food eaten, and some foods can leave the stomach in ½ hour whereas other may take as long as 7 hours. Carbohydrates take the least time to be processed; proteins, slightly more; and fats require the longest digestion time—which explains their high satiety value, or feeling of "fullness." The more food one consumes, the longer it will take to process this food in the stomach. Once the work of the stomach is finished, the chyme is flushed by peristalsis out of the stomach through a valve called the pyloric sphincter and into the duodenum, the upper section of the small intestine.

The most important digestive processes take place in the small intestine and involve three types of secretions. The pancreas secretes pancreatic juice, which contains many enzymes that split proteins, starches, fats, and other food components as well as bicarbonate that neutralizes the gastric acid in the chyme as it comes from the stomach. The liver secretes bile, which is concentrated and stored in the gallbladder; the bile helps to digest fats in the small intestine by emulsifying them and making them more accessible to digestive enzymes. And finally the cells of the intestinal lining itself produce intestinal juice, which contains a number of enzymes, most for processing carbohydrates, two for protein, and one for fats. While this is going on, the villi—small, fingerlike projections that line the wall of the small intestine—go to work to absorb and transport nutrients to the bloodstream. Peristaltic and rhythmic actions mix the food and carry it through the small intestine, causing it to brush against the villi, which are constantly in motion and are able to "pick out" molecules of nutrients with such efficiency that by the time the chyme has passed through

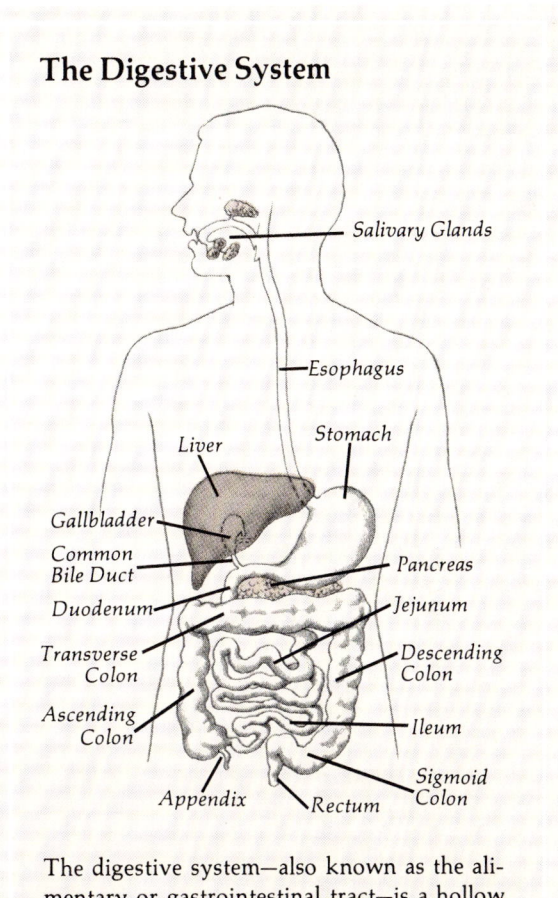

The Digestive System

The digestive system—also known as the alimentary or gastrointestinal tract—is a hollow tube, about 30 feet long, that is open to the environment at each end. Technically, digestion takes place outside the body. It is not until digested nutrients enter the bloodstream that they can be used by the cells. The entire process involves the passing of food through five principal digestive organs: mouth, esophagus, stomach, small and large intestines.

the small intestine, nearly 95 percent of some nutrients will have been absorbed.

The process of absorption itself operates in a number of physical and chemical ways, both active and passive. Vitamins, minerals, and the end products of carbohydrate and protein digestion are absorbed mainly into the blood of the capillaries, and the end products of fat digestion first mainly enter ducts known as lymphatic ducts and are then transported to the bloodsteam. Only at this point are the

Necessary Nutrients
Food and Your Body

nutrients from the food we have eaten ready to be transported to the cells where they will be utilized for energy; for building and repairing tissue or for regulating body functions; converted to storage forms for future use; or transported elsewhere in the body for elimination. Any material present in the small intestine that has not been absorbed for use in the cells is passed into the large intestine.

The large intestine, so-called because it is wider than the small intestine, is the final reservoir of the digestive tract. Its main job is to actively reabsorb excess fluid and dissolve mineral salts from the digested food mass to help maintain the body's fluid balance. Water not used in other processes is excreted by being flushed (along with waste products) through the kidneys.

The large intestine also helps form the body's solid waste, the feces. Fecal matter is approximately two-thirds water and one-third cellulose (fiber that must be present in adequate amounts for intestinal muscle tone), and large amounts of bacteria, as well as sloughed cells from the small intestine lining, which replaces itself every 48 hours.

The intestinal flora—a population of microbes found mainly in the large intestine—are also important to nutrition. These flora synthesize vitamins K, biotin, and pantothenic acid, thereby preventing serious deficiency of any of these three vitamins.

Calories Equal Energy

The food we eat has two main purposes: to act as fuel and building blocks for the activities and life-sustaining functions of the body. Similar to other fuels, when food is oxidized (in this case, burned) it produces energy, or heat. This energy is measured in units known as calories. In the field of human nutrition the caloric, or energy, values of food are actually measured in kilocalories (1,000 of these units), but in popular usage the "kilo" has been dropped. The accepted international unit of energy is the joule (1 calorie = 4.184 joules).

Different foods supply different amounts of energy, and so have different caloric values. Fat supplies 9 calories per gram, carbohydrates and proteins supply 4 calories per gram, and water and cellulose (fiber) no calories. That is why foods high in fat are highest in calories, and foods high in cellulose and water (such as fresh vegetables) are lowest.

When a diet supplies just the amount of fuel or calories the body needs, all the food energy will be used. But when the diet supplies more calories than are needed, the excess fuel is stored in the body as fat. This is also true when the excess is carbohydrate or protein; the liver converts the excess to fat. When the diet supplies fewer calories than are needed, the body converts its fat stores to energy to make up the difference—and weight is lost.

A desirable body weight depends on balancing energy intake—determined by food choices—with energy output—determined by one's basal metabolism (energy needs of the body at rest) plus one's level of physical activity. The number of calories an individual will need every day depends on age, sex, size, and level of physical activity.

The energy allowances, or recommended calorie intakes for men and women (see charts on page 299, derived from the Recommended Dietary Allowances), take these factors into account to establish a level "consonant with good health of average persons in each age group within a given activity." (Pregnant and breastfeeding women, however, have greater needs, approximately 300 and 500 additional calories per day respectively, especially if the woman is also an adolescent and must satisfy her own growth requirements as well as those of the fetus.) In setting the RDA for energy, the pervasive problem of overweight in the United States was taken into account, and the following recommendations were made.

We should not only stay within optimum calorie levels to maintain ideal body weight, but if we are cutting down on calories, we should also select foods of greater nutrient density (most nutrients per calorie). The way to control body weight is by balancing food intake against physical activity. This is especially important for children, whose weight problems may set a pattern for life, and for the elderly, whose low energy needs may lead to a diet deficient in many of the nutrients needed for good health if nutrient-dense foods are not adequately used.

The Underrated Carbohydrates

All living beings need energy in order to function. Carbohydrates, fats, and proteins, in any reasonable combination, are the sources of energy, or fuel, for the human body.

Despite their importance to the body as the dominant source of energy, foods rich in carbohydrates are regarded by many people in our society as inferior. Yet they are enjoyable to eat and are the most economical of all nutrients to produce, to store, and to buy. With the high cost of meat and other protein foods, money-saving carbohydrate foods will probably continue to gain in popularity. Most nutrition scientists agree that the 12 percent of daily calories obtained by Americans from protein is about the right amount but that the 42 percent obtained from fat should perhaps drop toward 30 to 35 percent, and the 46 percent obtained from carbohydrates should increase. They suggest including more complex carbohydrates in the diet while reducing refined sugar intake.

To many people, the word "carbohydrate" is synonymous with certain foods: bread, rice, potatoes, or spaghetti, for example. However, no one food is a source of a single nutrient. Also, carbohydrates are present in varying amounts in many foods, including fruits, vegetables, and some dairy products. The sugars, starches, pectins, cellulose, and glycogen in foods are all carbohydrates.

It is important to learn about high-carbohydrate foods—those containing large amounts of sugars and starches that can be broken down in the body into glucose. Sugars are in foods such as table sugar, honey, jam, jelly, syrup, and fruits. Starches are a major component of cereals, flour, potatoes, beans, squash, and other vegetables.

Glucose is a simple sugar, the main one known to exist in a pure state in the body during fasting, and the body's preferred source of energy. The carbohydrates found in most of our foods are broken down during digestion to release glucose for fuel. This fuel supplies the energy specifically needed for the operation of the brain and nervous system as well as the energy for physical activity and the inner workings of the body such as tissue building and repair and the absorption and transport of nutrients.

The Chemistry of Carbohydrates

The life cycle of plants helps to explain the chemistry of carbohydrates. All forms of life on this planet get their energy, directly or indirectly, from the sun. Through photosynthesis, plants are able to use the energy of sunlight to combine water and carbon dioxide from the air into a molecule that stores energy—a carbohydrate. When plants are eaten and digested, this molecule is broken down and its energy is released.

All living matter contains carbon and other elements attached to the carbon. The shape of the carbon-containing molecule and the other elements joined with the carbon determine the nature of this living matter. Carbohydrates link carbon with oxygen and hydrogen in single molecules, or in groups ranging up to hundreds of molecules.

The three types of carbohydrates are monosaccharides, disaccharides, and polysaccharides. The simplest group are monosaccharides—single molecules of sugar. These are glucose (sometimes known as dextrose, corn sugar, or grape sugar); fructose, found in fruits, vegetables, and honey; and galactose, usually combined with glucose to form the lactose found in milk.

Disaccharides are the double sugar molecules: sucrose, from sugarcane or sugar beets; maltose, from grain; and lactose. Although most people can safely eat all carbohydrate foods, some individuals have a problem with lactose because they have low amounts of the enzyme lactase. Because their digestive systems cannot break down lactose, drinking too much milk can cause these people to experience cramps, diarrhea, and other symptoms. Lactase deficiency symptoms are most common in children from 11 months to 11 years old; the condition appears to be inherited, and it is found to a large degree among certain ethnic groups such as blacks, Arabs, and Orientals (see pages 371-372).

Complex carbohydrates, or polysaccharides, are made up of molecules that break down into two or more sugars during digestion or other chemical processes. (Complex carbohydrates are discussed further on page 15). These polysaccharides include starch, dextrin, glycogen, and glucose. Starch is the most important polysaccharide for human nutrition and is found in staple foods such as cereals, grains, potatoes, carrots, turnips, beets, and squash. Fresh starch granules are insoluble and practically indigestible, but cooking causes them to swell and break down, thus forming a digestible solution. Cooked carrots, therefore, are a better source of carbohydrate

Necessary Nutrients
The Underrated Carbohydrates

than are raw carrots, though they are not quite as good a source of vitamins.

How Carbohydrates Work

In the human body, a series of complex chemical steps allows all carbohydrates (except for fiber) to be metabolized—separated into their basic molecules and used for energy. Our need for energy is constant. The amount rises and falls depending on our level of activity, but the basic processes of life, such as the working of the heart and lungs and the controlling of body temperature, continue even when we are completely at rest. To fuel these functions, the cells must send out a steady stream of energy, even though there may not be a steady supply of nutrients from the digestive system.

Because the body has a very efficient storage system, the amount of energy—glucose—in the bloodstream remains fairly constant, no matter when or how much we eat. (Although most people have high blood-glucose levels soon after eating, it drops within one or two hours.) The amount of glucose available in the bloodstream is usually sufficient for about 10 to 15 minutes of normal activity.

When there is extra glucose in the blood, it is transported to the liver, where it is converted to the complex carbohydrate glycogen, for short-term storage. Glycogen, which is stored in the liver and the muscles, can be held by the body in only limited amounts; when the body's stores are filled, extra energy will be converted to body fat.

Providing the body with energy is not the only role of carbohydrates. When converted to glycogen, this nutrient helps the liver to protect the body against toxins and to control the breakdown of protein. Although protein can be used by the body for fuel, its greater value is in the function of cell growth and repair. A sufficient intake of carbohydrates reduces the use of protein for energy and is said to be "protein sparing." By preventing the breakdown of protein, carbohydrates also protect the body from an excess of the nitrogenous waste that is a by-product of this breakdown.

The breakdown of fat can also cause a buildup of waste products, in this case ketone bodies. High levels of ketone bodies in the blood (the condition ketosis) can cause the nausea, headache, fatigue, and other ill effects associated with low-carbohydrate diets (see page 286).

Your Carbohydrate Requirement

Carbohydrates should be a larger part of your diet than any other nutrient. Probably about 55 percent of our daily calories should come from carbohydrate foods, 30 to 35 percent from fat, and 10 to 15 percent from protein foods. Currently, fats contribute nearly as many calories (42 percent) to the daily diet as do carbohydrates (46 percent).

Because humans are able to convert protein and fat to glucose for energy, there is no specific dietary requirement for carbohydrate. However, nutrition experts agree that a reasonable proportion of total daily calories should come from this nutrient to prevent the ketosis (protein waste), loss of sodium, and dehydration that accompany a severe lack of carbohydrates.

An ideal diet is neither too high nor too low in carbohydrates. Too high a level may not supply enough high-quality protein for proper growth and body maintenance—especially for children. A low-carbohydrate diet, on the other hand, is automatically high in fat—usually the saturated fat found in animal foods. Fat is high in calories, and obesity results from eating more calories each day than we burn up. Populations in countries where most people eat high-carbohydrate diets show a lower proportion of overweight and other health problems related to overweight.

To increase your carbohydrate intake and to assure yourself many other valuable nutrients as well, choose fruits, low-fat milk products, and complex carbohydrates such as vegetables, cereals, grains, and legumes. Avoid concentrated sweets, which are devoid of the nutrients present in other carbohydrate foods. Sugars, syrups, candy, and the like contribute almost nothing but sweet flavor and calories to the diet.

Because they supply little else besides energy, concentrated sweets are often known as "empty calories." The same designation might be given to alcohol, which is even higher in calories than sugar: 7 calories for each gram, as compared to 4 calories for each gram of sugar (or any other carbohydrate). Government information notes that persons who drink alcoholic beverages may derive 5 to 10 percent of their total energy intake from alcohol and that some persons consume as much as 1,800 calories in alcohol per day.

For people who normally eat a nutritionally well-balanced diet, alcoholic beverages, in moderation, pose no health problems as long as their caloric content is kept in mind. Several studies have shown that small amounts of alcohol can aid circulation in healthy people. However, overconsumption can damage the heart muscle and liver and may be associated with vitamin and mineral deficiencies. What do the experts recommend? Most agree that a small amount of alcohol can be good for the healthy person, especially before or with a meal, to improve

Complex Carbohydrates

All carbohydrates are not created equal. Although some are wonderful sources of energy and essential nutrients, others are simply a sweet waste of calories. What are the best carbohydrates and how should you choose them? This simple guide can help you decide.

Understanding the Difference. The health benefits of complex carbohydrates—foods high in starch—are well established. So is the absence of vitamins and minerals in sweets and refined carbohydrates such as candy, cakes, and soft drinks. The important difference between these two types of carbohydrates is the range of nutrition they provide.

Complex carbohydrates are found in nearly all foods of plant origin: fruits, vegetables, grains, and legumes. These foods, especially when they are only slightly refined, are often high in "nutrient density." This term compares the overall nutritive value of the ingredients contained in a food to its energy (calorie) content. Because they contain vitamins, minerals, protein, and fiber, in addition to energy, complex carbohydrates are a highly recommended part of a healthful diet. On the other hand, foods that have had most of their natural goodness refined away are low in nutrient density, supply little or nothing besides calories, and should be avoided in large quantity.

Nutrition experts stress that our sedentary life-style and national tendency toward overweight mean most of us cannot afford too many calories unaccompanied by essential nutrients—the so-called empty calories. Eating low-density foods may either prevent us from meeting our nutritional needs, or may cause us to go over our limit in calories to achieve needed levels of nutrients.

A preference for sweetened and refined foods seems to be a major factor in many of our diets. Even though, as a general rule, complex carbohydrates are nutritionally superior to simple sugars, there are "good" and "poor" choices to be made in either category. For example, although the carbohydrate in milk products (lactose) and that in fruits (fructose or glucose) is considered a simple sugar, these sugars are outweighed by the presence of many other important nutrients. Milk contains calcium, high-quality protein, vitamins A, D, and B_{12}, and other nutrients as well. Fruits and vegetables are excellent food choices in terms of the vitamins, minerals, and fiber they provide.

Simple sugars are absorbed into the blood more rapidly, causing a quicker but less sustained rise in blood sugar. There is also a rapid increase in insulin secretion and a related tendency toward the formation of fat. The drop in blood sugar that follows this rapid rise is the well-known sensation associated with returning hunger.

Making Your Choice. The following are some of the "good" carbohydrate foods from which you should choose:

Fruits and vegetables. Be sure to include those high in vitamin C and vitamin A (citrus, cantaloupe, strawberries, peaches, carrots, turnips, broccoli, spinach, and so forth). If you are trying to lose weight, baked and boiled potatoes are better than French-fried, which add calories because of the oil in which they are cooked. The skins of baked potatoes or boiled new potatoes provide fiber.

Corn. Fresh corn, grits, and cornmeal are good for you; popcorn (without salt, butter, or oil) is a filling low-calorie snack.

Legumes. Dried peas and beans provide excellent protein when eaten with grain products.

Cereals and breads. Whole grains are slightly preferred, but enriched varieties are also healthful and usually will better resist spoilage.

Rice and pasta. Brown rice may be slightly more nutritious than converted rice; however, converted rice is also fine. Pasta is available in many varieties, including high-protein and whole-wheat kinds.

Necessary Nutrients
The Underrated Carbohydrates

the appetite and enhance enjoyment of the meal. Pregnancy is a special condition during which extreme moderation in alcohol consumption is probably a good idea.

About Blood Sugar

A discussion of carbohydrates would be incomplete without some mention of the highly publicized issue of blood sugar. The presence of sugar (glucose) in the blood, the rising and falling of blood-sugar levels in response to foods, and the relationship between carbohydrates and sugar has raised many questions in people's minds. Some people erroneously believe that sugar causes diabetes; others, that it causes hypoglycemia (low blood sugar). Here is what the experts say.

Diabetes. Most experts today believe that diabetes is an inherited problem, the symptoms of which are related to the diet, but which is not caused by the diet. The inability to process glucose causes the disease's most obvious symptom: sugar in the urine. Contrary to popular opinion, the most accurate test for the presence of diabetes is not the glucose tolerance test, which is performed after giving a test dose of glucose by serial sampling of the blood and analyzing its glucose content. Rather, the most accurate test measures fasting blood sugar and insulin levels.

The cause of diabetes is not yet known. Insulin, the hormone that sets off key bodily reactions in the processing of glucose, was once thought to be missing in the diabetic, but doctors now know that this simple explanation is not correct. They also know that the control of obesity and eating a balanced diet that contains a good proportion of complex carbohydrates is helpful in managing the disease. Complex carbohydrates are recommended rather than simple sugars, which cause the rapid rising of blood-sugar levels that trouble the diabetic.

Hypoglycemia. The media have made hypoglycemia a popular diagnosis for such symptoms as nervousness, fatigue, depression, headache, and numerous other problems, which have been erroneously linked to the consumption of sugar and other simple carbohydrates.

A glucose tolerance test will uncover hypoglycemia where it truly exists. But if the symptoms do not appear when the blood sugar is low, and the blood sugar is not low each time the symptoms appear, hypoglycemia is rarely the correct diagnosis. Although this test is given to hundreds of people, most responsible doctors find few cases. Many experts have pointed out that the symptoms so offhandedly attributed to this disease might just as well result from anxiety reaction. There is no evidence that this psychological condition and others, such as childhood behavior problems or depression, are related to low blood sugar.

What Dieters Should Know

Of all health issues related to carbohydrates, that of weight loss is probably the most misunderstood. Most dieters are aware of the disastrous effects of too much of the wrong carbohydrates—principally sweets—on a weight-loss plan. Sweets are high in

---

The American Sweet Tooth

Sugar is a popular part of our everyday lives. We spoon it into coffee, stir it into cakes, and enjoy it in hundreds of foods we *know* to be high in sugar as well as in many others containing sweeteners in hidden form. Sucrose—99 percent pure and obtained from sugar cane or sugar beets—is what we call sugar, but it is far from being the only sweetener in our lives. There are also dextrose, fructose, mannose, maltose, and more. (For a list of sugars and other sweeteners, see page 196.)

Are you concerned about the sugar in your diet? Then here are some facts you probably want to know.

- Sugar is found in many processed foods. If you read the label on the products you buy, you may be surprised to note its presence—as dextrose, or under some other lesser known name—in beans, soups, yogurt, baby food, canned ham, vegetables, bread, even nonsugar-coated cereals, catsup, peanut butter, salad dressing, chili, and many other foods.
- The average American consumes an astonishing ¼ pound (½ cup) of sugar per day—more than 100 pounds per year when other sweeteners are included. Average consumption of sugar has remained fairly stable over the past 50 years, though much of what was once added in the kitchen now shows up in processed food purchased at the supermarket. Adding 4 extra teaspoons of sugar to your diet every day, one expert

ABC'S OF NUTRITION

points out, will necessitate walking 1 mile per day to work it off—or you will gain 6 pounds in one year.

- All sweeteners—brown and white sugar, molasses, honey, and pure maple syrup—are equal in caloric content. Corn syrup is a more concentrated sweetener and is about 30 percent higher in calories.
- There is no specific dietary need for sugar, as such. The body's nutritional need for glucose can be met by many other carbohydrates, as well as by protein or fat (which are not preferred sources).
- Our attraction to sweet taste is believed to be inborn. When a sweet solution is injected into the amniotic fluid of a pregnant woman, the fetus will swallow actively, a reaction considered instinctive.
- Most dentists agree that sticky sweets are a major source of dental caries (cavities) in children. Sweet foods that are part of a meal are less cavity producing than between-meal snacks. The total amount of sugar eaten is not as important in the formation of dental decay as is the type of sugary food eaten, how often it is eaten, and how long it sticks to the teeth. Brushing and/or flossing teeth and rinsing the mouth after meals and snacks is recommended.
- Sugar and other sweets do not really provide "quick energy"; they just provide a quick rise in blood-sugar level. The body has energy reserves it can call on when needed for activity and does not need, or particularly profit from, an outside food source such as a candy bar or high-sugar drink for "instant fuel" just prior to activity.
- While some popular writers link sugar and heart disease, there is no scientific support for such speculation. However, a diet high in sugar (or, of course, high in any other source of calories) may lead to obesity, which *is* often associated with heart disease as well as various other health problems.

To cut down on sugar consumption, try the following.

- Always read the label on processed foods and avoid those with sugar (or other sweeteners such as dextrose, fructose, or corn syrup) high on the list of ingredients.
- Switch from soft drinks to fruit juices or water.
- Reduce the amount of sugar you use in coffee or tea—or eliminate it altogether.
- Do not keep sweet foods in the house, or use them to reward children.
- Serve more fresh fruit and fewer baked goods for snacks and dessert. Beware of the high sugar content in the syrup of many canned fruits.
- Experiment with gradually cutting down on the amount of sweetener in recipes. Adding a grated carrot to a recipe can replace some of the sugar in tomato sauce, salads, and even cookies.

calories, essentially devoid of nutrients, though they may take the edge off the appetite. But most people are unaware of the benefits of moderate amounts of the right carbohydrates, such as fruits, vegetables, and whole-grains.

Despite their popularity, high-protein, low-carbohydrate diets are neither healthful nor truly effective. Since low-carbohydrate diets are not meant for long-term use, they do little to improve eating habits. In fact, these unbalanced regimens are more likely to cause the repeated cycles of weight loss and weight gain that experts consider dangerous. Fad diets are discussed on pages 282-292.

The promotion of low-carbohydrate diets leads many weight watchers to make misguided food choices. For example, many will choose a 5-ounce steak (about 500 calories) over a serving of spaghetti with meat sauce—at about half the calories.

One experiment has shown that a diet including 12 slices of bread per day can result in weight loss because the dieter feels satisfied without consuming an excess of calories. And carbohydrates such as fruits can provide the healthful solution to a craving for sweets. Foods such as dried beans and peas, which many people criticize as "starchy and fattening," are excellent sources of protein, fiber, and other nutrients that dieters—and all people—need.

When you are tempted to turn down carbohydrate foods on your diet, remember this: ounce per ounce, carbohydrates and proteins supply the same number of calories (4 calories per gram), whereas fats supply twice as many (9 calories per gram). Carbohydrate foods can also help stave off between-meal hunger since they are high in fiber and water. Considering their many benefits, carbohydrates might be the best friend a dieter could ever have.

Necessary Nutrients
The Underrated Carbohydrates

Facts About Fiber

Although most people are aware of the role fiber plays in helping to maintain good health, questions remain as to the best types of fiber, how much is needed, and how it works. Here are some of the answers:

Q. What is fiber and where is it found?

A. Simply defined, fiber is the structural part of plants—the framework that supports and holds a plant together. Sometimes called roughage or bulk, fiber is a strandlike material that cannot be digested by the human stomach because it is resistant to digestive enzymes. It can, however, be partly digested by some bacteria in the lower intestines.

Although the term "fiber" suggests a solid or stringlike substance, much of our dietary fiber is more in the nature of a gelatin or mucilage.

Fiber is found only in plant foods such as fruits and vegetables, beans, and grains. Plants contain different kinds and amounts of fiber, depending on the species, the variety, the growing conditions, the age of the plant when harvested, and the degree to which it has been processed. Fiber is made up of the nondigestible carbohydrates and carbohydratelike components cellulose, hemicellulose, pectin, and lignin.

The amount of fiber found in foods is often expressed as "crude fiber," a scientific measurement of the organic material left after chemical digestion of food in the laboratory. Because this process digests much more than the natural chemical digestion that occurs in the body, most experts prefer the measure expressed as "total dietary fiber," which is usually two to three times higher than crude fiber.

The list on the opposite pages gives the percentage of total dietary fiber per 100 grams (or 3½ ounces) of food. Any food that contain 6 or more percent fiber is considered to be a high-fiber food.

Q. What can fiber do for health?

A. Many benefits of fiber—particularly its value in aiding elimination and treating constipation—are well established. It is also generally accepted as a factor in lowering the risk of hemorrhoids and diverticulosis. The possible role of fiber in helping to prevent diseases such as cardiovascular disease, cancer of the colon, and diabetes is still under study. Current findings suggest that moderate amounts of fiber are good for your health, an association that may be stronger with the fibers in fruits and vegetables than with those in grains.

Q. How does fiber work?

A. Fiber is sometimes called "nature's broom" because it helps to sweep the products of digestion through the body and eliminate them. Fiber absorbs moisture, thereby adding bulk to food materials as they pass through the intestinal tract. Bulk stimulates muscles, helping the waste products to move along quickly and to be eliminated regularly, reducing strain on blood vessels and the lower bowel.

Theories relating fiber consumption to disease prevention suggest that a fast intestinal "transit time" can remove harmful substances from the body before they can cause disease, and that absorption of cholesterol by fiber may prevent its absorption into the blood. However, fiber also absorbs significant amounts of iron and zinc, thus reducing the percentage of these two important nutrients going into the blood.

Studies have shown that diabetics on a high-fiber diet (that is also low in fat and sugar) have improved control of blood-sugar levels. In this case, researchers have evidence that fiber actually delays digestion and thus delays conversion of starches to glucose. This slowdown—which works only when fiber is included as part of a meal and not as a between-meal snack or supplement—helps to control the rise in blood sugar that can be a problem for diabetics.

Fiber is a proven aid to dieters too. It requires chewing, and also tends to satisfy hunger without providing calories because it swells up in the body and creates a feeling of fullness.

Q. How much fiber should be eaten every day?

A. As with most dietary recommendations, moderation is the key to the healthful use of fiber. It is not a cure-all, and adding fiber to an unbalanced diet will do little or no good. While research into its full impact on the human diet continues, fiber should form just one important part of a balanced diet chosen from a variety of wholesome foods.

Q. What are some recommended ways to add fiber to meals?

A. A gradual increase in high-fiber foods—particularly complex carbohydrates—along with a decrease in the amount of animal fats and refined sugars is the recommended way to improve fiber intake. To benefit from all types of fiber, eat a wide variety of foods, and remember it is essential to drink liquids. Have raw vegetables and, where possible, unpeeled fruits as snacks, desserts, or in meals, and try to eat a salad every day. For even more fiber, look for whole-grain breads, cereals, and other baked goods and use whole-grain flours whenever possible for homebaking.

Q. Is it possible to eat too much fiber?
A. Too much fiber in the diet can do more harm than good. Symptoms ranging from painful gas, nausea, and vomiting to an inability to absorb essential vitamins and minerals are possible results of a sudden switch to a diet very high in fiber. People with sensitive digestive tracts can be especially affected by too much fiber, and even normal digestion needs a period of adjustment to less refined foods.

Experts remind us that not all forms of fiber are the same. Bran, the outer cover of a grain kernel, is mostly cellulose, and is sometimes an effective treatment for constipation. However, eating bran dry can have the opposite of the desired effect and may instead help to clog the intestine.

High-fiber breads are relatively new on the market and contain many times more fiber and about 30 percent fewer calories than most white breads. High-fiber breads contain wood cellulose, as well as wheat bran and other types of fiber. While these products may be more filling and less "fattening" than other breads, wood-pulp fiber is not the same as the dietary fiber in bran, grains, fruits, and vegetables—foods considered the best sources of dietary fiber.

Nutrition scientists worry about the adverse effects on the health of people who fill up on foods containing large amounts of wood cellulose and therefore cut back on their consumption of more nutritious foods.

Percent of Total Dietary Fiber in Foods (per 100 grams)

Food	Fiber	Food	Fiber	Food	Fiber
Apple, cooked	2.4	wheat, puffed	16.6	peanuts, roasted	9.3
Apple, fresh	2.4	wheat, shredded	13.3	walnuts	5.2
Asparagus, cooked	1.7	Cherries, fresh	1.7	Onion, raw	2.1
Avocado, fresh	2.0	Coconut, fresh	13.6	Orange, fresh	2.0
Banana	2.7	Corn, sweet, cooked	5.7	Peach, fresh	2.3
Beans		Crackers		Peanut butter, smooth	7.6
kidney, cooked	10.4	Graham	10.1	Pear, fresh	2.4
lima, cooked	9.3	rye wafer	11.7	Peas	
string, fresh	3.4	whole wheat	11.1	chick, cooked	6.0
Bean sprouts	1.8	Dates, dried	8.7	garden, cooked	6.3
Blackberries, fresh	6.2	Figs, dried	18.5	Plums, fresh	2.1
Bread		Flour		Popcorn, popped	16.5
pumpernickel	5.8	oat, milled	3.8	Prunes, dried	16.1
rye	3.0	oat, whole grain	14.0	Radishes, raw	2.2
white	2.7	rye, dark	12.7	Raisins, dried	6.8
whole wheat	5.1	white	3.0	Raspberries, red, fresh	7.4
Broccoli, fresh	3.9	whole wheat (100%)	9.6	Rice	
Cabbage, white, raw	3.4	Grapefruit, fresh	.9	brown, cooked	2.4
Carrots, fresh	3.3	Grapes, fresh	.9	white, cooked	.8
Cereal		Lentils, cooked	3.7	Spinach, cooked	6.3
bran, 100%	30.1	Lettuce	1.5	Spinach, fresh	3.5
bran, other	15.9-26.0	Mushrooms, fresh	2.5	Squash, winter, cooked	2.9
corn flakes	12.3	Nuts		Strawberries, fresh	2.2
oatflakes, fortified	12.0	almonds	14.3	Tomatoes, fresh	1.5
oat, whole, dry	14.0	chestnuts	6.8	Watermelon	.9

Necessary Nutrients
The Unavoidable Fats

The word "fat" has several meanings, and its relationship to health is often misunderstood. Many people feel that fat—whether body size, type of food, or nutrient—is something to be avoided at all costs. But fat is an essential part of the diet, necessary to the health of people of all ages, and a principal source of energy. In recognition of the body's need for fat, the U.S. Department of Agriculture has added to the Basic Four Food Groups a fifth group, which includes fats (see page 97).

Why Our Bodies Need Fat

All extra energy contained in the body (other than a small amount of glucose stored as glycogen) becomes fat. Some of this fat is found in blood plasma and other cells throughout the body, but the greatest amount is in the body's adipose—fat storage—cells. This body fat is the storage form for all the extra energy (calories) taken in, regardless of the source: fat, carbohydrate, protein, or alcohol.

Adipose tissue is active—continually changing in response to our energy needs. Cells throughout the body, other than erythrocytes (red blood corpuscles) and the cells in the central nervous system, are able to use fatty acids directly for energy.

In addition to storing energy, adipose tissue insulates the body. About one half of body fat is the layer just below the skin that protects us from changes in external temperature and helps to maintain a fairly constant internal temperature. Other adipose deposits surround and cushion such vital organs as the kidneys and those of the reproductive system. There are also fat pads in the cheeks, palms of the hands, and balls of the feet.

Importance of Dietary Fat

The fats in our food are important because they are carriers of the fat-soluble vitamins: A, D, E, and K. In addition, dietary fat includes and supplies essential fatty acids, particularly linoleic acid.

All animal life requires polyunsaturated fatty acids, and linoleic acid is of primary importance to humans. The adult requirement is low, and easily met by a well-rounded diet, but children have a greater need for linoleic acid for growth. The essential fatty acids are important in preventing drying and flaking of the skin and have several metabolic roles: maintaining cell membranes, regulating cholesterol metabolism, and helping to create hormone-like substances needed for many body processes. But what, in fact, are these fatty acids?

The fats in our body contain the same substances as the fats in our food: fatty acids and fatlike compounds called phospholipids (such as lecithin) and cholesterol.

Fats are made up of the same three elements as carbohydrates: carbon, hydrogen, and oxygen. Fat differs from carbohydrate in that the former is a more concentrated form of fuel and contains proportionately more carbon and less oxygen than does carbohydrate. This difference causes fat to supply 9 calories per gram, whereas carbohydrate supplies only 4.

When one molecule of fat is broken down, it becomes three molecules of fatty acids and one molecule of glycerol. These molecules are known as triglycerides. You may have heard of "serum triglycerides," a medical term used to describe the level of fat molecules in the blood.

Fatty acids are straight chains of carbon atoms ranging in number from 2 to 20. Each of these carbon atoms may be linked to hydrogen atoms, also in varying numbers from 0 to 3. The number of carbon and hydrogen atoms in a fatty acid, as well as the different combinations of fatty acids found in a particular fat, will determine what type of fat it will be and how it will taste. Some of the many fatty acids may be familiar to you from the labels on food packages: acetic, butyric, myristic, palmitic, stearic, and linoleic.

Fatty acids are either saturated or unsaturated—terms that refer to the number of hydrogen atoms attached to the carbon atoms. When all the carbon atoms are linked to hydrogen atoms on both sides, the fatty acid is considered saturated, or filled with hydrogen. If any of the carbon atoms are free, that is, not linked to a pair of hydrogen atoms, the fatty acid is unsaturated. Monounsaturated fatty acids lack only one pair of hydrogen atoms, while polyunsaturated fatty acids lack many such pairs.

The Fats in Our Foods

The fats we consume come from many sources, both visible and invisible. Visible fats are ingredients such as olive oil or shortening, which are used in preparing foods, or extras such as butter, salad dressing, or cream cheese, added at the table. The fat you trim from your steak is also the visible variety. Invisible fats are an integral part of foods, including the fat found in meat, nuts, fish, or eggs, the butterfat in whole milk or cheese, and fat added in processing.

Fats contained in foods improve the texture (the marbling in a steak, for instance) and absorb and retain flavors, making meals more palatable. Fats have characteristics that cause them to remain in the stomach longer and prolong the "good-and-full" feeling. Most fats of either animal or vegetable origin are easily digested by healthy persons.

All of the fats naturally found in foods are made of mixtures of saturated and unsaturated fatty acids. In general, fats containing mainly saturated fatty acids do not melt at room temperature and are found in animal foods such as beef or lamb, lard, butter, and other dairy products. Fats containing mainly polyunsaturated fatty acids are usually liquid at room temperature and include corn, cottonseed, and safflower oils. Exceptions include poultry and fish oils, which come from animal sources but are high in unsaturated fatty acids despite being solid, and coconut oil, a vegetable oil high in saturated fatty acids despite being a liquid.

Some fat products such as shortening and margarine, are hydrogenated. This process adds hydrogen atoms to polyunsaturated fatty acids, creating a solid fat which is more stable and which can be stored at room temperature.

How Much Do We Need?

The dietary role of fats is not a simple one. Although a moderate amount of fat is needed in everyone's diet, many people go overboard. The consumption of too much fat, and fat of the "wrong" type, may be linked to two of this country's greatest health problems: obesity and cardiovascular disease.

Good nutrition depends on as little as one tablespoon of dietary fat each day. Most people exceed that amount many times over. While holding off on butter and mayonnaise, they may still be eating large amounts of hidden fat in foods.

For most essential nutrients there is a recommended minimum daily amount. Some nutritionists feel that a recommended maximum would help people keep their fat intake down to levels more consistent with good health. The U.S. Dietary Guidelines (see pages 96-97) recommend a reduction in the percentage of total daily calories consumed as fat—from the national average of almost 45 percent to no more

Cutting Down on Fats

The following suggestions may help reduce your fat intake:

- Include more fruits and vegetables, breads and whole-grain cereals, and dried beans and peas in your diet.
- Switch to leaner meats and other sources of protein. Instead of ground beef, sausage, or fatty steaks, choose beef round or rump, or veal and, above all, try to include more fish and poultry (without skin) in menus.
- Substitute skim milk and low-fat milk products in recipes and for drinking. Instead of whole milk, cream, ice cream, and hard cheese, try skim buttermilk, 1 or 2-percent milk, yogurt, and low-fat cottage cheese.
- Cut down on peanut butter, coconut, olives, avocados, and cream cheese.
- Learn low-fat cooking methods such as poaching, steaming, roasting, or broiling instead of frying. Drain off as much fat as possible after cooking. Instead of high-fat gravies or butter for flavoring, serve foods with broth, lemon juice, vinegar, and spices and herbs.
- Learn to distinguish among the different types of fats: *saturated*—butter, lard, shortening, coconut oil; *monounsaturated*—olive oil, peanut oil; *polyunsaturated*—corn, cottonseed, safflower, soybean, and sunflower oil; most margarines.

than 35 percent; of the 35 percent, 8 to 10 percent should be essential fatty acids.

The American Academy of Pediatrics recommended allowance for essential fatty acids is 3 percent of total dietary calories for infants and, according to the Food and Nutrition Board of the National Academy of Sciences, 2 percent, in the form of linoleic acid, for adults. Vegetable sources, especially vegetable oils, contribute the largest quantities of linoleic acid as well as arachidonic and linolenic acids, the other two primary fatty acids.

All fats, no matter what their source, have the same caloric value, but whether you eat more saturated or polyunsaturated fats may make a difference in your blood cholesterol. A number of nutrition experts recommend a reduction of saturated fats and an increase in polyunsaturated fats in the diet.

Necessary Nutrients
The Unavoidable Fats

Cholesterol

The media have made us all familiar with the term "cholesterol." Although most people tend to believe that there is a link between the cholesterol in their diet and heart disease, the experts consider this topic a controversial one because the scientifically established link is between *blood*, or serum, cholesterol and heart disease, not *dietary* cholesterol and heart disease. Only about 15 percent of blood cholesterol is from the diet; the rest we make in our own liver and in other cells. Research into fat, cholesterol, and heart disease is destined to continue for years to come. Meanwhile, here is what is known—so far.

Cholesterol is a complex, waxlike substance that the body needs for many vital processes. The brain, the nervous system, and all cell walls require some cholesterol. It is also important in creating hormones and vitamin D, and in aiding the digestion of fats.

The primary source of dietary cholesterol are foods of animal origin, with the greatest amounts of cholesterol found in red meats, eggs, dairy products, and some shellfish. Regardless of the amount you consume in your diet, your body continues to produce cholesterol every day. Your body will attempt to balance the cholesterol it manufactures with what it takes in, tending to produce less and to eliminate more in response to a high cholesterol diet. However, in some people the amounts of cholesterol in the bloodstream cannot adjust to overcome the effects of a high cholesterol diet.

Most healthy people maintain a fairly constant level of cholesterol in the bloodstream, although this level may rise with age. A diet high in polyunsaturated fats is associated with lower levels of blood cholesterol, whereas a diet high in saturated fats tends to increase the amount of cholesterol circulating in the blood—a condition that is a risk factor for heart disease.

Cholesterol appears in the fat deposits that form in the linings of the arteries, causing these vessels to become less elastic. The role of blood-cholesterol level in forming these deposits is unknown. This process, known as atherosclerosis, takes place gradually, in any artery of the body, beginning at any time from childhood on. When the fatty deposits in the arteries are heavy and irregular, they are known as plaques. These plaques can restrict or even stop the flow of blood through the arteries or can cause rough spots that may break loose and create blood clots. When this occurs in one of the major blood vessels of the heart or brain, it causes a coronary or a stroke.

Medical experts stress that diet alone does not create a high risk of heart disease. Your heredity, physical activity, smoking habits, body weight, and even your personality may all play a part. New discoveries are continually changing the medical community's views of cholesterol and heart disease. Most recently, two types of cholesterol-carrying lipoproteins have been linked to protection against or promotion of the disease process. Though both of these lipoproteins contain cholesterol, the "protective" higher density ones (HDL) are found in greater amounts in people who exercise, drink only moderately, and do not smoke; while the "promoting" lower density ones (LDL) are more prevalent in obese people, smokers, and sedentary people. This research has not proven a connection between diet and these lipoproteins, but it does provide further evidence that there is a wide variety in the way people do and do not respond to diet, in the composition of their blood, and in their tendency to develop heart disease.

The latest Recommended Dietary Allowances state that changes in diet only, without consideration of measures to alter other risk factors, will probably have minimal desirable effects toward reducing risk of this disease. Many experts *do* find the evidence linking fats, cholesterol, and heart disease convincing enough to warrant changes in diet; many others do not. One of the seemingly most impressive studies in this area was a long-term analysis of 1,900 middle-aged American men, the results of which were published in a January 1981 issue of the *New England Journal of Medicine*, and which was taken to task in a May 1981 issue of the same journal.

This study claimed that the consumption of large amounts of cholesterol increased the risk that these men would die prematurely from heart attack, and that a higher intake of polyunsaturated fats helped to protect against this early death, without increasing the risk of dying from cancer or other causes. Between 1957, when these men were first examined, and 1977, when the study was concluded, the men in the group with the lowest dietary intake of saturated fats and cholesterol had a 33 percent lower death rate from coronary heart disease than the men in the group with the highest intakes. Contrary to expectations, however, the lowest death rate from coronary heart disease occurred among the group of men with the *middle* intake of cholesterol.

Saturated fat intake alone was not found directly

related to coronary risk, which was contrary to most other studies and caused some consternation in the scientific community. When dietary fats and cholesterol were analyzed independently of other factors such as age, weight, smoking habits, blood pressure, and alcohol intake, they were found to be directly related to coronary risk for one part of the group but not for another part—again raising scientific eyebrows.

The authors of this study were among leading experts recommending prudent decreases in the amount of saturated fats and cholesterol in the diet. Changes already made since 1965 by a significant portion of the population may have accounted for a lowering of the coronary death rate for Americans by about 3 percent per year. But another scientific group concluded that no necessary relationship could be established between the lowering of the coronary death rate and dietary changes because of concurrent improvements in medical care. Dietary changes cannot be recommended to the entire population, but combined with changes in lifestyle such as quitting smoking and increasing exercise, they are considered desirable to those at risk because of overweight, family history of heart disease, or a tendency toward high levels of serum cholesterol.

Cholesterol Content of Foods (milligrams per 100 grams)

Food	Cholesterol	Food	Cholesterol	Food	Cholesterol
Cheeses		Eggs		Frankfurter, cooked	70
American	96	Boiled	548	Lamb	70
Cheddar	106	Omelet, plain	388	Organ meats	
Cottage, creamed	15	Poached	545	brains	2,100
Cream	120	Substitute, frozen	2	giblets, chicken, simmered	195
Mozzarella	78	Fats and Oils		hearts	
Mozzarella, part skim	57	Butter		calf, braised	180
Parmesan, hard	68	salted	220	chicken, simmered	231
Swiss	93	sweet	260	kidneys, braised	375
Desserts		Margarine	0	tongue, beef, smoked	210
Cakes		Vegetable oils	0	Turkey	82
chocolate with chocolate icing	43	Fish and Shellfish		Veal	90
gingerbread	1	Clams, raw	50	Milk and Milk Products	
pound	99	Crab, canned	101	Cream	
sponge	246	Fish sticks, frozen	70	half and half	40
white with chocolate icing	2	Haddock, fried	60	heavy whip, fluid	133
yellow with chocolate icing	48	Halibut, broiled	60	sour, cultured	60
Cookies		Oysters, canned	230	Ice Cream (12% fat)	
chocolate chip	60	Salmon, broiled or baked	47	Ice milk, vanilla	14
molasses	45	Scallops, steamed	53	Milk	
oatmeal with raisins	52	Shrimp, canned	150	evaporated, unsweetened, canned	31
peanut	55	Shrimp, French fried	120	low fat (1% fat)	4
Doughnut, cake type	83	Tuna, canned in oil or water	63	low fat (2% fat)	8
Pies		Meats and Poultry		skim	2
apple, frozen	10	Bacon, cooked	81	whole	14
Boston cream pie	48	Beef	70	Yogurt	
mince, frozen	10	Chicken	60	low fat with nonfat milk solids, plain	6
		Duck	70		

Necessary Nutrients
The Powerful Proteins

Protein is an indispensable part of the diet—involved in thousands of the body's vital functions and found in every living cell. Once energy needs are met, protein is your body's most important requirement.

Most people value protein foods above all others—an attitude that has a long history. From ancient Greece, where the rich ate poultry and game and the poor ate grains and honey, to 19th-century England, where the aristocracy dined on fish and roasts while the common folk ate bread and potatoes, to contemporary America, protein foods have been considered status foods.

The word protein is taken from the Greek word for "primary," a term chosen by a 19th-century Dutch scientist who believed he had found the "essential substance of animal matter." This researcher was on the right track, but many more years of investigation were needed to determine the true biochemical nature of protein and to uncover its wide range of functions in the human body.

The Functions of Protein

Proteins play a variety of important roles in the body. They are needed for the growth, maintenance, and repair of cells, and for the production of enzymes, hormones, and the chemicals that control our heredity. Proteins are the main components of muscle tissue and are important to the internal organs, bones, skin, and hair. They also play a role in the working of the memory and the transmission of impulses through the nerves.

Proteins are important regulators—involved in maintaining the body's osmotic pressure and fluid balance, its acidity (PH), blood pressure, growth, blood-sugar level, and metabolism. Some proteins act as antibodies, some enable the blood to clot, and others transport nutrients and oxygen throughout the bloodstream. Proteins also make up all enzymes, the catalytic substances that control almost all of the chemical processes in our bodies.

Proteins can be a source of energy, supplying the body with 4 calories per gram of protein. When the body does not get enough carbohydrate or fat to meet its energy need, proteins will be broken down to supply these calories. However, proteins that are used for energy are not available for other vital functions that can be carried out only by proteins. This energy-protein relationship explains why a diet that supplies adequate calories from carbohydrates or fats is considered to be protein sparing.

On the other hand, when there is more protein in the body than is needed, this energy must be stored. The body has no provisions for storing extra amounts of proteins in their original form, so protein molecules are altered by the body in order to be stored as fat.

Protein Chemistry

Proteins are the most complex substances known to science. They are large molecules composed of the same elements—carbon, hydrogen, and oxygen—that make up carbohydrates and fats. In addition, proteins contain nitrogen—an element needed by all living plants and animals—and sometimes sulfur, phosphorus, and iron as well. Plants can create protein by combining the nitrogen in the soil, or in some cases air, with carbon dioxide and water, whereas animals get their protein from eating plants or other plant-eating animals.

Every protein is made up of amino acids—smaller molecules known as the building blocks of protein. These molecules can be combined in many different ways, much as the letters of the alphabet are combined to make words. We do not really need to eat proteins themselves, but rather the amino acids from which the body makes its own proteins.

There may be hundreds or thousands of amino-acid compounds in a protein, held together by peptide linkages—unique chemical bonds—in shapes that are coiled, straight, folded, or globular. The complex molecular structure of proteins permits thousands of variations, each one designed to play a specific role in the cell of a plant or animal. The number of amino acids, the order in which they are joined, and the shape of the molecule are directly related to the protein's function. For example, one insoluble shape of protein molecule is part of your hair and nails, whereas a different, soluble shape of molecule carries nutrients through the bloodstream. The order of amino acids in a protein may be a matter of life and death; if just one of the hundreds of amino-acid compounds in hemoglobin—the oxygen-carrying protein of the blood—is out of order, the very serious disease called sickle cell anemia occurs.

It is principally through the process of digestion that the amino acids in foods reach the cells where they are needed. For proteins, unlike carbohydrates and fats, this process begins in the stomach, where large protein molecules are broken down into smaller groups called polypeptides, and continues in the small intestine. Here polypeptides are broken down into amino acids that are absorbed through the intestinal wall into the blood for transport to the liver and to cells throughout the body. Some of these amino acids are used to synthesize new proteins, and some are returned to the liver for energy use, for storage, or for elimination.

DNA and Your Protein Needs

DNA is the material that lets your cells "know" which proteins are needed and how to synthesize them. You may be aware of DNA (deoxyribonucleic acid) as the genetic material that controls inherited traits. DNA is the blueprint that contains the information to duplicate all the cells, tissues, and organs of any human being. The complex structure of this substance was discovered in 1962 by James D. Watson, Francis H. Crick, and Maurice H. F. Wilkins, who received the Nobel Prize for their work. A review of the way DNA works helps to explain the difference in quality among proteins.

DNA is found in every reproducing cell. Although it does not actually take part in protein synthesis, DNA does establish the "code" that enables the amino acids in a particular cell to combine in the correct order and shape—from one generation of cells to the next. Although it is a very complicated process, the linking of amino acids to create a new protein in a cell occurs quickly—and it depends on a full supply of all the "coded" amino acids specified by DNA. These amino acids must be present in the specified quantities, all at the same time.

The human body needs a total of about 22 amino acids to form all its proteins. Your cells can make many of these amino acids, but 8 of them (9 for children) can only be obtained through the food you eat, and are delivered to your cells through the bloodstream. The amino acids that cannot be created in the body, and thus must be present in the diet, are the so-called essential amino acids: leucine, isoleucine, threonine, valine, methionine, lysine, tryptophan, phenylalanine, and (for children) histidine. Although most nutrition scientists agree on the basic designations of essential and nonessential amino acids, the dividing line between the groups is not always precise. Dietary recommendations for pro-

The Remarkable Soybean

Soybeans have been used as a source of protein since ancient times. First cultivated in China more than 2,000 years ago, they were brought to the United States early in the 19th century as animal fodder. Although soybeans are still most frequently used for animal fodder in this country, their versatility and nutritional value, as well as their low cost, are making them increasingly popular.

The dried soybean is a legume that has a higher proportion of protein (30 to 40 percent) than any other vegetable and also contains a generous supply of carbohydrates. Soybean crops yield many "calories per acre" and are an economic source of high protein to produce and to buy.

Soybeans lend themselves to many cooking techniques and, in fact, must always be cooked in order to be digested. Soybeans can also be roasted as a snack or sprouted for use in salads and sandwiches.

Soy protein may be ground into flour, which can be used in baking or for making pasta. Soy protein is also processed and textured to be used as a meat extender or as analogs—to be eaten in place of meat. Soy analogs, formed into shapes and flavored to resemble bacon, ham, fish, chicken, or beef, have limited appeal for most people, although they may satisfy the cravings of some who are forced to give up meat or help with a transition from a conventional to a vegetarian diet.

The most popular soy-protein product today is bean curd, also known by its Japanese name, "tofu." Looking something like cheese, tofu is made by soaking, cooking, and curdling the soybeans to create a food that is mild in taste and easy to use in cooking. Tofu and many other soy-based products are also discussed on page 163.

It should be remembered, however, that no vegetable protein is as complete in essential amino acids as is animal protein—and even soy is no exception. It is low in the essential amino acid methionine, and must be supplemented with a food containing methionine. Modest amounts of eggs, cheese, milk, and other sources of animal protein supply this lack.

Necessary Nutrients
The Powerful Proteins

tein emphasize the importance of a wide variety of foods in order to ensure an adequate supply of each of the essential amino acids.

The quality of a protein food is primarily determined by the amounts of essential amino acids it contains. Since most animal foods contain some amount of all the amino acids, it is the difference in the quantity of each essential amino acid that makes one food a "better" protein source than another. Most proteins of animal origin such as meat, milk, and eggs contain all of the essential amino acids. These proteins are able to maintain body cells and promote growth and are therefore considered complete, or high-quality, proteins.

Proteins from plant or vegetable sources are usually lacking sufficient amounts of one or more of the essential amino acids (except for soybeans, which are considered nearly the equal of animal protein); these are called incomplete, or partially incomplete, proteins. Each such lower quality protein food is lacking more of one particular essential amino acid than the others. Wheat, corn, and rice, for example, are most lacking in lysine, and beans in methionine. This deficient amino acid is known as the limiting one in that protein food.

The classification of proteins as complete or incomplete helps in choosing a diet that provides all the essential amino acids. When two incomplete proteins are combined in one meal, they may produce complete protein if the right foods are chosen and are eaten in the right amounts. Red kidney beans and corn, when combined, supplement each other in lysine and methionine. Not all incomplete protein combinations are this effective, however, and careful, informed selection is needed to assure an adequate intake of protein.

Nutrition scientists use another classification of protein foods—one that assigns them a chemical value based on how closely they match the exact pattern of amino acids needed for protein synthesis within the human body. Although your body is able to take proteins from any source and use them to reconstruct the proteins it needs, some foods provide a combination of amino acids in proportions very close to your body's exact needs. In this classification a whole egg gets the highest rating (100 percent), whereas foods that are lacking in one or more amino acids are rated lower.

Yet another system of protein evaluation—a bio-

Amino Acid Patterns

Proteins are complex molecules constructed of about 22 amino acids—9 of which are essential in the diet and the rest of which we make in our liver. Generally, protein foods of animal origin are "complete" because they contain sufficient amounts of all the essential amino acids, whereas plant proteins are "incomplete" because they lack one or more of these amino acids. The diagram at right shows that milk is a high-quality protein food since it fills the protein pattern. Rice, on the other hand, is lacking a sufficient amount of lysine, making it incomplete. However, when these two foods are combined, the protein pattern of rice can be improved because the additional lysine in milk complements the missing lysine in rice. In the same way, some plant proteins can complement other plant proteins, as in beans and rice.

logical one—rates not only amino acid content but efficiency of use: how much of the protein is actually digested by the body. This standard of protein quality is called net protein utilization.

The fourth, and most widely used, standard is the "protein efficiency ratio," which uses the relationship between intake and growth to compare the protein values of individual foods. By this system, whole egg, again, and milk proteins are given a value of 100, whereas wheat gluten is given a value of 20, signifying that five times the amount of wheat gluten would need to be consumed to achieve the same growth rate and gain in body weight as are achieved by consuming an egg, under the same conditions.

Experts stress that there is a great deal of complex information to be considered in determining the value of protein foods to your body, of which these four classifications form only a small part. Even more important than ratings of individual foods, as well as the way in which the foods are prepared (which affects their digestibility), is a person's full diet with its complex interactions. All these factors are considered in establishing the Recommended Dietary Allowances for protein.

Meeting Your Protein Needs

The Recommended Dietary Allowances for protein are based on body size, with extra amounts recom-

ABC'S OF NUTRITION

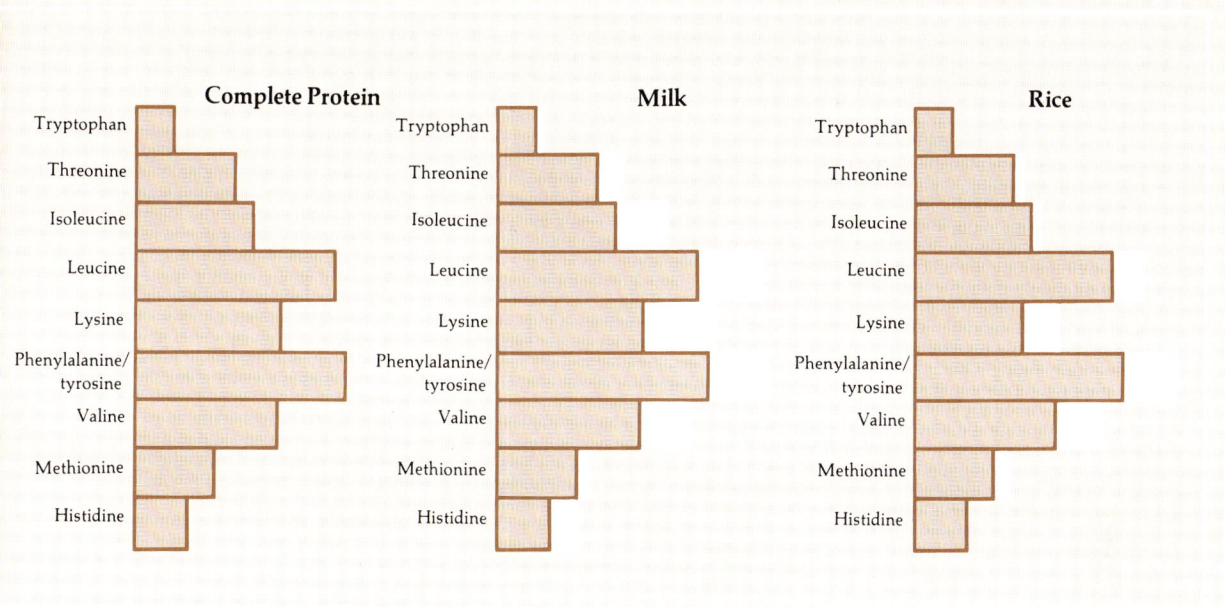

mended for growth, pregnancy, and breast-feeding. More protein may be needed under conditions of stress such as fever, surgery, or shock, and extra amounts may be advised by a physician.

The ideal level of protein intake allows the body to be in a state of nitrogen equilibrium—a condition nutrition scientists determine by measuring the amount of nitrogen waste resulting from use of body protein. In theory, consumption of protein in the diet in amounts equal to those used, or "lost," in the body would create this equilibrium, and would enable researchers to determine the exact protein requirements of certain groups of people. Protein intake that is too high would result in "positive nitrogen balance"—more consumed than excreted—whereas protein intake that is too low would result in "negative nitrogen balance"—more excreted than consumed.

Studies of nitrogen balance are not completely precise. Measurements are subject to error, and the calorie intake of subjects must be neither too high nor too low for true equilibrium to be established. Nonetheless, nutrition experts find these studies useful in determining protein needs.

A recommendation of 0.8 grams of protein per kilogram of body weight has been established, based on the mixed proteins that make up the typical American diet, and allows a generous amount (30 percent) above the proven minimum need to cover individual differences. This amount allows 56 grams of protein per day for a man of average size, and 44 grams per day for a woman. This requirement is easily met by two 3-ounce servings of lean meat, fish, or poultry, a cup of milk, and an egg (although this may not be the ideal diet for some people, who would have to look elsewhere for their protein). For the protein content of foods, see the nutritive value charts on pages 51-93.

Protein Undernutrition

Most people in the United States have little or no trouble meeting their need for protein. However, some individuals with lower standards of living, such as the elderly and certain ethnic groups, and others with higher protein needs, such as pregnant teenagers or women who are breast-feeding, may be deficient in this nutrient. For them, the addition to the diet of low-cost, high-quality protein foods such as poultry or nonfat dry milk, or the substitution of yogurt, cheese, or milk for less nutritious snacks may make up for missing protein.

Serious protein deficiencies, found in environments of extreme deprivation, are usually protein-calorie deficiencies caused by a lack of all types of good food, not just protein. In order for people to exist on low levels of protein, their diets must supply

Necessary Nutrients
The Powerful Proteins

sufficient energy (calories) from other sources—namely carbohydrates and fats. The symptoms of protein-calorie malnutrition include fatigue, lowered body resistance to infection, stunted growth, and mental retardation.

Eating for Protein

You can meet your need for protein with a wide variety of foods: from animal sources alone, from both plant and animal sources, or from specific plant-protein combinations. This variety is possible because the body's need for protein is not a need for a particular food—or a particular nutrient—but is a combined need for various amounts of 22 different amino acids. The combinations in which protein foods are eaten are just as important as the foods themselves.

While high-quality protein foods such as milk, eggs, meat, poultry, and fish will supply all the amino acids you need for protein synthesis in a single food, these are not the only contributors of dietary protein. Grains such as wheat, rice, and corn, potatoes, and leafy vegetables provide lesser quality protein that is an important source of all amino acids as well as vitamins, minerals, and fiber.

By supplementing a vegetable-source protein food with animal-source protein food, you obtain a total amount of dietary protein equal to the dietary protein from a large amount of animal protein alone. Some studies have suggested that combinations of foods from different sources are more beneficial than single protein foods. Apparently, the more different amino acids you eat, the better off you are.

You can also obtain high-quality, or complete, protein without any animal foods—by pairing two specific incomplete proteins in a meal, such as the corn and beans mentioned earlier—a method used by many vegetarians. Although this diet can be a healthful one, vegetarians must carefully choose from a wide variety of foods to meet their full need for high-quality protein. In addition, they must bear in mind that relatively large quantities of plant foods have to be eaten to match the amount of protein one would get from animal sources.

Lacto-ovo vegetarians, who eat milk and eggs in addition to plant foods, have an easier time achieving a well-balanced, complete diet than do vegans, who eat no foods of animal origin. Vegans must rely on meals that supply precise amounts of grains such as wheat, rice, corn, or oats with legumes such as peanuts, chick-peas, kidney beans, black-eyed peas, or soybeans. Meals of this type are popular in many cultures throughout the world. Pasta and beans are eaten in Italy, rice and beans in Latin America, and rice and soybean curd in the Orient—as well as many other healthful combinations.

These meals have provided the necessary protein for millions of people for generations—without the high levels of saturated fat and cholesterol, and the expense, of some of the protein foods favored in the United States. Some nutritionists recommend that we incorporate occasional meatless main meals into our diet—but that we do not make them the sole components of our diets without knowing the drawbacks of vegetarian eating.

For children, the amount of plant food necessary to fulfill the protein requirements of growth may be almost impossible to consume. Some adults may have the same problem, but most likely involving proportions. Since the average person is unlikely to know the amino acid content of many grains or legumes, incorrectly matching up low-quality protein foods may create an amino acid imbalance or deficiency. It is also important to understand that these foods must be eaten at the same meal to be of maximum benefit. For a further discussion of vegetarianism, see pages 390–394.

In general, the best way to assure adequate protein is to include some animal protein in each meal. A glass of milk, a slice of cheese, some yogurt, or a small amount of meat, fish, or poultry will suffice. Many popular dishes such as macaroni and cheese, cereal and milk, spaghetti with meat sauce, or Chinese dishes made with a small amount of fish and a large amount of vegetables and rice are good choices.

In keeping with the U.S. Dietary Guidelines (see pages 96–97), a number of nutrition experts recommend rethinking of protein selection, with greater emphasis on foods such as fish, poultry, low-fat milk products, and legumes. Although many of us have grown up with the idea of meat as the foremost protein food, we should remember that more than half the calories in almost all meats come from fat.

Economics are another consideration in choosing protein foods. Although some foods may seem to be money savers, large amounts of fats or fillers may make sausages, luncheon meats, cold cuts, or very fatty meats relatively high-priced protein per pound. Oversized portions of protein foods can also be wasteful, since extra protein calories are a costly form of bodily energy and, more important from a nutrition standpoint, excess dietary protein may in turn help create larger needs for calcium and other nutrients.

Here are two important reminders in choosing protein foods: foods should not be thought of in terms of a single nutrient, but in terms of their full contribution to the diet; the best way to get protein, and all other nutrients, is by eating a wide variety of healthful foods carefully selected from each of the Basic Four Food Groups.

Protein Myths

Over the years protein has been the subject of much misunderstanding. As a result, a body of myths has arisen regarding the power of proteins. Here are 10 popular fallacies about protein—and the facts to set them straight.

- *Large amounts of protein are needed every day for good health.*

The body uses protein very efficiently, and a little goes a long way. The amount of protein in two chicken breasts will supply an average person's daily need.

- *Athletes need extra protein for strength and endurance.*

Research shows that no extra protein is used by the body during exercise. Protein supplements and high-protein diets promoted for many athletes are expensive and can be stressful to the body. A balanced diet, with extra carbohydrates for needed calories, and a controlled training schedule are recommended for strength and endurance.

- *Red meats build muscle.*

The body has a complex system for using the proteins in all the foods it takes in and for all the functions it carries out. Meat protein does not go directly to the muscles, but is processed in the body in the same way as all other proteins. The body can make protein from carbohydrates and, conversely, can take stored protein to use as an energy source for the carbohydrates missing from the diet.

- *Protein foods are low in calories.*

Proteins supply the same number of calories as carbohydrates—4 per gram. Protein foods such as beef can be high in fat and calories, whereas protein foods such as chicken or skim milk are low in fat and therefore low in calories.

- *Extra protein provides extra energy.*

The body's most efficient energy source is carbohydrate—especially starch. For fighting fatigue, a balanced diet, adequate rest, and regular exercise are recommended.

- *A high-protein diet is the best way to lose weight.*

Proteins do not have the power to burn fat, as some people claim. High-protein diets are not balanced, can put a strain on the kidneys, and do not really change eating habits for the better. Experts recommend a balanced, low-calorie diet for weight loss. Liquid protein diets, it should be noted, can be dangerous, especially to the heart, and should only be followed under a physician's close supervision.

- *Vegetables have no protein.*

Most vegetables contain some amount of protein; dried peas and beans contain very good amounts. However, vegetable protein is not as high quality as animal protein, although it can be made so by balancing vegetables in the diet.

- *Older people do not need protein because they are no longer growing.*

While infants and children need the most protein per pound of body weight, everyone needs some protein for good health. Experts recommend that older people eat no less than 12 percent of their calories as protein foods, which is similar to the amount recommended for younger people.

- *Cosmetics containing protein nourish the skin and hair.*

Proteins cannot be absorbed into living cells through the skin and hair. These products have only a surface effect on the skin and hair.

Necessary Nutrients
What You Should Know About Vitamins

People long suspected that certain foods would prevent or cure illnesses; but proof was lacking until modern times. During the 14th and 15th centuries, sailors at sea died by the hundreds from the vitamin C-deficiency disease scurvy, and ships often returned to port with only a third of their crew. In 1601, however, when the English East India Company sent out its first ship, most of the seamen survived the arduous voyage because the captain had seen to it that each of them received three teaspoons of lemon juice daily. Although many sea captains probably knew that citrus cured scurvy, they did not know why and thus went on experimenting with cheaper and less perishable foods while lives continued to be lost. Finally, at the end of the 18th century, the British Admiralty made it a rule that lemon juice be given to sailors each day, starting with the fifth or sixth week at sea, and mortality rates dropped dramatically. When limes from the West Indies were substituted for lemons in the mid-19th century, British sailors acquired their famous nickname "limeys." However, people still did not know that it was the vitamin C content of lemons (or limes) that prevented or cured scurvy; indeed, no one had ever heard of vitamins.

It wasn't until 1913 that two American biochemists actually isolated the first vitamin. In the course of experimenting with the effects of a specific type of diet on young rats, E.V. McCollum and his associate Marguerite Davis discovered a substance they called simply "fat-soluble A." Just a year earlier, across the Atlantic in England, Casimir Funk, a Polish biochemist who became an American citizen, had partially isolated one of the B vitamins. For this substance he coined the word *vitamine* (for *vital amine*), amine being the group of chemical compounds that Funk believed essential for the prevention or cure of such diseases as scurvy, beriberi, pellagra, and rickets. Although Funk was proved wrong about the chemical compounds (some subsequently isolated vitamins contained no amine), the word caught on and continued to be used, but without the *e*.

In 1922 McCollum identified vitamin D, and from that time on discoveries came in rapid succession. By 1948 scientists had identified the 13 vitamins now considered essential to good human health (see chart on pages 36-37). This was great progress indeed, considering the special challenges of vitamin research: because the amounts of vitamins in the body are so small, they are extremely difficult to detect and track.

The discovery of vitamins was linked at the very beginning to the prevention of disease. In fact, shortly after the turn of the century, Funk and the Englishman Frederick G. Hopkins enunciated the theory of vitamin deficiency disease. And scientists quickly accepted the idea that certain substances in food could prevent disease, adding to the knowledge, learned a century earlier, that diseases were caused by food-borne germs or by infections. Vitamin deficiency diseases are now almost entirely wiped out in this country. Nonetheless, health scientists continue to stress the preventive role vitamins play in warding off deficiency diseases.

What Is a Vitamin?

Vitamins are organic chemical compounds vital in tiny amounts to life and growth. ("Organic" is a chemical term designating compounds containing a carbon skeleton; the molecules of vitamins are made up of carbon, hydrogen, oxygen, and sometimes nitrogen.) They are essential nutrients and must be supplied through diet, since they either are not made in the body or are made in insufficient quantity. A prolonged shortage of any of the vitamins can lead to a deficiency disease. However, all 13 vitamins can be obtained in adequate quantity from a well-chosen diet containing the Basic Four Food Groups (see pages 96–107). The work of vitamins is to help bring about the body's chemical responses. They act as catalysts in the processing of other nutrients (proteins, fats, and carbohydrates), help form red blood cells and hormones, create genetic materials, and regulate the nervous system.

Vitamins fall into two groups: the water-soluble vitamins (B complex and C) and the fat-soluble vitamins (A, D, E, and K). The water-soluble ones are widely found in plant and animal tissues, but some of them are destroyed to a variable degree during the processing of foods and in cooking. Being water-soluble, these vitamins are easily eliminated from the body in sweat or urine; since only small amounts are stored, they must be steadily present in the diet. Fat-soluble vitamins, on the other hand, are less widely distributed in nature. Being fat-soluble and *not* soluble in water, they are not easily excreted and can even build up to toxic levels over a period of time if substantially more than the Recommended

A Nutrition Glossary

Organic. Compounds that contain carbon, such as vitamins, carbohydrates, proteins, fats.

Inorganic. Compounds that do not contain carbon, such as minerals and water. "Inorganic" is not synonymous with "synthetic," as it is sometimes erroneously suggested.

Macronutrients. Vitamins or minerals that are needed in daily amounts of hundreds of milligrams.

Micronutrients. Vitamins or minerals that are needed in daily amounts up to a few milligrams.

Enzymes. These protein molecules, produced by cells, act as catalysts in breaking down carbohydrates, protein, and fats during digestion so that these products can be absorbed; the enzymes remain unchanged in the process. Within all living body cells there are also enzymes that catalyze body metabolism.

Coenzymes or cofactors. Nonprotein substances necessary for the function of some enzymes.

Absorption. A process by which nutrients move from the digestive tract (stomach, small and large intestines) into the bloodstream to be utilized by the body.

Metabolism. A process by which digested nutrients are converted into energy and building blocks for vital processes or body cells.

Nucleic acids. The collective name for the DNA and RNA molecules found in the nucleus of every cell; they are involved in reproduction and cell division.

Hormones. These are substances created in the body and secreted by the endocrine or ductless glands; they regulate enzyme activity of the digestive system and much other cell activity. Hormones are often unfairly blamed for a person being overweight.

Dietary Allowances are consumed daily. A deficiency in a fat-soluble vitamin may take many more months to develop than a deficiency of a water-soluble vitamin.

Although vitamins are needed for thousands of bodily reactions every day, they are required in very small amounts. The total amount of vitamins one person needs each day for maintaining good health measures less than ⅛ teaspoon. Such small amounts are sufficient because vitamins are not usually depleted in doing their work for the body. Instead, the body "recycles" vitamins, releasing and reutilizing them until they are replaced by new ones.

The two units of measure commonly used to express vitamin amounts are milligrams and micrograms. To understand these units, think of an ounce—which equals 28.3 grams. A milligram is 1/1,000 of a gram, or slightly less than .03 ounces. The recommended allowance for the average adult is only 60 milligrams of vitamin C per day, for example. The recommended allowance of some vitamins, such as B_{12}, is even smaller. These are measured in micrograms, that is 1/1,000 of a milligram or 1 millionth of a gram. Thus, a single ounce of B_{12} would be enough to supply one day's requirement for nearly 9 million people. Until recently, international units (IU) were the common measure used to express the biological activity of fat-soluble vitamins. But since these vitamins are found in nature in different forms, with varying degrees of biological effect, this imprecise system has created confusion. To help clear matters, fat-soluble vitamins are now measured in their pure form according to weight (micrograms and milligrams). However, during this period of transition, both systems of measurement will continue to be employed simultaneously.

Recommended Dietary Allowances—RDA

Your vitamin needs depend on your age, sex, weight, level of activity, and state of health. The Recommended Dietary Allowances (RDA), published by the National Academy of Sciences since the 1940s and revised at approximately five-year intervals, provide guidelines that take these factors into account. The RDA are based on "available scientific knowledge" and the amounts of every essential nutrient that should be consumed each day to supply the needs of practically all healthy people.

Necessary Nutrients
What You Should Know About Vitamins

Experts on the National Academy of Sciences' Food and Nutrition Board, who set up the RDA, stress that these recommendations are intended for *groups* rather than for individuals. They tend to be more than any individual needs, since they are amounts to meet the greatest need of any person in any group. However, the RDA are the only reliable and clear-cut set of nutrient recommendations available to most people. They are used in ways that affect each of us. Utilizing the findings of the National Academy of Sciences, the U.S. Food and Drug Administration (FDA) developed the U.S. Recommended Daily Allowances as a standard for labeling the nutrient content of products. The USRDA is now used instead of the MDR, or Minimum Daily Requirements. For a discussion of how the USRDA works in labeling, see page 198.

If your diet is a balanced one and you have no special medical needs, you can be confident that your vitamin intake is adequate. By eating each day four servings of bread and cereal products, four or more servings of fruits and vegetables (including one fresh fruit or fruit juice or one uncooked vegetable), two servings of dairy products, and two servings of meat, fish, or poultry, a healthy adult will obtain all needed nutrients. (Guidelines for selecting food from these Basic Four Food Groups are discussed on pages 96-107.) Even if the quality of your diet varies, your body can adapt accordingly. Although the RDA are based on daily intake, you can achieve nutritional balance over a period of a week or so. Bear in mind, however, that prolonged vitamin shortages can cause health problems, and prolonged avoidance of one or more of the Basic Four Food Groups can produce such a vitamin shortage.

People on weight-loss or other diets containing less than 1,200 calories may not be eating enough food to meet their vitamin needs. Increased physical activity would allow these individuals to consume substantially more calories without weight gain. Mild exercise such as walking would stimulate the appetite of elderly people, whereas more vigorous exercise for the dieters would burn off the additional calories and avoid weight gain. Improved food choices, especially foods of high nutrient density, also boost vitamin levels. Fruits and vegetables, fish and poultry, skim milk, and whole-grain breads are examples of foods that supply substantial amounts of vitamins per calorie.

The choice of how to meet your nutritional requirements is really up to you. Nutrition is a science, and individuals vary widely in their needs and habits. In developing the RDA, nutrition scientists allow for a safety margin in addition to determining the amounts needed to prevent deficiency. Some circumstances can create needs which tap this margin but almost never exceed it. The controversial subject of vitamin supplements is discussed on pages 42-43.

Fat-Soluble Vitamins
Vitamin A, also called retinol, is most important to the health of our eyes. The retina, that part of the eye which reacts to light, changes when we see colors and light or dark. After each reaction the eye needs vitamin A to restore the retina so we can continue to see. An inadequate supply of vitamin A leads to night blindness, causing the eyes to readjust slowly, making it difficult to see in dim light or when changing from light to dark.

In a related role, vitamin A helps maintain the body's epithelial tissues. These are the skin and the linings of the nose, mouth, and throat, the eyes, ears,

Recommended Daily Dietary Allowances

Designed for the maintenance of good nutrition of practically all healthy people in the U.S.A.

	Age	Protein (grams)	Vitamin A (micrograms)[a]	Vitamin D (micrograms)[b]	Vitamin E (milli...)
Infants	to 6 mos.	kg × 2.2	420	10	3
	6-12 mos.	kg × 2.0	400	10	4
Children	1-3 yrs	23	400	10	5
	4-6	30	500	10	6
	7-10	34	700	10	7
Males	11-14	45	1000	10	8
	15-18	56	1000	10	10
	19-22	56	1000	7.5	10
	23-50	56	1000	5	10
	51+	56	1000	5	10
Females	11-14	46	800	10	8
	15-18	46	800	10	8
	19-22	44	800	7.5	8
	23-50	44	800	5	8
	51+	44	800	5	8
Pregnant		+30	+200	+5	+2
Nursing		+20	+400	+5	+3

ABC'S OF NUTRITION

and lungs, and the digestive and urinary tracts. Healthy epithelial tissues are smooth and soft, and are resistant to infection.

Normal growth and development of bones during childhood and their continued soundness in the adult years depend on vitamin A. It also plays a part in the reproductive process and in the creation of hormones.

A shortage of this vitamin can have serious consequences. Xerophthalmia, the advanced stage of night blindness that could lead to permanent loss of vision, is widespread in the Third World. Other symptoms of deficiency include hardening and drying of skin, partial loss of the senses of taste and smell, increased vulnerability to respiratory infections, and faulty development of bones and teeth in children. Serious deficiencies are almost unheard of in this country, even though one-third of children get less than the Recommended Dietary Allowance level of vitamin A. This is because the RDA for vitamin A, as for all vitamins, is well above actual daily need to allow for substantial shortage.

In the United States, overdosage of vitamin A is a serious medical problem. Vitamin A, like all fat-soluble vitamins, can be stored in the body. The question of the minimum human requirement for vitamin A is a cloudy issue because the liver can keep amounts for more than a year.

Infants, children, and teenagers need more vitamin A than adults to help their developing bones and teeth. However, recommended amounts of the vitamin are based on body weight, and increase from 400 micrograms of retinol equivalents for an average one-year-old child to 1,000 micrograms for teenage boys and 800 for teenage girls. Excess amounts of this vitamin can cause glare blindness, loss of appetite, irritability, loss of hair, headaches, joint pain, and nausea. Prolonged megadosing can lead to an increase in pressure inside the skull and even to death. Most vitamin A overdoses occur when children are given a high-potency vitamin supplement. No one should take more than the RDA of vitamin A except on the advice of his physician, after proper evaluation by that physician. Anyone taking 25,000 or more units of vitamin A daily should have his blood vitamin-A level measured at regular intervals

	WATER-SOLUBLE VITAMINS							MINERALS						
Vitamin C (milligrams)	Thiamin (milligrams)	Riboflavin (milligrams)	Niacin (milligrams)[d]	Vitamin B$_6$ (milligrams)	Folacin (micrograms)	Vitamin B$_{12}$ (micrograms)	Calcium (milligrams)	Phosphorus (milligrams)	Magnesium (milligrams)	Iron (milligrams)	Zinc (milligrams)	Iodine (micrograms)		
35	0.3	0.4	6	0.3	30	0.5	360	240	50	10	3	40	Infants	
35	0.5	0.6	8	0.6	45	1.5	540	360	70	15	5	50		
45	0.7	0.8	9	0.9	100	2.0	800	800	150	15	10	70	Children	
45	0.9	1.0	11	1.3	200	2.5	800	800	200	10	10	90		
45	1.2	1.4	16	1.6	300	3.0	800	800	250	10	10	120		
50	1.4	1.6	18	1.8	400	3.0	1200	1200	350	18	15	150	Males	
60	1.4	1.7	18	2.0	400	3.0	1200	1200	400	18	15	150		
60	1.5	1.7	19	2.2	400	3.0	800	800	350	10	15	150		
60	1.4	1.6	18	2.2	400	3.0	800	800	350	10	15	150		
60	1.2	1.4	16	2.2	400	3.0	800	800	350	10	15	150		
50	1.1	1.3	15	1.8	400	3.0	1200	1200	300	18	15	150	Females	
60	1.1	1.3	14	2.0	400	3.0	1200	1200	300	18	15	150		
60	1.1	1.3	14	2.0	400	3.0	800	800	300	18	15	150		
60	1.0	1.2	13	2.0	400	3.0	800	800	300	18	15	150		
60	1.0	1.2	13	2.0	400	3.0	800	800	300	10	15	150		
+20	+0.4	+0.3	+2	+0.6	+400	+1.0	+400	+400	+150	[e]	+5	+25	Pregnant	
+40	+0.5	+0.5	+5	+0.5	+100	+1.0	+400	+400	+150	[e]	+10	+50	Nursing	

[a] Retinol equivalents. [b] As cholecalciferol. [c] Alpha-tocopherol equivalents. [d] Niacin equivalents. [e] The increased requirement during pregnancy cannot be met by the iron content of habitual American diets nor by the existing iron stores of many women. Therefore the use of 30 to 60 milligrams of supplemental iron is recommended.

Necessary Nutrients
What You Should Know About Vitamins

to determine if the blood vitamin A is rising to toxic levels.

True vitamin A, or retinol, is supplied by animal products such as liver, fish oils, milk, and butter. Carotene, found in many fruits and vegetables, is a provitamin, or a vitamin precursor, which the body converts into vitamin A. Too much carotene, while it can cause yellowing of the skin, does not lead to vitamin A poisoning. Foods fortified with vitamin A contain the same form of the vitamin as found in vitamin pills, and eating excessive amounts of vitamin A in any product can be toxic.

Deep-yellow vegetables such as pumpkin, squash, carrots, or yams, and leafy greens such as spinach and broccoli are excellent sources of vitamin A. Cantaloupe, apricots, and mangoes are also high in vitamin A.

Vitamin D is needed for growth and for the forming of bones. It controls the amount and placement of calcium and phosphorus (bone-building minerals) throughout the body. The popular name for vitamin D is "the sunshine vitamin." When your body is exposed to the ultraviolet rays of the sun, an oily substance in the skin is converted to vitamin D and subsequently transferred to the blood stream. However, according to one study, people with heavily pigmented skins may be prevented from assimilating up to 95 percent of vitamin D. It is the only vitamin that is also created in the body from another bodily substance. Vitamin D is unique in being not only a vitamin but also a hormone.

Our greatest need for vitamin D is during the growth years. To assure that children, teenagers, and pregnant and breast-feeding women meet their needs, milk is fortified with 400 IUs of vitamin D per quart, equivalent to 10 micrograms of cholecalciferol. Since milk also supplies calcium and phosphorus, and contains fat to help the body utilize vitamin D, it is the ideal food to promote the development of strong, healthy bones. Children who are strict vegetarians and eat no animal protein (including milk products) are particularly prone to rickets.

The end of childhood does not mean the end of our need for vitamin D. Most adults who live in moderate climates and spend part of their time outdoors can meet this need through some daily exposure to the sun. But people who are dark skinned, who spend all their time indoors, or who live in smoggy regions should be careful to get some vitamin D from their diets.

The two vitamin D-deficiency diseases are rickets, which causes bone deformities in children, and osteomalacia, a condition characterized by softened bones in adults. Much of the groundwork in curing these diseases was done in England early in the 20th century. When a thick blanket of smog created by industrial pollution kept the sun from reaching the workers' tenements, the children in that area developed large joints, knock-knees, and the deformed spine that are characteristic of rickets. Regular dosages of cod-liver oil—one of the few food sources of vitamin D—subsequently prevented the condition.

As with vitamin A, excess doses of vitamin D can create serious health problems. Weight loss, weakness, vomiting, and diarrhea are signs of hypervitaminosis D. Since these symptoms can be caused by other factors, it is always wise to check with your doctor. In advanced stages, toxic amounts of this vitamin can cause calcium deposits in the soft tissues such as the kidneys, eventually causing death.

Amounts of vitamin D as small as 3 to 5 times the RDA are dangerous for children, while 10 times this amount is dangerous for adults. A daily intake of 10 micrograms of cholecalciferol (or 400 international units—the amount in one quart of milk) is considered safe for people of all ages. Natural sources of vitamin D are few. It is found in egg yolk, liver, and oily fish such as tuna or herring. Fish liver oils, the richest concentrated source, are considered a supplement rather than a food.

Vitamin E is a scientific puzzle because it is "a vitamin in search of a disease." It was discovered in 1922 in the course of experiments on fertility in rats. It was named *tocopherol*, from the Greek "to bear young." The results of other animal experiments have led vitamin E enthusiasts to claim benefits to humans ranging from increased sexual potency to prevention of heart disease and the cure of burns. But studies of vitamin E in humans have not substantiated these claims.

Biochemically, vitamin E acts as an antioxidant, meaning that it prevents the oxidation of other substances where oxidation should not occur. It helps to maintain cell membranes and to protect vitamin A and polyunsaturated fatty acids as they are transported in the bloodstream. Vitamin E also helps keep red blood cells from being ruptured by oxidizing agents, thereby leading to blood disorders.

When vitamin E is added to oils, it prevents them from becoming rancid. Its role as a preservative and a protector of cell membranes has led to unsubstantiated claims that vitamin E can prevent the effects of aging. Although vitamin E cosmetics and supplements are popular, there is no evidence that they prolong youth.

The average Recommended Dietary Allowance for vitamin E as alpha-tocopherol equivalents is 10 milligrams for men and 8 for women. This amount is easily met by a balanced diet. If your diet contains considerable amounts of polyunsaturated fats, which accelerate the rate of oxidation of vitamin E, your vitamin E needs rise. However, since high polyunsaturated foods nearly always contain more vitamin E, supplemental vitamin E is unnecessary.

Cases of vitamin E deficiency are almost nonexistent. They are difficult to create even in the laboratory. Premature infants on iron supplements sometimes need vitamin E medication to counteract the oxidant effect of the iron in their red blood cells.

The use of vitamin E supplements is of highly questionable value. The toxic effects that have been reported tend to be mild and have included headache, fatigue, and nausea. As a fat-soluble vitamin, E is stored in the body. If people continue to use the great amounts of E that are popular today, some other harmful effects of excess doses may be further established.

There are many sources of vitamin E in the average diet. These include oils such as peanut, soy, and corn; margarine; whole-grain breads and cereals, especially wheat germ; leafy green vegetables; egg yolks; and liver.

Vitamin K must be present for the proper clotting of the blood. In cases of injury, vitamin K acts as a catalyst, helping to create the clotting factors in blood that prevent hemorrhages. There are a number of chemical forms of vitamin K. K_1 occurs in leafy green vegetables, and K_2 is formed in the human intestinal tract by bacteria normally present there. Synthetic vitamin K, meniadone, is available only by prescription. Because vitamin K is so readily available no recommended allowance has been set. Nonetheless, certain individuals may need extra vitamin K. Newborn infants may not have the necessary intestinal bacteria that aid in formation of the vitamin. People undergoing long-term treatment with antibiotics that kill intestinal bacteria, or those with liver disease, may develop shortages, resulting in prolonged clotting time or liver damage.

Vitamin K deficiencies occur only under severe circumstances and should be treated by a physician. Excessive use of K supplements can be toxic. People with low levels of prothrombin (a blood-clotting factor) may be given vitamin K prior to surgery. To protect a newborn infant, the vitamin may be given to the mother prior to delivery and later to the infant.

The main source of vitamin K is the bacteria in the intestine. Good food sources include green leafy vegetables such as spinach, kale, and darker lettuce, as well as cauliflower, cabbage, egg yolks, and liver.

Water-Soluble Vitamins

Although many people think of the eight B vitamins separately, all of them belong in the B complex group. They are found in many of the same foods and carry out related functions in the body. Most are involved in carbohydrate metabolism: the conversion of sugars and starches to energy. It is important to remember that some of the B complex vitamins are interdependent. If one is missing, the function of others will be affected. Increased intake of a single B vitamin may create a greater need for certain others. In general, moderately excess amounts of B vitamins are not toxic because they are easily eliminated. However, excesses (10 or more times the RDA) should be considered unsafe until proved otherwise.

The B complex vitamins are fragile, since they are soluble in water, and some are easily destroyed by heat and light. Food processing also takes a toll of some of these vitamins.

Thiamin, vitamin B_1, functions in energy production, growth, appetite, digestion, and nerve activity. Nearly half the thiamin in your body is used by the muscles. Thiamin acts as a coenzyme in the energy cycle, enabling a working muscle to operate continuously.

Because thiamin is directly related to the conversion of carbohydrates to energy, thiamin requirements are based on the calorie, or food energy, content of the diet. The recommended allowance is

Necessary Nutrients
What You Should Know About Vitamins

.5 milligrams for every 1,000 calories consumed. If your calorie intake is restricted because of special health problems, a minimal intake of 1 milligram per day is recommended.

Severe thiamin shortages cause beriberi, a serious disease of the nervous system and the heart. Symptoms of this disease are numbness, confusion, apathy, muscular weakness, and swelling of the heart. Beriberi is rarely seen in the United States. However, deficiency symptoms may appear among the populace in areas where the diet depends mainly on unenriched rice and white flour or large amounts of raw fish, the latter of which contains a thiamin-destroying enzyme. Heavy drinkers, who tend to eat poorly, can develop thiamin shortages.

Thiamin is found in a variety of foods, but few contain large amounts. Whereas wheat germ is one of the richest plant sources, pork is one of the best meat sources (one 3-ounce serving supplies about one-half the recommended allowance for an adult male). Legumes are another good source, along with whole grains, liver, and other organ meats.

Riboflavin, vitamin B_2, is a close relative of thiamin. It was discovered during experiments with thiamin: when food was heated, thiamin was destroyed but riboflavin was not.

In the body, riboflavin is used to form a coenzyme that helps to release energy from carbohydrates and fats. This vitamin is also used in protein metabolism, helping the body to metabolize amino acids—the building blocks of protein—in the process of growth and repair. Your body needs riboflavin in amounts based on your calorie intake: .6 milligrams per 1,000 calories of food. Children and pregnant and breast-feeding women, however, need more.

Riboflavin shortages in the body can cause a disease called ariboflavinosis. The symptoms include skin problems such as scaling sores and cracks of the mouth, dim vision, and in children, slowed growth. Severe riboflavin deficiencies are rare because the vitamin is present in various foods. Yet some people may not meet their riboflavin requirement because of poor food choices.

Organ meats (liver, kidney, heart) are the best sources of riboflavin. Milk and cheese are good sources as are whole-grain bread and cereals, dark-green leafy vegetables, legumes, yeast, and eggs. Since riboflavin can be destroyed by light, store

Guide to Vitamins

	VITAMIN	MAIN ROLES
WATER-SOLUBLE VITAMINS	Thiamin (B_1)	Release of energy from carbohydrates; synthesis of nerve-regulating substance.
	Riboflavin (B_2)	Release of energy to cells from carbohydrates, proteins, and fats; maintenance of mucous membranes.
	Niacin	Works with thiamin and riboflavin in energy-producing reactions in cells.
	Pyridoxine (B_6)	Absorption and metabolism of proteins; use of fats; formation of red blood cells.
	Cobalamin (B_{12})	Building of genetic material; formation of red blood cells; functioning of nervous system.
	Folacin (Folic acid)	Assists in forming body proteins and genetic material; formation of red blood cells.
	Pantothenic acid	Metabolism of carbohydrates, proteins, and fats; formation of hormones and nerve-regulating substances.
	Biotin	Formation of fatty acids; release of energy from carbohydrates.
	C (Ascorbic acid)	Maintenance of health of bones, teeth, blood vessels; formation of collagen, which supports body structure; antioxidant.
FAT-SOLUBLE VITAMINS	A (Retinol)	Formation and maintenance of skin and mucous membranes; bone growth; vision; reproduction; teeth.
	D (Calciferol)	Essential for normal bone growth and maintenance of strong bones.
	E (Tocopherol)	Prevents oxidation of polyunsaturated fatty acids.
	K	Essential for normal blood clotting.

ABC'S OF NUTRITION

DEFICIENCY SYMPTOMS*	GOOD SOURCES	REDUCED BY	OVERCONSUMPTION SYMPTOMS
Beriberi: mental confusion; muscular weakness; swelling of heart; leg cramps.	Pork (especially ham); liver; oysters; whole-grain and enriched cereals; pasta and bread; wheat germ; brewers yeast; green peas.	Cooking; baking soda.	Shock from megadoses 1,000 times the RDA.
Skin disorders, especially around nose and lips; eyes very sensitive to light.	Liver; milk; meat; dark-green vegetables; cereals, pasta, bread; mushrooms.	Light.	None reported.
Pellagra: skin disorders, especially parts exposed to sun; smooth tongue; diarrhea; mental confusion; irritability.	Liver; poultry; meat; tuna; cereals, pasta, bread; nuts, legumes. Made in body from amino acid tryptophan.	Cooking.	Flushing, headache, cramps, nausea, itching, liver damage, intestinal problems.
Skin disorders; cracks at mouth corners; smooth tongue; convulsions; dizziness; anemia; kidney stones.	Whole-grain (but not enriched) cereals and bread; liver; avocados; spinach; green beans; bananas.	Cooking; oral contraceptives.	Liver damage in rats.
Pernicious anemia; anemia; degeneration of peripheral nerves.	Liver; kidneys; meat; fish; eggs; milk; oysters.	Grilling on intense heat.	None reported.
Anemia with large red blood cells; smooth tongue; diarrhea.	Liver; kidneys; dark-green leafy vegetables; wheat germ; brewers yeast.	Cooking.	May obscure the existence of pernicious anemia. May be harmful to epileptics taking anticonvulsants.
Not known except experimentally in man: vomiting; abdominal pain; fatigue; sleep problems.	Liver; kidneys; whole-grain bread and cereal; nuts; eggs; dark-green vegetables; yeast.	Not established.	None reported
Known only experimentally in man: fatigue; depression; nausea; pains; appetite loss.	Egg yolk; liver; kidneys; dark-green vegetables; green beans. Made in intestinal tract.	Prolonged treatment with antibiotics and sulfa drugs; raw egg whites.	None reported.
Scurvy: gums bleed; muscles degenerate; wounds don't heal; skin rough, brown, and dry; teeth loosen.	Many fruits and vegetables, including citrus, tomato, strawberries, melon, green pepper, potato, dark-green vegetables.	Heat, light.	When megadose is discontinued, deficiency symptoms may briefly appear until the body adapts. Possible kidney stones. Damage to vitamin B_{12}.
Night blindness; rough skin and mucous membranes; no bone growth; cracked, decayed teeth; drying of eyes.	Liver; eggs; cheese; butter, fortified margarine, and milk; yellow, orange, and dark-green vegetables (e.g. carrots, broccoli, squash, spinach).	Strong light.	**Mild:** nausea, irritability, blurred vision. **Severe:** growth retardation, damage to liver and spleen, loss of hair, rheumatic pain, increased pressure in skull.
Rickets (in children): retarded growth; bowed legs; protruding abdomen. Osteomalacia (in adults): bones soften, deform and fracture easily; muscular twitching and spasms.	Milk; egg yolk; liver; tuna, salmon. Made on skin in sunlight.	Oral contraceptives.	**Mild:** nausea, weight loss, irritability. **Severe:** mental and physical growth retardation, kidney damage, calcium drawn from bony tissue and deposited in soft tissues.
Mild damage to blood cells.	Vegetable oils; margarine; whole-grain cereal and bread; wheat germ; liver; dried beans; green leafy vegetables.	Heat.	Headaches, nausea, tiredness, increased bleeding tendency.
Hemorrhage (especially in newborns).	Green leafy vegetables; vegetables in cabbage family; milk. Made in intestinal tract.	Prolonged treatment with antibiotics and sulfa drugs.	**Newborns:** anemia, jaundice. **Adults:** thrombosis, vomiting.

*The presence of a symptom does not diagnose a deficiency. Many things other than deficiencies produce symptoms similar to those produced by deficiencies. Vitamin deficiencies are diagnosed only by blood and tissue analysis.

Necessary Nutrients
What You Should Know About Vitamins

these foods in opaque containers. And, since a substantial amount of this vitamin can be lost in cooking, using a small amount of water is preferable.

Niacin, sometimes referred to as B_3, is needed for the health of all cells. It works in two ways: to release energy from fats and carbohydrates and to store energy in the body. As part of two coenzymes, it helps to synthesize the body's fat and cholesterol.

Niacin, known until 1971 as nicotinic acid, was first found in yeast. It was recognized as a cure for pellagra, a disease caused by a diet deficient not only in niacin but also in thiamin, riboflavin, and in the amino acid tryptophan, some of which the body converts to niacin. A diet that includes some high-quality protein—the source of tryptophan—will rarely be deficient in niacin. Since the discovery of niacin, pellagra and its accompanying skin disorders and mental confusion is almost never seen today in this country. The role of niacin in curing pellagra-caused mental problems has led some people to speculate that niacin can help in treating schizophrenia. But this has never been demonstrated and has been condemned as misleading.

Your need for niacin is between 13 and 19 milligrams per day, depending on your calorie consumption. Liver and yeast are rich in niacin. Meats, poultry, fish, legumes, wheat germ, whole grains, and nuts supply both niacin and tryptophan. Peanuts and legumes are important niacin sources for vegetarians who eat no animal products.

Pyridoxine, vitamin B_6, is essential for the metabolism and absorption of proteins, the proper use of fats and carbohydrates, and for the maintenance of the central nervous system and red blood cells. There are three forms of B_6 and all are involved with the conversion of tryptophan to niacin; changing of amino acids from one type to another; building of red blood cells; and use of protein for energy.

The need for B_6 was made clear by finding a deficiency among infants fed on a commercial formula

FDA on Food and Drug Interactions

Drugs may act in various ways to impair proper nutrition: by hastening excretion of certain nutrients, or by interfering with the body's ability to convert nutrients into usable forms. Nutrient depletion of the body occurs gradually, but for those taking drugs over long periods of time, these interactions can lead to deficiencies of certain vitamins and minerals, especially in children, the elderly, those with poor diets, and the chronically ill.

Some drugs inhibit nutrient absorption by their effect on the bowel wall. Among these are colchicine, a drug prescribed for gout, and mineral oil, an ingredient used in some over-the-counter laxatives.

A number of drugs affect specific vitamins and minerals. The antihypertension drug hydralazine and the antituberculosis drug INH can deplete the body's supply of vitamin B_6 by inhibiting production of the enzyme necessary to convert the vitamin into a form the body can use, or by combining with the vitamin to form a compound that is excreted.

Similarly, anticonvulsant drugs that are used to control epilepsy can lead to deficiencies of vitamin D and folic acid because they increase the turnover rate of these vitamins in the body.

Quite a few drugs—for example, colchicine, oral antidiabetic agents, and the antibiotic neomycin—can impair absorption of vitamin B_{12}. But because most Americans have good stores of B_{12} in their livers, it takes prolonged ingestion of these drugs to cause a deficiency.

Long-term use of diuretics, or "water pills," to treat such conditions as congestive heart failure, can lead to serious potassium depletion. If the potassium loss is not corrected in heart patients taking digitalis, the heart may become more sensitive to the effects of the drug. People taking diuretics regularly should eat foods which are good sources of potassium. These include tomatoes and tomato juice, oranges and orange juice, dried apricots, cantaloupes, figs, raisins, bananas, prunes, potatoes, sweet potatoes, and winter squash.

Modifying the diet to include more foods rich in the vitamins and minerals that may be depleted by certain drugs generally is preferable to taking vitamin or mineral supplements. In fact, supplements of some vitamins can counter the effectiveness of certain drugs.

Fortunately, the diets of most Americans are sufficiently well balanced so that the threat of drug-related nutritional deficiencies can be easily overcome.

lacking the vitamins. The heat processing of the formula destroyed all the B_6, and some infants became so ill that they developed convulsions. B_6 added to the formula quickly eliminated the problem.

For adults on well-balanced diets, symptoms of B_6 deficiency are rare. Experiments have created a deficiency disease with symptoms similar to those caused by a lack of other B vitamins. The need for vitamin B_6 apparently increases when a high-protein diet is eaten. The recommended allowance for B_6 is thus based on the amount of protein consumed. One's need for B_6 can increase slightly under certain circumstances: pregnancy, use of certain drugs such as birth-control pills, heavy consumption of alcohol, or eating of a high-protein diet. In no case does this increase exceed the RDA.

Liver, fish, poultry, whole-grain breads and cereals, seeds, wheat germ, potatoes, soybeans, yeast, avocados, and spinach are good sources of vitamin B_6. Foods high in other B vitamins are usually high in B_6 as well. Enriched flour, however, does not have the same B_6 value as whole-grain flour, since processing destroys some of this vitamin. Vegetarians should be aware of their B_6 intake, since nonmeat protein foods such as eggs and dairy products do not contain the levels of vitamin B_6 found in meats.

Folacin, or folic acid, is one of the most important of all vitamins. Folacin helps to manufacture red blood cells, to promote normal amino-acid metabolism, and to foster the renewal of all the cells in the body.

The amount of folacin needed by the body is actually quite small—only 400 micrograms is the RDA for average adults. The need rises during pregnancy, when there is greater cell division and production of nucleic acids. The RDA is set higher than most people's needs partly to protect against losses of folacin in cooking and storage, to allow for variability among individuals, and also to allow for storage of a supply sufficient for a few months.

Folacin deficiency can lead to many health problems. There can be disorders of the digestive tract,

Because oral contraceptives are used so widely, their effect on nutrition has been getting increasing attention. The Pill is known to deplete the blood's content of certain vitamins, notably folic acid and vitamin B_6, but usually the vitamin depletion is not serious enough to cause overt symptoms. In most healthy women with good diets, these vitamin levels do not fall to an alarming level, says Dr. Daphne Roe of Cornell University. "But in a poverty group of young women who are trying to make do with very little and who have limited nutritional knowledge, you may find a different situation," Dr. Roe notes. "It is this group we are most concerned about."

Because her requirements for several vitamins may be increased, it is especially important for any woman on the Pill to eat a nutritionally balanced diet. In particular, if a woman on the Pill is living on snack foods, she is more likely to develop folate deficiency than her neighbor who eats such good sources of folic acid as green, leafy vegetables.

Drugs readily available without prescription also can lead to nutritional problems. The worst offenders are antacids, Dr. Roe says, because they are so widely abused by the public. Chronic use of these remedies without a doctor's supervision can cause phosphate depletion, a condition that in its milder form produces muscle weakness and in more severe form leads to a vitamin D deficiency.

"Unfortunately," says Dr. Roe, "some people get into the habit of taking enormous amounts of these drugs to treat gastric upset that in itself is due to their abuse of some other substance, such as alcohol, coffee, or food."

Mineral oil, an old-fashioned laxative still widely used by elderly people and in nursing homes, can hinder absorption of vitamin D. One study reported that as little as 20 milliliters (4 teaspoons) of mineral oil twice daily can interfere with absorption of vitamin D, vitamin K, and carotene, a substance the body converts to vitamin A.

Don't be afraid to ask how drugs might interact with your favorite edibles, especially if you consume large amounts of certain foods and beverages. While taking drugs, be sure to tell your doctor about any unusual symptoms that follow eating particular foods.

If you are eating a nutritionally well-balanced diet from a wide variety of foods, use of a needed drug, even on a long-term basis, is less likely to cause depletion of vitamins and minerals.

Necessary Nutrients
What You Should Know About Vitamins

which affect the body's ability to take in other essential nutrients. The most serious disease resulting from a lack of folacin is macroovalocytic anemia, during which red blood cells become too large and too few. In the United States, folacin deficiencies are sometimes found in women in the last months of pregnancy and while breast-feeding. The deficiency is also seen among alcoholics and in persons who have diets lacking one fresh fruit or vegetable or fruit juice each day.

Liver, green leafy vegetables, yeast, legumes, nuts, eggs, fish, and whole grains are good sources. Oranges have a substantial folacin content. The amount of folacin in nutrient supplements is limited by law, since the taking of folacin-containing vitamin pills can mask the symptoms of pernicious anemia, a serious disease.

Vitamin B_{12}, cobalamin, forms coenzymes used in the metabolism of all reproducing cells, particularly in the bone marrow, where blood is produced. Other important functions are the formation of genetic material and the maintenance of the nervous system.

The RDA for B_{12} is only 3 micrograms. If deficiency of B_{12} occurs, sore tongue, weakness, and disorders of the nervous system can result. Long-term B_{12} deficiency can bring on pernicious anemia: new blood cells develop abnormally, eventually leading to severe anemia. Permanent damage to the spinal cord may finally appear. Pernicious anemia stems from an inability to assimilate B_{12} from food, and appears late in life, in fact, rarely before age 50. People who develop this affliction must have regular B_{12} injections. Fatigue or emotional problems that are not the result of B_{12} deficiency will not be helped by vitamin B_{12} injections.

Only foods of animal origin and certain bacteria supply vitamin B_{12}. Vegetarians who eat no dairy products or eggs will develop a deficiency unless they take a supplement—ideally one that meets the RDA of 3 micrograms. Users of soy "meat substitutes" should look for products fortified with vitamin B_{12}. The best food sources of vitamin B_{12} are liver, meats, poultry, eggs, fish, and milk.

Pantothenic acid is part of coenzyme A, one of the most important enzymes in the body. Coenzyme A has been called a master-control enzyme, taking part in the metabolism of protein, fat, and carbohydrates. Its name is taken from the Greek word *panthos*, meaning "everywhere."

Pantothenic acid is probably the easiest of all vitamins to obtain. It is found in varying degrees in all naturally occurring foods and is manufactured by intestinal bacteria as well. No deficiency of pantothenic acid has been reported outside the laboratory except as part of a deficiency of all B vitamins, and a Recommended Dietary Allowance has not been set. The best sources of pantothenic acid are those foods containing the greatest amounts of the other B vitamins. Processing of foods can destroy some pantothenic acid, but you probably are getting all you need from your intestinal bacteria.

Biotin, once called vitamin H, is needed for growth, energy, and the metabolism of proteins, fats, and carbohydrates. Along with pantothenic acid, biotin is used to form coenzyme A. Biotin is also manufactured by intestinal bacteria.

There is no Recommended Dietary Allowance for biotin. A deficiency, produced experimentally, causes symptoms like those of other B vitamin deficiencies. The protein avidin, found only in raw egg-whites can block the body's use of biotin. Deficiency in adults will only occur if a dozen raw egg-whites are consumed daily over a long period of time.

Vitamin C, ascorbic acid, is the most talked about vitamin. Many spectacular claims are made for this vitamin but none has so far been substantiated.

Most animals produce their own vitamin C from chemicals within their bodies, but humans must rely on food sources. Because the body's ability to store vitamin C is limited, regular intake is important.

Vitamin C is vital to the formation of collagen, the connective tissue that holds cells together. This vitamin helps to maintain the blood vessels, to form the dentine of the teeth, to harden bones, to heal burns and wounds, and form hemoglobin. Vitamin C also helps to make key hormones, to protect other nutrients within the body, and to fight infections.

A prolonged lack of vitamin C leads to scurvy. This disease is practically eliminated in the adult population of the United States, but is sometimes seen in infants six months to one year of age who have had no vitamin C because of their limited diet. True scurvy causes breakdown of blood vessels, muscles, teeth, gums, bone, and skin. A less severe

Vitamin C Questions and Answers

Q. Does vitamin C cure the common cold?
A. Vitamin C *may* help to alleviate the severity of the common cold symptoms such as body aches and chills and fever, but it will not cure or prevent colds.

Q. How much vitamin C do adults need daily?
A. A 4-ounce serving of orange juice provides roughly 60 milligrams of vitamin C—the Recommended Dietary Allowance (RDA) for people over 15 years old. The same amount of vitamin C is supplied by ½ cup of green pepper or cooked broccoli.

Q. Will smoking cause vitamin C loss?
A. Although this has not been proved, a study done in Canada suggested that those who smoked more than a pack of cigarettes a day had approximately 40 percent less vitamin C in their blood than nonsmokers.

Q. Are massive doses of vitamin C harmful?
A. It has been shown that in susceptible people megadoses of vitamin C (10 times the RDA) can lead to the formation of kidney stones. In addition, excessive intake of vitamin C can increase the body's need for this nutrient.

Q. Why is vitamin C added to foods?
A. Vitamin C, or ascorbic acid, is an antioxidant, an agent that prevents foods from becoming rancid or turning brown. Since it is also a nutrient, it can be used to enrich or fortify foods.

Q. Is vitamin C effective in treating cancer?
A. This matter is still under study and no generally accepted conclusion can be drawn.

Q. Can vitamin C be destroyed in cooking?
A. This water-soluble vitamin is one of the most fragile of all nutrients. Foods rich in vitamin C should be cooked in as little water as possible in a stainless steel, aluminum, or enamel pan rather than a glass pan because vitamin C is susceptible to light.

---

shortage of vitamin C causes bleeding gums, a tendency to bruise easily, and pain in the joints, as well as reduced resistance to infection.

To protect the body from scurvy, a minimum of 10 milligrams of vitamin C is needed daily. However, to maintain a desirable level of vitamin C in the body at all times, the RDA is set at 60 milligrams to include everyone. This amount is enough to allow the body to store a five-month supply of vitamin C as a reserve against those days and weeks when the intake of vitamin C may be low.

Very high levels of vitamin C have been recommended for curing the common cold, for preventing cancer, and for various other purposes. A number of carefully controlled studies have shown that vitamin C supplements do not prevent viral colds and flu, although they may slightly lessen the severity of the symptoms. There is some evidence that stress such as infection may slightly increase your need for vitamin C. Many people "under stress" consume large doses of vitamin C "just to be safe." The body uses only the amount of the vitamin it needs, and must eliminate most of the rest through the kidneys, storing only a small percentage. Moderate increases in vitamin C intake are probably harmless, but experts warn against the hazards of large doses, 10 or more times the RDA. Studies relate vitamin C megadoses to problems in treating blood diseases, risk of termination of pregnancy, formation of bladder and kidney stones, destruction of B_{12} in pills and in the body, and loss of calcium from the blood. Large doses can create a dependency that causes deficiency symptoms if dosages are lowered. Pregnant women taking megadoses of vitamin C may give birth to infants who show symptoms of scurvy and whose vitamin C requirements are abnormally high.

Recent research on animals has related vitamin C to a reduction of some forms of cancer and an increase in others. What this information means is not yet known, and nutrition experts recommend a "wait and see" approach.

Everyone knows that citrus fruits are good sources of vitamin C. Strawberries, melons, papayas, and tomatoes are also high in vitamin C, along with broccoli, spinach and other leafy greens, sweet potatoes, raw cabbage, white potatoes, and raw green peppers. It's among the least stable of all the vitamins, easily destroyed by light, air, and heat.

Necessary Nutrients
What You Should Know About Vitamins

Over-the-Counter Vitamins

The pursuit of vitamins has become a national pastime. Many people think of a daily multiple-vitamin pill as nutritional money in the bank. Breakfast cereals that claim to supply "100 percent of your daily allowance for 10 essential vitamins and minerals" are popular, despite their relatively high cost. Some people have been led to believe that our basic diet is inadequate and that they need vitamin and mineral pills to supply their needs and cure their ills. Whatever their reasons for doing so, Americans, it is estimated, spend as much as $5 billion a year on vitamin supplements.

Nutrition scientists know that a well-balanced diet, including choices from each of the Basic Four Food Groups, does not need supplements. When the blood and tissue vitamin levels of people on such diets are measured, they are normal. Vitamin deficiencies can not be diagnosed by hair analyses because there are no vitamins above the root; as for minerals, there is no generally recognized standard for below-normal mineral content of hair.

Although the nutritional needs of individuals differ based on their genetic inheritance, medical needs, lifestyle, and habits, the Recommended Dietary Allowances encompass the entire range of normal needs. People on balanced weight-losing diets below 1,200 calories a day may not be getting enough vitamins. Of course, people on unbalanced diets (see pages 282–292) run the risk of not getting their essential nutrients, including vitamins. Vegetarians, too, may miss out on essential nutrients if they eat no milk products or eggs. Alcohol consumption and prolonged treatment with certain medicines may affect vitamin stores or your ability to absorb vitamins. There is no clear evidence of more than a trivial loss of nutrients by smokers and those who consume quantities of caffeine-containing products. Picky eaters and those who are "too busy to eat" also run risks with their health if they do not follow the rules of moderation and variety which underlie the Basic Four Food Groups.

If maintaining a balanced diet or upgrading your present diet to a balanced one is not possible, then daily multivitamin pills—preferably taken on the advice of a physician—may help you meet your needs. In most cases, a multivitamin pill that supplies no more than the Recommended Dietary Allowance of six essential vitamins is the best choice. Supplements of the fat-soluble vitamins (A,D,E,K) are rarely needed, and our intestinal bacteria supply biotin and pantothenic acid.

If you find it necessary to meet your vitamin and mineral needs with supplements, you may wonder whether to opt for "natural" or "synthetic" vitamins. They are identical, though natural vitamins are extracted from foods, whereas synthetic vitamins are manufactured in the laboratory. Claims that natural vitamins are superior have no basis in fact, though natural vitamins are generally higher in price.

Vitamin research has uncovered much important information, but some remains to be discovered. Many people wish to improve their health through new developments in nutrition, but they are wary, fortunately, of fads and false claims. Nutrition scientists recommend a moderate approach of awareness and "healthy skepticism." This means knowing the credentials of vitamin enthusiasts. For example, to qualify as a professional nutritionist, a person has to complete four years of study in science, nutrition, and other relevant courses at a college or university recognized by the U.S. Department of Education. Registered dietitians have completed a special curriculum in dietetics or nutrition as well as an internship in the field, or have earned a master's degree in nutrition plus work experience in the field. Beware of self-styled nutritionists who write fad-diet books and appear on television to promote them.

Scientifically sound research projects in nutrition are one of the hopes of the future. Meanwhile, government agencies such as the Food and Drug Administration warn consumers of unsubstantiated claims and bring hazards to our attention. Nutrition experts and consumer protectors are especially concerned about two current issues in nutrition: food supplementation and nutrient megadosing.

Food supplementation takes two forms: enrichment and fortification. *Enrichment* is the addition of one or more nutrients to food at higher levels than already present and/or adding back nutrients depleted by processing. This process was originated in the interest of public health. *Fortification*, on the other hand, is the addition of nutrients whether or not they were present in the original food. Fortification has become a profit booster for manufacturers, and large amounts of nutrients are added to products ranging from breakfast cereal to soft drinks.

Consumers may believe they are meeting their nutritional needs while actually eating foods higher in fat or sugar than necessary. A diet based exclusively on highly fortified foods can cause unnecessarily high intakes of certain nutrients and inadequate intakes of others.

Megadoses are vitamin supplements taken in amounts 10 or more times above the Recommended Dietary Allowances. In these amounts, vitamins are being used as drugs rather than as traditional nutrients.

Much of the popularity of megadosage is due to the belief that "if a small amount of a vitamin is good for you, then a large amount is even better." The truth, one nutrition scientist says, is "more is sometimes good, sometimes bad, often irrelevant, and always more expensive." Enthusiasts of megadosage claim cures of diseases ranging from colds to mental illness, but none of these claims has withstood scientific evaluation. The committee that formulates the Recommended Dietary Allowances maintains, as do nearly all nutrition scientists, however, that there is no direct scientific evidence that megadoses are helpful, while there is direct evidence that they may be quite harmful.

There are many promising new developments in vitamin therapy, and these should be noted. Research (still in the early stages) links folic acid deficiency to increased risk of some forms of cervical cancer. Another project suggests a possible relation of vitamin D deficiencies to some forms of diabetes. Large doses of these nutrients may someday be involved in disease prevention or cure—but not all the evidence is in. Moreover, it is known that large doses of these vitamins can be harmful.

Using large doses of vitamins as a guarantee of good health can lead instead to harmful overdoses as well as to undervaluing rest, exercise, and proper diet. Self-treatment of any illness can prevent a person from seeking needed medical help until it is too late. Large doses of vitamins A and D are toxic; niacin can create heart and digestive problems; and vitamin C can promote development of kidney stones. (For symptoms of vitamin overconsumption, see chart on pages 36–37.) Clearly, do-it-yourself vitamin dosing is something to be approached with caution and should never involve megadoses of either vitamins or minerals.

Nonvitamins

The following substances are sometimes incorrectly referred to as vitamins.

Choline. A substance manufactured in the body, choline is a component of lecithin, essential to cell membrane structure; it is a precursor of acetylcholine, which is essential in the transmission of nerve impulses. Although choline is found in organ meats, such as liver, and egg yolks, there is no daily dietary requirement because it is manufactured in the body.

Pangamic acid or pangamate (also but incorrectly called vitamin B_{15}). This is not legal for sale as either a dietary supplement or a drug because the Food and Drug Administration has found that there is no standard of identity for it—that is, it is not a specific substance and each seller can put any substance he chooses in bottles labeled pangamic acid, pangamate, or B_{15}. No dietary need for any product labeled pangamic acid, pangamate, or B_{15} has been demonstrated.

Inositol. A compound adequately produced in the cells, inositol has not been found to be essential in the diets of humans.

Laetrile or amygdalin (incorrectly called vitamin B_{17}). This substance, found in apricot pits as well as pits of other fruits and in bitter almonds, is harmful to human metabolism because it is 6 percent cyanide by weight. Recent laboratory tests have confirmed that it is ineffective in curing cancer. Laboratory studies also show that a dose of laetrile high enough to kill human cancer cells always kills normal cells, so it is too toxic to be used as chemotherapy. The body "detoxifies" laetrile to thiocyanate, which is also a poison.

PABA (para-aminobenzoic acid). A vitamin for some microorganisms but not for humans, PABA has no known value when added to the human diet and may be harmful to a person who is taking a sulfa drug.

Necessary Nutrients
Minerals Your Body Needs

Essential for health and growth, minerals perform many important functions in the body. Among these are: formation of bones and teeth; regulation of body fluids; participation in the life processes of cells, including many chemical reactions.

Essential minerals are divided into two groups: *macrominerals*—needed in amounts from 100 milligrams to 1 gram—including calcium, phosphorus, magnesium, sodium, potassium, chloride, and sulfur; and *trace minerals*—needed in far smaller amounts—including iron, manganese, copper, iodine, zinc, cobalt, fluoride, selenium, and others not yet identified as having specific major health roles.

Experts tell us that the same minerals that are essential to good health can be harmful in excess. Too much of one mineral may interfere with the function of other minerals, or may even be poisonous. Excess minerals pose a special health risk for children, pregnant or breast-feeding women, the elderly, or people with poor diets or diseases.

Animal foods are generally the best sources of minerals, because they tend to contain minerals in the proportions humans need. Large amounts of plant foods tend to pull minerals like iron and zinc out in the stool with excess fiber. Unlike vitamins, minerals are not damaged by heat or light, but some can be lost in excess cooking water. Mineral supplements are seldom needed except for iron. Supplemental iron is needed by many infants, about 10 percent of early adolescents, and about 20 percent of women in the child-bearing years. Taking iron if you don't have a proven iron deficiency is unwise, since it can produce iron overload that can damage the liver, pancreas, and heart.

Calcium is the major building material of bones and teeth. The skeleton holds about 98 percent of the body's calcium and the teeth 1 percent. The remaining 1 percent is used throughout the body for the regulation of muscles—especially the heart—the clotting of blood, nourishment of cells, release of energy, and transmission of nerve impulses. All these bodily functions call for calcium. For this reason, calcium can be considered one of the most essential minerals. The skeleton—often thought of as a solid, static structure—is really living tissue made up of protein and minerals. There is a continuous exchange of materials between the bones and the rest of the body, an exchange controlled by hormones. The amount of the mineral held in storage and the amount drawn on for bodily functions depends on your needs as well as the balance among the calcium and other nutrients in your body. The greatest need for calcium exists during childhood and adolescence and for women during pregnancy and breast-feeding. Infants and children require two to four times more calcium than adults per pound of body weight. The Recommended Dietary Allowance (RDA) for calcium for adults is 800 milligrams; 1,200 milligrams is the recommended intake for adolescents, and 1,600 for pregnant teenagers. The amounts encompass the entire range of need of essentially all members of these three groups.

Calcium deficiency can bring about the same bone problems as those caused by lack of vitamin D. Older adults may develop osteoporosis—brittle, porous bones—from a prolonged shortage of calcium, protein, and vitamins A and C, the group of nutrients involved in maintaining the basic bone structure. For calcium to be properly assimilated, vitamin D must be present. A shortage of calcium can produce nervousness, cramps and muscle spasms, and insomnia. However, these symptoms are much more frequently due to causes that have nothing to do with calcium deficiency.

Calcium is transported from the skeleton to maintain a wide range of body processes. Prolonged "borrowing" of calcium from the bones, without replacement of losses, may cause demineralization of the bones. Studies are now being carried out to determine if demineralization—as well as the many broken bones of old age—can be avoided by diet or hormone treatment to alter the mineral balance. Exercise retards demineralization and helps keep the skeleton appropriately dense. Milk and milk products are the best sources of calcium. Small fish such as sardines, eaten with the bones, green leafy vegetables (except for spinach and Swiss chard), citrus fruits, dried peas and beans, and sesame seeds supply good amounts of calcium.

Phosphorus, the nutritional co-worker of calcium, is also found mainly in the bones and teeth. Phosphorus is a reactive substance that—in addition to building bones—helps to release energy from carbohydrates and build protein, and also forms part of nucleic acid.

The adult RDA for phosphorus is set at 800

milligrams, to equal calcium intake. This amount is intended to limit phosphorus intake to the level of calcium as much as to ward off shortages. Widely unbalanced levels of calcium and phosphorus can have the same effect in the body as a calcium deficiency and lead to bone demineralization.

It is not generally known that phosphorus is added to processed foods, to hams for water retention, and to cola drinks. Although some calcium/phosphorus imbalance is tolerated by the body, high phosphorus levels, such as those associated with excessively high protein diet, should be avoided.

Since most foods contain phosphorus, deficiencies are unlikely to occur in people with normal diets. Meat, poultry, fish, eggs, whole grains, legumes, milk, and cheese are good sources of this mineral.

Magnesium is needed for bone structure, nerve and muscle activity, release of energy, regulation of body temperature, fat metabolism, and protein synthesis. Most adults need about 300 to 350 milligrams of magnesium each day. Nearly all foods contain this mineral, so meeting the RDA presents few problems. However, some alcoholics and postsurgical patients may develop a magnesium deficiency.

The amount of magnesium the body can obtain from food depends on the levels of calcium, protein, phosphorus, and vitamin D in the diet. Some magnesium found in fresh foods can also be lost during some forms of processing. Good sources of magnesium such as whole grains, nuts, beans, leafy vegetables, and milk should be eaten as part of a diet that is adequate in all other nutrients as well. More magnesium is found in hard water than in soft.

Sodium, potassium, and chloride are the regulators of the body fluids. In order for each cell to produce energy or to rebuild its structure, it must obtain needed nutrients from the fluids that surround it. Concentrations of sodium, potassium, and chloride control this exchange across the cell membrane. Sodium is involved in regulating water balance, in muscle contractions, and in nerve reactions. Potassium aids in these functions as well as in protein synthesis and the formation of glucose. Chloride combines with the other two, or with water, to form hydrochloric acid in the stomach for digestion.

Shortages of sodium, potassium, or chloride are unlikely under normal conditions. There are no RDA for these three minerals. Amounts of sodium in the diet are often much higher than we need, and in some people are associated with high blood pressure (see pages 48-49). Sodium is found in table salt, salted foods, and most protein foods. Potassium is contained in almost all foods, especially fruits such as bananas, oranges, or dates, cooked dry beans, winter squash, and in meats. Chloride is supplied almost entirely by sodium chloride.

Sulfur is found in all body tissues. It is important to the forming of cartilage and of hair and nails. Major sources of sulfur are three of the amino acids that make up protein. We also get small amounts from pantothenic acid, thiamin, and biotin. There is no RDA for this mineral. If your diet contains adequate animal protein, there will be no sulfur deficiency, since it is easily obtained from such foods. Sulfur content of vegetable protein varies widely.

Trace Minerals

There are 11 trace minerals now considered essential to human health. Recommended Dietary Allowances have been established for the three that are essential for life: iron, zinc, and iodine. Six other minerals have been found in living creatures to be sufficiently important for the Food and Nutritional Board of the National Academy of Sciences to establish for them estimated safe and adequate dietary intakes. These six are: copper, manganese, fluoride, chromium, selenium, and molybdenum. Very small amounts of these trace minerals are necessary for health and growth. If taken in large amounts, most can become deadly poisons.

Iron is needed to form the compounds that use and transport oxygen in the body. Part of hemoglobin, the oxygen-carrying part of the red blood cell, iron is also a component of certain enzymes used in energy metabolism.

The RDA for iron for most children and males is 10 milligrams. Male adolescents and women of child-bearing age need 18 milligrams of iron per day—an amount that can be difficult to obtain from an average American diet. This explains why iron deficiency occurs frequently among these segments of the population. To meet this increased need for iron during pregnancy, 30 to 60 milligrams daily of supplementary iron is recommended.

Necessary Nutrients
Minerals Your Body Needs

Iron deficiency anemia is the most prevalent nutritional deficiency in this country. In common with anemias of other causes, its symptoms are fatigue, shortness of breath, headaches, and paleness. True iron deficiency should be diagnosed by a doctor through a blood test. You may wind up with iron overload disease if you take iron supplements for an anemia that is not traceable to iron deficiency.

The high rate of iron deficiency is caused in part by the body's ability to absorb only an average of about 10 percent of the iron we consume. Also to blame is the trend away from good dietary sources of iron such as meat, fish, and poultry—20 percent of iron from these sources can be absorbed—toward vegetarian diets—only 2 to 5 percent of iron from plant foods can be absorbed. When we eat a balanced

Guide to Minerals

MINERAL	MAIN ROLES	DEFICIENCY SYMPTOMS*	GOOD SOURCES
Calcium	Formation of bones and teeth; blood clotting; transmission of nerve impulses.	Stunted growth; rickets; osteoporosis; convulsions.	Milk; cheese; dark-green vegetables; sardines; clams; oysters.
Phosphorus	Formation of bones and teeth; acid-base balance.	Weakness; bone demineralization; calcium loss.	Milk; cheese; meat; fish; poultry; grains; legumes; nuts.
Magnesium	Activation of enzymes; protein synthesis.	Failure to grow; behavioral disturbances; weakness; spasms.	Whole-grain cereals; green leafy vegetables; nuts; meat; milk; legumes.
Sodium	Acid-base balance; body-water balance; nerve function.	Muscle cramps; mental apathy; reduced appetite.	Most foods except fruit.
Potassium	Acid-base balance; body-water balance; nerve function.	Muscle weakness; paralysis	Meat; milk; many fruits; cereals; legumes; vegetables.
Chloride	Gastric juice formation; acid-base balance.	Muscle cramps; mental apathy; reduced appetite.	Table salt; seafood; milk; meat; eggs.
Sulfur	Component of active tissue compounds, and cartilage.	Related to deficiency of sulfur amino acids.	Protein foods.
Iron	Component of hemoglobin and enzymes involved in energy metabolism.	Iron-deficiency anemia (weakness, shortness of breath).	Liver; lean meats; legumes; whole grains; dark-green vegetables; eggs; dark molasses; shrimp; oysters.
Zinc	Component of enzymes involved in digestion.	Growth failure; lack of sexual maturation; loss of appetite; abnormal glucose tolerance.	Milk; liver; shellfish; herring; wheat bran.
Iodine	Component of thyroid hormones.	Decreased metabolic rate (hypothyroidism).	Fish and shellfish; dairy products; vegetables; iodized salt.
Copper	Component of enzymes involved in digestion.	Anemia; rarely, bone changes.	Drinking water; liver; shellfish; whole grains; cherries; legumes; kidney; poultry; oysters; nuts; cookies.
Manganese	Component of enzymes involved in fat synthesis.	Not clearly established.	Beet greens; blueberries; grains; legumes; fruit; tea.
Fluoride (Fluorine)	Maintenance of bone and tooth structure.	Higher frequency of tooth decay.	Drinking water; tea; coffee; seafood; rice; soybeans; spinach; gelatin; onions; lettuce.
Chromium	Involved in glucose and energy metabolism.	Moderately reduced ability to metabolize glucose.	Fats; vegetable oils; meats; clams; whole-grain cereals.
Selenium	Can function in association with vitamin E.	Not clearly established.	Fish; poultry; meats; grains; milk; vegetables (depending on selenium in the soil).
Molybdenum	Component of some enzymes.	Not clearly established.	Legumes; cereals; organ meats; dark-green leafy vegetables.

*The presence of a symptom does not diagnose a deficiency. Many things other than deficiencies produce symptoms similar to those produced by deficiencies. Mineral deficiencies are diagnosed by analysis of blood and tissues (other than hair). They cannot be diagnosed by hair analysis because there is no generally recognized lower limit of normal for mineral content of hair.

diet of animal and plant foods, the animal foods increase the absorbability of iron in the plant foods, and the plant food reduces the absorbability of the iron in the animal foods. Thus, we wind up with an average of about 10 percent of the iron absorbed from a balanced meal.

Zinc is used as part of many enzymes in the body. Zinc is important for growth, good appetite, and digestion. The average adult requirement for zinc is 15 milligrams, an amount most people can obtain through diet. Slight zinc deficiencies can be caused by low soil levels of this mineral, which means that zinc is not passed along in the food chain. Symptoms may include decreased sense of taste and slower healing of wounds. Severe zinc deficiencies, however, can stop growth.

Most animal protein foods such as fish, meat, egg yolk, and milk are good sources of zinc. Supplements are not generally recommended except as medical treatment for long-term illnesses, since excessive intake may aggravate marginal copper deficiency. If you need a supplement, do not take more than 100 percent of the RDA (a good rule for any self-administered vitamin or mineral supplement).

Iodine is found in the hormones produced by the thyroid gland. The body's basal metabolism is controlled by these hormones, which are critical to a normal rate of growth from conception to adulthood. A lack of iodine leads to goiter, an enlargement of the thyroid gland in the neck, and to a generally slowed metabolism. Deficiencies before or soon after birth can cause cretinism, which retards physical and mental development.

The adult RDA for iodine is 150 micrograms. The RDA is higher for pregnant and breast-feeding women. The use of iodized table salt in the home can completely prevent iodine deficiency. However, recent studies by the Food and Drug Administration reveal that Americans may be getting several times the iodine they need from a number of unexpected sources. Dairy products, for example, have been found to contain as much as 180 micrograms of iodine per cup. How does the iodine get there? To prevent goiter in cattle, farmers provide their herds with iodine salt licks; some of this iodine is subsequently passed on in the food supply. Another source is iodophors, an iodine-containing chemical used widely by the food-processing industry to disinfect equipment; again, some of this iodine enters the food chain. Finally, of course, seafood is a direct, rich source of iodine. Excessive intakes of iodine can lead to goiter by interfering with the work of the thyroid gland. To deal with the situation, the Food and Nutrition Board in 1980 recommended that the many unexpected sources of iodine in the American food system—such as iodophors in the dairy industry, alginates, coloring dyes, and dough conditioners—be replaced wherever possible by compounds containing less or no iodine.

Other Trace Minerals

Copper is needed for respiratory enzymes and development of red blood cells. Deficiency can cause problems in blood and blood vessels, skeletal defects, and changes in hair color and texture. However, these are highly unlikely in persons who eat a varied diet. Good dietary sources of copper are organ meats, shellfish, nuts, cocoa, and dried legumes.

Fluoride is vital to the formation and strength of teeth and bones. Fluoridated water is the best source of this mineral, also found in canned fish and tea. In those areas where natural fluoride levels in the water are low, fluoridation is recommended by public health authorities.

Manganese is needed for normal bone structure, reproduction, and growth. Deficiencies have never been reported among people who are eating balanced diets, and excesses can be dangerous. Good natural sources include nuts, whole grains, vegetables, and fruits.

Chromium is an aid to normal glucose metabolism and is usually in adequate supply in a balanced diet. The estimated safe and adequate daily dietary intake is from 0.05 to 0.2 milligrams for adults. The upper level (0.2 milligrams) should not be habitually exceeded, because toxic levels for many trace elements may be only several times the usual intakes. Good sources of available chromium are brewer's yeast (a glass of beer, for example), meat products, cheeses, whole grains, and condiments. Vegetables are a poor source of chromium.

Molybdenum, nickel, selenium, silicon, tin, and *vanadium* have all been found in the cells of the human body. Research on the function of these minerals is incomplete. All can be found in foods, and all are poisonous when used to excess.

Necessary Nutrients
Minerals Your Body Needs

Sodium in Your Diet

The indiscriminate use of salt by Americans has concerned health experts as well as the FDA, which issued the following article excerpted here:

Salt—or sodium chloride—was probably the first food additive ever used by man to flavor and preserve meat and fish. Salt is still one of the most popular additives, second only to sugar in the total quantity added to food in the American diet.

The addition of iodine to salt was instituted years ago as a public health measure to prevent goiter, an enlargement of the thyroid gland in the neck as a result of insufficient iodine. Salt manufacturers are not required to add iodine, so consumers should check labels to determine what type of salt they are buying.

Americans like salt. Each of us eats an average of 2 to 2½ teaspoons of it a day—or about 8½ pounds a year. "Not me," you say. "I don't put that much salt on my food!" But what comes pouring out of your salt shaker at dinner or during cooking tells only part of the story. It accounts for only about a third of all the salt in your diet. According to a panel of independent scientists, one-fourth to one-half comes from processed food. The remaining salt you eat occurs naturally in food and in some drinking water.

Many people are confused by the difference between sodium and salt. It is the sodium content of foods that is of health concern to some people. Sodium occurs naturally in many foods and is also added via salt and other sodium-containing ingredients.

To keep sodium in perspective, it's important to understand both its positive and negative aspects. Sodium is an essential nutrient—in fact, we could not survive without it. A healthy person's system can normally handle a wide range of sodium by conserving it when it is scarce and excreting any excess through the urine. However the amount of sodium Americans consume has become a source of increasing concern to nutritionists, health professionals, and others who keep watch on the American diet. More and more evidence is linking excessive sodium intake with hypertension—high blood pressure—a disease that affects 10 to 20 percent of all Americans (estimates vary). Hypertension has been called a silent killer because it rarely produces warning signals, yet it can lead to stroke, heart disease, and kidney failure.

Although the body normally maintains a balance of sodium and other minerals at the proper level, evidence suggests that individuals who are genetically predisposed to hypertension may be increasing their risk by eating a diet high in sodium.

From 10 to 30 percent of all Americans are born with a genetic predisposition to hypertension, according to one estimate. Evidence suggests that when this genetic factor is present, a diet high in sodium will increase the risk of hypertension. It is not widely accepted that sodium actually causes hypertension. Many experts feel that if sodium consumption is high, the effects of other factors that are associated with high blood pressure might be intensified.

For people who are trying to restrict their intake of sodium, eating is somewhat of a guessing game. At present there is no requirement that labels of food products state how much sodium they contain, except for foods claimed to be "low-sodium" or that are otherwise represented as being useful in sodium or salt-restricted diets.

Substantial amounts of sodium are regularly added to processed foods, but not just in the form of salt. Some other common ingredients are sodium nitrite (a curing agent and preservative), sodium benzoate (preservative), monosodium glutamate (MSG, a flavor enhancer), sodium bicarbonate (baking soda, a leavening agent), and sodium phosphate (a wetting agent for quick-cooking cereals).

The "hidden sodium" in processed foods can create difficulties for some people. Consider the predicament of a hypertensive patient who has been told by a physician to keep his or her sodium consumption down to 2,000 milligrams (2 grams) a day. A single serving of canned chicken-noodle soup (about 1¼ cups) would use up more than half the day's allowance of sodium. Besides canned and dried soups and bouillon cubes, some other processed foods that contain large amounts of sodium are canned vegetables, cheese, tomato juice, dill pickles, olives, canned tuna and crab, sauerkraut, frozen dinners, and condiments such as soy sauce, catsup, and salad dressing. Items such as instant pudding, breakfast cereals, ice cream, cookies, cakes, and bread also contain significant quantities of sodium.

Salt substitutes with little or no sodium are available, but these should be used only under advice of a doctor because they contain substantially large amounts of potassium or other substances that may not be desirable for some individuals. Consumers can also buy low-sodium foods that offer enormous reductions in sodium content (for example, most low-sodium versions of the soups mentioned above contain less than 100 milligrams of sodium). These products are regulated as special dietary foods and must state their sodium content. Consumers should read the labels carefully because some of these foods may contain more sodium than the purchaser realizes.

There is one drawback to low-sodium foods that most dieters will mention—the taste. There is just no denying it: to most people salt makes food more palatable. However, gourmet cooks with hypertension (for example, Craig Claiborne) have written cookbooks on how to avoid salt by substituting a wide range of tasty condiments, herbs and spices, and other flavorings such as lemon juice.

Sodium Content of Foods

Food	Sodium (in milligrams)
Beverages	
Beer, 12 fl oz	25
Cocoa with water, 1 c	232
Coffee, 1 c	2
Club soda, 8 fl oz	39
Cola, 8 fl oz	16
Cola, low calorie, 8 fl oz	21
Juices, 1 c	
apple, orange, prune	5
tomato	878
Soda, fruit flavored	34
Wine, white, 4 fl oz	19
Cheeses, 1 oz	
American, process	406
Blue	396
Brie	158
Camembert	239
Cheddar	176
Cottage, low fat	457
Cream	84
Parmesan, grated	528
Swiss	213
Eggs	
Egg	59
Egg substitute, ¼ c	120
Fast Foods	
Cheeseburger	709
Chicken dinner	2,243
French fries, 2½ oz	146
Hamburger, regular	461
Pizza, cheese, ¼ pie	599
Taco	401
Fish and Shellfish, 3 oz	
Clams, raw	174

Food	Sodium (in milligrams)
Bluefish, baked with butter	87
Flounder, baked with butter	201
Salmon, broiled	99
Salmon, pink, canned	443
Sardines, canned	552
Shrimp, canned	1,195
Shrimp, fried	159
Tuna, light meat, canned in oil	303
Grains and Grain Products	
Bran (40%), ⅔ c	251
Crackers	
Graham	48
rye	70
whole wheat	30
Cream of wheat, quick, ¾ c	126
Rice, brown, cooked, 1 c	10
Rice, white, cooked, 1 c	6
Fats and Oils, 1 tbsp	
Butter, salted	116
Margarine, salted	140
Vegetable oil	0
Legumes and Nuts, 1 c	
Almonds	311
Cashews, dry roasted, salted	1,200
Cashews, roasted	21
Beans	
kidney, canned, 1 c	844
kidney or navy, dry, cooked	3-4
Miso, white, ¼ c	2,126

Food	Sodium (in milligrams)
Meats and Poultry	
Bacon, 2 slices	274
Beef, cooked, lean, 3 oz	55
Bologna, beef, 1 slice	220
Chicken, roasted, ½ breast	69
Frankfurter	639
Ham, 3 oz	1,114
Liver, calves, 1 oz	33
Pork, cooked, lean, 3 oz	69
Pork sausage, cooked	168
Salami, beef, 1 slice	255
Milk and Milk Products	
Ice cream, chocolate, 1 c	75
Ice cream, vanilla, 1 c	153
Milk, dry, nonfat, ½ c	322
Milk, whole or low fat	122
Sherbet, orange, 1 c	89
Yogurt, low fat, 8 oz	159
Vegetables	
Asparagus, canned, 4 spears	298
Asparagus, fresh, 4 spears	4
Beets, canned, 1 c	479
Beets, fresh, 1 c	73
Broccoli, fresh, 1 stalk	23
Cabbage, raw, 1 c	8
Celery, raw, 1 stalk	25
Peas, canned, 1 c	493
Peas, frozen, 3 oz	80
Tomato, raw	14
Tomatoes, stewed, canned, 1 c	584

Necessary Nutrients
The Importance of Water

The human body is about 60 percent water, an amount that varies with age, sex, and the proportion of muscle tissue and fat. Infants have the largest percentage of water in their bodies, men have more than women, and athletes more than nonathletes. Approximately 45 quarts of water are distributed throughout the cells of the average adult body. Some parts are more water than anything else: muscles contain about 75 percent water, and blood plasma is almost all water (more than 90 percent). Water also plays an important role in cushioning the joints and internal organs, lubricating body tissues such as eyes, lungs, and air passages, and protecting the fetus during pregnancy.

Of all the essential nutrients, water is the most critical. We can survive on our body's store of food for as long as 10 weeks, but without water, life would be over in a matter of days.

Every function of the body uses water. It is needed for digestion, absorption, circulation, and excretion; for transporting nutrients, helping to build tissue, and maintaining body temperature.

Through perspiration and other bodily functions, large amounts of water are steadily being lost from the body each day. For example, as much as ⅓ of a quart may be exhaled from the lungs every day, and about 1 pint may be lost through perspiration—an amount that increases noticeably in warm weather or during exercise. In very hot, dry climates the water loss may be anywhere from 50 to 100 percent. Perspiration acts as a thermostat for controlling the temperature of the body. The cooling effect of the evaporation of water from the skin allows the inner body to maintain an even temperature regardless of the ambient, or environmental, temperature. Humid weather inhibits this natural evaporation and makes a person feel uncomfortable.

The body's control mechanism for assuring an adequate water intake is thirst. Inadequate replacement of water can result in water depletion heat exhaustion. Never ignore thirst. In fact, you should drink more than to just satisfy your thirst. Most experts agree that the liquid equivalent of six to eight 8-ounce glasses of water per day is sufficient for adults. Alcohol does not count in this equation. Alcohol intake also affects water requirements: 2 ounces of whisky (1 ounce of pure alcohol) requires 8 ounces of water to help metabolize it.

Your individual requirement, though, will be affected by such things as your age, activity level, diet, and the climate in which you live. In general, infants, active people, and those living in the hotter climates need more water than do adults, sedentary people, or those living in the colder zones. If you are on a low-carbohydrate diet you will need large amounts of water to wash out the nitrogen wastes through the urine (see pages 286-287).

The question of adequate water intake is especially important for athletes and others involved in strenuous physical activity. The relatively large amount of weight an athlete may lose during competition is largely a loss of water, in amounts up to 4 or 5 quarts. Failure to replace this water can mean fatigue, salt depletion, and eventually more severe damage to the body. "Sports drinks" are considered of little value, and salt pills should be used only on the advice of a physician.

While liquids such as water, tea, coffee, juices, soups, and the like are the largest suppliers of water to the body, solid foods make a contribution too. Most fruits and vegetables are about 80 percent water; cooked spaghetti is more than 60 percent water; meats are about 50 percent water; and bread is almost 30 percent water by weight. Since water is the one item in the diet that has no calories, its presence in a food is an advantage for the weight-loss dieter. Many crunchy foods such as cucumbers, lettuce, or celery are very high in water and are therefore filling, but are low in calories. These foods also contain fiber, which requires chewing, a factor that adds to their value as low-calorie, satisfying snack foods. Other foods such as bananas, apples, tomatoes, and even spaghetti also can be considered diet aids for weight loss because of their high water content.

There is no reason to avoid drinking water with meals. In fact the practice has no known ill effects just as long as the food is chewed sufficiently and the temperature and amount of water ingested is moderate. Excessive amounts of water, though, can dilute the digestive juices.

Water's role in the body is so vital that experts strongly recommend and urge you to consume adequate amounts, especially if you are active, live in a hot climate, or are suffering from a fever. No matter what your condition, frequent water breaks will improve your performance and health; a cool glass of water will pick you up at the end of a busy day.

Nutritive Value of Foods

ABC'S OF NUTRITION

In 1896 the U.S. Department of Agriculture issued the first general table of food composition for the United States entitled *The Chemical Composition of American Food Materials*. It provided the calorie counts for 1,000 then-common foods plus their water content and the percentage of protein, fat, carbohydrate, and ash (a term then used to include minerals) they contained. At that time the presence of vitamins in foods and the role they play in nutrition were still unrecognized.

Since the publication of that first bulletin, the Department of Agriculture has periodically issued updated and revised food charts. As we learn more about nutrition and the foods we eat, the need for data keeps expanding. Over the years the charts have become increasingly more complex, providing up-to-date information on our food content. The most detailed composition tables appear in a series of books that constitute an ongoing revision of USDA *Agriculture Handbook No. 8 Composition of Foods: Raw, Processed, Prepared*. These are technical publications that are of particular interest to nutritionists and other scientists who are concerned with people's health.

The nutritive value charts presented on the following pages are adapted from *Home and Garden Bulletin 72*, a consumer-oriented brochure that gives a nutrition profile of commonly used foods in household measures and market units. The table of contents to these charts appears at the bottom right of this page.

Generally the foods in each group are listed in alphabetical order; one exception is Dairy Products, where the items are listed according to the category of food, such as cream, milk, and so forth. The approximate measure of each food is given in cups, ounces, pounds, or in another measure that applies to that particular food, such as the number of crackers or cookies or fruits of a specific size. For each item the weight also appears in grams. Remember, though, that the weight of a fluid ounce varies according to the food measured.

The nutritive values for which data are given are as follows: water, food energy (calories), protein, fat, carbohydrate, four minerals (calcium, phosphorus, iron, potassium), and five vitamins (vitamin A, thiamin, riboflavin, niacin, and ascorbic acid, or vitamin C). The total fat content is given as well as the amount of saturated fatty acids and unsaturated fatty acids. Oleic acid is a monounsaturated fatty acid, whereas linoleic acid is a polyunsatuarated fatty acid and the most essential fatty acid needed in the human diet. Monounsaturated fatty acids do not affect the level of blood cholesterol, whereas, according to some experts, the substitution of polyunsaturated fatty acids for saturated fatty acids tends to lower blood cholesterol.

Each of the foods in these tables has been chemically analyzed. The information is collected from various sources such as unpublished data from the food industry, from independent laboratories, and from government research facilities. Since the same foods vary according to the season, the climate, and the soil in which they grow, many variables have to be taken into account. The values given in these charts are representative for the foods all year round, raw or cooked, throughout the country as a whole.

In broad terms these charts can be used to evaluate your diet and how it compares with generally accepted nutritional needs. The tables are also helpful in planning meals and figuring out calorie intake. You can compare many food items and choose suitable alternates. One important fact to keep in mind, however, is that since the figures represent mean values, you cannot be assured that each food you eat actually contains exactly the amount of nutrients specified in the chart. For this reason it is advisable to use these figures in estimating the quality of your diet over a period of time.

Table of Contents

Dairy Products	52
Eggs	58
Fats and Oils; Related Products	58
Fish, Shellfish, Meat, and Poultry; Related Products	60
Fruits and Fruit Products	64
Grain Products	72
Legumes (dry), Nuts, and Seeds	80
Sugars and Sweets	82
Vegetables and Vegetable Products	84

Nutritive Value of Foods

Foods, approximate measures, units, and weight (in grams)		Water	Food energy	Protein	Fat
DAIRY PRODUCTS (BUTTER, CHEESE, CREAM, IMITATION CREAM, MILK; RELATED PRODUCTS)	Grams	Percent	Calories	Grams	Grams
Butter					
Regular (1 brick or 4 sticks per lb)					
Stick (½ cup) . . . . 1 stick	113	16	815	1	92
Tablespoon (about 1/8 stick) . . . . 1 tbsp	14	16	100	Trace	12
Pat (1 in square, 1/3 in high; 90 per lb) . . . . 1 pat	5	16	35	Trace	4
Whipped (6 sticks or two 8-oz containers per lb)					
Stick (½ cup) . . . . 1 stick	76	16	540	1	61
Tablespoon (about 1/8 stick) . . . . 1 tbsp	9	16	65	Trace	8
Pat (1¼ in square, 1/3 in high; 120 per lb) . . . . . 1 pat	4	16	25	Trace	3
Cheese, natural					
Blue . . . . 1 oz	28	42	100	6	8
Camembert, wedge (1.3 oz) . . . . 1 wedge	38	52	115	8	9
Cheddar					
Cut pieces . . . . 1 oz	28	37	115	7	9
Shredded . . . . 1 cup	113	37	455	28	37
Cottage					
Creamed (4% fat)					
Large curd . . . . 1 cup	225	79	235	28	10
Small curd . . . . 1 cup	210	79	220	26	9
Low fat (2%) . . . . 1 cup	226	79	205	31	4
Low fat (1%) . . . . 1 cup	226	82	165	28	2
Uncreamed (dry curd, less than 0.5% fat) . . . . . 1 cup	145	80	125	25	1
Cream . . . . 1 oz	28	54	100	2	10
Mozzarella					
Whole milk . . . . 1 oz	28	48	90	6	7
Part skim milk . . . . 1 oz	28	49	80	8	5
Parmesan, grated					
Cup . . . . 1 cup	100	18	455	42	30
Tablespoon . . . . 1 tbsp	5	18	25	2	2
Ounce . . . . 1 oz	28	18	130	12	9
Provolone . . . . 1 oz	28	41	100	7	8
Ricotta					
Whole milk . . . . 1 cup	246	72	430	28	32
Part skim milk . . . . 1 cup	246	74	340	28	19
Swiss . . . . 1 oz	28	37	105	8	8
Cheese, pasteurized process					
American . . . . 1 oz	28	39	105	6	9
Swiss . . . . 1 oz	28	42	95	7	7
Cream, sweet					
Half-and-half (cream and milk) . . . . 1 cup	242	81	315	7	28
. . . . 1 tbsp	15	81	20	Trace	2
Light, coffee, or table . . . . 1 cup	240	74	470	6	46
. . . . 1 tbsp	15	74	30	Trace	3

ABC'S OF NUTRITION

Dashes — — in the columns for nutrients denotes lack of reliable data for a constituent believed to be present in measurable amounts.

Fatty Acids			Carbo-hydrate	Calcium	Phos-phorus	Iron	Potas-sium	Vitamin A value	Thiamin	Ribo-flavin	Niacin	Ascorbic acid
Satu-rated (total)	Unsaturated											
	Oleic	Linoleic										
Grams	Grams	Grams	Grams	Milligrams	Milligrams	Milligrams	Milligrams	International units	Milligrams	Milligrams	Milligrams	Milligrams
57.3	23.1	2.1	Trace	27	26	.2	29	3,470	.01	.04	Trace	0
7.2	2.9	.3	Trace	3	3	Trace	4	430	Trace	Trace	Trace	0
2.5	1.0	.1	Trace	1	1	Trace	1	150	Trace	Trace	Trace	0
38.2	15.4	1.4	Trace	18	17	.1	20	2,310	Trace	.03	Trace	0
4.7	1.9	.2	Trace	2	2	Trace	2	290	Trace	Trace	Trace	0
1.9	.8	.1	Trace	1	1	Trace	1	120	0	Trace	Trace	0
5.3	1.9	0.2	1	150	110	0.1	73	200	0.01	0.11	0.3	0
5.8	2.2	.2	Trace	147	132	.1	71	350	.01	.19	.2	0
6.1	2.1	.2	Trace	204	145	.2	28	300	.01	.11	Trace	0
24.2	8.5	.7	1	815	579	.8	111	1,200	.03	.42	.1	0
6.4	2.4	.2	6	135	297	.3	190	370	.05	.37	.3	Trace
6.0	2.2	.2	6	126	277	.3	177	340	.04	.34	.3	Trace
2.8	1.0	.1	8	155	340	.4	217	160	.05	.42	.3	Trace
1.5	.5	.1	6	138	302	.3	193	80	.05	.37	.3	Trace
.4	.1	Trace	3	46	151	.3	47	40	.04	.21	.2	0
6.2	2.4	.2	1	23	30	.3	34	400	Trace	.06	Trace	0
4.4	1.7	.2	1	163	117	.1	21	260	Trace	.08	Trace	0
3.1	1.2	.1	1	207	149	1	27	180	.01	.10	Trace	0
19.1	7.7	.3	4	1,376	807	1.0	107	700	.05	.39	.3	0
1.0	4	Trace	Trace	69	40	Trace	5	40	Trace	.02	Trace	0
5.4	2.2	.1	1	390	229	.3	30	200	.01	.11	.1	0
4.8	1.7	.1	1	214	141	.1	39	230	.01	.09	Trace	0
20.4	7.1	.7	7	509	389	.9	257	1,210	.03	.48	.3	0
12.1	4.7	.5	13	669	449	1.1	308	1,060	.05	.46	.2	0
5.0	1.7	.2	1	272	171	Trace	31	240	.01	.10	Trace	0
5.6	2.1	.2	Trace	174	211	.1	46	340	.01	.10	Trace	0
4.5	1.7	.1	1	219	216	.2	61	230	Trace	.08	Trace	0
17.3	7.0	.6	10	254	230	.2	314	260	.08	.36	.2	2
1.1	.4	Trace	1	16	14	Trace	19	20	.01	.02	Trace	Trace
28.8	11.7	1.0	9	231	192	.1	292	1,730	.08	.36	.1	2
1.8	.7	.1	1	14	12	Trace	18	110	Trace	.02	Trace	Trace

53

Nutritive Value of Foods

Foods, approximate measures, units, and weight (in grams)		Water	Food energy	Protein	Fat
	Grams	Percent	Calories	Grams	Grams
DAIRY PRODUCTS—Continued					
Cream, sweet-Continued					
Whipping, unwhipped (volume about double when whipped)					
Light .... 1 cup	239	64	700	5	74
1 tbsp	15	64	45	Trace	5
Heavy .... 1 cup	238	58	820	5	88
1 tbsp	15	58	80	Trace	6
Whipped topping (pressurized) .... 1 cup	60	61	155	2	13
1 tbsp	3	61	10	Trace	1
Cream, sour .... 1 tbsp	12	71	25	Trace	3
Cream products, imitation					
Creamers, sweet					
Liquid (frozen) .... 1 tbsp	15	77	20	Trace	1
Powdered .... 1 tsp	2	2	10	Trace	1
Whipped topping, sweet					
Frozen .... 1 cup	75	50	240	1	19
1 tbsp	4	50	15	Trace	1
Pressurized .... 1 cup	70	60	185	1	16
1 tbsp	4	60	10	Trace	1
Sour dressing (imitation sour cream) .... 1 tbsp	12	75	20	Trace	2
Ice cream and ice milk. See **Milk desserts, frozen.**					
Milk, fluid					
Whole (3.3% fat) .... 1 cup	244	88	150	8	8
Low fat (2%)					
No milk solids added .... 1 cup	244	89	120	8	5
Milk solids added					
Less than 10 grams of protein per cup ..... 1 cup	245	89	125	9	5
10 or more grams of protein per cup ...... 1 cup	246	88	135	10	5
Low fat (1%)					
No milk solids added .... 1 cup	244	90	100	8	3
Milk solids added					
Less than 10 grams of protein per cup ..... 1 cup	245	90	105	9	2
10 or more grams of protein per cup ...... 1 cup	246	89	120	10	3
Nonfat (skim)					
No milk solids added .... 1 cup	245	91	85	8	Trace
Milk solids added					
Less than 10 grams of protein per cup ..... 1 cup	245	90	90	9	1
10 or more grams of protein per cup ...... 1 cup	246	89	100	10	1
Buttermilk .... 1 cup	245	90	100	8	2
Milk, canned					
Evaporated, unsweetened					
Whole milk .... 1 cup	252	74	340	17	19
Skim milk .... 1 cup	255	79	200	19	1

[1] Vitamin A value is largely from beta-carotene used for coloring. [2] Applies to product without added vitamin A.

ABC'S OF NUTRITION

Dashes — — in the columns for nutrients denotes lack of reliable data for a constituent believed to be present in measurable amounts.

Fatty Acids			Carbo-hydrate	Calcium	Phos-phorus	Iron	Potas-sium	Vitamin A value	Thiamin	Ribo-flavin	Niacin	Ascorbic acid
Satu-rated (total)	Unsaturated											
	Oleic	Linoleic										
Grams	Grams	Grams	Grams	Milligrams	Milligrams	Milligrams	Milligrams	Inter-national units	Milligrams	Milligrams	Milligrams	Milligrams
46.2	18.3	1.5	7	166	146	0.1	231	2,690	0.06	0.30	0.1	1
2.9	1.1	.1	Trace	10	9	Trace	15	170	Trace	.02	Trace	Trace
54.8	22.2	2.0	7	154	149	.1	179	3,500	.05	.26	.1	1
3.5	1.4	.1	Trace	10	9	Trace	11	220	Trace	.02	Trace	Trace
8.3	3.4	.3	7	61	54	Trace	88	550	.02	.04	Trace	0
.4	.2	Trace	Trace	3	3	Trace	4	30	Trace	Trace	Trace	0
1.6	.6	.1	1	14	10	Trace	17	90	Trace	.02	Trace	Trace
1.4	Trace	0	2	1	10	Trace	29	[1]10	0	0	0	0
.7	Trace	0	1	Trace	8	Trace	16	[1]Trace	0	[1]Trace	0	0
16.3	1.0	.2	17	5	6	.1	14	[1]650	0	0	0	0
.9	.1	Trace	1	Trace	Trace	Trace	1	[1]30	0	0	0	0
13.2	1.4	.2	11	4	13	Trace	13	[1]330	0	0	0	0
.8	.1	Trace	1	Trace	1	Trace	1	[1]20	0	0	0	0
1.6	.2	.1	1	14	10	Trace	19	[1]Trace	.01	.02	Trace	Trace
5.1	2.1	.2	11	291	228	.1	370	[2]310	.09	.40	.2	2
2.9	1.2	.1	12	297	232	.1	377	500	.10	.40	.2	2
2.9	1.2	.1	12	313	245	.1	397	500	.10	.42	.2	2
3.0	1.2	.1	14	352	276	.1	447	500	.11	.48	.2	3
1.6	.7	.1	12	300	235	.1	381	500	.10	.41	.2	2
1.5	.6	.1	12	313	245	.1	397	500	.10	.42	.2	2
1.8	.7	.1	14	349	273	.1	444	500	.11	.47	.2	3
.3	.1	Trace	12	302	247	.1	406	500	.09	.34	.2	2
0.4	0.1	Trace	12	316	255	0.1	418	500	0.10	0.43	0.2	2
.4	.1	Trace	14	352	275	.1	446	500	.11	.48	.2	3
1.3	.5	Trace	12	285	219	.1	371	[2]80	.08	.38	.1	2
11.6	5.3	0.4	25	657	510	.5	764	[2]610	.12	.80	.5	5
.3	.1	Trace	29	738	497	.7	845	[3]1,000	.11	.79	.4	3

[3] Applies to product with added vitamin A.

Nutritive Value of Foods

Foods, approximate measures, units, and weight (in grams)	Water	Food energy	Protein	Fat
DAIRY PRODUCTS—Continued	Grams	Percent	Calories	Grams	Grams
Milk, canned-Continued					
Sweetened, condensed .... 1 cup	306	27	980	24	27
Milk, dried, nonfat instant					
Envelope, net wt, 3.2 oz (yields 1 qt) .... 1 qt	91	4	325	32	1
Cup .... 1 cup	68	4	245	24	Trace
Milk beverages					
Chocolate milk (commercial)					
Regular .... 1 cup	250	82	210	8	8
Low fat (2%) .... 1 cup	250	84	180	8	5
Low fat (1%) .... 1 cup	250	85	160	8	3
Eggnog (commercial) .... 1 cup	254	74	340	10	19
Milk desserts, frozen					
Ice cream					
Regular (about 11% fat)					
Hardened .... ½ gal	1,064	61	2,155	38	115
.... 1 cup	133	61	270	5	14
Soft serve (frozen custard) .... 1 cup	173	60	375	7	23
Rich (about 16% fat), hardened .... ½ gal	1,188	59	2,805	33	190
.... 1 cup	148	59	350	4	24
Ice milk					
Hardened (about 4.3% fat) .... ½ gal	1,048	69	1,470	41	45
.... 1 cup	131	69	185	5	6
Soft serve (about 2.6% fat) .... 1 cup	175	70	225	8	5
Sherbet (about 2% fat) .... 1 cup	193	66	270	2	4
Milk desserts, other					
Custard, baked .... 1 cup	265	77	305	14	15
Puddings					
From home recipe					
Starch base					
Chocolate .... 1 cup	260	66	385	8	12
Vanilla (blancmange) .... 1 cup	255	76	285	9	10
Tapioca cream .... 1 cup	165	72	220	8	8
From mix (chocolate) and milk					
Regular (cooked) .... 1 cup	260	70	320	9	8
Instant .... 1 cup	260	69	325	8	7
Yogurt					
With added milk solids					
Made with low-fat milk					
Fruit flavored[6] .... 8-oz container	227	75	230	10	3
Plain .... 8-oz container	227	85	145	12	4
Made with nonfat milk .... 8-oz container	227	85	125	13	Trace
Without added milk solids					
Made with whole milk .... 8-oz container	227	88	140	8	7

[4] Applies to product without added vitamin A. [5] Applies to product with added vitamin A.

ABC'S OF NUTRITION

Dashes — — in the columns for nutrients denotes lack of reliable data for a constituent believed to be present in measurable amounts.

Fatty Acids			Carbo-hydrate	Calcium	Phos-phorus	Iron	Potas-sium	Vitamin A value	Thiamin	Ribo-flavin	Niacin	Ascorbic acid
Satu-rated (total)	Unsaturated											
	Oleic	Linoleic										
Grams	Grams	Grams	Grams	Milligrams	Milligrams	Milligrams	Milligrams	International units	Milligrams	Milligrams	Milligrams	Milligrams
16.8	6.7	.7	166	868	775	.6	1,136	[4]1,000	.28	1.27	.6	8
.4	.1	Trace	47	1,120	896	.3	1,552	[5]2,160	.28	1.19	.6	4
.3	.1	Trace	35	837	670	.2	1,160	[5]1,610	.28	1.19	.6	4
5.3	2.2	.2	26	280	251	.6	417	[4]300	.09	.41	.3	2
3.1	1.3	.1	26	284	254	.6	422	500	.10	.42	.3	2
1.5	.7	.1	26	287	257	.6	426	500	.10	.40	.2	2
11.3	5.0	.6	34	330	278	.5	420	890	.09	.48	.3	4
71.3	28.8	2.6	254	1,406	1,075	1.0	2,052	4,340	.42	2.63	1.1	6
8.9	3.6	.3	32	176	134	.1	257	540	.05	.33	.1	1
13.5	5.9	.6	38	236	199	.4	338	790	.08	.45	.2	1
118.3	47.8	4.3	256	1,213	927	.8	1,771	7,200	.36	2.27	.9	5
14.7	6.0	.5	32	151	115	.1	221	900	.04	.28	.1	1
28.1	11.3	1.0	232	1,409	1,035	1.5	2,117	1,710	.61	2.78	.9	6
3.5	1.4	.1	29	176	129	.1	265	210	.08	.35	.1	1
2.9	1.2	0.1	38	274	202	0.3	412	180	0.12	0.54	0.2	1
2.4	1.0	.1	59	103	74	.3	198	190	.03	.09	.1	4
6.8	5.4	.7	29	297	1.1	310	387	930	.11	.50	.3	1
7.6	3.3	.3	67	250	1.3	255	445	390	.05	.36	.3	1
6.2	2.5	.2	41	298	Trace	232	352	410	.08	.41	.3	2
4.1	2.5	.5	28	173	.7	180	223	480	.07	.30	.2	2
4.3	2.6	.2	59	265	.8	247	354	340	.05	.39	.3	2
3.6	2.2	.3	63	374	1.3	237	335	340	.08	.39	.3	2
1.8	.6	.1	42	343	.2	269	439	[7]120	.08	.40	.2	1
2.3	.8	.1	16	415	.2	326	531	[7]150	.10	.49	.3	2
.3	.1	Trace	17	452	.2	355	579	[7]20	.11	.53	.3	2
4.8	1.7	.1	11	274	.1	215	351	280	.07	.32	.2	1

[6] Content of fat, vitamin A, and carbohydrate varies. Consult the label when precise values are needed for special diets.
[7] Applies to product made with milk containing no added vitamin A.

Nutritive Value of Foods

Foods, approximate measures, units, and weight (in grams)		Water	Food energy	Protein	Fat
EGGS	Grams	Percent	Calories	Grams	Grams
Eggs, large (24 oz per dozen)					
Raw					
Whole, without shell . . . . 1 egg	50	75	80	6	6
White . . . . 1 white	33	88	15	3	Trace
Yolk . . . . 1 yolk	17	49	65	3	6
Cooked					
Fried in butter . . . . 1 egg	46	72	85	5	6
Hard-cooked, shell removed . . . . 1 egg	50	75	80	6	6
Poached . . . . 1 egg	50	74	80	6	6
Scrambled (milk added) in butter. . . . . 1 egg	64	76	95	6	7
FATS, OILS; RELATED PRODUCTS					
Fats, cooking (vegetable shortenings) . . . . 1 tbsp	13	0	110	0	13
Lard . . . . 1 tbsp	13	0	115	0	13
Margarine					
Regular (1 brick or 4 sticks per lb)					
Stick (½ cup) . . . . 1 stick	113	16	815	1	92
Tablespoon (about 1/8 stick) . . . . 1 tbsp	14	16	100	Trace	12
Pat (1 in square, 1/3 in high) . . . . 1 pat	5	16	35	Trace	4
Soft (two 8-oz containers per lb) . . . . 1 container	227	16	1,635	1	184
1 tbsp	14	16	100	Trace	12
Whipped (6 sticks per lb)					
Stick (½ cup) . . . . 1 stick	76	16	545	Trace	61
Tablespoon (about 1/8 stick) . . . . 1 tbsp	9	16	70	Trace	8
Oils, salad or cooking					
Corn . . . . 1 tbsp	14	0	120	0	14
Olive . . . . 1 tbsp	14	0	120	0	14
Peanut . . . . 1 tbsp	14	0	120	0	14
Safflower . . . . 1 tbsp	14	0	120	0	14
Soybean, hydrogenated (partially hardened) . . . . . 1 tbsp	14	0	120	0	14
Soybean-cottonseed blend, hydrogenated . . . . 1 tbsp	14	0	120	0	14
Salad dressings, commercial					
Blue cheese					
Regular . . . . 1 tbsp	15	32	75	1	8
Low calorie (5 cal per tsp) . . . . 1 tbsp	16	84	10	Trace	1
French					
Regular . . . . 1 tbsp	16	39	65	Trace	6
Low calorie (5 cal per tsp) . . . . 1 tbsp	16	77	15	Trace	1
Italian					
Regular . . . . 1 tbsp	15	28	85	Trace	9
Low calorie (2 cal per tsp) . . . . 1 tbsp	15	90	10	Trace	1

[8] Based on average vitamin A content of fortified margarine.

ABC'S OF NUTRITION

Dashes — — in the columns for nutrients denotes lack of reliable data for a constituent believed to be present in measurable amounts.

Fatty Acids			Carbo-hydrate	Calcium	Phos-phorus	Iron	Potas-sium	Vitamin A value	Thiamin	Ribo-flavin	Niacin	Ascorbic acid
Satu-rated (total)	Unsaturated											
	Oleic	Linoleic										
Grams	Grams	Grams	Grams	Milligrams	Milligrams	Milligrams	Milligrams	International units	Milligrams	Milligrams	Milligrams	Milligrams
1.7	2.0	.6	1	28	90	1.0	65	260	.04	.15	Trace	0
0	0	0	Trace	4	4	Trace	45	0	Trace	.09	Trace	0
1.7	2.1	.6	Trace	26	86	.9	15	310	.04	.07	Trace	0
2.4	2.2	.6	1	26	80	.9	58	290	.03	.13	Trace	0
1.7	2.0	.6	1	28	90	1.0	65	260	.04	.14	Trace	0
1.7	2.0	.6	1	28	90	1.0	65	260	.04	.13	Trace	0
2.8	2.3	.6	1	47	97	.9	85	310	.04	.16	Trace	0
3.2	5.7	3.1	0	0	0	0	0	— —	0	0	0	0
5.1	5.3	1.3	0	0	0	0	0	0	0	0	0	0
16.7	42.9	24.9	Trace	27	26	.2	29	[8]3,750	.01	.04	Trace	0
2.1	5.3	3.1	Trace	3	3	Trace	4	[8]470	Trace	Trace	Trace	0
.7	1.9	1.1	Trace	1	1	Trace	1	[8]170	Trace	Trace	Trace	0
32.5	71.5	65.4	Trace	53	52	.4	59	[8]7,500	.01	.08	.1	0
2.0	4.5	4.1	Trace	3	3	Trace	4	[8]470	Trace	Trace	Trace	0
11.2	28.7	16.7	Trace	18	17	.1	20	[8]2,500	Trace	.03	Trace	0
1.4	3.6	2.1	Trace	2	2	Trace	2	[8]310	Trace	Trace	Trace	0
1.7	3.3	7.8	0	0	0	0	0	— —	0	0	0	0
1.9	9.7	1.1	0	0	0	0	0	— —	0	0	0	0
2.3	6.2	4.2	0	0	0	0	0	— —	0	0	0	0
1.3	1.6	10.0	0	0	0	0	0	— —	0	0	0	0
2.0	5.8	4.7	0	0	0	0	0	— —	0	0	0	0
2.4	3.9	6.2	0	0	0	0	0	— —	0	0	0	0
1.6	1.7	3.8	1	12	11	Trace	6	30	Trace	.02	Trace	Trace
.5	.3	Trace	1	10	8	Trace	5	30	Trace	.01	Trace	Trace
1.1	1.3	3.2	3	2	2	.1	13	— —	— —	— —	— —	— —
.1	.1	.4	2	2	2	.1	13	— —	— —	— —	— —	— —
1.6	1.9	4.7	1	2	1	Trace	2	Trace	Trace	Trace	Trace	— —
.1	.1	.4	Trace	Trace	1	Trace	2	Trace	Trace	Trace	Trace	— —

Nutritive Value of Foods

Foods, approximate measures, units, and weight (in grams)		Water	Food energy	Protein	Fat
	Grams	Percent	Calories	Grams	Grams
FATS, OILS; RELATED PRODUCTS—Continued					
Salad dressings, commercial-Continued					
Mayonnaise . . . . 1 tbsp	14	15	100	Trace	11
Mayonnaise type					
Regular . . . . 1 tbsp	15	41	65	Trace	6
Low calorie (8 cal per tsp) . . . . 1 tbsp	16	81	20	Trace	2
Tartar sauce, regular . . . . 1 tbsp	14	34	75	Trace	8
Thousand Island					
Regular . . . . 1 tbsp	16	32	80	Trace	8
Low calorie (10 cal per tsp) . . . . 1 tbsp	15	68	25	Trace	2
FISH, SHELLFISH, MEAT, POULTRY; RELATED PRODUCTS					
Fish and Shellfish					
Bluefish, baked with butter or margarine . . . . 3 oz	85	68	135	22	4
Clams					
Raw, meat only . . . . 3 oz	85	82	65	11	1
Canned, meat and liquid . . . . 3 oz	85	86	45	7	1
Crabmeat (white or king), canned . . . . 1 cup	135	77	135	24	3
Fish sticks, frozen, breaded, cooked, reheated . . . . . . 1 stick (stick, 4 by 1 by ½ in)	28	66	50	5	3
Haddock, breaded, fried . . . . 3 oz	85	66	140	17	5
Ocean perch, breaded, fried . . . . 1 fillet	85	59	195	16	11
Oysters, raw (13-19 medium) . . . . 1 cup	240	85	160	20	4
Salmon, pink, canned, meat, bones, and liquid . . . . . . 3 oz	85	71	120	17	5
Sardines, Atlantic, canned in oil, drained . . . . 3 oz	85	62	175	20	9
Scallops, frozen, breaded, fried, reheated . . . . 6 scallops	90	60	175	16	8
Shad, baked with butter or margarine, bacon . . . . 3 oz	85	64	170	20	10
Shrimp					
Breaded, French fried . . . . 3 oz	85	57	190	17	9
Canned . . . . 3 oz	85	70	100	21	1
Tuna, canned in oil, drained . . . . 3 oz	85	61	170	24	7
Meat and Meat Products					
Bacon (20 slices per lb) broiled or fried, crisp . . . . . . 2 slices	15	8	85	4	8
Beef, trimmed, cooked					
Cuts, braised, simmered, or pot roasted					
Lean and fat (piece, 2½ by 2½ by ¾ in) . . . . . . 3 oz	85	53	245	23	16
Lean only . . . . 2.5 oz	72	62	140	22	5
Ground beef, broiled					
Lean with 10% fat (patty, 3 by 5/8 in) . . . . 1 patty	85	60	185	23	10
Lean with 21% fat (patty, 3 by 5/8 in) . . . . 1 patty	82	54	235	20	17

ABC'S OF NUTRITION

Dashes — — in the columns for nutrients denotes lack of reliable data for a constituent believed to be present in measurable amounts.

Fatty Acids			Carbo-hydrate	Calcium	Phos-phorus	Iron	Potas-sium	Vitamin A value	Thiamin	Ribo-flavin	Niacin	Ascorbic acid
Satu-rated (total)	Unsaturated											
	Oleic	Linoleic										
Grams	Grams	Grams	Grams	Milligrams	Milligrams	Milligrams	Milligrams	International units	Milligrams	Milligrams	Milligrams	Milligrams
2.0	2.4	5.6	Trace	3	4	.1	5	40	Trace	.01	Trace	——
1.1	1.4	3.2	2	2	4	Trace	1	30	Trace	Trace	Trace	——
.4	.4	1.0	2	3	4	Trace	1	40	Trace	Trace	Trace	——
1.5	1.8	4.1	1	3	4	.1	11	30	Trace	Trace	Trace	Trace
1.4	1.7	4.0	2	2	3	.1	18	50	Trace	Trace	Trace	Trace
.4	.4	1.0	2	2	3	.1	17	50	Trace	Trace	Trace	Trace
——	——	——	0	25	244	0.6	——	40	0.09	0.08	1.6	——
——	——	——	2	59	138	5.2	154	90	.08	.15	1.1	8
0.2	Trace	Trace	2	47	116	3.5	119	——	.01	.09	.9	——
.6	0.4	0.1	1	61	246	1.1	149	——	.11	.11	2.6	——
——	——	——	2	3	47	.1	——	0	.01	.02	.5	——
1.4	2.2	1.2	5	34	210	1.0	296	——	.03	.06	2.7	2
2.7	4.4	2.3	6	28	192	1.1	242	——	.10	.10	1.6	——
1.3	.2	.1	8	226	343	13.2	290	740	.34	.43	6.0	——
.9	.8	.1	0	167	243	.7	307	60	.03	.16	6.8	——
3.0	2.5	.5	0	372	424	2.5	502	190	.02	.17	4.6	——
——	——	——	9	——	——	——	——	——	——	——	——	——
——	——	——	0	20	266	.5	320	30	.11	.22	7.3	——
2.3	3.7	2.0	9	61	162	1.7	195	——	.03	.07	2.3	——
.1	.1	Trace	1	98	224	2.6	104	50	.01	.03	1.5	——
1.7	1.7	.7	0	7	199	1.6	——	70	.04	.10	10.1	——
2.5	3.7	.7	Trace	2	34	.5	35	0	.08	.05	.8	——
6.8	6.5	.4	0	10	114	2.9	184	30	.04	.18	3.6	——
2.1	1.8	.2	0	10	108	2.7	176	10	.04	.17	3.3	——
4.0	3.9	.3	0	10	196	3.0	261	20	.08	.20	5.1	——
7.0	6.7	.4	0	9	159	2.6	221	30	.07	.17	4.4	——

Nutritive Value of Foods

Foods, approximate measures, units, and weight (in grams)		Water	Food energy	Protein	Fat
FISH, SHELLFISH, MEAT, POULTRY; RELATED PRODUCTS—Continued	Grams	Percent	Calories	Grams	Grams
Beef, trimmed, cooked-Continued					
Roast, oven cooked					
Relatively fat, such as rib					
Lean and fat (2 pieces, 4 by 2¼ by ¼ in) .... 3 oz	85	40	375	17	33
Lean only .... 1.8 oz	51	57	125	14	7
Relatively lean, such as heel of round					
Lean and fat (2 pieces, 4 by 2¼ by ¼ in) .... 3 oz	85	62	165	25	7
Lean only .... 2.8 oz	78	65	125	24	3
Steak					
Relatively fat, sirloin, broiled					
Lean and fat (piece, 2½ by 2½ by ¾ in) .... 3 oz	85	44	330	20	27
Lean only .... 2 oz	56	59	115	18	4
Relatively lean, round, braised					
Lean and fat (piece, 4 by 2¼ by ½ in) ...... 3 oz	85	55	220	24	13
Lean only .... 2.4 oz	68	61	130	21	4
Beef, corned, canned					
Hash .... 1 cup	220	67	400	19	25
Meat .... 3 oz	85	59	185	22	10
Beef, dried, chipped (2½-oz jar) .... 1 jar	71	48	145	24	4
Lamb, cooked					
Chop, rib (cut 3 per lb with bone), broiled					
Lean and fat .... 3.1 oz	89	43	360	18	32
Lean only .... 2 oz	57	60	120	16	6
Leg, roasted					
Lean and fat (2 pieces, 4 by 2¼ by ¼ in) ...... 3 oz	85	54	235	22	16
Lean only .... 2.5 oz	71	62	130	20	5
Shoulder, roasted					
Lean and fat (3 pieces, 2½ by 2½ by ¼ in) .... 3 oz	85	50	285	18	23
Lean only .... 2.3 oz	64	61	130	17	6
Liver, beef, fried in margarine (slice, 6½ by .... 3 oz 2½ by ½ in)	85	56	195	22	9
Pork, cured, cooked					
Ham, light cure, trimmed, lean and fat, ... 3 oz roasted (2 pieces, 4 by 2¼ by ¼ in)	85	54	245	18	19
Luncheon meat. See also **Sausage.**					
Boiled ham, slice (8 per 8-oz pkg) .... 1 oz	28	59	65	5	5
Canned, spiced or unspiced, slice .... 1 slice (approx 3 by 2 by ½ in)	60	55	175	9	15
Pork, fresh, trimmed, cooked					
Chop, loin (cut 3 per lb with bone), broiled					
Lean and fat .... 2.7 oz	78	42	305	19	25
Lean only .... 2 oz	56	53	150	17	9

[9] Value varies widely.

ABC'S OF NUTRITION

Dashes — — in the columns for nutrients denotes lack of reliable data for a constituent believed to be present in measurable amounts.

Fatty Acids			Carbo-hydrate	Calcium	Phos-phorus	Iron	Potas-sium	Vitamin A value	Thiamin	Ribo-flavin	Niacin	Ascorbic acid
Satu-rated (total)	Unsaturated											
	Oleic	Linoleic										
Grams	Grams	Grams	Grams	Milligrams	Milligrams	Milligrams	Milligrams	International units	Milligrams	Milligrams	Milligrams	Milligrams
14.0	13.6	.8	0	8	158	2.2	189	70	.05	.13	3.1	— —
3.0	2.5	.3	0	6	131	1.8	161	10	.04	.11	2.6	— —
2.8	2.7	.2	0	11	208	3.2	279	10	.06	.19	4.5	— —
1.2	1.0	0.1	0	10	199	3.0	268	Trace	0.06	0.18	4.3	— —
11.3	11.1	.6	0	9	162	2.5	220	50	.05	.15	4.0	— —
1.8	1.6	.2	0	7	146	2.2	202	10	.05	.14	3.6	— —
5.5	5.2	.4	0	10	213	3.0	272	20	.07	.19	4.8	— —
1.7	1.5	.2	0	9	182	2.5	238	10	.05	.16	4.1	— —
11.9	10.9	.5	24	29	147	4.4	440	— —	.02	.20	4.6	— —
4.9	4.5	.2	0	17	90	3.7	— —	— —	.01	.20	2.9	— —
2.1	2.0	.1	0	14	287	3.6	142	— —	.05	.23	2.7	0
14.8	12.1	1.2	0	8	139	1.0	200	— —	.11	.19	4.1	— —
2.5	2.1	.2	0	6	121	1.1	174	— —	.09	.15	3.4	— —
7.3	6.0	.6	0	9	177	1.4	241	— —	.13	.23	4.7	— —
2.1	1.8	.2	0	9	169	1.4	227	— —	.12	.21	4.4	— —
10.8	8.8	.9	0	9	146	1.0	206	— —	.11	.20	4.0	— —
3.6	2.3	.2	0	8	140	1.0	193	— —	.10	.18	3.7	— —
2.5	3.5	.9	5	9	405	7.5	323	[9]45,390	.22	3.56	14.0	23
6.8	7.9	1.7	0	8	146	2.2	199	0	.40	.15	3.1	— —
1.7	2.0	.4	0	3	47	.8	— —	0	.12	.04	.7	— —
5.4	6.7	1.0	1	5	65	1.3	133	0	.19	.13	1.8	— —
8.9	10.4	2.2	0	9	209	2.7	216	0	0.75	0.22	4.5	— —
3.1	3.6	.8	0	7	181	2.2	192	0	.63	.18	3.8	— —

Nutritive Value of Foods

Foods, approximate measures, units, and weight (in grams)		Water	Food energy	Protein	Fat
	Grams	Percent	Calories	Grams	Grams
FISH, SHELLFISH, MEAT, POULTRY; RELATED PRODUCTS —Continued					
Pork, fresh, trimmed, cooked-Continued					
Roast, oven cooked					
Lean and fat (piece, 2½ by 2½ by ¾ in) ...... 3 oz	85	46	310	21	24
Lean only .... 2.4 oz	68	55	175	20	10
Shoulder cut, simmered					
Lean and fat (3 pieces, 2½ by 2½ by ¼ in) ..... 3 oz	85	46	320	20	26
Lean only .... 2.2 oz	63	60	135	18	6
Sausage. See also **Pork, cured** Luncheon meat.					
Bologna, slice (8 per 8-oz pkg) .... 1 slice	28	56	85	3	8
Braunschweiger, slice (6 per 6-oz pkg) .... 1 slice	28	53	90	4	8
Brown and serve (10-11 per 8-oz pkg), cooked .... 1 link	17	40	70	3	6
Deviled ham, canned .... 1 tbsp	13	51	45	2	4
Frankfurter (8 per 1-lb pkg), heated .... 1 frankfurter	56	57	170	7	15
Pork link (16 per 1-lb pkg), cooked .... 1 link	13	35	60	2	6
Salami					
Dry, slice (12 per 4-oz pkg) .... 1 slice	10	30	45	2	4
Cooked, slice (8 per 8-oz pkg) .... 1 slice	28	51	90	5	7
Vienna sausage (7 per 4-oz can) .... 1 sausage	16	63	40	2	3
Veal, medium fat, cooked, bone removed					
Cutlet (4 by 2¼ by ½ in), braised or broiled ...... 3 oz	85	60	185	23	9
Rib (2 pieces, 4 by 2¼ by ¼ in), roasted .... 3 oz	85	55	230	23	14
Poultry and Poultry Products					
Chicken, cooked					
Breast, fried in vegetable shortening .... 2.8 oz	79	58	160	26	5
½ breast (3.3 oz with bones)					
Drumstick, fried in vegetable shortening .... 1.3 oz	38	55	90	12	4
(2 oz with bones)					
Half broiler, broiled (10.4 oz with bones) .... 6.2 oz	176	71	240	42	7
Turkey, roasted					
Dark meat (4 pieces, 2½ by 1 5/8 by ¼ in) ...... 3 oz	85	61	175	26	7
Light meat (2 pieces, 4 by 2 by ¼ in) .... 3 oz	85	62	150	28	3
Light and dark meat, chopped or diced .... 1 cup	140	61	265	44	9
FRUITS AND FRUIT PRODUCTS					
Apples, fresh, unpeeled, cored					
2¾-in diam (about 3 per lb with cores) .... 1 apple	138	84	80	Trace	1
3¼-in diam (about 2 per lb with cores) .... 1 apple	212	84	125	Trace	1
Apple juice, bottled or canned .... 1 cup	248	88	120	Trace	Trace
Applesauce, canned					
Sweetened .... 1 cup	255	76	230	1	Trace
Unsweetened .... 1 cup	244	89	100	Trace	Trace

[10] Applies to product without added ascorbic acid.

ABC'S OF NUTRITION

Dashes — — in the columns for nutrients denotes lack of reliable data for a constituent believed to be present in measurable amounts.

Fatty Acids			Carbo-hydrate	Calcium	Phos-phorus	Iron	Potas-sium	Vitamin A value	Thiamin	Ribo-flavin	Niacin	Ascorbic acid
Satu-rated (total)	Unsaturated											
	Oleic	Linoleic										
Grams	Grams	Grams	Grams	Milligrams	Milligrams	Milligrams	Milligrams	International units	Milligrams	Milligrams	Milligrams	Milligrams
8.7	10.2	2.2	0	9	218	2.7	233	0	.78	.22	4.8	— —
3.5	4.1	.8	0	9	211	2.6	224	0	.73	.21	4.4	— —
9.3	10.9	2.3	0	9	118	2.6	158	0	.46	.21	4.1	— —
2.2	2.6	.6	0	8	111	2.3	146	0	.42	.19	3.7	— —
3.0	3.4	.5	Trace	2	36	.5	65	— —	.05	.06	.7	— —
2.6	3.4	.8	1	3	69	1.7	— —	1,850	.05	.41	2.3	— —
2.3	2.8	.7	Trace	— —	— —	— —	— —	— —	— —	— —	— —	— —
1.5	1.8	.4	0	1	12	.3	— —	0	.02	.01	.2	— —
5.6	6.5	1.2	1	3	57	.8	— —	— —	.08	.11	1.4	— —
2.1	2.4	.5	Trace	1	21	.3	35	0	.10	.04	.5	— —
1.6	1.6	.1	Trace	1	28	.4	— —	— —	.04	.03	.5	— —
3.1	3.0	.2	Trace	3	57	.7	— —	— —	.07	.07	1.2	— —
1.2	1.4	.2	Trace	1	24	.3	— —	— —	.01	.02	.4	— —
4.0	3.4	.4	0	9	196	2.7	258	— —	.06	.21	4.6	— —
6.1	5.1	.6	0	10	211	2.9	259	— —	.11	.26	6.6	— —
1.4	1.8	1.1	1	9	218	1.3	— —	70	.04	.17	11.6	— —
1.1	1.3	.9	Trace	6	89	.9	— —	50	.03	.15	2.7	— —
2.2	2.5	1.3	0	16	355	3.0	483	160	.09	.34	15.5	— —
2.1	1.5	1.5	0	— —	— —	2.0	338	— —	.03	.20	3.6	— —
.9	.6	.7	0	— —	— —	1.0	349	— —	.04	.12	9.4	— —
2.5	1.7	1.8	0	11	351	2.5	514	— —	.07	.25	10.8	— —
— —	— —	— —	20	10	14	.4	152	120	.04	.03	.1	6
— —	— —	— —	31	15	21	.6	233	190	.06	.04	.2	8
— —	— —	— —	30	15	22	1.5	250	— —	.02	.05	.2	[10]2
— —	— —	— —	61	10	13	1.3	166	100	.05	.03	.1	[10]3
— —	— —	— —	26	10	12	1.2	190	100	.05	.02	.1	[10]2

Nutritive Value of Foods

Foods, approximate measures, units, and weight (in grams)		Water	Food energy	Protein	Fat
FRUITS AND FRUIT PRODUCTS—Continued	Grams	Percent	Calories	Grams	Grams
Apricots					
Fresh, without pits (about 12 per lb with pits) .... 3 apricots	107	85	55	1	Trace
Canned in heavy syrup (halves and syrup) .... 1 cup	258	77	220	2	Trace
Dried (28 large or 37 medium halves per cup)					
Uncooked .... 1 cup	130	25	340	7	1
Cooked, unsweetened (fruit and liquid) ...... 1 cup	250	76	215	4	1
Apricot nectar, canned .... 1 cup	251	85	145	1	Trace
Avocados, fresh, whole, without skins and pits					
California, mid and late winter (3-in diam) .... 1 avocado	216	74	370	5	37
Florida, late summer and fall (4-in diam) .... 1 avocado	304	78	390	4	33
Bananas (about 2-6 per lb) .... 1 banana	119	76	100	1	Trace
Blackberries, fresh .... 1 cup	144	85	85	2	1
Blueberries, fresh .... 1 cup	145	83	90	1	1
Cantaloupe. See **Muskmelons.**					
Cherries					
Sour, canned, pitted, water pack .... 1 cup	244	88	105	2	Trace
Sweet, fresh, without pits .... 10 cherries	68	80	45	1	Trace
Cranberry juice cocktail, bottled, sweetened .... 1 cup	253	83	165	Trace	Trace
Cranberry sauce, canned, sweetened .... 1 cup	277	62	405	Trace	1
Dates					
Whole, without pits..................... 10 dates	80	23	220	2	Trace
Chopped .... 1 cup	178	23	490	4	1
Fruit cocktail, canned in heavy syrup .... 1 cup	255	80	195	1	Trace
Grapefruit					
Fresh, medium, 3¾-in diam, with peel					
Pink or red .... ½ grapefruit	241	89	50	1	Trace
White .... ½ grapefruit	241	89	45	1	Trace
Canned, sections with syrup .... 1 cup	254	81	180	2	Trace
Grapefruit juice					
Fresh, pink, red, or white .... 1 cup	246	90	95	1	Trace
Canned, white					
Unsweetened .... 1 cup	247	89	100	1	Trace
Sweetened .... 1 cup	250	86	135	1	Trace
Frozen concentrate, unsweetened, diluted .... 1 cup	247	89	100	1	Trace
with 3 parts water by volume					
Grapes, fresh					
Thompson Seedless (green) .... 10 grapes	50	81	35	Trace	Trace
Tokay and Emperor (red), seeded .... 10 grapes	60	81	40	Trace	Trace
Grape juice					
Bottled or canned .... 1 cup	253	83	165	1	Trace
Frozen concentrate, sweetened, diluted .... 1 cup	250	86	135	1	Trace
with 3 parts water by volume					
Grape drink, canned .... 1 cup	250	86	135	Trace	Trace

[11] For white-fleshed varieties, value is about 20 International Units (I.U.) per cup; for red-fleshed varieties, 1,080 I.U.

ABC'S OF NUTRITION

Dashes — — in the columns for nutrients denotes lack of reliable data for a constituent believed to be present in measurable amounts.

Fatty Acids			Carbo-hydrate	Calcium	Phos-phorus	Iron	Potas-sium	Vitamin A value	Thiamin	Ribo-flavin	Niacin	Ascorbic acid
Satu-rated (total)	Unsaturated											
	Oleic	Linoleic										
Grams	Grams	Grams	Grams	Milligrams	Milligrams	Milligrams	Milligrams	International units	Milligrams	Milligrams	Milligrams	Milligrams
— —	— —	— —	14	18	25	.5	301	2,890	.03	.04	.6	11
— —	— —	— —	57	28	39	.8	604	4,490	.05	.05	1.0	10
— —	— —	— —	86	87	140	7.2	1,273	14,170	.01	.21	4.3	16
— —	— —	— —	54	55	88	4.5	795	7,500	.01	.13	2.5	8
— —	— —	— —	37	23	30	.5	379	2,380	.03	.03	.5	36
5.5	22.0	3.7	13	22	91	1.3	1,303	630	.24	.43	3.5	30
6.7	15.7	5.3	27	30	128	1.8	1,836	880	.33	.61	4.9	43
— —	— —	— —	26	10	31	.8	440	230	.06	.07	.8	12
— —	— —	— —	19	46	27	1.3	245	290	0.04	0.06	0.6	30
— —	— —	— —	22	22	19	1.5	117	150	.04	.09	.7	20
— —	— —	— —	26	37	32	.7	317	1,660	.07	.05	.5	12
— —	— —	— —	12	15	13	.3	129	70	.03	.04	.3	7
— —	— —	— —	42	13	8	.8	25	Trace	.03	.03	.1	81
— —	— —	— —	104	17	11	.6	83	60	.03	.03	.1	6
— —	— —	— —	58	47	50	2.4	518	40	.07	.08	1.8	0
— —	— —	— —	130	105	112	5.3	1,153	90	.16	.18	3.9	0
— —	— —	— —	50	23	31	1.0	411	360	.05	.03	1.0	5
— —	— —	— —	13	20	20	.5	166	540	.05	.02	.2	44
— —	— —	— —	12	19	19	.5	159	10	.05	.02	.2	44
— —	— —	— —	45	33	36	.8	343	30	.08	.05	.5	76
— —	— —	— —	23	22	37	.5	399	([11])	.10	.05	.5	93
— —	— —	— —	24	20	35	1.0	400	20	.07	.05	.5	84
— —	— —	— —	32	20	35	1.0	405	30	.08	.05	.5	78
— —	— —	— —	24	25	42	.2	420	20	.10	.04	.5	96
— —	— —	— —	9	6	10	.2	87	50	.03	.02	.2	2
— —	— —	— —	10	7	11	.2	99	60	.03	.02	.2	2
— —	— —	— —	42	28	30	.8	293	— —	.10	.05	.5	[12]Trace
— —	— —	— —	33	8	10	.3	85	10	.05	.08	.5	[12]10
— —	— —	— —	35	8	10	.3	88	— —	([13])	([13])	.3	11

[12] Applies to product without added ascorbic acid.   [13] Value varies with brand. Consult the label.

Nutritive Value of Foods

Foods, approximate measures, units, and weight (in grams)		Water	Food energy	Protein	Fat
		Grams	Percent	Calories	Grams	Grams
FRUITS AND FRUIT PRODUCTS—Continued						
Lemon, fresh, without peel and seeds . . . . 1 lemon	74	90	20	1	Trace
Lemon juice					
Fresh . . . . 1 cup	244	91	60	1	Trace
Bottled or canned, unsweetened . . . . 1 cup	244	92	55	1	Trace
Lemonade, frozen concentrate, diluted . . . . 1 cup with 4 1/3 parts water by volume	248	89	105	Trace	Trace
Limeade, frozen concentrate, diluted . . . . 1 cup with 4 1/3 parts water by volume	247	89	100	Trace	Trace
Lime juice					
Fresh . . . . 1 cup	246	90	65	1	Trace
Canned, unsweetened . . . . 1 cup	246	90	65	1	Trace
Muskmelons, fresh, with rind, without seed cavity					
Cantaloupe, orange-fleshed (5-in diam) . . . . ½ melon	477	91	80	2	Trace
Honeydew (6½-in diam) . . . . 1/10 melon	226	91	50	1	Trace
Oranges, all varieties, fresh					
Whole, 3-in diam, without peel and seeds . . . . . . 1 orange	131	86	65	1	Trace
Sections, without membranes . . . . 1 cup	180	86	90	2	Trace
Orange juice					
Fresh, all varieties . . . . 1 cup	248	88	110	2	Trace
Canned, unsweetened . . . . 1 cup	249	87	120	2	Trace
Frozen concentrate, unsweetened, diluted with . . . 1 cup 3 parts water by volume	249	87	120	2	Trace
Papayas, fresh, ½-in cubes . . . . 1 cup	140	89	55	1	Trace
Peaches					
Fresh, yellow-fleshed					
Whole, 2½-in diam, peeled, pitted (about . . . . . 1 peach 4 per lb with peels and pits)	100	89	40	1	Trace
Sliced . . . . 1 cup	170	89	65	1	Trace
Canned, fruit and liquid (halves or slices)					
Syrup pack . . . . 1 cup	256	79	200	1	Trace
Water pack . . . . 1 cup	244	91	75	1	Trace
Dried					
Uncooked . . . . 1 cup	160	25	420	5	1
Cooked, unsweetened, halves and liquid . . . . . . 1 cup	250	77	205	3	1
Frozen, sliced, sweetened, ascorbic acid added					
10-oz container . . . . 1 container	284	77	250	1	Trace
Cup . . . . 1 cup	250	77	220	1	Trace
Pears					
Fresh, with skin, cored					
Bartlett, 2½-in diam (about 2½ per lb . . . . 1 pear with cores and stems)	164	83	100	1	1

ABC'S OF NUTRITION

Dashes — — in the columns for nutrients denotes lack of reliable data for a constituent believed to be present in measurable amounts.

Fatty Acids			Carbo-hydrate	Calcium	Phos-phorus	Iron	Potas-sium	Vitamin A value	Thiamin	Ribo-flavin	Niacin	Ascorbic acid
Satu-rated (total)	Unsaturated											
	Oleic	Linoleic										
Grams	Grams	Grams	Grams	Milligrams	Milligrams	Milligrams	Milligrams	Inter-national units	Milligrams	Milligrams	Milligrams	Milligrams
— —	— —	— —	6	19	12	.4	102	10	.03	.01	.1	39
— —	— —	— —	20	17	24	.5	344	50	.07	.02	.2	112
— —	— —	— —	19	17	24	.5	344	50	.07	.02	.2	102
— —	— —	— —	28	2	3	.1	40	10	.01	.02	.2	17
— —	— —	— —	27	3	3	Trace	32	Trace	Trace	Trace	Trace	6
— —	— —	— —	22	22	27	.5	256	20	.05	.02	.2	79
— —	— —	— —	22	22	27	.5	256	20	.05	.02	.2	52
— —	— —	— —	20	38	44	1.1	682	9,240	.11	.08	1.6	90
— —	— —	— —	11	21	24	.6	374	60	.06	.04	.9	34
— —	— —	— —	16	54	26	.5	263	260	.13	.05	.5	66
— —	— —	— —	22	74	36	.7	360	360	.18	.07	.7	90
— —	— —	— —	26	27	42	.5	496	500	.22	.07	1.0	124
— —	— —	— —	28	25	45	1.0	496	500	.17	.05	.7	100
— —	— —	— —	29	25	42	.2	503	540	.23	.03	.9	120
— —	— —	— —	14	28	22	.4	328	2,450	.06	.06	.4	78
— —	— —	— —	10	9	19	.5	202	1,330	.02	.05	1.0	7
— —	— —	— —	16	15	32	.9	343	2,260	.03	.09	1.7	12
— —	— —	— —	51	10	31	.8	333	1,100	.03	.05	1.5	8
— —	— —	— —	20	10	32	.7	334	1,100	.02	.07	1.5	7
— —	— —	— —	109	77	187	9.6	1,520	6,240	.02	.30	8.5	29
— —	— —	— —	54	38	93	4.8	743	3,050	.01	.15	3.8	5
— —	— —	— —	64	11	37	1.4	352	1,850	0.03	0.11	2.0	116
— —	— —	— —	57	10	33	1.3	310	1,630	.03	.10	1.8	103
— —	— —	— —	25	13	18	.5	213	30	.03	.07	.2	7

Nutritive Value of Foods

Foods, approximate measures, units, and weight (in grams)		Water	Food energy	Protein	Fat
	Grams	Percent	Calories	Grams	Grams
FRUITS AND FRUIT PRODUCTS—Continued					
Pears-Continued					
Bosc, 2½-in diam (about 3 per lb with cores and stems) .... 1 pear	141	83	85	1	1
D'Anjou, 3-in diam (about 2 per lb with cores and stems) .... 1 pear	200	83	120	1	1
Canned in heavy syrup (fruit and liquid) .... 1 cup	255	80	195	1	1
Pineapple					
Fresh, diced .... 1 cup	155	85	80	1	Trace
Canned in heavy syrup (fruit and liquid)					
Crushed, chunks, tidbits .... 1 cup	255	80	190	1	Trace
Slices and liquid, medium .... 1 slice	58	80	45	Trace	Trace
Pineapple juice, unsweetened, canned .... 1 cup	250	86	140	1	Trace
Plums					
Fresh, without pits					
Japanese and hybrid (2-in diam, about 6½ per lb with pits) .... 1 plum	66	87	30	Trace	Trace
Prune-type (1½-in diam, about 15 per lb with pits) .... 1 plum	28	79	20	Trace	Trace
Canned in heavy syrup					
Cup .... 1 cup	272	77	215	1	Trace
Portion .... 3 plums	140	77	110	1	Trace
Prunes, dried, "softenized," with pits					
Uncooked, large .... 5 prunes	49	28	110	1	Trace
Cooked, unsweetened, all sizes, fruit and liquid .. 1 cup	250	66	255	2	1
Prune juice, bottled or canned .... 1 cup	256	80	195	1	Trace
Raisins, seedless					
Cup .... 1 cup	145	18	420	4	Trace
Packet, ½ oz (1½ tbsp) .... 1 packet	14	18	40	Trace	Trace
Raspberries, red					
Fresh, hulled, whole .... 1 cup	123	84	70	1	1
Frozen, sweetened, 10-oz container .... 1 container	284	74	280	2	1
Rhubarb, cooked, added sugar					
Fresh .... 1 cup	270	63	380	1	Trace
Frozen, sweetened .... 1 cup	270	63	385	1	1
Strawberries					
Fresh, whole berries, hulled .... 1 cup	149	90	55	1	1
Frozen, sweetened					
Sliced, 10-oz container .... 1 container	284	71	310	1	1
Whole, 1-lb container .... 1 container	454	76	415	2	1
Tangerine, fresh, 2½-in diam .... 1 tangerine	86	87	40	1	Trace
Tangerine juice, canned, sweetened .... 1 cup	249	87	125	1	Trace
Watermelon, fresh, with rind and seeds, ... 1 wedge 4 by 8 in wedge	926	93	110	2	1

ABC'S OF NUTRITION

Dashes — — in the columns for nutrients denotes lack of reliable data for a constituent believed to be present in measurable amounts.

Fatty Acids			Carbo-hydrate	Calcium	Phos-phorus	Iron	Potas-sium	Vitamin A value	Thiamin	Ribo-flavin	Niacin	Ascorbic acid
Satu-rated (total)	Unsaturated											
	Oleic	Linoleic										
Grams	Grams	Grams	Grams	Milligrams	Milligrams	Milligrams	Milligrams	International units	Milligrams	Milligrams	Milligrams	Milligrams
—	—	—	22	11	16	.4	83	30	.03	.06	.1	6
—	—	—	31	16	22	.6	260	40	.04	.08	.2	8
—	—	—	50	13	18	.5	214	10	.03	.05	.3	3
—	—	—	21	26	12	.8	226	110	.14	.05	.3	26
—	—	—	49	28	13	.8	245	130	.20	.05	.5	18
—	—	—	11	6	3	.2	56	30	.05	.01	.1	4
—	—	—	34	38	23	.8	373	130	.13	.05	.5	80
—	—	—	8	8	12	.3	112	160	.02	.02	.3	4
—	—	—	6	3	5	.1	48	80	.01	.01	.1	1
—	—	—	56	23	26	2.3	367	3,130	.05	.05	1.0	5
—	—	—	29	12	13	1.2	189	1,610	.03	.03	.5	3
—	—	—	29	22	34	1.7	298	690	.04	.07	.7	1
—	—	—	67	51	79	3.8	695	1,590	.07	.15	1.5	2
—	—	—	49	36	51	1.8	602	—	.03	.03	1.0	5
—	—	—	112	90	146	5.1	1,106	30	.16	.12	.7	1
—	—	—	11	9	14	.5	107	Trace	.02	.01	.1	Trace
—	—	—	17	27	27	1.1	207	160	.04	.11	1.1	31
—	—	—	70	37	48	1.7	284	200	.06	.17	1.7	60
—	—	—	97	211	41	1.6	548	220	.05	.14	.8	16
—	—	—	98	211	32	1.9	475	190	.05	.11	.5	16
—	—	—	13	31	31	1.5	244	90	0.04	0.10	0.9	88
—	—	—	79	40	48	2.0	318	90	.06	.17	1.4	151
—	—	—	107	59	73	2.7	472	140	.09	.27	2.3	249
—	—	—	10	34	15	.3	108	360	.05	.02	.1	27
—	—	—	30	44	35	.5	440	1,040	.15	.05	.2	54
—	—	—	27	30	43	2.1	426	2,510	.13	.13	.9	30

Nutritive Value of Foods

Foods, approximate measures, units, and weight (in grams)		Water	Food energy	Protein	Fat
GRAIN PRODUCTS		Grams	Percent	Calories	Grams	Grams
Bagel, 3-in diam						
Egg	1 bagel	55	32	165	6	2
Water	1 bagel	55	29	165	6	1
Biscuits, baking powder, 2-in diam (enriched flour, vegetable shortening)						
From home recipe	1 biscuit	28	27	105	2	5
From mix	1 biscuit	28	29	90	2	3
Breadcrumbs (enriched)						
Dry, grated	1 cup	100	7	390	13	5
Soft	1 cup	45	36	120	4	1
Breads						
Boston brown bread (white cornmeal), canned, slice (½-in)	1 slice	45	45	95	2	1
Cracked-wheat bread (¾ enriched wheat flour, ¼ cracked wheat), slice (18 per 1-lb loaf)	1 slice	25	35	65	2	1
French bread (enriched), slice (5 by 2½ in)	1 slice	35	31	100	3	1
Raisin bread (enriched), slice (18 per 1-lb loaf)	1 slice	25	35	65	2	1
Rye bread						
American, light (2/3 enriched wheat flour, 1/3 rye flour), slice (4¾ by 3¾ in)	1 slice	25	36	60	2	Trace
Pumpernickel (2/3 rye flour, 1/3 enriched wheat flour), slice (5 by 4 in)	1 slice	32	34	80	3	Trace
White bread (enriched)						
Soft-crumb type						
Slice (18 per 1-lb loaf)	1 slice	25	36	70	2	1
Slice (22 per 1-lb loaf)	1 slice	20	36	55	2	1
Cubes	1 cup	30	36	80	3	1
Firm-crumb type						
Slice (20 per 1-lb loaf)	1 slice	23	35	65	2	1
Slice (34 per 2-lb loaf)	1 slice	27	35	75	2	1
Whole-wheat bread						
Soft-crumb type						
Slice (16 per 1-lb loaf)	1 slice	28	36	65	3	1
Firm-crumb type						
Slice (18 per 1-lb loaf)	1 slice	25	36	60	3	1
Breakfast cereals						
Hot, cooked						
Corn (hominy) grits, white variety, degermed						
Enriched	1 cup	245	87	125	3	Trace
Unenriched	1 cup	245	87	125	3	Trace
Farina, quick cooking, enriched, without disodium phosphate	1 cup	245	89	105	3	Trace
Oatmeal or rolled oats	1 cup	240	87	130	5	2
Wheat, rolled	1 cup	240	80	180	5	1
Wheat, whole meal	1 cup	245	88	110	4	1

[14] Value varies with brand. Consult the label.

ABC'S OF NUTRITION

Dashes — — in the columns for nutrients denotes lack of reliable data for a constituent believed to be present in measurable amounts.

Fatty Acids			Carbo-hydrate	Calcium	Phos-phorus	Iron	Potas-sium	Vitamin A value	Thiamin	Ribo-flavin	Niacin	Ascorbic acid
Satu-rated (total)	Unsaturated											
	Oleic	Linoleic										
Grams	Grams	Grams	Grams	Milligrams	Milligrams	Milligrams	Milligrams	International units	Milligrams	Milligrams	Milligrams	Milligrams
0.5	0.9	0.8	28	9	43	1.2	41	30	.14	.10	1.2	0
.2	.4	.6	30	8	41	1.2	42	0	.15	.11	1.4	0
1.2	2.0	1.2	13	34	49	.4	33	Trace	.08	.08	.7	Trace
.6	1.1	.7	15	19	65	.6	32	Trace	.09	.08	.8	Trace
1.0	1.6	1.4	73	122	141	3.6	152	Trace	.35	.35	4.8	Trace
.3	.5	.5	23	38	44	1.1	47	Trace	.18	.11	1.5	Trace
.1	.2	.2	21	41	72	.9	131	0	.06	.04	.7	0
.1	.2	.2	13	22	32	.5	34	Trace	.08	.06	.8	Trace
.2	.4	.4	19	15	30	.8	32	Trace	.14	.08	1.2	Trace
.2	.3	.2	13	18	22	.6	58	Trace	.09	.06	.6	Trace
Trace	Trace	.1	13	19	37	.5	36	0	.07	.05	.7	0
.1	Trace	.2	17	27	73	.8	145	0	.09	.07	.6	0
.2	.3	.3	13	21	24	.6	26	Trace	.10	.06	.8	Trace
.2	.2	.2	10	17	19	.5	21	Trace	.08	.05	.7	Trace
.2	.3	.3	15	25	29	.8	32	Trace	.12	.07	1.0	Trace
.2	.3	.3	12	22	23	.6	28	Trace	.09	.06	.8	Trace
.2	.3	.3	14	26	28	.7	33	Trace	.11	.06	.9	Trace
.1	.2	.2	14	24	71	.8	72	Trace	.09	.03	.8	Trace
.1	.2	.3	12	25	57	.8	68	Trace	.06	.03	.7	Trace
Trace	Trace	.1	27	2	25	.7	27	Trace	.10	.07	1.0	0
Trace	Trace	.1	27	2	25	.2	27	Trace	.05	.02	.5	0
Trace	Trace	.1	22	147	113	12	25	0	(14)	.07	1.0	0
.4	.8	.9	23	22	137	1.4	146	0	.19	.05	.2	0
— —	— —	— —	41	19	182	1.7	202	0	.17	.07	2.2	0
— —	— —	— —	23	17	127	1.2	118	0	.15	.05	1.5	0

Nutritive Value of Foods

Foods, approximate measures, units, and weight (in grams)		Water	Food energy	Protein	Fat
	Grams	Percent	Calories	Grams	Grams
GRAIN PRODUCTS—Continued					
Breakfast cereals-Continued					
Ready to eat					
Bran flakes (40% bran), added sugar, salt, iron, vitamins . . . . 1 cup	35	3	105	4	1
Bran flakes with raisins, added sugar, salt, iron, vitamins, added nutrients . . . . 1 cup	50	7	145	4	1
Corn flakes					
Plain, added sugar, salt, iron, vitamins . . . . . . 1 cup	25	4	95	2	Trace
Sugar coated, added salt, iron, vitamins . . . . . 1 cup	40	2	155	2	Trace
Corn, puffed, plain, added sugar, salt, iron, vitamins . . . . 1 cup	20	4	80	2	1
Corn, shredded, added sugar, salt, iron, thiamin, niacin . . . . 1 cup	25	3	95	2	Trace
Oats, puffed, added sugar, salt, minerals, vitamins . . . . 1 cup	25	3	100	3	1
Rice, puffed					
Plain, added iron, thiamin, niacin . . . . 1 cup	15	4	60	1	Trace
Presweetened, added salt, iron, vitamins . . . . 1 cup	28	3	115	1	0
Wheat flakes, added sugar, salt, iron, vitamins . . . . 1 cup	30	4	105	3	Trace
Wheat, puffed					
Plain, added iron, thiamin, niacin . . . . 1 cup	15	3	55	2	Trace
Presweetened, added salt, iron, vitamins . . . . 1 cup	38	3	140	3	Trace
Wheat, shredded, plain . . . . 1 biscuit	25	7	90	2	1
Wheat germ, without salt and sugar, toasted . . . . 1 tbsp	6	4	25	2	1
Buckwheat flour, light, sifted . . . . 1 cup	98	12	340	6	1
Bulgur (parboiled wheat), canned, seasoned . . . . 1 cup	135	56	245	8	4
Cake icings. See **Sugars and Sweets.**					
Cakes, made from cake mixes (enriched flour)					
Angel food (9¾-in diam tube cake), piece (1/12 of cake) . . . . 1 piece	53	34	135	3	Trace
Coffee cake (7¾ by 6 in), piece (1/6 of cake) . . . . . 1 piece	72	30	230	5	7
Cupcakes, made with egg, milk (2½-in diam)					
Without icing . . . . 1 cupcake	25	26	90	1	3
With chocolate icing . . . . 1 cupcake	36	22	130	2	5
Devil's food with chocolate icing (2-layer cake, 8- or 9-in diam)					
Piece (1/16 of cake) . . . . 1 piece	69	24	235	3	8
Cupcake (2½-in diam) . . . . 1 cupcake	35	24	120	2	4
Gingerbread (8-in square), piece (1/9 of cake) . . . . 1 piece	63	37	175	2	4
White (2-layer with chocolate icing, 8- or 9-in diam), piece (1/16 of cake) . . . . 1 piece	71	21	250	3	8
Yellow (2-layer with chocolate icing, 8- or 9-in diam), piece (1/16 of cake) . . . . 1 piece	69	26	235	3	8

[15] Applies to product with added nutrient. Without added nutrient value is trace.

ABC'S OF NUTRITION

Dashes — — in the columns for nutrients denotes lack of reliable data for a constituent believed to be present in measurable amounts.

Fatty Acids			Carbo-hydrate	Calcium	Phos-phorus	Iron	Potas-sium	Vitamin A value	Thiamin	Ribo-flavin	Niacin	Ascorbic acid
Satu-rated (total)	Unsaturated											
	Oleic	Linoleic										
Grams	Grams	Grams	Grams	Milligrams	Milligrams	Milligrams	Milligrams	International units	Milligrams	Milligrams	Milligrams	Milligrams
— —	— —	— —	28	19	125	5.6	137	1,540	.46	.52	6.2	0
— —	— —	— —	40	28	146	7.9	154	[15]2,200	([16])	([16])	([16])	0
— —	— —	— —	21	([16])	9	([16])	30	([16])	([16])	([16])	([16])	[15]13
— —	— —	— —	37	1	10	([16])	27	1,760	.53	.60	7.1	21
— —	— —	— —	16	4	18	5.7	— —	880	.26	.30	3.5	11
— —	— —	— —	22	1	10	.6	— —	0	.33	.05	4.4	13
— —	— —	— —	19	44	102	4.0	— —	1,100	.33	.38	4.4	13
— —	— —	— —	13	3	14	.3	15	0	.07	.01	.7	0
— —	— —	— —	26	3	14	([16])	43	1,240	([16])	([16])	([16])	[15]15
— —	— —	— —	24	12	83	4.8	81	1,320	.40	.45	5.3	16
— —	— —	— —	12	4	48	.6	51	0	.08	.03	1.2	0
— —	— —	— —	33	7	52	([16])	63	1,680	.50	.57	6.7	[15]20
— —	— —	— —	20	11	97	.9	87	0	.06	.03	1.1	0
— —	— —	— —	3	3	70	.5	57	10	.11	.05	.3	1
0.2	0.4	0.4	78	11	86	1.0	314	0	.08	.04	.4	0
— —	— —	— —	44	27	263	1.9	151	0	.08	.05	4.1	0
— —	— —	— —	32	50	63	.2	32	0	.03	.08	.3	0
2.0	2.7	1.5	38	44	125	1.2	78	120	.14	.15	1.3	Trace
.8	1.2	.7	14	40	59	.3	21	40	.05	.05	.4	Trace
2.0	1.6	.6	21	47	71	.4	42	60	.05	.06	.4	Trace
3.1	2.8	1.1	40	41	72	1.0	90	100	.07	.10	.6	Trace
1.6	1.4	.5	20	21	37	.5	46	50	.03	.05	.3	Trace
1.1	1.8	1.1	32	57	63	.9	173	Trace	.09	.11	.8	Trace
3.0	2.9	1.2	45	70	127	.7	82	40	.09	.11	.8	Trace
3.0	3.0	1.3	40	63	126	.8	75	100	.08	.10	.7	Trace

[16] Value varies with brand. Consult the label.

Nutritive Value of Foods

Foods, approximate measures, units, and weight (in grams)		Water	Food energy	Protein	Fat
	Grams	Percent	Calories	Grams	Grams
GRAIN PRODUCTS—Continued					
Cakes, made from home recipes (enriched flour)					
Boston cream pie with custard filling (8-in diam), piece (1/12 of cake) .... 1 piece	69	35	210	3	6
Fruitcake, dark (loaf, 1-lb, 7½ by 2 by 1½ in), slice (1/30 of loaf) .... 1 slice	15	18	55	1	2
Plain, sheet cake (9-in square)					
Without icing, piece (1/9 of cake) .... 1 piece	86	25	315	4	12
With uncooked white icing, piece........... 1 piece (1/9 of cake)	121	21	445	4	14
Pound (loaf, 8½ by 3½ by 3¼ in), slice .... 1 slice (1/17 of loaf)	33	16	160	2	10
Sponge cake with butter icing (9¾-in diam ...... 1 piece tube cake), piece (1/12 of cake)	66	32	195	5	4
Cookies (enriched flour, except for macaroons)					
Brownies, with nuts (1¾ by 1¾ by 1 in)					
From home recipe .... 1 brownie	20	10	95	1	6
From mix .... 1 brownie	20	11	85	1	4
Frozen, with chocolate icing made with ...... 1 brownie butter (1½ by 1¾ by 1 in)	25	13	105	1	5
Chocolate chip					
Commercial (2½-in diam, 3/8 in thick) .... 4 cookies	42	3	200	2	9
From home recipe (2 1/3-in diam) .... 4 cookies	40	3	205	2	12
Fig bars, square (1 5/8 by 1 5/8 by 3/8 in) ..... 4 cookies	56	14	200	2	3
Gingersnaps (2-in diam, ¼ in thick) .... 4 cookies	28	3	90	2	2
Macaroons (2¾-in diam, ¼ in thick) .... 2 cookies	38	4	180	2	9
Oatmeal, with raisins (3-in diam, ¼ in thick) ..... 4 cookies	52	3	235	3	8
Plain, from commercial chilled dough .... 4 cookies (2½-in diam, ¼ in thick)	48	5	240	2	12
Sandwich type (chocolate or vanilla, ... 4 cookies 1¾-in diam, 3/8 in thick)	40	2	200	2	9
Vanilla wafers (1¾-in diam, ¼ in thick) .... 10 cookies	40	3	185	2	6
Cornmeal, yellow variety					
Whole ground, unbolted, dry form .... 1 cup	122	12	435	11	5
Bolted (nearly whole grain), dry form .... 1 cup	122	12	440	11	4
Degermed, enriched					
Dry form .... 1 cup	138	12	500	11	2
Cooked .... 1 cup	240	88	120	3	Trace
Degermed, unenriched					
Dry form .... 1 cup	138	12	500	11	2
Cooked .... 1 cup	240	88	120	3	Trace
Crackers, made with vegetable shortening					
Graham, plain (2½-in square) .... 2 crackers	14	6	55	1	1
Rye wafers, whole grain (1 7/8 by 3½ in) .... 2 wafers	13	6	45	2	Trace
Saltines, made with enriched flour .... 4 crackers	11	4	50	1	1

ABC'S OF NUTRITION

Dashes — — in the columns for nutrients denotes lack of reliable data for a constituent believed to be present in measurable amounts.

Fatty Acids			Carbo-hydrate	Calcium	Phos-phorus	Iron	Potas-sium	Vitamin A value	Thiamin	Ribo-flavin	Niacin	Ascorbic acid
Satu-rated (total)	Unsaturated											
	Oleic	Linoleic										
Grams	Grams	Grams	Grams	Milligrams	Milligrams	Milligrams	Milligrams	International units	Milligrams	Milligrams	Milligrams	Milligrams
1.9	2.5	1.3	34	46	70	.7	61	140	.09	.11	.8	Trace
.5	1.1	.5	9	11	17	.4	74	20	.02	.02	.2	Trace
3.3	4.9	2.6	48	55	88	.9	68	150	.13	.15	1.1	Trace
4.7	5.5	2.7	77	61	91	.8	74	240	.14	.16	1.1	Trace
2.5	4.3	2.3	16	6	24	.5	20	80	.05	.06	.4	0
1.1	1.3	.5	36	20	74	1.1	57	300	.09	.14	.6	Trace
1.5	3.0	1.2	10	8	30	.4	38	40	.04	.03	.2	Trace
.9	1.4	1.3	13	9	27	.4	34	20	.03	.02	.2	Trace
2.0	2.2	.7	15	10	31	.4	44	50	.03	.03	.2	Trace
2.8	2.9	2.2	29	16	48	1.0	56	50	.10	.17	.9	Trace
3.5	4.5	2.9	24	14	40	.8	47	40	.06	.06	.5	Trace
.8	1.2	.7	42	44	34	1.0	111	60	.04	.14	.9	Trace
.7	1.0	.6	22	20	13	.7	129	20	.08	.06	.7	0
— —	— —	— —	25	10	32	.3	176	0	.02	.06	.2	0
2.0	3.3	2.0	38	11	53	1.4	192	30	.15	.10	1.0	Trace
3.0	5.2	2.9	31	17	35	0.6	23	30	0.10	0.08	0.9	0
2.2	3.9	2.2	28	10	96	.7	15	0	.06	.10	.7	0
— —	— —	— —	30	16	25	.6	29	50	.10	.09	.8	0
.5	1.0	2.5	90	24	312	2.9	346	620	.46	.13	2.4	0
.5	.9	2.1	91	21	272	2.2	303	590	.37	.10	2.3	0
.2	.4	.9	108	8	137	4.0	166	610	.61	.36	4.8	0
Trace	.1	.2	26	2	34	1.0	38	140	.14	.10	1.2	0
.2	.4	.9	108	8	137	1.5	166	610	.19	.07	1.4	0
Trace	.1	.2	26	2	34	.5	38	140	.05	.02	.2	0
.3	.5	.3	10	6	21	.5	55	0	.02	.08	.5	0
— —	— —	— —	10	7	50	.5	78	0	.04	.03	.2	0
.3	.5	.4	8	2	10	.5	13	0	.05	.05	.4	0

Nutritive Value of Foods

Foods, approximate measures, units, and weight (in grams)		Water	Food energy	Protein	Fat
GRAIN PRODUCTS—Continued	Grams	Percent	Calories	Grams	Grams
Danish pastry, plain, without fruit or nuts .... 1 pastry (enriched flour, vegetable shortening, butter), round piece (about 4¼-in diam by 1 in)	65	22	275	5	15
Doughnuts, made with enriched flour and vegetable shortening					
Cake type, plain (2½-in diam, 1 in high) .... 1 doughnut	25	24	100	1	5
Yeast leavened, glazed (3¾-in diam, ... 1 doughnut 1¼ in high)	50	26	205	3	11
Macaroni, cut lengths, elbows, shells (enriched)					
Cooked, firm stage, "al dente" .... 1 cup	130	64	190	7	1
Cooked, tender stage .... 1 cup	140	73	155	5	1
Muffins, made with enriched flour and vegetable shortening					
From home recipe					
Blueberry (2-in diam, 1½ in high) .... 1 muffin	40	39	110	3	4
Bran .... 1 muffin	40	35	105	3	4
Corn (enriched, degermed yellow corn- .... 1 muffin meal and flour, 3-in diam, 1½ in high)	40	33	125	3	4
Plain (3-in diam, 1½ in high) .... 1 muffin	40	38	120	3	4
From mix (degermed yellow cornmeal, enriched flour), egg, milk					
Corn (3-in diam, 1½ in high) .... 1 muffin	40	30	130	3	4
Noodles (egg noodles), enriched, cooked .... 1 cup	160	71	200	7	2
Pancakes, made with vegetable shortening (4 in diam)					
Buckwheat, made from mix (buckwheat .... 1 cake and enriched flours), egg, milk	27	58	55	2	2
Plain					
From home recipe (enriched flour) .... 1 cake	27	50	60	2	2
From mix (enriched flour), egg, milk .... 1 cake	27	51	60	2	2
Pies, piecrust made with enriched flour, vegetable shortening (9-in diam)					
Apple, sector (1/7 of pie) .... 1 sector	135	48	345	3	15
Banana cream, sector (1/7 of pie) .... 1 sector	130	54	285	6	12
Blueberry, sector (1/7 of pie) .... 1 sector	135	51	325	3	15
Cherry, sector (1/7 of pie) .... 1 sector	135	47	350	4	15
Custard, sector (1/7 of pie) .... 1 sector	130	58	285	8	14
Lemon meringue, sector (1/7 of pie) .... 1 sector	120	47	305	4	12
Mince, sector (1/7 of pie) .... 1 sector	135	43	365	3	16
Peach, sector (1/7 of pie) .... 1 sector	135	48	345	3	14
Pecan, sector (1/7 of pie) .... 1 sector	118	20	495	6	27
Pumpkin, sector (1/7 of pie) .... 1 sector	130	59	275	5	15
Piecrust, home recipe, made with enriched .... 1 pie shell flour and vegetable shortening (9-in diam)	180	15	900	11	60
Piecrust mix, made with enriched flour and .... Piecrust for vegetable shortening, 10-oz pkg (9-in diam) 2-crust pie	320	19	1,485	20	93

Dashes — — in the columns for nutrients denotes lack of reliable data for a constituent believed to be present in measurable amounts.

Fatty Acids			Carbo-hydrate	Calcium	Phos-phorus	Iron	Potas-sium	Vitamin A value	Thiamin	Ribo-flavin	Niacin	Ascorbic acid
Satu-rated (total)	Unsaturated											
	Oleic	Linoleic										
Grams	Grams	Grams	Grams	Milligrams	Milligrams	Milligrams	Milligrams	International units	Milligrams	Milligrams	Milligrams	Milligrams
4.7	6.1	3.2	30	33	71	1.2	73	200	.18	.19	1.7	Trace
1.2	2.0	1.1	13	10	48	.4	23	20	.05	.05	.4	Trace
3.3	5.8	3.3	22	16	33	.6	34	25	.10	.10	.8	0
——	——	——	39	14	85	1.4	103	0	.23	.13	1.8	0
——	——	——	32	11	70	1.3	85	0	.20	.11	1.5	0
1.1	1.4	.7	17	34	53	.6	46	90	.09	.10	.7	Trace
1.2	1.4	.8	17	57	162	1.5	172	90	.07	.10	1.7	Trace
1.2	1.6	.9	19	42	68	.7	54	120	.10	.10	.7	Trace
1.0	1.7	1.0	17	42	60	0.6	50	40	0.09	0.12	0.9	Trace
1.2	1.7	.9	20	96	152	.6	44	100	.08	.09	.7	Trace
——	——	——	37	16	94	1.4	70	110	.22	.13	1.9	0
.8	.9	.4	6	59	91	.4	66	60	.04	.05	.2	Trace
.5	.8	.5	9	27	38	.4	33	30	.06	.07	.5	Trace
.7	.7	.3	9	58	70	.3	42	70	.04	.06	.2	Trace
3.9	6.4	3.6	51	11	30	.9	108	40	.15	.11	1.3	2
3.8	4.7	2.3	40	86	107	1.0	264	330	.11	.22	1.0	1
3.5	6.2	3.6	47	15	31	1.4	88	40	.15	.11	1.4	4
4.0	6.4	3.6	52	19	34	.9	142	590	.16	.12	1.4	Trace
4.8	5.5	2.5	30	125	147	1.2	178	300	.11	.27	.8	0
3.7	4.8	2.3	45	17	59	1.0	60	200	.09	.12	.7	4
4.0	6.6	3.6	56	38	51	1.9	240	Trace	.14	.12	1.4	1
3.5	6.2	3.6	52	14	39	1.2	201	990	.15	.14	2.0	4
4.0	14.4	6.3	61	55	122	3.7	145	190	.26	.14	1.0	Trace
5.4	5.4	2.4	32	66	90	1.0	208	3,210	.11	.18	1.0	Trace
14.8	26.1	14.9	79	25	90	3.1	89	0	.47	.40	5.0	0
22.7	39.7	23.4	141	131	272	6.1	179	0	1.07	.79	9.9	0

Nutritive Value of Foods

Foods, approximate measures, units, and weight (in grams)		Water	Food energy	Protein	Fat
	Grams	Percent	Calories	Grams	Grams
GRAIN PRODUCTS —Continued					
Pizza, cheese (4¾-in sector) .... 1 sector	60	45	145	6	4
Popcorn, popped					
Plain, large kernel .... 1 cup	6	4	25	1	Trace
With oil (coconut) and salt added, large kernel .... 1 cup	9	3	40	1	2
Sugar coated .... 1 cup	35	4	135	2	1
Pretzels (enriched flour)					
Dutch, twisted (2¾ by 2 5/8 in) .... 1 pretzel	16	5	60	2	1
Thin, twisted (3¼ by 2¼ by ¼ in) .... 10 pretzels	60	5	235	6	3
Stick (2¼ in long) .... 10 pretzels	3	5	10	Trace	Trace
Rice (white, enriched)					
Instant, ready-to-serve .... 1 cup	165	73	180	4	Trace
Long grain, cooked .... 1 cup	205	73	225	4	Trace
Parboiled, cooked .... 1 cup	175	73	185	4	Trace
Rolls (enriched, made with vegetable shortening)					
Commercial					
Brown-and-serve (12 per 12-oz pkg), browned .. 1 roll	26	27	85	2	2
Cloverleaf or pan (2½-in diam) .... 1 roll	28	31	85	2	2
Frankfurter and hamburger (8 per 11½-oz pkg) . 1 roll	40	31	120	3	2
Hard (3¾-in diam) .... 1 roll	50	25	155	5	2
Hoagie or submarine (11½ by 3 by 2½ in) ..... 1 roll	135	31	390	12	4
From home recipe					
Cloverleaf (2½-in diam) .... 1 roll	35	26	120	3	3
Spaghetti (enriched)					
Cooked, firm stage, "al dente" .... 1 cup	130	64	190	7	1
Cooked, tender stage .... 1 cup	140	73	155	5	1
Waffles (enriched, made with vegetable shortening, 7-in diam)					
From home recipe .... 1 waffle	75	41	210	7	7
From mix, egg and milk added .... 1 waffle	75	42	205	7	8
Wheat flours					
All purpose or family flour, enriched					
Sifted, spooned .... 1 cup	115	12	420	12	1
Unsifted, spooned .... 1 cup	125	12	455	13	1
Cake or pastry flour, enriched, sifted, spooned .... 1 cup	96	12	350	7	1
Self-rising, enriched, unsifted, spooned .... 1 cup	125	12	440	12	1
Whole wheat, from hard wheats, stirred .... 1 cup	120	12	400	16	2
LEGUMES, NUTS, SEEDS; RELATED PRODUCTS					
Almonds, shelled					
Chopped (about 130 almonds) .... 1 cup	130	5	775	24	70
Slivered (about 115 almonds) .... 1 cup	115	5	690	21	62

[17] Value varies with brand. Consult the label.

ABC'S OF NUTRITION

Dashes — — in the columns for nutrients denotes lack of reliable data for a constituent believed to be present in measurable amounts.

Fatty Acids			Carbo-hydrate	Calcium	Phos-phorus	Iron	Potas-sium	Vitamin A value	Thiamin	Ribo-flavin	Niacin	Ascorbic acid
Satu-rated (total)	Unsaturated											
	Oleic	Linoleic										
Grams	Grams	Grams	Grams	Milligrams	Milligrams	Milligrams	Milligrams	International units	Milligrams	Milligrams	Milligrams	Milligrams
1.7	1.5	0.6	22	86	89	1.1	67	230	0.16	0.18	1.6	4
Trace	.1	.2	5	1	17	.2	— —	— —	— —	.01	.1	0
1.5	.2	.2	5	1	19	.2	— —	— —	— —	.01	.2	0
.5	.2	.4	30	2	47	.5	— —	— —	— —	.02	.4	0
— —	— —	— —	12	4	21	.2	21	0	.05	.04	.7	0
— —	— —	— —	46	13	79	.9	78	0	.20	.15	2.5	0
— —	— —	— —	2	1	4	Trace	4	0	.01	.01	.1	0
Trace	Trace	Trace	40	5	31	1.3	— —	0	.21	(17)	1.7	0
.1	.1	.1	50	21	57	1.8	57	0	.23	.02	2.1	0
.1	.1	.1	41	33	100	1.4	75	0	.19	.02	2.1	0
.4	.7	.5	14	20	23	.5	25	Trace	.10	.06	.9	Trace
.4	.6	.4	15	21	24	.5	27	Trace	.11	.07	.9	Trace
.5	.8	.6	21	30	34	.8	38	Trace	.16	.10	1.3	Trace
.4	.6	.5	30	24	46	1.2	49	Trace	.20	.12	1.7	Trace
.9	1.4	1.4	75	58	115	3.0	122	Trace	.54	.32	4.5	Trace
.8	1.1	.7	20	16	36	.7	41	30	.12	.12	1.2	Trace
— —	— —	— —	39	14	85	1.4	103	0	.23	.13	1.8	0
— —	— —	— —	32	11	70	1.3	85	0	.20	.11	1.5	0
2.3	2.8	1.4	28	85	130	1.3	109	250	.17	.23	1.4	Trace
2.8	2.9	1.2	27	179	257	1.0	146	170	.14	.22	.9	Trace
0.2	0.1	0.5	88	18	100	3.3	109	0	0.74	0.46	6.1	0
.2	.1	.5	95	20	109	3.6	119	0	.80	.50	6.6	0
.1	.1	.3	76	16	70	2.8	91	0	.61	.38	5.1	0
.2	.1	.5	93	331	583	3.6	— —	0	.80	.50	6.6	0
.4	.2	1.0	85	49	446	4.0	444	0	.66	.14	5.2	0
5.6	47.7	12.8	25	304	655	6.1	1,005	0	.31	1.20	4.6	Trace
5.0	42.2	11.3	22	269	580	5.4	889	0	.28	1.06	4.0	Trace

Nutritive Value of Foods

Foods, approximate measures, units, and weight (in grams)		Water	Food energy	Protein	Fat
LEGUMES, NUTS, SEEDS; RELATED PRODUCTS—Continued	Grams	Percent	Calories	Grams	Grams
Beans					
Dry, cooked, drained					
Great Northern .... 1 cup	180	69	210	14	1
Lima .... 1 cup	190	64	260	16	1
Navy (pea) .... 1 cup	190	69	225	15	1
Canned, beans and liquid					
White, with pork and tomato sauce .... 1 cup	255	71	310	16	7
Red kidney .... 1 cup	255	76	230	15	1
Black-eyed peas, dry, cooked .... 1 cup	250	80	190	13	1
Brazil nuts, shelled (6-8 large kernels) .... 1 oz	28	5	185	4	19
Cashew nuts, roasted in oil .... 1 cup	140	5	785	24	64
Coconut meat, fresh					
Piece (about 2 by 2 by ½ in) .... 1 piece	45	51	155	2	16
Shredded or grated .... 1 cup	80	51	275	3	28
Filberts (hazelnuts), chopped (about 80 kernels) .... 1 cup	115	6	730	14	72
Lentils, whole, cooked .... 1 cup	200	72	210	16	Trace
Peanuts, roasted in oil, salted, chopped .... 1 cup	144	2	840	37	72
Peanut butter .... 1 tbsp	16	2	95	4	8
Peas, split, dry, cooked .... 1 cup	200	70	230	16	1
Pecans, chopped or pieces (about 120 large halves) ... 1 cup	118	3	810	11	84
Pumpkin and squash seeds, dry, hulled .... 1 cup	140	4	775	41	65
Sunflower seeds, dry, hulled .... 1 cup	145	5	810	35	69
Walnuts					
Black					
Chopped or broken kernels .... 1 cup	125	3	785	26	74
Ground (finely) .... 1 cup	80	3	500	16	47
Persian or English, chopped (about 60 halves) .... 1 cup	120	4	780	18	77
SUGARS AND SWEETS					
Cake icings					
Boiled, white					
Plain .... 1 cup	94	18	295	1	0
With coconut .... 1 cup	166	15	605	3	13
Uncooked					
Chocolate, made with milk and butter .... 1 cup	275	14	1,035	9	38
Creamy fudge, from mix and water .... 1 cup	245	15	830	7	16
White .... 1 cup	319	11	1,200	2	21
Candy					
Caramels, plain or chocolate .... 1 oz	28	8	115	1	3
Chocolate					
Milk, plain .... 1 oz	28	1	145	2	9
Semisweet, small pieces (60 per oz) .... 1 cup	170	1	860	7	61

ABC'S OF NUTRITION

Dashes — — in the columns for nutrients denotes lack of reliable data for a constituent believed to be present in measurable amounts.

Fatty Acids			Carbo-hydrate	Calcium	Phos-phorus	Iron	Potas-sium	Vitamin A value	Thiamin	Ribo-flavin	Niacin	Ascorbic acid
Satu-rated (total)	Unsaturated											
	Oleic	Linoleic										
Grams	Grams	Grams	Grams	Milligrams	Milligrams	Milligrams	Milligrams	International units	Milligrams	Milligrams	Milligrams	Milligrams
— —	— —	— —	38	90	266	4.9	749	0	.25	.13	1.3	0
— —	— —	— —	49	55	293	5.9	1,163	— —	.25	.11	1.3	— —
— —	— —	— —	40	95	281	5.1	790	0	.27	.13	1.3	0
2.4	2.8	.6	48	138	235	4.6	536	330	.20	.08	1.5	5
— —	— —	— —	42	74	278	4.6	673	10	.13	.10	1.5	— —
— —	— —	— —	35	43	238	3.3	573	30	.40	.10	1.0	— —
4.8	6.2	7.1	3	53	196	1.0	203	Trace	.27	.03	.5	— —
12.9	36.8	10.2	41	53	522	5.3	650	140	.60	.35	2.5	— —
14.0	.9	.3	4	6	43	.8	115	0	.02	.01	.2	1
24.8	1.6	.5	8	10	76	1.4	205	0	.04	.02	.4	2
5.1	55.2	7.3	19	240	388	3.9	810	— —	.53	— —	1.0	Trace
— —	— —	— —	39	50	238	4.2	498	40	.14	.12	1.2	0
13.7	33.0	20.7	27	107	577	3.0	971	— —	.46	.19	24.8	0
1.5	3.7	2.3	3	9	61	.3	100	— —	.02	.02	2.4	0
— —	— —	— —	42	22	178	3.4	592	80	.30	.18	1.8	— —
7.2	50.5	20.0	17	86	341	2.8	712	150	1.01	.15	1.1	2
11.8	23.5	27.5	21	71	1,602	15.7	1,386	100	.34	.27	3.4	— —
8.2	13.7	43.2	29	174	1,214	10.3	1,334	70	2.84	.33	7.8	— —
6.3	13.3	45.7	19	Trace	713	7.5	575	380	.28	.14	.9	— —
4.0	8.5	29.2	12	Trace	456	4.8	368	240	.18	.09	.6	— —
8.4	11.8	42.2	19	119	456	3.7	540	40	.40	.16	1.1	2
0	0	0	75	2	2	Trace	17	0	Trace	0.03	Trace	0
11.0	.9	Trace	124	10	50	0.8	277	0	0.02	.07	0.3	0
23.4	11.7	1.0	185	165	305	3.3	536	580	.06	.28	.6	1
5.1	6.7	3.1	183	96	218	2.7	238	Trace	.05	.20	.7	Trace
12.7	5.1	.5	260	48	38	Trace	57	860	Trace	.06	Trace	Trace
1.6	1.1	.1	22	42	35	.4	54	Trace	.01	.05	.1	Trace
5.5	3.0	.3	16	65	65	.3	109	80	.02	.10	.1	Trace
36.2	19.8	1.7	97	51	255	4.4	553	30	.02	.14	.9	0

83

Nutritive Value of Foods

Foods, approximate measures, units, and weight (in grams)		Water	Food energy	Protein	Fat
		Grams	Percent	Calories	Grams	Grams
SUGARS AND SWEETS—Continued						
Candy-Continued						
Chocolate-coated peanuts	1 oz	28	1	160	5	12
Fondant, uncoated (mints, candy corn, other)	1 oz	28	8	105	Trace	1
Fudge, chocolate, plain	1 oz	28	8	115	1	3
Gumdrops	1 oz	28	12	100	Trace	Trace
Hard	1 oz	28	1	110	0	Trace
Marshmallows	1 oz	28	17	90	1	Trace
Chocolate-flavored beverage powders (about 4 heaping tsp per oz)						
With nonfat dry milk	1 oz	28	2	100	5	1
Without milk	1 oz	28	1	100	1	1
Honey, strained or extracted	1 tbsp	21	17	65	Trace	0
Jams and preserves	1 tbsp	20	29	55	Trace	Trace
Jellies	1 tbsp	18	29	50	Trace	Trace
	1 packet	14	29	40	Trace	Trace
Syrups						
Chocolate-flavored syrup or topping						
Thin type	1 fl oz or 2 tbsp	38	32	90	1	1
Fudge type	1 fl oz or 2 tbsp	38	25	125	2	5
Molasses, cane						
Light (first extraction)	1 tbsp	20	24	50	--	--
Blackstrap (third extraction)	1 tbsp	20	24	45	--	--
Sorghum	1 tbsp	21	23	55	--	--
Table blends, chiefly corn, light and dark	1 tbsp	21	24	60	0	0
Sugars						
Brown, pressed down	1 cup	220	2	820	0	0
White						
Granulated	1 cup	200	1	770	0	0
	1 tbsp	12	1	45	0	0
Powdered, sifted, spooned into cup	1 cup	100	1	385	0	0
VEGETABLES AND VEGETABLE PRODUCTS						
Asparagus						
Cooked, drained						
Cuts and tips, 1½- to 2-in lengths						
Fresh	1 cup	145	94	30	3	Trace
Frozen	1 cup	180	93	40	6	Trace
Spears, ½-in diam at base						
Fresh	4 spears	60	94	10	1	Trace
Frozen	4 spears	60	92	15	2	Trace
Canned, spears, ½-in diam at base	4 spears	80	93	15	2	Trace

ABC'S OF NUTRITION

Dashes — — in the columns for nutrients denotes lack of reliable data for a constituent believed to be present in measurable amounts.

Fatty Acids			Carbo-hydrate	Calcium	Phos-phorus	Iron	Potas-sium	Vitamin A value	Thiamin	Ribo-flavin	Niacin	Ascorbic acid
Satu-rated (total)	Unsaturated											
	Oleic	Linoleic										
Grams	Grams	Grams	Grams	Milligrams	Milligrams	Milligrams	Milligrams	International units	Milligrams	Milligrams	Milligrams	Milligrams
4.0	4.7	2.1	11	33	84	.4	143	Trace	.10	.05	2.1	Trace
.1	.3	.1	25	4	2	.3	1	0	Trace	Trace	Trace	0
1.3	1.4	.6	21	22	24	.3	42	Trace	.01	.03	.1	Trace
——	——	——	25	2	Trace	.1	1	0	0	Trace	Trace	0
——	——	——	28	6	2	.5	1	0	0	0	0	0
——	——	——	23	5	2	.5	2	0	0	Trace	Trace	0
.5	.3	Trace	20	167	155	.5	227	10	.04	.21	.2	1
.4	.2	Trace	25	9	48	.6	142	——	.01	.03	.1	0
0	0	0	17	1	1	.1	11	0	Trace	.01	.1	Trace
——	——	——	14	4	2	.2	18	Trace	Trace	.01	Trace	Trace
——	——	——	13	4	1	.3	14	Trace	Trace	.01	Trace	1
——	——	——	10	3	1	.2	11	Trace	Trace	Trace	Trace	1
.5	.3	Trace	24	6	35	.6	106	Trace	.01	.03	.2	0
3.1	1.6	.1	20	48	60	.5	107	60	.02	.08	.2	Trace
——	——	——	13	33	9	.9	183	——	.01	.01	Trace	——
——	——	——	11	137	17	3.2	585	——	.02	.04	.4	——
——	——	——	14	35	5	2.6	——	——	——	.02	Trace	——
0	0	0	15	9	3	.8	1	0	0	0	0	0
0	0	0	212	187	42	7.5	757	0	.02	.07	.4	0
0	0	0	199	0	0	.2	6	0	0	0	0	0
0	0	0	12	0	0	Trace	Trace	0	0	0	0	0
0	0	0	100	0	0	.1	3	0	0	0	0	0
——	——	——	5	30	73	0.9	265	1,310	0.23	0.26	2.0	38
——	——	——	6	40	115	2.2	396	1,530	.25	.23	1.8	41
——	——	——	2	13	30	.4	110	540	.10	.11	.8	16
——	——	——	2	13	40	.7	143	470	.10	.08	.7	16
——	——	——	3	15	42	1.5	133	640	.05	.08	.6	12

Nutritive Value of Foods

Foods, approximate measures, units, and weight (in grams)	Water	Food energy	Protein	Fat
VEGETABLES AND VEGETABLE PRODUCTS —Continued	Grams	Percent	Calories	Grams	Grams
Beans					
Lima, frozen, cooked, drained					
Thick-seeded types (Fordhooks) .... 1 cup	170	74	170	10	Trace
Thin-seeded types (baby limas) .... 1 cup	180	69	210	13	Trace
Snap, green					
Cooked, drained					
Fresh (cuts and French style) .... 1 cup	125	92	30	2	Trace
Frozen, (French style) .... 1 cup	130	92	35	2	Trace
Canned, drained vegetables .... 1 cup	135	92	30	2	Trace
Yellow or wax					
Cooked, drained					
Fresh (cuts and French style) .... 1 cup	125	93	30	2	Trace
Frozen (cuts) .... 1 cup	135	92	35	2	Trace
Canned, drained vegetables (cuts) .... 1 cup	135	92	30	2	Trace
Bean sprouts (mung)					
Raw .... 1 cup	105	89	35	4	Trace
Cooked, drained .... 1 cup	125	91	35	4	Trace
Beets					
Cooked, drained, peeled					
Whole beets, 2-in diam .... 2 beets	100	91	30	1	Trace
Diced or sliced .... 1 cup	170	91	55	2	Trace
Canned, drained vegetables					
Whole beets, small .... 1 cup	160	89	60	2	Trace
Diced or sliced .... 1 cup	170	89	65	2	Trace
Beet greens, leaves and stems, cooked, drained ...... 1 cup	145	94	25	2	Trace
Black-eyed peas, cooked and drained					
Fresh .... 1 cup	165	72	180	13	1
Frozen .... 1 cup	170	66	220	15	1
Broccoli, cooked, drained					
Fresh					
Stalk, medium size .... 1 stalk	180	91	45	6	1
Stalks cut into ½-in pieces .... 1 cup	155	91	40	5	Trace
Frozen					
Stalk, 4½ to 5 in long .... 1 stalk	30	91	10	1	Trace
Chopped .... 1 cup	185	92	50	5	1
Brussels sprouts, cooked, drained					
Fresh, 7-8 sprouts (1¼- to 1½-in diam) .... 1 cup	155	88	55	7	1
Frozen .... 1 cup	155	89	50	5	Trace
Cabbage					
Common varieties					
Raw, coarsely shredded or sliced .... 1 cup	70	92	15	1	Trace
Cooked, drained .... 1 cup	145	94	30	2	Trace
Red, raw, coarsely shredded or sliced .... 1 cup	70	90	20	1	Trace
Savoy, raw, coarsely shredded or sliced .... 1 cup	70	92	15	2	Trace

ABC'S OF NUTRITION

Dashes — — in the columns for nutrients denotes lack of reliable data for a constituent believed to be present in measurable amounts.

Fatty Acids			Carbo-hydrate	Calcium	Phos-phorus	Iron	Potas-sium	Vitamin A value	Thiamin	Ribo-flavin	Niacin	Ascorbic acid
Satu-rated (total)	Unsaturated											
	Oleic	Linoleic										
Grams	Grams	Grams	Grams	Milligrams	Milligrams	Milligrams	Milligrams	International units	Milligrams	Milligrams	Milligrams	Milligrams
--	--	--	32	34	153	2.9	724	390	.12	.09	1.7	29
--	--	--	40	63	227	4.7	709	400	.16	.09	2.2	22
--	--	--	7	63	46	.8	189	680	.09	.11	.6	15
--	--	--	8	49	39	1.2	177	690	.08	.10	.4	9
--	--	--	7	61	34	2.0	128	630	.04	.07	.4	5
--	--	--	6	63	46	.8	189	290	.09	.11	.6	16
--	--	--	8	47	42	.9	221	140	.09	.11	.5	8
--	--	--	7	61	34	2.0	128	140	.04	.07	.4	7
--	--	--	7	20	67	1.4	234	20	.14	.14	.8	20
--	--	--	7	21	60	1.1	195	30	.11	.13	.9	8
--	--	--	7	14	23	.5	208	20	.03	.04	.3	6
--	--	--	12	24	39	.9	354	30	.05	.07	.5	10
--	--	--	14	30	29	1.1	267	30	.02	.05	.2	5
--	--	--	15	32	31	1.2	284	30	.02	.05	.2	5
--	--	--	5	144	36	2.8	481	7,400	.10	.22	.4	22
--	--	--	30	40	241	3.5	625	580	.50	.18	2.3	28
--	--	--	40	43	286	4.8	573	290	.68	.19	2.4	15
--	--	--	8	158	112	1.4	481	4,500	.16	.36	1.4	162
--	--	--	7	136	96	1.2	414	3,880	.14	.31	1.2	140
--	--	--	1	12	17	.2	66	570	.02	.03	.2	22
--	--	--	9	100	104	1.3	392	4,810	.11	.22	.9	105
--	--	--	10	50	112	1.7	423	810	.12	.22	1.2	135
--	--	--	10	33	95	1.2	457	880	.12	.16	.9	126
--	--	--	4	34	20	0.3	163	90	0.04	0.04	0.2	33
--	--	--	6	64	29	.4	236	190	.06	.06	.4	48
--	--	--	5	29	25	.6	188	30	.06	.04	.3	43
--	--	--	3	47	38	.6	188	140	.04	.06	.2	39

Nutritive Value of Foods

Foods, approximate measures, units, and weight (in grams)	Water	Food energy	Protein	Fat
	Grams	Percent	Calories	Grams	Grams
VEGETABLES AND VEGETABLE PRODUCTS —Continued					
Cabbage, white mustard (also called bokchoy or pakchoy), cooked, drained ..... 1 cup	170	95	25	2	Trace
Carrots					
Raw, trimmed, scraped					
Whole, 7½ by 1 1/8 in .... 1 carrot	72	88	30	1	Trace
Grated .... 1 cup	110	88	45	1	Trace
Cooked (crosswise cuts), drained .... 1 cup	155	91	50	1	Trace
Canned, sliced, drained vegetables ..... 1 cup	155	91	45	1	Trace
Cauliflower					
Raw, chopped .... 1 cup	115	91	31	3	Trace
Cooked, drained					
Fresh (flower buds) .... 1 cup	125	93	30	3	Trace
Frozen (flowerets) .... 1 cup	180	94	30	3	Trace
Celery, Pascal, raw					
Stalk, large outer, 8 in long .... 1 stalk	40	94	5	Trace	Trace
Pieces, diced .... 1 cup	120	94	20	1	Trace
Collards, cooked, drained					
Fresh (leaves without stems) .... 1 cup	190	90	65	7	1
Frozen (chopped) .... 1 cup	170	90	50	5	1
Corn, yellow sweet					
Cooked, drained					
Fresh, ear 5 by 1¾ in .... 1 ear	140	74	70	2	1
Frozen					
Ear, 5 in long .... 1 ear	229	73	120	4	1
Kernels .... 1 cup	165	77	130	5	1
Canned					
Cream style .... 1 cup	256	76	210	5	2
Whole kernel					
Vacuum pack .... 1 cup	210	76	175	5	1
Wet pack, drained vegetables .... 1 cup	165	76	140	4	1
Cowpeas. See **Black-eyed peas.**					
Cucumber slices, 1/8 in thick (large, 2 1/8-in diam)					
With peel .... 8 slices	28	95	5	Trace	Trace
Without peel .... 6½ pieces	28	96	5	Trace	Trace
Dandelion greens, cooked, drained .... 1 cup	105	90	35	2	1
Endive, curly (including escarole), raw, small pieces .. 1 cup	50	93	10	1	Trace
Kale, cooked, drained					
Fresh (leaves without stems and midribs) .... 1 cup	110	88	45	5	1
Frozen (leaf style) .... 1 cup	130	91	40	4	1
Lettuce					
Butterhead, as Boston types					
Head, 5-in diam .... 1 head	220	95	25	2	Trace
Leaves, outer .... 1 leaf	15	95	Trace	Trace	Trace

ABC'S OF NUTRITION

Dashes — — in the columns for nutrients denotes lack of reliable data for a constituent believed to be present in measurable amounts.

Fatty Acids			Carbo-hydrate	Calcium	Phos-phorus	Iron	Potas-sium	Vitamin A value	Thiamin	Ribo-flavin	Niacin	Ascorbic acid
Satu-rated (total)	Unsaturated											
	Oleic	Linoleic										
Grams	Grams	Grams	Grams	Milligrams	Milligrams	Milligrams	Milligrams	International units	Milligrams	Milligrams	Milligrams	Milligrams
--	--	--	4	252	56	1.0	364	5,270	.07	.14	1.2	26
--	--	--	7	27	26	.5	246	7,930	.04	.04	.4	6
--	--	--	11	41	40	.8	375	12,100	.07	.06	.7	9
--	--	--	11	51	48	.9	344	16,280	.08	.08	.8	9
--	--	--	10	47	34	1.1	186	23,250	.03	.05	.6	3
--	--	--	6	29	64	1.3	339	70	.13	.12	.8	90
--	--	--	5	26	53	.9	258	80	.11	.10	.8	69
--	--	--	6	31	68	.9	373	50	.07	.09	.7	74
--	--	--	2	16	11	.1	136	110	.01	.01	.1	4
--	--	--	5	47	34	.4	409	320	.04	.04	.4	11
--	--	--	10	357	99	1.5	498	14,820	.21	.38	2.3	144
--	--	--	10	299	87	1.7	401	11,560	.10	.24	1.0	56
--	--	--	16	2	69	.5	151	310	.09	.08	1.1	7
--	--	--	27	4	121	1.0	291	440	.18	.10	2.1	9
--	--	--	31	5	120	1.3	304	580	.15	.10	2.5	8
--	--	--	51	8	143	1.5	248	840	.08	.13	2.6	13
--	--	--	43	6	153	1.1	204	740	.06	.13	2.3	11
--	--	--	33	8	81	.8	160	580	.05	.08	1.5	7
--	--	--	1	7	8	.3	45	70	.01	.01	.1	3
--	--	--	1	5	5	0.1	45	Trace	0.01	0.01	0.1	3
--	--	--	7	147	44	1.9	244	12,290	.14	.17	--	19
--	--	--	2	41	27	.9	147	1,650	.04	.07	.3	5
--	--	--	7	206	64	1.8	243	9,130	.11	.20	1.8	102
--	--	--	7	157	62	1.3	251	10,660	.08	.20	.9	49
--	--	--	4	57	42	3.3	430	1,580	.10	.10	.5	13
--	--	--	Trace	5	4	.3	40	150	.01	.01	Trace	1

Nutritive Value of Foods

Foods, approximate measures, units, and weight (in grams)		Water	Food energy	Protein	Fat
VEGETABLES AND VEGETABLE PRODUCTS —Continued	Grams	Percent	Calories	Grams	Grams
Lettuce-Continued					
Crisphead, as Iceberg					
Head, 6-in diam .... 1 head	567	96	70	5	1
Wedge, ¼ of head .... 1 wedge	135	96	20	1	Trace
Pieces, chopped or shredded .... 1 cup	55	96	5	Trace	Trace
Loose-leaf (bunching varieties including .... 1 cup Romaine), chopped or shredded	55	94	10	1	Trace
Mushrooms, raw, sliced or chopped .... 1 cup	70	90	20	2	Trace
Mustard greens, without stems and .... 1 cup midribs, cooked, drained	140	93	30	3	1
Okra pods, 3 in long, cooked .... 10 pods	106	91	30	2	Trace
Onions					
Mature, white-fleshed					
Raw					
Chopped .... 1 cup	170	89	65	3	Trace
Sliced .... 1 cup	115	89	45	2	Trace
Cooked (whole or sliced), drained ..... 1 cup	210	92	60	3	Trace
Young green, bulb and white portion of top ..... 6 onions	30	88	15	Trace	Trace
Parsley, fresh, chopped .... 1 tbsp	4	85	Trace	Trace	Trace
Parsnips, cooked, diced .... 1 cup	155	82	100	2	1
Peas, green					
Canned					
Whole, drained vegetables .... 1 cup	170	77	150	8	1
Frozen, cooked, drained .... 1 cup	160	82	110	8	Trace
Peppers, sweet (about 5 per lb, whole), stem and seeds removed					
Raw .... 1 pod	74	93	15	1	Trace
Cooked, boiled, drained .... 1 pod	73	95	15	1	Trace
Potatoes, cooked					
Baked, peeled after baking (about 2 per lb) .... 1 potato	156	75	145	4	Trace
Boiled (about 3 per lb)					
Peeled after boiling .... 1 potato	137	80	105	3	Trace
Peeled before boiling .... 1 potato	135	83	90	3	Trace
French-fried, strip, 2 to 3½ in long					
Prepared from raw .... 10 strips	50	45	135	2	7
Frozen, oven heated .... 10 strips	50	53	110	2	4
Hashed brown, prepared from frozen .... 1 cup	155	56	345	3	18
Mashed, prepared from raw					
Milk added .... 1 cup	210	83	135	4	2
Milk and butter added .... 1 cup	210	80	195	4	9
Dehydrated flakes (without milk), water, ... 1 cup milk, butter, and salt added	210	79	195	4	7
Potato chips, 1¾ by 2½ in .... 10 chips	20	2	115	1	8
Pumpkin, canned .... 1 cup	245	90	80	2	1

ABC'S OF NUTRITION

Dashes — — in the columns for nutrients denotes lack of reliable data for a constituent believed to be present in measurable amounts.

Fatty Acids			Carbo-hydrate	Calcium	Phos-phorus	Iron	Potas-sium	Vitamin A value	Thiamin	Ribo-flavin	Niacin	Ascorbic acid
Satu-rated (total)	Unsaturated											
	Oleic	Linoleic										
Grams	Grams	Grams	Grams	Milligrams	Milligrams	Milligrams	Milligrams	International units	Milligrams	Milligrams	Milligrams	Milligrams
— —	— —	— —	16	108	118	2.7	943	1,780	.32	.32	1.6	32
— —	— —	— —	4	27	30	.7	236	450	.08	.08	.4	8
— —	— —	— —	2	11	12	.3	96	180	.03	.03	.2	3
— —	— —	— —	2	37	14	.8	145	1,050	.03	.04	.2	10
— —	— —	— —	3	4	81	.6	290	Trace	.07	.32	2.9	2
— —	— —	— —	6	193	45	2.5	308	8,120	.11	.20	.8	67
— —	— —	— —	6	98	43	.5	184	520	.14	.19	1.0	21
— —	— —	— —	15	46	61	.9	267	Trace	.05	.07	.3	17
— —	— —	— —	10	31	41	.6	181	Trace	.03	.05	.2	12
— —	— —	— —	14	50	61	.8	231	Trace	.06	.06	.4	15
— —	— —	— —	3	12	12	.2	69	Trace	.02	.01	.1	8
— —	— —	— —	Trace	7	2	.2	25	300	Trace	.01	Trace	6
— —	— —	— —	23	70	96	.9	587	50	.11	.12	.2	16
— —	— —	— —	29	44	129	3.2	163	1,170	.15	.10	1.4	14
			19	30	138	3.0	216	960	.43	.14	2.7	21
— —	— —	— —	4	7	16	.5	157	310	.06	.06	.4	94
— —	— —	— —	3	7	12	.4	109	310	.05	.05	.4	70
— —	— —	— —	33	14	101	1.1	782	Trace	.15	.07	2.7	31
— —	— —	— —	23	10	72	.8	556	Trace	.12	.05	2.0	22
— —	— —	— —	20	8	57	.7	385	Trace	.12	.05	1.6	22
1.7	1.2	3.3	18	8	56	.7	427	Trace	.07	.04	1.6	11
1.1	.8	2.1	17	5	43	.9	326	Trace	.07	.01	1.3	11
4.6	3.2	9.0	45	28	78	1.9	439	Trace	.11	.03	1.6	12
.7	.4	Trace	27	50	103	.8	548	40	.17	.11	2.1	21
5.6	2.3	0.2	26	50	101	0.8	525	360	0.17	0.11	2.1	19
3.6	2.1	.2	30	65	99	.6	601	270	.08	.08	1.9	11
2.1	1.4	4.0	10	8	28	.4	226	Trace	.04	.01	1.0	3
— —	— —	— —	19	61	64	1.0	588	15,680	.07	.12	1.5	12

Nutritive Value of Foods

Foods, approximate measures, units, and weight (in grams)		Water	Food energy	Protein	Fat
VEGETABLES AND VEGETABLE PRODUCTS —Continued	Grams	Percent	Calories	Grams	Grams
Radishes, raw (prepackaged), trimmed .... 4 radishes	18	95	5	Trace	Trace
Sauerkraut, canned, solids and liquid .... 1 cup	235	93	40	2	Trace
Southern peas. See **Black-eyed peas.**					
Spinach					
Fresh, chopped .... 1 cup	55	91	15	2	Trace
Cooked, drained					
Fresh .... 1 cup	180	92	40	5	1
Frozen					
Chopped .... 1 cup	205	92	45	6	1
Leaf .... 1 cup	190	92	45	6	1
Canned, drained .... 1 cup	205	91	50	6	1
Squash, cooked					
Summer (all varieties), diced, drained .... 1 cup	210	96	30	2	Trace
Winter (all varieties), baked, mashed .... 1 cup	205	81	130	4	1
Sweet potatoes					
Cooked (raw, 5 by 2 in)					
Baked in skin, peeled .... 1 potato	114	64	160	2	1
Boiled in skin, peeled .... 1 potato	151	71	170	3	1
Candied, 2½ by 2-in piece .... 1 piece	105	60	175	1	3
Canned					
Solid pack (mashed) .... 1 cup	255	72	275	5	1
Vacuum pack, 2¾ by 1-in piece .... 1 piece	40	72	45	1	Trace
Tomatoes					
Fresh, including cores and stem ends, ... 1 tomato	135	94	25	1	Trace
2½-in diam					
Canned, solids and liquid .... 1 cup	241	94	50	2	Trace
Tomato catsup .... 1 tbsp	15	69	15	Trace	Trace
Tomato juice, canned .... 1 cup	243	94	45	2	Trace
Turnips, cooked, diced .... 1 cup	155	94	35	1	Trace
Turnip greens, cooked, drained					
Fresh (leaves and stems) .... 1 cup	145	94	30	3	Trace
Frozen (chopped) .... 1 cup	165	93	40	4	Trace
Vegetables, mixed, frozen, cooked .... 1 cup	182	83	115	6	1

[18] Without calcium salts added.

ABC'S OF NUTRITION

Dashes — — in the columns for nutrients denotes lack of reliable data for a constituent believed to be present in measurable amounts.

Fatty Acids			Carbo-hydrate	Calcium	Phos-phorus	Iron	Potas-sium	Vitamin A value	Thiamin	Ribo-flavin	Niacin	Ascorbic acid
Satu-rated (total)	Unsaturated											
	Oleic	Linoleic										
Grams	Grams	Grams	Grams	Milligrams	Milligrams	Milligrams	Milligrams	International units	Milligrams	Milligrams	Milligrams	Milligrams
——	——	——	1	5	6	.2	58	Trace	.01	.01	.1	5
——	——	——	9	85	42	1.2	329	120	.07	.09	.5	33
——	——	——	2	51	28	1.7	259	4,460	.06	.11	.3	28
——	——	——	6	167	68	4.0	583	14,580	.13	.25	.9	50
——	——	——	8	232	90	4.3	683	16,200	.14	.31	.8	39
——	——	——	7	200	84	4.8	688	15,390	.15	.27	1.0	53
——	——	——	7	242	53	5.3	513	16,400	.04	.25	.6	29
——	——	——	7	53	53	.8	296	820	.11	.17	1.7	21
——	——	——	32	57	98	1.6	945	8,610	.10	.27	1.4	27
——	——	——	37	46	66	1.0	342	9,230	.10	.08	.8	25
——	——	——	40	48	71	1.1	367	11,940	.14	.09	.9	26
2.0	.8	.1	36	39	45	.9	200	6,620	.06	.04	.4	11
——	——	——	63	64	105	2.0	510	19,890	.13	.10	1.5	36
——	——	——	10	10	16	.3	80	3,120	.02	.02	.2	6
——	——	——	6	16	33	.6	300	1,110	.07	.05	.9	28
——	——	——	10	[18]14	46	1.2	523	2,170	.12	.07	1.7	41
——	——	——	4	3	8	.1	54	210	.01	.01	.2	2
——	——	——	10	17	44	2.2	552	1,940	.12	.07	1.9	39
——	——	——	8	54	37	.6	291	Trace	.06	.08	.5	34
——	——	——	5	252	49	1.5	——	8,270	.15	.33	.7	68
——	——	——	6	195	64	2.6	246	11,390	.08	.15	.7	31
——	——	——	24	46	115	2.4	348	9,010	.22	.13	2.0	15

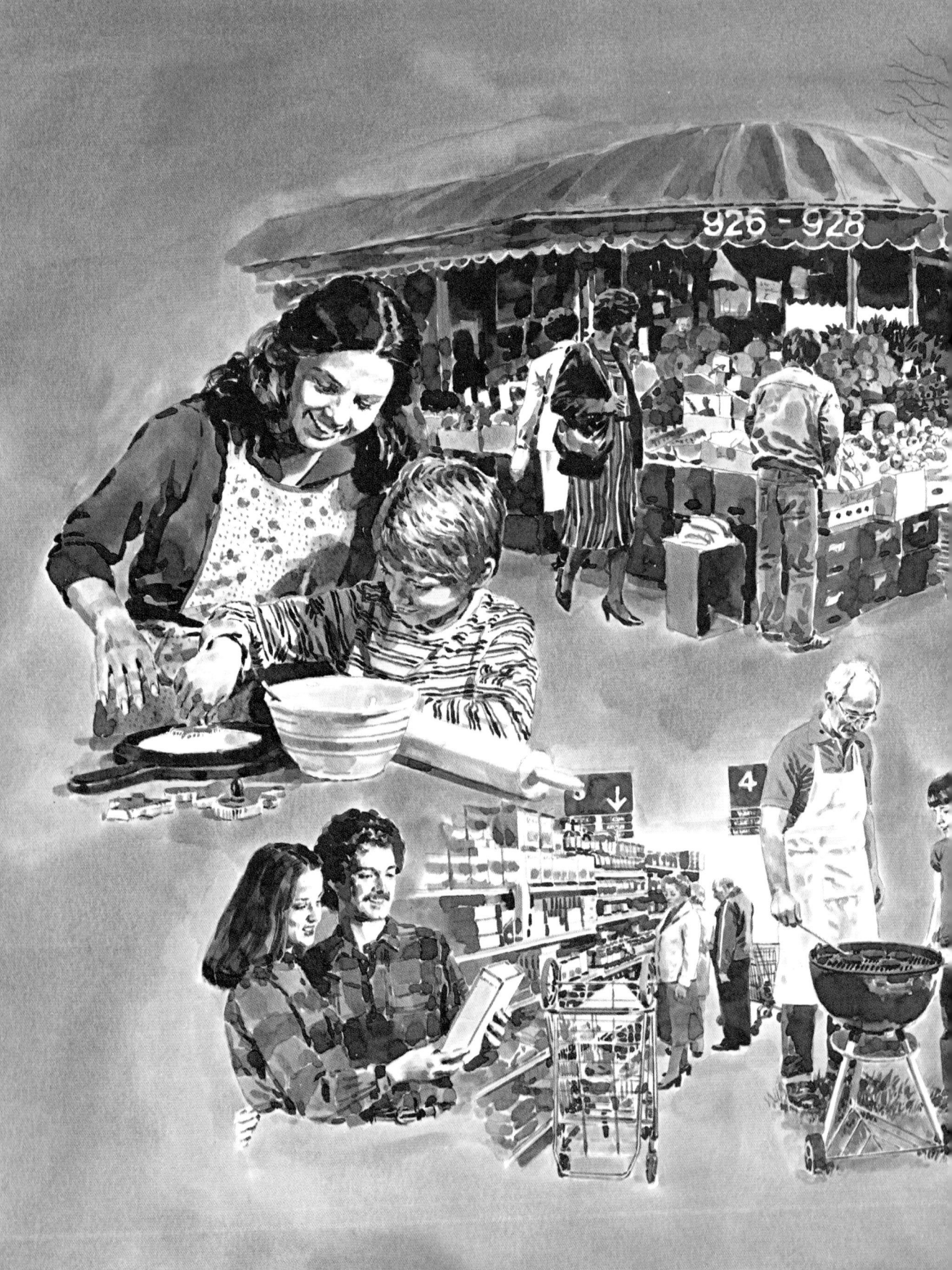

2. FAMILY FOOD GUIDE

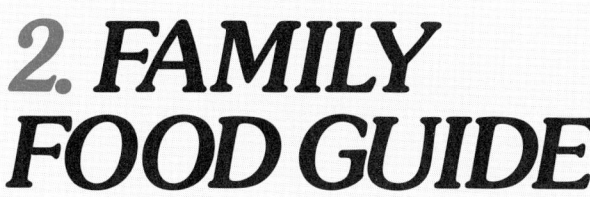

A detailed guide to selecting foods and beverages with nutrition in mind. The latest information on how to store foods safely and preserve quality. Practical tips for food preparation, plus more than 200 delicious recipes: Cooking the Nutritious Way.

The Basic Four Food Groups .. 96
   Fruits and Vegetables 98
   Breads, Cereals, and Grains . 100
   Milk and Milk Products 102
   Poultry, Fish, Meat, Eggs,
      Legumes, Nuts, and Seeds 104
   An Eating Quiz 106
Buying Guide
   Vegetables 108
   Fruits 124
   Freshwater Fish 136
   Saltwater Fish 138
   Shellfish 140
   Beef 142
   Veal 144
   Lamb 146
   Pork 148
   Variety Meats 150
   Sausages 151
   Poultry 152
   Eggs 153
   Milk Products 154
   Cheese 155
   Legumes 160
      The Versatile Soybean ... 163
      Sprouting Your Own 164
   Nuts and Seeds 166

Grains and Grain Products .. 168
   Cereals 172
   Flours 173
   Pasta 175
   Herbs and Spices 176
Gathering Foods from the Wild 180
Beverages 182
Market Basket
   A Guide to Shopping 192
   Food Standards 194
   Food Grades and Inspection
      Stamps 195
   Food Labels 196
   Nutrition Labels 198
   Additives to Foods 199
Keeping Foods Fresh
   On the Shelf 202
   In the Refrigerator 204
   In the Freezer 206
   Other Long-term Storage ... 211
Preparation Techniques
   Handle with Care 212
   Choosing a Cooking Method 213
   Useful Facts and Figures 216
Cooking the Nutritious Way .. 218
   Baking Yeast Breads 270
   Adding Variety to Meals 277

The Basic Four Food Groups

If you are like most people, when you make up a shopping list, go to the supermarket, or order food at a restaurant, you don't want to think about proteins, carbohydrates, vitamins, or minerals. You think about what tastes good, what your family likes, and what's reasonably priced because it's in season or on sale.

To simplify meal planning and ensure that people eat a balanced diet, the U.S. Department of Agriculture has divided foods into five groups. The first four—the Basic Four—comprise a foundation diet, with a recommended number of servings to be eaten daily from each group. A fifth group (see box opposite) provides additional calories but fewer nutrients. In the following pages the Basic Four are described and pictured in detail. In brief they are:

Group 1. Fruits and vegetables
    4 or more servings per day
Group 2. Breads, cereals, and other grains
    4 or more servings per day
Group 3. Milk and milk products
    Adults—2 servings per day
    Children—3 to 4 servings per day
Group 4. Poultry, fish, meat, eggs, legumes, nuts, and seeds
    2 servings per day

By eating a variety of foods from the Basic Four, you should obtain the nutrients you need. The number and size of servings is intended to be the foundation for meal planning. The total of 12 servings for adults provides approximately 1,200 calories. Most people want—and need—more than that. Calorie intake can be increased by eating more or larger servings from the Basic Four or by eating other foods from the fifth group, for which no number of servings is recommended.

The Basic Four has the advantages of simplicity and flexibility, but as a system for meal planning, it has its critics who argue that it overemphasizes animal foods (two out of four groups) and that it is entirely possible to have a poor diet by eating indiscriminately from the Basic Four. For example, a fast-food chain could claim that this meal fulfills the Basic Four requirements: French fries (vegetable), white roll (bread), hamburger (meat), and milk shake (milk products). While nutritious enough once in a while, a steady diet of such meals with their extra load of fat, sugar, and salt could be a nutritional disaster. By changing some elements of the meal, however, it could become a nutritious one: a salad of lettuce and tomato, whole-wheat bread, a lean-meat hamburger, and a glass of milk.

The text and lists on the following eight pages are designed to help you make better food choices by rating the foods as to whether they should be included in the diet anytime (every day), in moderation (two to three times a week), or only now and then (once a week or less).

Foods in the anytime columns contain less than 30 percent fat and are usually low in salt and sugar. Foods that may be eaten in moderation usually contain somewhat more fat and may also contain somewhat more salt or sugar. Foods in the now-and-then columns usually contain more than 50 percent fat and may be high in salt and sugar as well.

Start the day right. To provide balance, each meal ideally should include foods from at least three of the four groups. With a total of 12 or more servings to be divided among three meals, it's hard to get in all the necessary servings unless you start with a good breakfast. From this standpoint and also because your body, like an engine, needs refueling for the day ahead, breakfast is the most important meal of the day. People often skip it because they can't find the time or don't like eating first thing in the morning. But many easily prepared foods besides ready-to-eat cereals can make a quick and easy breakfast—for example, cheese and crackers or bread, yogurt, cottage cheese, fresh fruits, or leftover casserole dishes such as macaroni and cheese. If you're unaccustomed to breakfast and your stomach rebels against food early in the morning, try eating just one item. When you're used to that, add a second item, and so on. The same goes for finicky eaters: try adding one new food at a time to the diet. Don't try to reform a confirmed steak-and-potato person overnight.

Don't undervalue snacks. Another way of getting in the 12 servings of the Basic Four is by eating some of them as snacks. Fresh fruits or raw vegetable sticks, two or three whole-meal crackers, a glass of milk or fruit juice, homemade custard or pudding, plain popcorn—all are nutritious snacks. Try them instead of such oversweetened, nutritionally empty snacks as soft drinks, candy, and most cookies.

Dietary Guidelines. In the foreword to this book (pages 5–6), you read about the Senate Select Committee on Nutrition and Human Needs and its controversial Dietary Goals report. In 1980 the Departments of Agriculture and Health and Human Services jointly issued a set of "Dietary Guidelines for Americans." They are seven in number, like the goals:

1. Eat a variety of foods
2. Maintain ideal weight
3. Avoid too much fat, saturated fat, and cholesterol
4. Eat foods with adequate starch and fiber
5. Avoid too much sugar
6. Avoid too much sodium
7. If you drink alcohol, do so in moderation

Items 2 through 6 are substantially the same as the Senate Select Committee's Dietary Goals, but items 1 and 7 are additions.

Alcoholic beverages lack nutrients but are high in calories (see table showing calorie counts on page 191). Excessive consumption, besides impairing mental and physical processes, can lead to vitamin and mineral deficiencies when alcohol rather than nutritious food accounts for too high a percentage of a person's calorie budget. However, in the opinion of many doctors, a drink or two a day is harmless and may even be beneficial.

Most important is the advice to eat a variety of foods. The body requires some 40 nutrients to maintain health and vigor. No average person is going to keep track of even a fraction of these nutrients. But it is a fairly safe bet that eating a wide range of foods will ensure that the body gets enough or close to the required amounts of those nutrients. It is also a good idea to eat as much fresh food as you can and avoid too much reliance on processed convenience foods. For further advice in reforming your eating habits, see pages 296–319.

Fats, Sweets, and Alcohol

If the foods of the Basic Four form a good foundation for your diet, the fifth group of foods—which includes those high in fats, sweets, or alcohol and little else—are extra trimmings. No number of servings is recommended because it's all too easy to eat from this group in excess.

Fats. A component of all animal foods, fats are also present in lesser amounts in some plant foods: nuts, avocados, olives, seeds, grains, cocoa. Fats are an integral part of these foods, and we generally are unaware of eating fat. Other fats are added to foods in the form of butter, margarine, salad dressings, and cooking oils. You can reduce fat intake by cutting down on visible fats, shunning fried foods, and choosing lean forms of meat and fat-free or low-fat dairy products.

Sweets. Aside from filling you up with nutritionally empty calories and taking the place of foods offering essential nutrients, sweets contribute to obesity and dental caries (cavities). Tooth decay is caused in part by bacteria that feed on sweets fermenting in the mouth; that's why brushing the teeth right after a meal is a good preventive measure.

Everyone knows that candy and soft drinks are sweet, but few realize just how sweet. A 5-ounce candy bar may contain as much as 20 teaspoons of sugar; a 12-ounce can of soda, 8 teaspoons. Other sources of sweets are jam, jelly, syrups, chewing gum, cookies, cake, pie, and presweetened breakfast cereals. The latter sometimes contain more sugar than any other ingredient; check labels for such words as "sucrose," "dextrose," and "corn syrup." They are all forms of sugar.

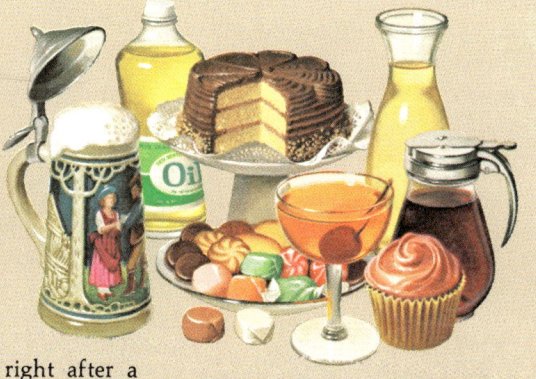

Alcohol. Like other foods in this group, alcohol in moderation is all right; in excess, harmful. Four to five drinks a day can lead to fatty deposits in the liver and eventually to cirrhosis of the liver, a serious nonreversible condition. On the other hand, a drink or two a day is believed by some medical researchers to beneficially stimulate the coronary arteries. This is not to suggest that you take up drinking as a health measure, but if you enjoy a predinner cocktail or a glass of wine with your meal, it is not a cause for concern.

The Basic Four Food Groups
Fruits and Vegetables

For adding variety to the diet, you can't beat fruits and vegetables. High in nutrients (and many low in calories), fruits and vegetables provide vitamins—particularly A and C—minerals, and fiber, the last of which is now thought by some scientists to help prevent certain diseases of the digestive tract.

There are several ways of sorting out the fruits and vegetables. Fruits are the ripened seed-bearing ovaries of plants. Vegetables, on the other hand, come from all parts of plants. Some are flowers (broccoli, cauliflower, Brussels sprouts, artichokes); some are leaves (lettuce, cabbage); some are stems (celery, asparagus); and some, like Swiss chard, spinach, and beet greens, are both leaf and stem. Then there are roots and tubers (potatoes, beets, carrots, turnips) and immature seeds (peas, corn, lima beans); all of these are high in starch. Still others are unsweet fruits. These include eggplant, tomatoes, squash, cucumbers, peppers, and okra.

A traditional way of categorizing vegetables is by color and nutritional character. Dark-green vegetables form one group; deep-yellow vegetables, such as carrots, winter squashes, pumpkins, another group; and starchy vegetables still another. You can choose from each of these groups plus a range of fruits, especially citrus fruits.

But the real plus for fruits and vegetables is their nutrient content. It is often recommended that we eat one fruit (for vitamin C) every day and a dark-green or dark-yellow vegetable (for vitamin A) at least every other day. (See the section on vitamins, pages 30–41, for fruits and vegetables containing those vitamins.) The rest of the four or more servings a day can be of any fruit or vegetable, including other sources of vitamins A and C. Broccoli, cantaloupe, tomatoes, and the various salad greens score high, being rich in both vitamins.

Because cooking often destroys some of the vitamin content, you should eat some fruits and vegetables raw. Some unsweetened fruit and vegetable juices will give you the vitamins, but whole fruits contain fiber and are usually less expensive. To increase your fruit and vegetable intake: keep your refrigerator stocked with raw vegetable sticks; add fruit to plain yogurt or vanilla ice cream.

What's a serving? According to the U.S. Department of Agriculture, a serving is any one of the following:

1 whole fruit (apple, orange, banana, etc.)
½ grapefruit or cantaloupe
½ cup raw or cooked vegetable
½ cup sliced or cooked fruit or berries
¾ cup of fruit or vegetable juice
Juice of one lemon
3 to 4 dried fruits
1 small salad
1 medium-size potato

There are almost no vegetables and fruits that you shouldn't eat regularly. Those in the in-moderation and now-and-then columns are there mostly because during processing or cooking they have gained sugar or salt. The exception is an avocado which is high in calories and fat, although it is low in sodium.

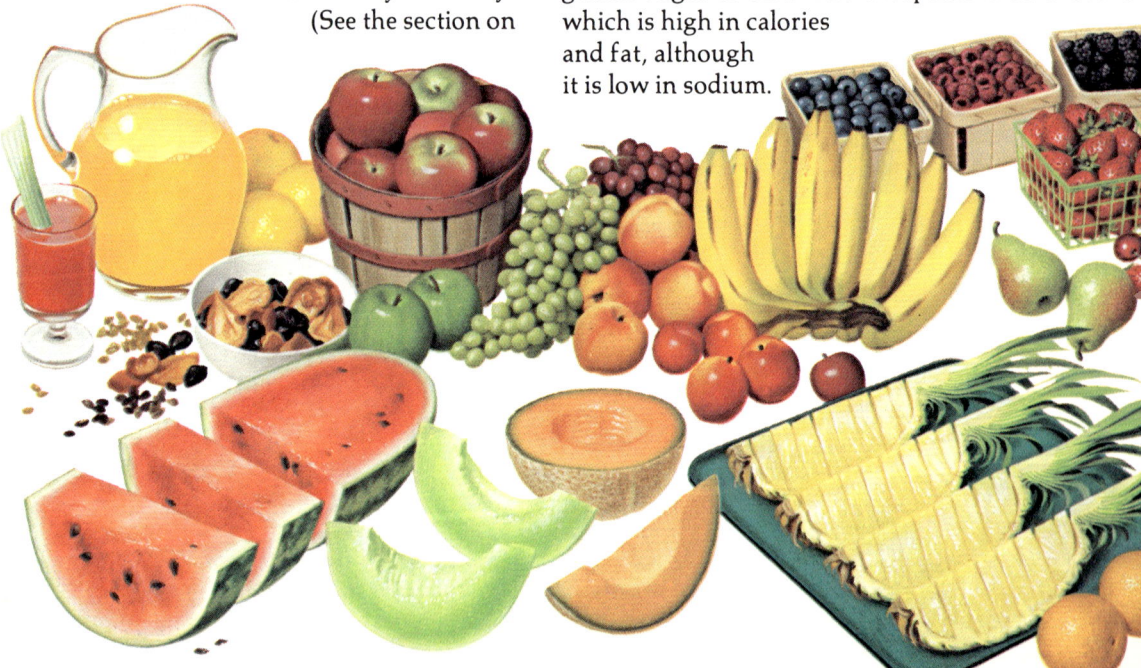

FAMILY FOOD GUIDE

4 Servings per Day

ANYTIME
(everyday)

most fruits and vegetables, raw or cooked, except those listed in other two columns
unsweetened applesauce
unsweetened fruit juices
unsalted vegetable juices
potatoes, white or sweet, boiled or baked

IN MODERATION
(two to three times a week)

avocado
coleslaw
cranberry sauce
dried fruits
eggplant, fried in vegetable oil
fruits canned in syrup
glazed carrots
potatoes au gratin or French-fried in vegetable oil
salted vegetable juices
sweetened fruit juices
vegetables canned with salt

NOW AND THEN
(once a week or less)

pickles
olives

The Basic Four Food Groups
Breads, Cereals, and Other Grains

Throughout most of the world, the foods in this group are truly the staff of life. They are the staples in the diet; everything else revolves around them. For example, the rice of the Far East, the bulgur of the Middle East, the pasta of Italy, the kasha and black breads of Russia, the tortillas of Mexico—all are central to their people's cuisine.

In America, with the exception of breakfast cereal, these foods are often passed by and even purposely avoided under the misguided notion that they are fattening. In fact, breads and cereals contain no more calories per gram than meats and far less than fats. They provide complex carbohydrates, some incomplete protein, B vitamins, iron, magnesium, traces of other minerals, folacin, and all-important fiber. The protein in breads, cereals, and other grains becomes complete when they are eaten with foods containing the missing amino acids, such as legumes or milk. Foods from this group can replace the calories you might otherwise be getting from sweets and fats and will better satisfy your hunger.

Whole-grain versus refined products. When whole wheat is refined into white flour, it loses much of its bran and germ, the most nutritious parts. What remains is the white, starchy endosperm. However, most refined white flour (and the bread made with it) is enriched with thiamin, riboflavin, niacin, and iron. And refined cereals may be fortified with vitamins not normally found in grains, such as A, B_{12}, C, and D. It's a good idea to include in the diet some of each—whole grain and enriched, refined grain products. Rice undergoes a similar transformation, but to a lesser degree. Converted white rice is nutritionally close to brown rice but lacks much of the fiber. Therefore, converted (parboiled) rice is a second-best choice after brown. Enriched white rice is a third-best choice.

Grains are the seeds of food grasses. An exception is buckwheat, the seed of a different family of herbaceous plants. Of all the grains, buckwheat has the best quality protein, for it contains lysine, an essential amino acid found only in low amounts in other grains. Oats too are high in protein as well as iron, calcium, and phosphorus. Rye flour and whole-wheat products follow closely in nutritional value. Rice is less nutritious, and corn still less.

What's a serving? If you don't ordinarily include many foods in this group in your diet, four or more servings perhaps sounds like a lot. But the size of the servings is really rather modest:

1 slice of bread
1 pancake, muffin, roll, or tortilla
½ English muffin
½ to ¾ cup of cooked cereal, rice, or pasta
1 ounce (approximately ½ to 1 cup, according to density) ready-to-eat cereal

At least one serving should be a whole-grain product, and at least one a cereal. If no cereal is eaten, it is better to have five servings from the group. That's not difficult if you have a slice of bread with each meal, rice, and two whole-grain crackers.

In the chart some foods appear in the in-moderation and now-and-then columns solely because they are refined products, such as white rice. Others are there because they incorporate added fats and sugar, with their extra calories, or salt.

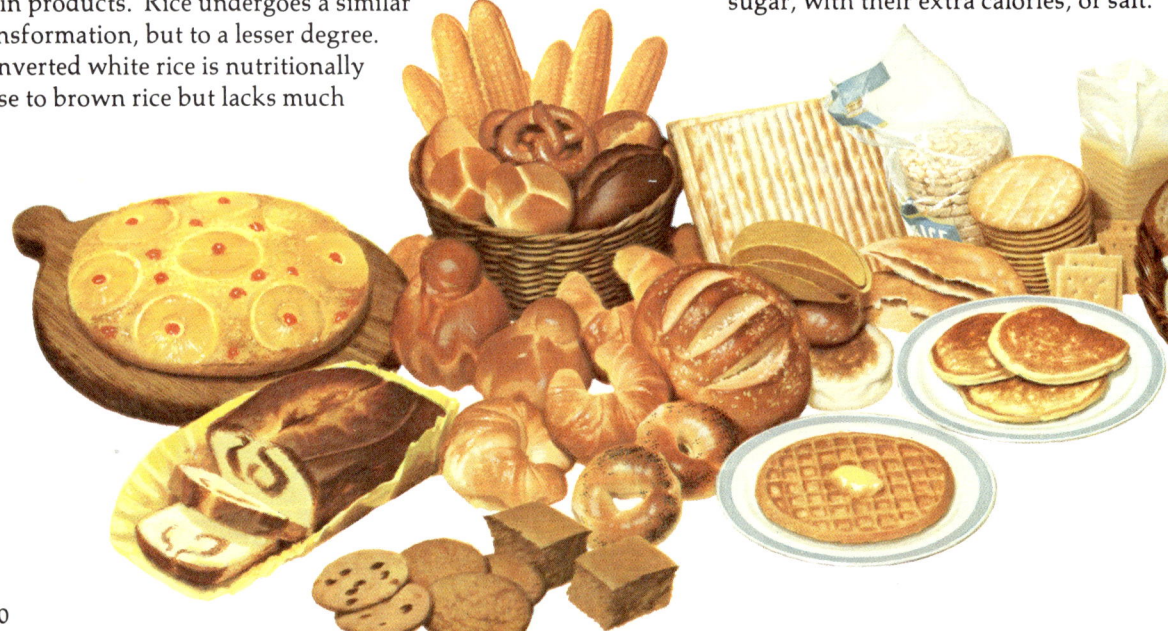

FAMILY FOOD GUIDE

4 Servings per Day

ANYTIME
(everyday)

whole-wheat bread and rolls
rye or pumpernickel bread
bulgur (parboiled wheat)
oatmeal
whole-grain hot and cold cereals
whole-wheat pasta
brown rice
whole-wheat matzoh

IN MODERATION
(two to three times a week)

cornbread
flour tortilla
granola cereals
hominy grits
refined, unsweetened cereals
matzoh
crackers
white bread and rolls
white rice
pasta, except whole wheat
macaroni and cheese
pizza
waffles or pancakes with syrup

NOW AND THEN
(once a week or less)

cake
cookies
croissant
doughnut
presweetened breakfast cereals
Danish pastry
stuffing made with butter

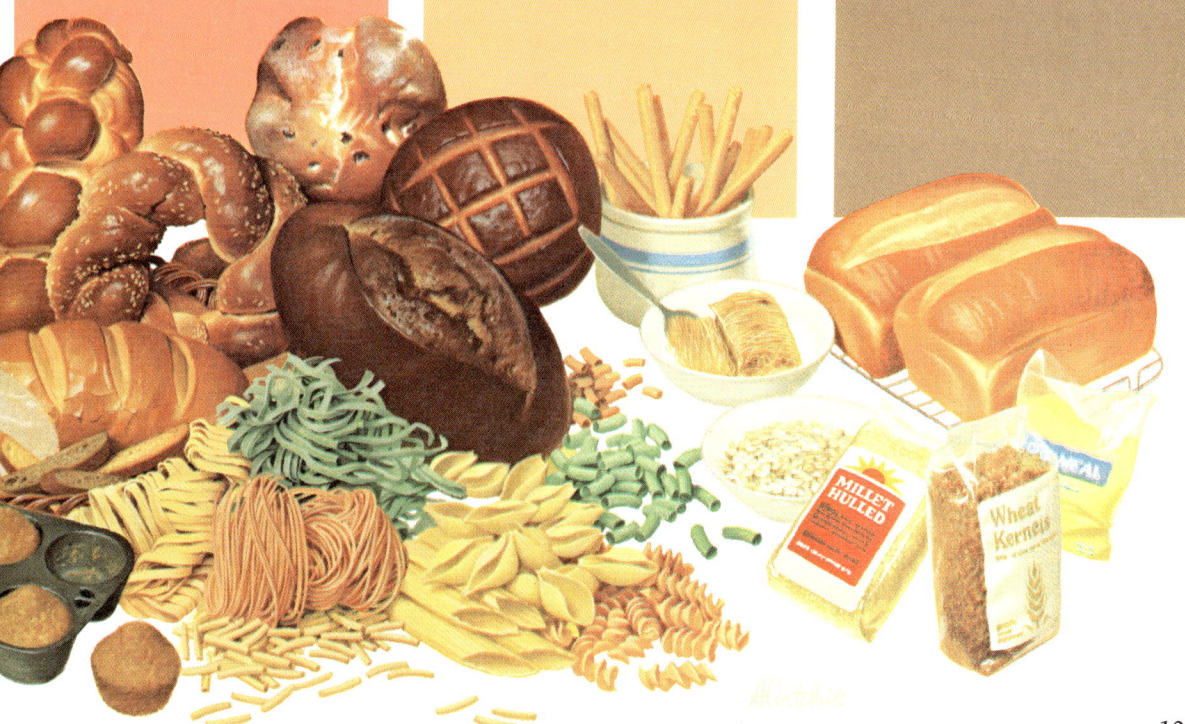

101

The Basic Four Food Groups
Milk and Milk Products

Of the four main food groups, this is the most limiting, for its products stem from one source: the cow. (In other cultures they might come from the goat, sheep, or yak.) Moreover, some people simply don't like milk and there are those whose digestive systems cannot tolerate some of the components of milk. The latter must be choosy in the type and amount of milk products they consume. If you think you have an intolerance, consult your doctor. After you have done so, you may want to read the section on milk-free diets (page 373- 375).

Everyone knows that babies and children need milk to grow. Not everyone recognizes that adults still need the nutrients most readily available in milk or milk products to keep their bones in a healthy condition. The mineral calcium, found in milk, is the significant nutrient in building and maintaining bone structure. Sometimes overlooked is the fact that milk also contains generous amounts of protein and vitamins—A, B_6, B_{12}, riboflavin, and (when fortified) D.

How much milk you need depends on your age and other factors. Adults should have 2 cups or the equivalent in milk products; children up to 9 years old, 2 to 3 cups; children 9 to 12 years old and pregnant women, 3 to 4 cups; 12- to 18-year-olds and nursing mothers require 4 cups or more. Although liquid milk is the simplest way to consume some or all of your daily quota, there are plenty of alternatives. The chart opposite lists some milk products and dishes that can substitute for milk itself in the diet. Yogurt is an acceptable substitute in the plain low-fat form. Any number of puddings are made with milk. Soufflés and quiches are often a bonus in that they contain both milk and cheese.

What's a serving? An 8-ounce cup of milk is one serving. The U.S. Department of Agriculture lists servings of milk products comparing the calcium contents with the amount of calcium in milk:

- 1 cup of plain low-fat yogurt = 1 cup of 2% milk
- 1-inch cube of Cheddar or Swiss cheese = ½ cup of whole milk
- ½ cup of cottage cheese = ¼ cup of whole milk
- 2 tablespoons processed cheese spread = ½ cup of whole milk
- ½ cup of ice cream or ice milk = ⅓ cup of whole milk

However, in addition to calcium, some milk and milk products contain fat and added sugar. To help you calculate how much fat and sugar you are getting along with calcium in your milk substitutes, here are some examples:

- 1 cup of whole milk = 1 cup of skim milk + 2 teaspoons of fat
- 1½ ounces of natural cheese = 1 cup of skim milk + 3 teaspoons of fat
- 1 cup of low-fat fruit yogurt = 1 cup of skim milk + 1 teaspoon of fat + 7 teaspoons of sugar
- ½ cup of ice cream = ⅓ cup of skim milk + 2 teaspoons of fat + 3 teaspoons of sugar

These lists show "tradeoffs," or approximations based on calories, calcium, protein, fat, and total carbohydrate content. Individual products vary.

Remember that a substitute for milk doesn't always contain the nutrients in a cup of milk and it may come burdened with fat and sugar.

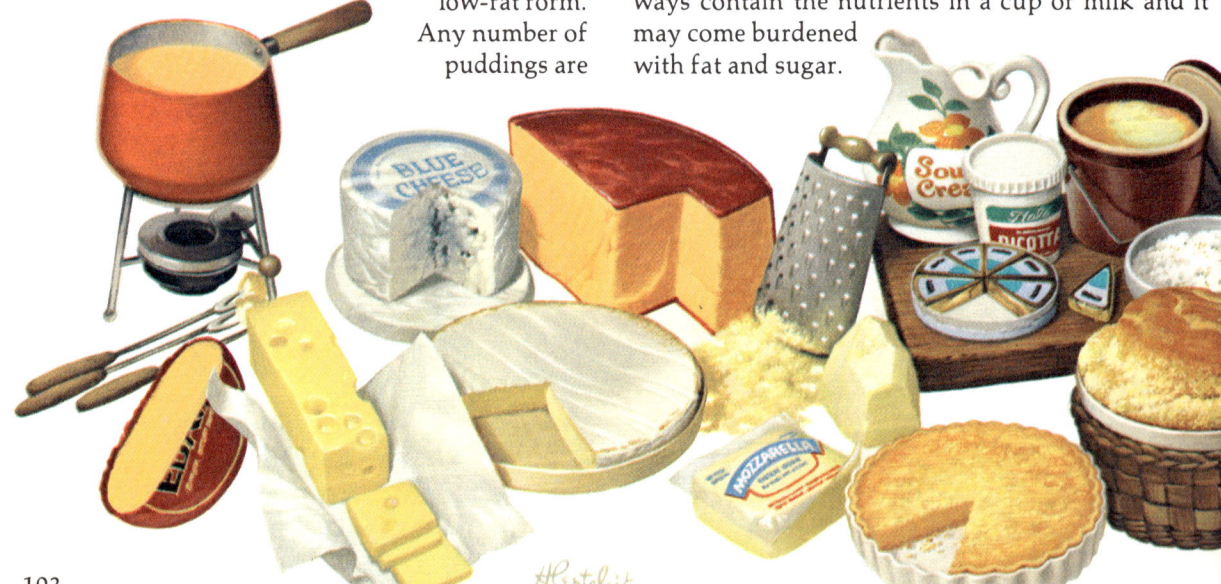

FAMILY FOOD GUIDE

2 Servings per Day

ANYTIME
(everyday)

skim milk
buttermilk (made from skim milk)
low-fat yogurt, plain
nonfat dry milk
low-fat milk (1% milk fat)
low-fat cottage cheese
skim milk and banana shake

IN MODERATION
(two to three times a week)

low-fat milk (2% milk fat)
frozen low-fat yogurt
low-fat yogurt, sweetened
cottage cheese, regular (4% milk fat)
ricotta and mozzarella cheeses made from part-skim milk
ice milk
cocoa made with skim milk

NOW AND THEN
(once a week or less)

whole milk
whole-milk yogurt
whole-milk cheeses, such as blue, brick, Camembert, Cheddar, Muenster, Parmesan, Swiss
processed cheeses
ice cream
cheese fondue
macaroni and cheese
cheese soufflé
cheesecake
caramel custard
puddings made with milk
eggnog
milk shake made with whole milk

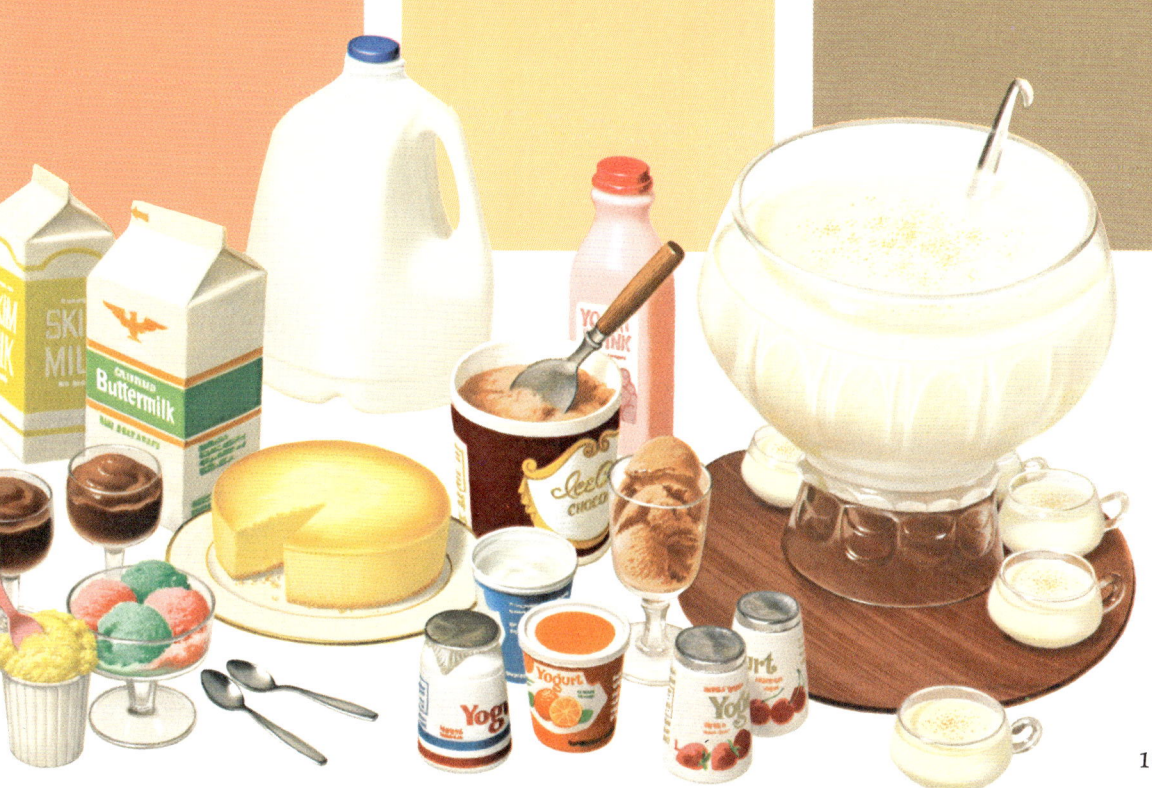

103

The Basic Four Food Groups
Poultry, Fish, Meat, Eggs, Legumes, Nuts, and Seeds

Usually thought of mainly as a source of protein, the foods in this group contain other important nutrients: vitamins, iron, phosphorus, other minerals, and in some cases substantial amounts of carbohydrates. Nor are they our only protein sources, for protein is found in milk and in lesser amounts in nearly all plant foods.

Most Americans eat ample meat and don't have to worry about getting enough protein. But many nutritionists recommend varying the sources of protein in the diet by eating more poultry and fish and by getting more protein from nonmeat sources, such as legumes, nuts, and seeds.

By themselves legumes do not provide complete protein. However, they can be made complete by combining them *in the same meal* with whole grains or with a little animal protein. The combination of tofu (soybean cake) and rice from the Orient is an example of the first way; chili beans with meat exemplifies the second way. Other nutritious and delicious combinations are nuts or seeds with cooked vegetables or in salads, macaroni and cheese (grain plus milk product), pasta or rice with bits of meat. For more such combinations see the section on vegetarian eating (pages 390-394).

What's a serving? Americans are so accustomed to large servings of poultry, fish, and meat that it may come as a surprise how small a serving of protein food is adequate to supply the body's needs.

According to the U.S. Department of Agriculture, a serving is 2 to 3 ounces of cooked poultry, fish, or meat. Partial servings are given for some other foods because they are closer to the amounts that people normally eat. Thus 1 egg, ½ to ¾ cup of cooked legumes, 2 tablespoons of peanut butter, or ¼ to ½ cup of nuts or seeds is considered a partial serving. Each of these items counts as 1 ounce of meat, poultry, or fish. In one day's meals, you might have an egg for breakfast and 2 tablespoons of peanut butter on whole-grain bread for lunch. (The combination of the peanut butter and whole-grain bread makes a complete protein.) A piece of cooked meat approximately 2 inches by 4 inches and ½-inch thick weighing about 3 ounces and a portion of cooked lentils or beans would complete the serving requirements for the day.

Note that the weight of a serving is specified in cooked foods. Foods shrink in cooking and some contain fat and bones, so you will need to buy more in raw foods. For example, a pound of trimmed shell steak or of whole fish yields about 7½ ounces of cooked meat. Even a pound of fish fillets when cooked yields only 10½ ounces.

Foods that should be eaten in moderation (see chart opposite) usually contain medium to high amounts of fat or cholesterol, and fish may be high in sodium and have medium or high amounts of fat. Foods in the now-and-then column are almost all high in saturated fat and sodium; beef, liver, and egg dishes are high in cholesterol.

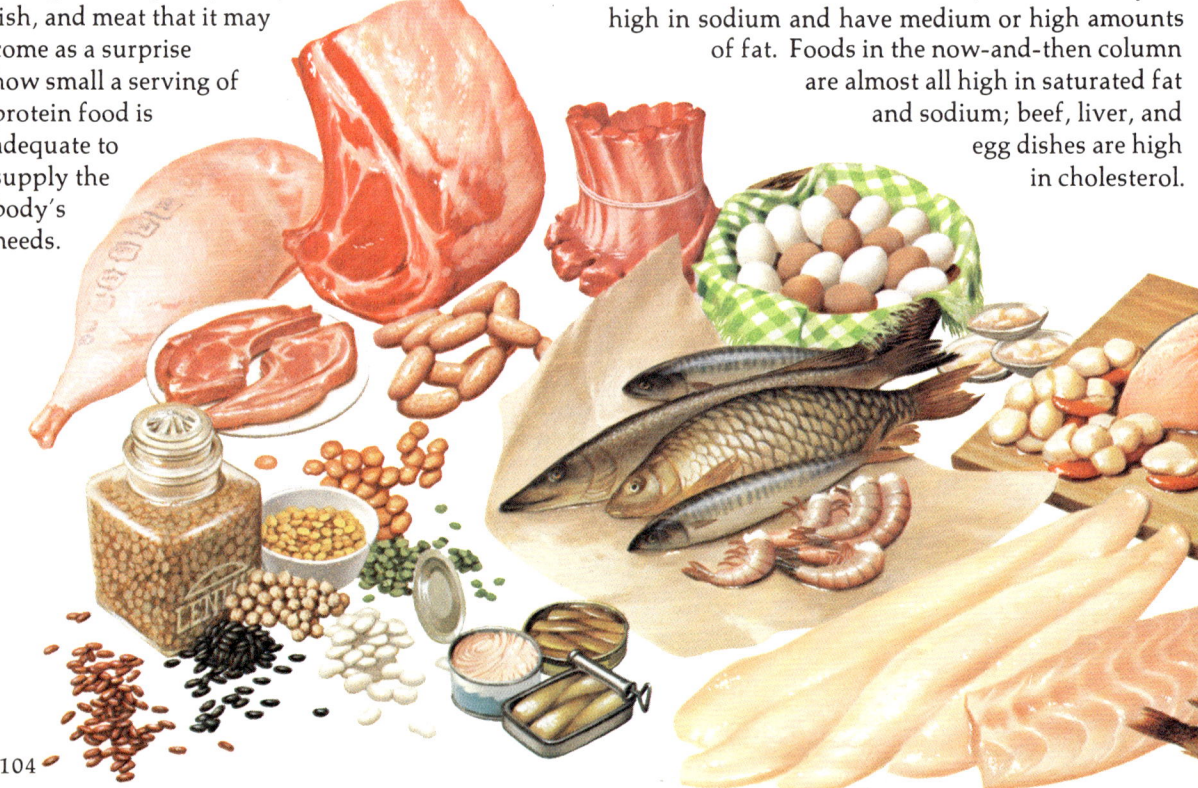

FAMILY FOOD GUIDE

2 Servings per Day

ANYTIME
(everyday)

POULTRY
chicken or turkey, boiled or roasted, without skin

FISH
cod
flounder
gefilte fish
haddock
halibut
perch
rockfish
shellfish, except shrimp
sole
tuna, packed in water

EGG PRODUCTS
egg whites only

LEGUMES
dried beans and peas
lentils
chick-peas

IN MODERATION
(two to three times a week)

POULTRY
chicken livers, baked or broiled
fried chicken, homemade, in vegetable oil
chicken or turkey, boiled or roasted, with skin

FISH
(drain well if canned)
fried fish
herring
salmon, pink, canned
sardines, canned
shrimp
tuna, packed in oil

EGG PRODUCTS
egg yolk or whole egg

MEATS
(trim off all outside fat)
leg or loin of lamb
pork shoulder or loin, lean
flank steak or ground round
rump roast

MISCELLANEOUS
seeds, such as sunflower
soybeans, tofu
peanut butter

NOW AND THEN
(once a week or less)

POULTRY
fried chicken, commercially prepared

FISH
frozen fish sticks

EGG DISHES
cheese omelet
quiche
souffle

MEATS
bacon
organ meats
cold cuts
corned beef
ground beef
ham, trimmed well
frankfurters
spareribs
untrimmed red meats
sirloin steak, lean
veal

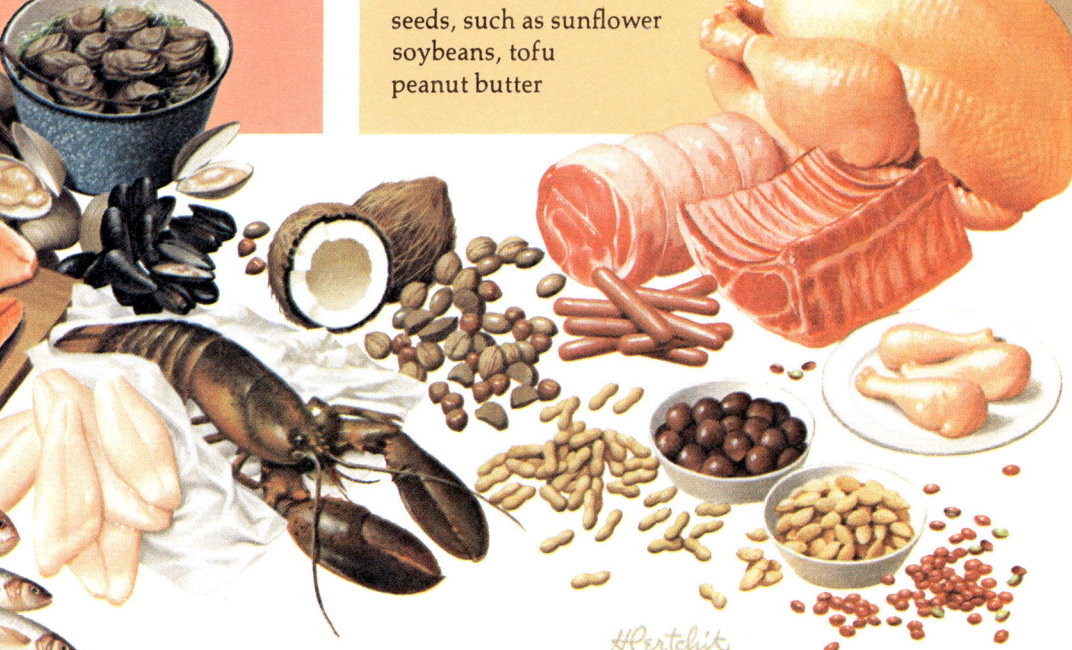

The Basic Four Food Groups
An Eating Quiz

How much has your food consciousness been raised? Americans' eating habits have indeed been changing. Supermarkets and greengrocers regularly stock food items that were hard to find not too many years ago. Street food—food sold in delicatessens and from pushcarts to be eaten on the run—has expanded to include hummus (chick-pea spread) and pita-bread sandwiches, vegetable and fruit salads, croissants with a variety of fillings, yogurt with toppings of all kinds, and even baked potatoes with a multitude of dressings. Many restaurants are serving smaller portions of meat, a happy coincidence of economy and their clientele's desire for fewer calories. And they are emphasizing fresh, lightly cooked vegetables and tossed green salads rather than rich dishes with calorie-laden sauces. This change in taste is reflected in recipes in the food columns of magazines and newspapers.

Many influences have brought about this slow revolution in Americans' tastes in food. Among them are the *nouvelle cuisine*, the emphasis on fitness and youthful looks, and a genuine concern for eating nutritionally adequate foods—helped, no doubt, by the wide publicity given the U.S. Senate Committee's Dietary Goals in 1977 and the Dietary Guidelines of 1980. Have you and your family taken part in this eating revolution, or are you still dining as you did 10 or 20 years ago?

Many of our dietary problems are simply a matter of longtime habit—habit that can be changed once you've become aware of the wide range of choices available in meal planning. The preceding pages on the food groups can serve as your guide to constructing a better diet. Don't, however, try to reform your family habits all at once. Change is accepted more readily if brought about gradually.

Here is a quiz that points up common failings in the average American diet and should help you evaluate your own and your family's eating habits. Its topics in general reflect the Dietary Guidelines. There's probably no such thing as a perfect score, for we all have our quirks when it comes to food. In fact, if you answer "yes" to more than half the questions, you can consider that you have a reasonably good diet—but that it could stand improvement. The "no" answers will tell you where that improvement is needed. That's the whole point of the quiz: to make you more aware of where in your diet you might have problems.

Eating a Variety of Foods. Do you usually:
1. look upon eating as an adventure?
2. read the labels of processed foods?
3. appreciate the natural flavors of foods as compared with overprocessed, highly seasoned foods?
4. experiment with unfamiliar foods from time to time?
5. start the day with a breakfast consisting of food from at least three food groups (for instance, fruit or fruit juice, milk or milk products, cereal or bread)?
6. have a meatless lunch or dinner at least two days a week?
7. use legumes (beans, lentils, peanuts, and dried peas) and whole grains in meatless meals?
8. have skim or low-fat milk or milk products every day?
9. tuck some extra nutrients into salads, vegetables, and desserts by sprinkling them with chopped nuts, seeds, or wheat germ?

Maintaining Ideal Weight. Do you usually:
1. know and keep track of the calories in the foods you eat regularly?
2. limit the size of your food portions?
3. avoid second servings?
4. eat slowly, allowing at least 20 minutes per meal?
5. try not to skip breakfast or lunch and try to avoid overeating at dinner?
6. avoid using food as a way of dealing with boredom, anger, fatigue, or anxiety?
7. know the danger periods during the day when you are likely to overeat?
8. consciously choose food with a view to its nutritive value?
9. try to limit the quantities of foods you tend to eat in excess?
10. avoid keeping high-calorie, low-nutrient snacks around the home?
11. confine your eating, including snacks, to one or two places in the house?
12. avoid nibbling as you put away leftovers from a meal?
13. buy and prepare only the amount of food needed for each meal?

Avoiding Too Much Fat, Saturated Fat, and Cholesterol. Do you usually:
1. have an average meat intake of no more than 21 to 28 ounces a week (3 to 4 ounces a day)?

2. have fish and poultry more often than red meat (beef, pork, lamb)?
3. limit cold cuts or frankfurters to 1 serving a week (or none at all)?
4. select lean meat with little visible fat?
5. eat broiled or roasted meats more often than fried ones?
6. trim visible fat from meats before cooking?
7. remove skin from poultry and eat just the meat?
8. limit yourself to 4 ounces of cheese a week (other than cottage cheese or low-fat cheese)?
9. make your own salad dressing and then apply it sparingly?
10. choose low-fat snacks, such as raw vegetables or fruits, whole-grain crackers, or plain yogurt, rather than potato chips, doughnuts, pastries, and other fatty foods?
11. use butter, margarine, and mayonnaise sparingly?
12. eat fruit for dessert more often than cakes, pies, ice cream, or cookies?
13. steam, boil, or bake vegetables rather than fry them in fat or oil?
14. season vegetables with lemon or lime juice or herbs rather than butter or margarine?
15. limit egg yolks to three or four a week?
16. drink skim or low-fat milk or buttermilk rather than whole milk?
17. have organ meats (liver, kidney, heart, brains) only once a week or less?
18. eat cheeses made from skim or partially skim milk rather than from cream or whole milk?
19. use milk (preferably skim) in tea or coffee rather than cream or nondairy coffee whitener?
20. skim the fat off stews and soups?
21. drain most of the fat from the pan before making gravy?
22. limit yourself to eating commercial cookies, cakes, or pies once a week or less?
23. ask for unbuttered popcorn at the movies?

Eating Foods with Adequate Starch and Fiber. Do you usually:
1. buy whole-grain breads and rolls rather than white-flour breads?
2. choose whole-grain or bran breakfast cereals?
3. eat at least two servings of raw or lightly steamed vegetables per day?
4. eat whole fruits more often than fruit juice?
5. eat at least 2 servings of fruit a day?
6. have 4 servings of whole-grain or enriched bread or cereal a day?
7. eat potatoes and apples with their skins?

Avoiding Too Much Sugar. Do you usually:
1. drink water, club soda, or fruit juices instead of sugar-sweetened beverages?
2. choose fruit juice rather than fruit "drink"?
3. drink tea or coffee without sugar?
4. limit sweet desserts to two or three times a week?
5. snack on fresh fruits and vegetables rather than sweetened foods?
6. avoid sugar-coated cereals?
7. read cereal labels and choose brands that contain less than 5 grams per ounce of sucrose and other sugars?
8. choose packaged and convenience foods with low amounts of sugar or other sweeteners?
9. eat fresh or water-packed fruits rather than fruits canned in syrup?
10. eat whole-grain breads, rolls, and crackers rather than doughnuts, sweet muffins, or pastries?
11. eat candy only once a week or less?

Avoiding Too Much Sodium. Do you usually:
1. taste your food before salting it?
2. use salt sparingly (if at all) at the table?
3. use salt sparingly in cooking?
4. read food labels to ascertain whether salt and/or other sodium compounds are included?
5. choose unsalted nuts, crackers, or pretzels?
6. use sparingly such salty sauces as catsup, soy sauce, barbecue sauce, Worcestershire sauce?
7. eat fresh or unsalted frozen vegetables more often than canned vegetables?
8. order Oriental food without monosodium glutamate (MSG)?
9. limit canned or frozen entrees containing salt to twice a week or less?
10. limit salty snacks, such as pickles, olives, anchovies, or herring?
11. limit yourself to 2 servings a week of commercially prepared bouillon, broth, and other soups?

Using Alcoholic Beverages in Moderation. Do you usually:
1. limit alcohol consumption to an average of 1 drink a day? (One drink equals 1½ ounces of hard liquor, 4 ounces of wine, or 12 ounces of beer.)

Buying Guide/*Vegetables*

A Buying Guide to a variety of foods begins here with vegetables and continues through page 179. The main consideration in choosing any food is quality, and this guide features suggestions for judging the freshness and wholesomeness of foods to enable you to get the most nutrition for your food dollars. Learning more about vegetables and introducing new ones to your diet is a good way to broaden your menus. Many fresh vegetables are available year round and they lend a variety of taste, texture, and color to meals. However, be ready to change your menu if the vegetables you need are not top quality. For tips on preserving valuable nutrients during cooking, see page 215.

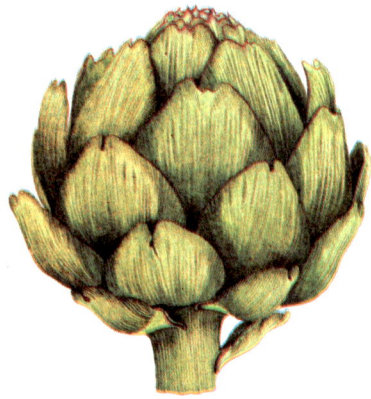

ARTICHOKE

Artichoke. The globe, or French, artichoke, is a native plant of the Mediterranean region. It was reputedly brought from Italy to France in the 16th century by King Henry II's bride, Catherine de Medicis. Despite their well-established popularity in Europe, where many varieties have long been cultivated, artichokes remained virtually unknown in the United States until the 20th century.

To eat a cooked artichoke, strip it petal by petal and eat the flesh from the base of each petal by pulling it off with your teeth. The pale inner leaves form the heart and hide the inedible choke, which must be scraped away to reach the meaty, sweet-tasting artichoke bottom.

When to buy. Available all year, but the peak season is March through May. The entire U.S. commercial crop comes from California.

What to look for. The artichoke is the unopened, leafy flower head of a plant related to the thistle. Look for plump, compact olive-green heads, heavy for their size, with full, fleshy, tightly closed scales, or leaves. Avoid those with spreading scales—they will be dry and tough—or extensive brown or gray discoloration.

How to keep. Buy one whole artichoke per person and use within a few days. To prevent drying, wrap unwashed artichokes in a damp towel and store in a plastic bag in the refrigerator.

Nutritive value. Artichokes provide potassium, calcium, and phosphorus as well as fiber. They are low in calories but are often served with high-calorie sauces.

Arugula. This peppery salad green, also known as rocket salad and rocket cress, belongs to the mustard family. Its flavor is much like that of cress but sharper; just a few leaves will add an exotic taste to a green salad. Arugula is available at many greengrocers and some supermarkets.

When to buy. May to October.

What to look for. Arugula is sold in small bunches, sometimes with the tiny roots still attached. The youngest plants have narrow, toothed leaves of a dark green color; larger leaves will be stronger flavored.

How to keep. Refrigerate greens in a plastic bag or a tightly covered container and use within a few days.

Nutritive value. Arugula contains vitamin C, phosphorus, calcium, and potassium.

Asparagus. The earliest mention of asparagus in American gardening annals appeared in 1775. But how the seed was brought—possibly from the eastern Mediterranean region—to the New World remains a mystery. The vegetable was a favorite with Romans—among them Julius Caesar and the satirist Juvenal.

When to buy. Asparagus is available as early as February in some areas, but the peak season is generally March through June.

What to look for. The most common variety of asparagus is a rich, bright green. (The color will be light green or whitish if the crop is harvested when most of the spear is still in the ground.) Choose straight spears of uniform thickness with compact, pointed tips. Round, plump spears are usually more tender than flat ones.

How to keep. Wrap bases in damp towel, and store in a plastic bag in the refrigerator.

Nutritive value. Asparagus is a good source of vitamins A and C; it is high in calcium, phosphorus, thiamin, potassium, and iron.

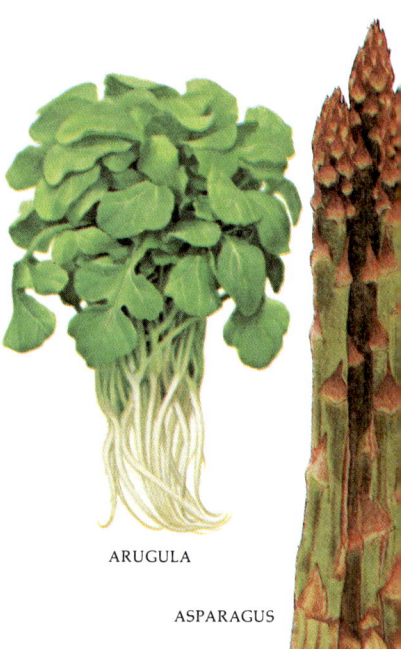

ARUGULA

ASPARAGUS

Avocado. Actually a fruit, the avocado is usually treated as a vegetable; its smooth, oily, pale-green flesh has none of the tartness or sweetness associated with fruit. Its popular nickname, "alligator pear," is something of a misnomer, since the many varieties of avocado differ dramatically in appearance: pear shaped to almost spherical, smooth skinned to rough and leathery, green to black.

Avocado culture probably started in the Americas—the 16th-century Spanish conquistadors encountered the fruit in places as widely scattered as Mexico, Colombia, and Peru—but it was nearly 400 years before California and Florida growers began to produce avocados commercially.

When to buy. Available all year.

What to look for. Avocados are usually sold slightly underripe, but ripe ones will yield to gentle pressure on the skin. Avoid those with dark, sunken spots or cracks; irregular light-brown surface markings do not affect quality.

How to keep. Use ripe avocados immediately. Firm ones will ripen at room temperature in three to five days. Coat cut avocados with lemon juice to prevent darkening.

Nutritive value. High in protein, fat, riboflavin, niacin, and potassium; also contains vitamins A and C.

Beans. These versatile vegetables, one of the world's major food crops since antiquity, are almost limitless in their varieties, characteristics, and even names. The three main groupings are: from the Americas, haricot, or green beans (also known as snap or string beans, though today's crops are largely stringless); from Europe, fava beans (broad or English beans); and from Asia, soybeans.

The haricot bean, whose name derives from the Aztec *ayacotl*, was grown in numerous forms by the prehistoric Indians of both North and South America; this category includes lima and yellow wax beans. The green

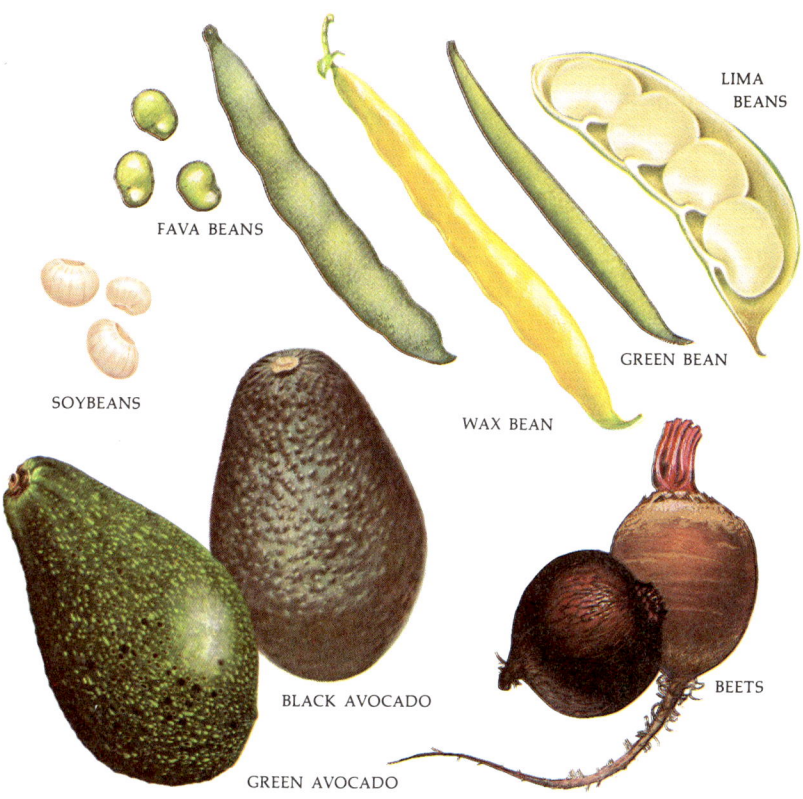

"French" haricots are now more popular in Europe than the native favas, whose major production center has shifted to China. In another shift, the United States has replaced China as the world's foremost grower and exporter of soybeans.

When to buy. Most beans are available all year, with peaks in late spring and summer. Soybeans peak in summer and early fall.

What to look for. Fresh beans are usually at their best when small and young. Haricots should snap easily and be slender, bright, and stringless; limas and the larger, thicker favas should be plump but not bulging, with smooth pods; soybeans should be plump and bright green. Avoid tough, rubbery, or discolored beans.

How to keep. Use within a few days. Refrigerate shell beans in their pods; wrap others in plastic bags before refrigerating. Cook snap beans until barely tender to preserve flavor.

Nutritive value. Soybeans have the highest protein content and are rich in potassium, iron, and calcium. Lima and snap beans are good sources of vitamin A.

Beets. Table or root beets are often sold in bunches, with their edible green tops attached. In fact, the early Romans ate only the beet greens and used the roots medicinally. Some table beets are almost white, but most are a deep, rich red. They can be served hot, cold, pickled, or in salads, or used in soups (notably in borscht).

What to look for. Firm, smooth, globular beets. Wilted tops, if attached, are acceptable if roots are still firm. Avoid flabby or elongated ones with scaly areas or soft spots.

When to buy. Available all year, with peak June to October.

How to keep. Tops are perishable, but tubers can be refrigerated in the vegetable crisper for up to two weeks.

Nutritive value. Beets provide potassium. The tops, cooked like other greens, are an excellent source of vitamin A and iron.

Buying Guide
Vegetables

Broccoli. This vitamin-packed vegetable, unjustly rejected by generations of American schoolchildren, is a member of the cabbage family, closely related to Brussels sprouts and cauliflower. It was first grown in its present form in Italy—the Etruscans or Romans may have developed it from cabbage, as cauliflower in turn was later bred from broccoli. The type most frequently found in U.S. markets, where broccoli was almost unknown until the early 1900s, is the Calabrese, with compact, dark-green to purplish flower buds on a lighter green stalk. It should be cooked lightly and quickly, as the Chinese and Italians do, to retain its crispness.

When to buy. All year, with availability highest October to May.

What to look for. Buy plants with firm, compact clusters of closed flower buds—sage green to purplish green—and firm, tender, lighter green stalks. Avoid those with open yellow buds (a sign of overmaturity) or soft wet spots. The young leaves can be cooked or added to salads.

How to keep. Wrap washed broccoli in plastic and refrigerate. Use within two or three days.

Nutritive value. Highest in nutrients of all the "flower" vegetables. Broccoli is rich in vitamin C and contains vitamin A, thiamin, riboflavin, calcium, and iron. It is also high in fiber and low in calories.

Brussels Sprouts. Like broccoli, these small descendants of the wild cabbage are victims of a bad press, brought about by many cooks' unfortunate tendency to boil them to a mushy pulp. Tradition has it that sprouts were first grown in Brussels in the 13th century, making them one of the few vegetables to have been developed in Northern Europe. The tightly rolled heads form along the stem at the bases of the leafstalks; they are extremely winter hardy and can be harvested long after freezing weather sets in, but they cannot tolerate heat. One way to preserve their flavor and crispness is to parboil them for about five minutes, then drain and sauté briefly.

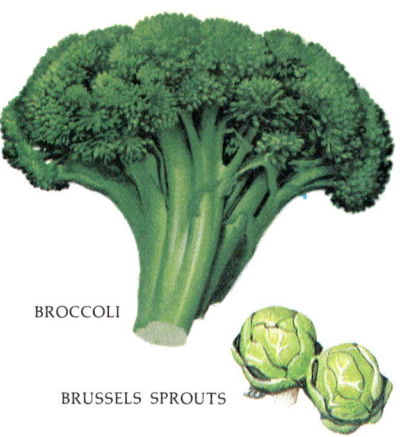

BROCCOLI

BRUSSELS SPROUTS

When to buy. The peak season is October through March; sprouts are seldom available in the hottest summer months.

What to look for. The heads are usually packed in small containers. Look for firm, compact, bright-green sprouts with tight outer leaves; avoid yellowing heads with holes or signs of puffiness.

How to keep. Refrigerate sprouts in an airtight plastic bag in the vegetable crisper; use as soon as possible.

Nutritive value. High in vitamin C, potassium, and iron.

Cabbage. One of the oldest cultivated vegetables, cabbage is also among the most varied in its forms. Many of the present varieties were probably developed in Italy by the farmers of ancient Rome. Besides the smooth green and red types and the crinkle-leafed Savoys, the cabbage family encompasses broccoli, Brussels sprouts, cauliflower, collards, kale, and kohlrabi (see individual entries). Two newer members of the cabbage family now available in American markets are bokchoy and Chinese cabbage, or celery cabbage (not shown), an elongated head of compact, greenish-white leaves.

When to buy. Available all year.

What to look for. Cabbage is marketed fresh ("new" cabbage) or from storage ("white" or "old" cabbage, usually sold with its outer leaves trimmed). New cabbages should have outer leaves of a fresh green or red color, depending on the variety. The crinkly Savoy and red cabbages are generally preferred for salads and coleslaw. Look for firm heads, heavy for their size (spring cabbage and bokchoy are softer, but the leaves should be crisp and fresh). There should be no signs of yellowing, wilting, or pest damage.

How to keep. Green and white cabbages keep as long as 10 days, but Savoys and Chinese cabbage should be used as soon as possible. If necessary, trim outermost "wrapper" leaves before storing heads in plastic bags in the refrigerator.

Nutritive value. Cabbage is rich in vitamins C and A (bokchoy is especially rich in the latter), calcium, phosphorus, and potassium.

Carrots. The familiar Queen Anne's lace that lines America's country roads is actually a form of wild carrot. Like other edible roots, carrots were probably one of man's earliest foods; they were first cultivated in Afghanistan but had spread to Southern Europe before the Christian era.

When to buy. Available all year.

What to look for. Firm, straight, bright-orange carrots with no green or yellow areas at the top. Young, tender ones (which need not be

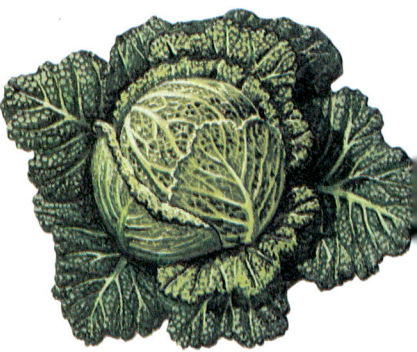

SAVOY CABBAGE

FAMILY FOOD GUIDE

scraped, merely scrubbed) are best for eating raw. The feathery green tops, if attached, may be cooked like other greens.

How to keep. Plastic-wrapped carrots (with greens removed) may be refrigerated for several weeks without loss of nutrients.

Nutritive value. Carrots are rich in carotene (a substance that converts to vitamin A).

Cauliflower. Like broccoli, cauliflower is basically a cabbage that has been bred for flower buds rather than leaves. In cauliflower, the immature buds form a dense mass called the "curd." Many varieties—white, green, and even purple—are grown in the Mediterranean region, but the most familiar kind in the United States, where cauliflower has been cultivated since the 17th century, has a curd that is creamy-white in color.

When to buy. Available all year; peak in September to November.

What to look for. Compact, solid, clean curds, white or cream colored. A newer green variety, produced by crossbreeding with broccoli, has a chartreuse-colored curd. If surrounding leaves are attached, they should be fresh and green; smaller green leaflets sometimes extend through the curd. (Though cooks often discard them, both leaves and flower stalks are edible.) A slightly granular texture is acceptable if the curd is dense and compact.

How to keep. Wrap curds in plastic and refrigerate in the vegetable crisper; use within a few days. Wash well before using.

Nutritive value. Cauliflower is high in vitamin C and potassium, and contains calcium and phosphorus.

Celeriac. First cultivated in Europe during the Renaissance, this vegetable is sometimes called knob celery or celery root. It is not, as some suppose, the root of the familiar stalk celery. Celeriac has a tough, fibrous outer skin that must be peeled and creamy-white flesh. Its flavor is similar to that of stalk celery but stronger. It can be served raw or cooked.

When to buy. Peak availability is from October through April.

What to look for. Outwardly, celeriac is unprepossessing; its coarse, brownish skin is often covered with small rootlets. Knobs are sold singly or in bunches. They should be relatively small (larger ones may be woody), firm, clean, and undamaged.

How to keep. Trim rootlets and green tops, if any, and refrigerate.

Nutritive value. Celeriac is high in phosphorus, iron, and sodium.

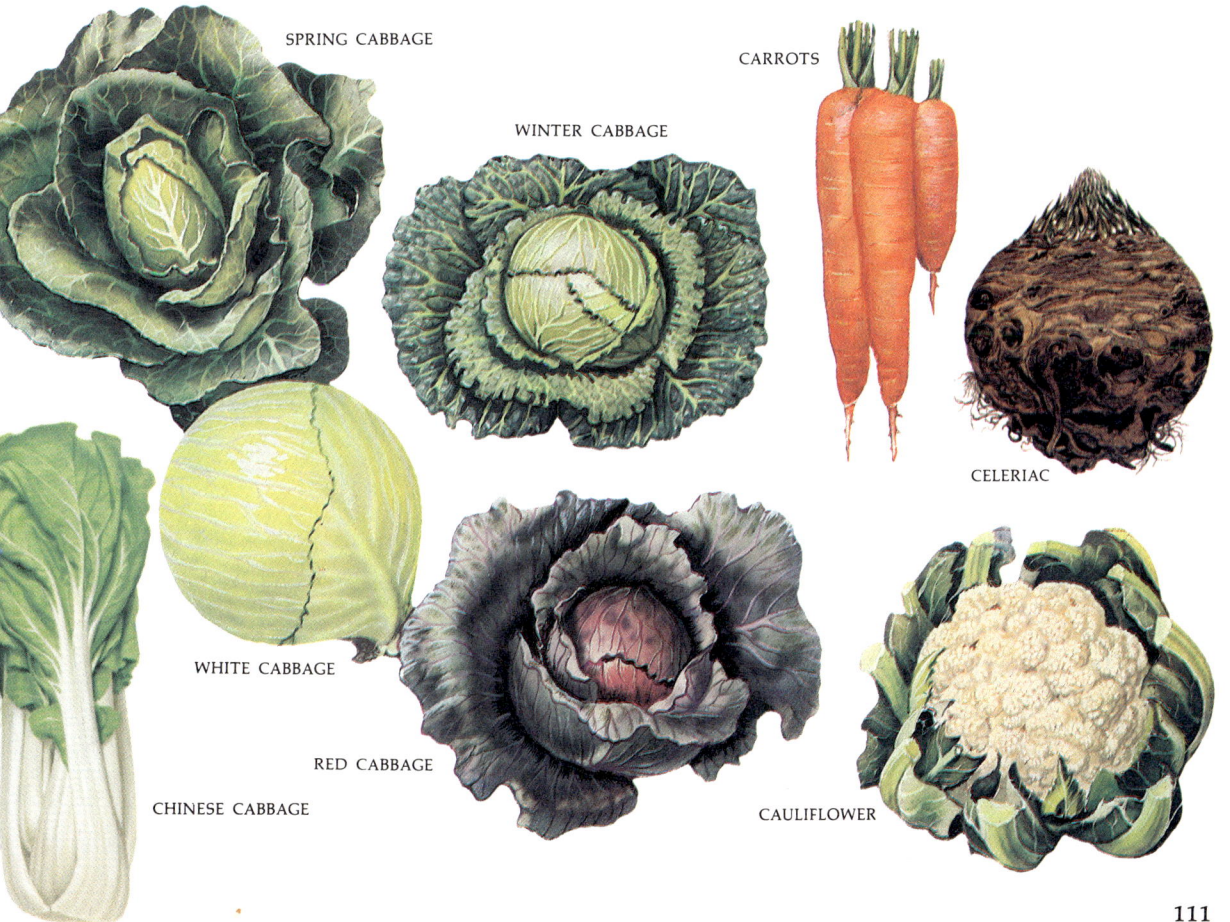

SPRING CABBAGE
WINTER CABBAGE
CARROTS
CELERIAC
WHITE CABBAGE
RED CABBAGE
CHINESE CABBAGE
CAULIFLOWER

111

Buying Guide
Vegetables

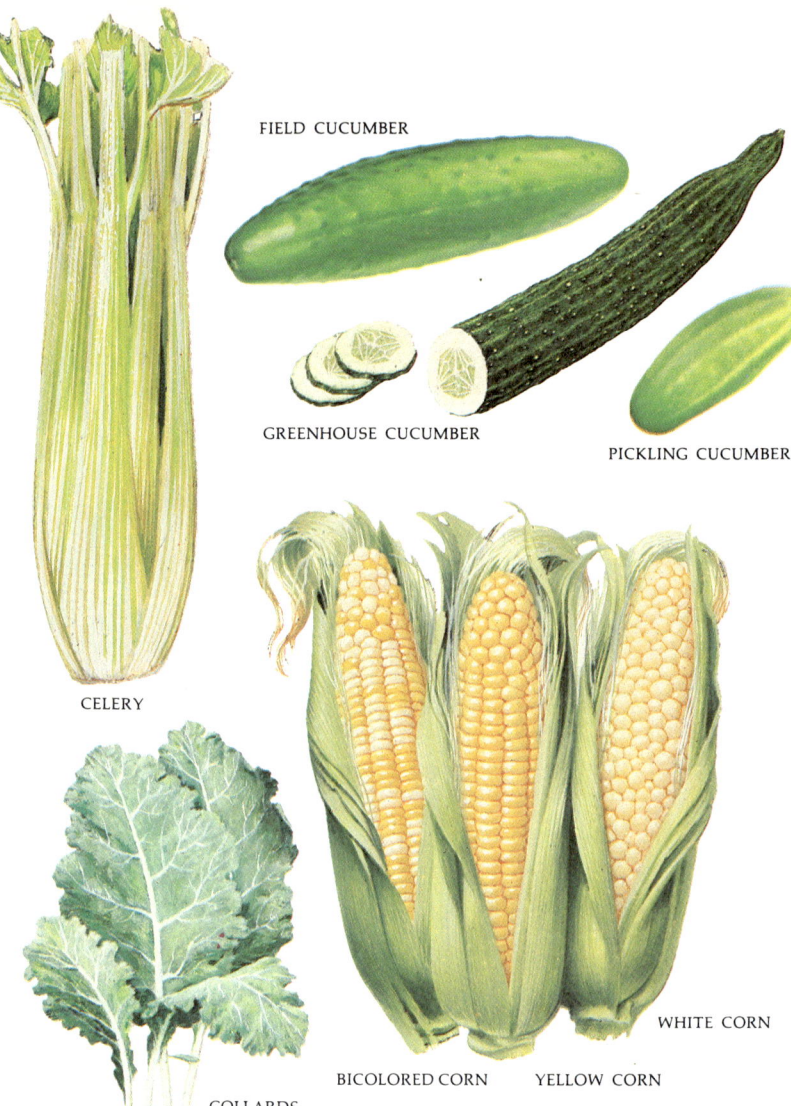

Celery. The ancient Egyptians gathered wild celery, which grew freely in marshy seaside areas, for food. The Romans, who apparently believed that they could ward off hangovers by wearing wreaths made of celery, developed cultivated varieties, but they preferred the more pungent wild plant for culinary use. (Even today, the Italians often add wild celery to cooked dishes.) The plant was used largely for seasoning until the 17th century, when the French acquired a taste for celery hearts; French growers were also the first to blanch celery by piling earth around the growing stalks.

Celery is a plant of many uses and little waste: the leaves and dried seeds make flavorful seasonings; the outer ribs are best cooked; and the inner ribs, or hearts, can be eaten raw.

When to buy. Available all year.

What to look for. The variety most commonly available is the light-green to medium-green Pascal celery. Stalks should be firm and solid with a maximum of fresh green leaves; they should also have a glossy surface and snap easily. Avoid celery with wilted, flabby upper branches, overly hard, woody stalks, or discolored areas in the central branches.

How to keep. Rinse well, shake off moisture, and refrigerate in a plastic bag in the vegetable crisper. Use within one or two weeks.

Nutritive value. High in sodium; also contains potassium.

Collard Greens. A favorite "soul food" of the American South, collard greens are one of the most vitamin-packed, nutritious foods on earth—and, when properly cooked and seasoned, extremely flavorful. Collards may have been brought to the South by African slaves; their name derives from "colewort," an old English word for cabbage.

When to buy. Available all year; peak from October through April.

What to look for. Crisp green leaves with no yellowing, wilting, or insect damage. Avoid those with coarse, fibrous stems. Since collards are highly perishable, they should be cold and moist when sold.

How to keep. Refrigerate in a plastic bag and use as soon as possible. Wash well before cooking.

Nutritive value. High in vitamins A, C, calcium, and potassium.

Corn. For North Americans, the word "corn" conjures up a vision of one of summer's major delights—fresh-picked local corn on the cob, its plump, sweet kernels drenched in butter. Historically, however, the word has meant many things to many people: in the Bible, it meant grain of all kinds; in England it usually means wheat; in Germany, rye; in Africa, millet. The original form of American corn, or maize, was Indian corn—the multicolored, small-kerneled ancestor of today's many hybrids.

Most of the sweet or table corn marketed in the United States is yellow; it has considerably more vitamin A than the white or bicolored ("butter and sugar") varieties.

When to buy. Available in winter months from California and Florida, but the peak season is May through September, depending on the area.

What to look for. Freshness is critical, because time and warmth soon convert sugar in the corn into starch. Ideally, corn should be kept cold from the moment it is harvested until cooking. If possible, avoid buying warm corn unless you know it is newly picked. Look for fresh green husks and stems, with no signs of decay in the silk ends. Avoid ears without husks or with dry, straw-colored husks, and signs of worm damage.

How to keep. Store immediately, unhusked and uncovered, in the refrigerator. Use as soon as possible.

Nutritive value. Vitamin A (yellow corn), potassium, and other minerals.

Cucumbers.
This ancient plant is a native of southwestern Asia, where cultivated seeds almost 12,000 years old have been found. The cucumber is related to melons and, like them, has a high water content, which keeps its interior flesh cool in the hottest weather—hence the expression "cool as a cucumber."

Cucumbers are divided into three classes, according to their use: the standard field-grown slicing cucumbers; the smaller pickling cucumbers, also field grown; and the newer greenhouse varieties, some of which are seedless. Of the first two classes the smaller slicing cucumbers can be pickled, and the pickling ones sliced.

When to buy. Available all year; peak season is April through August.

What to look for. Firm, well-shaped cucumbers of a strong green color, with no yellowing or shriveling. Some varieties are smooth skinned, but most have small surface bumps. They should be relatively slender; the largest ones are overly mature. To remove the wax that has been added as a protective coating, see instructions on page 212.

How to keep. Refrigerate cucumbers in the vegetable crisper; they are best used in a day or two.

Nutritive value. Cucumbers are low in calories.

Eggplant.
This dark, satiny fruit, always used as a vegetable, is prepared in hundreds of ways in Southern Europe and the Middle East. It was first imported from India by Arab caravans. Also known by its French name, *aubergine*, the eggplant was introduced to the United States by Thomas Jefferson, who experimented with seeds and cuttings of many foreign plants. Recently, American cooks have begun adapting traditional eggplant-based dishes of the Mediterranean—such as the French *ratatouille*, the Greek *moussaka*, the Italian *caponata*.

When to buy. Available all year.

What to look for. Eggplant can be red, yellow, or even white, but the most common variety is purple and pear shaped. Choose firm, smooth eggplants, heavy for their size, of a uniform dark purple, with no scars, flabbiness, or shriveling. Small fruits will have tenderer skins and fewer seeds than the larger ones, and those that have been waxed must be peeled.

How to keep. Store eggplant in a cool room (60°F) or refrigerate; use within a week. If it is to be cooked unpeeled, wash it first and cut off stems and tops.

Endive.
The names of the three salad plants in this family—endive, chicory, and escarole—are sometimes used interchangeably and often confusingly. In the United States, however, the name *endive* (or *Belgian endive*) usually refers to the small, pale, cigar-shaped plant; *escarole* to the broad, bushy head with wavy leaves; and *chicory* to the one with narrow, very curly, ragged-edged leaves. Endives have a slightly bitter taste, and because they were first cultivated in ancient Egypt, food expert Waverley Root has suggested that they might have been one of the original "bitter herbs" Jews ate during Passover.

When to buy. Chicory and escarole are available all year; Belgian endive, October through May.

What to look for. In endive, firm, tight stalks with white to pale-yellow leaves; in chicory and escarole, crisp, fresh heads with vivid-green outer leaves and no discolorations.

How to keep. Trim outer leaves of endive if bruised. Refrigerate all three types, wrapped in plastic, in the vegetable crisper, and use as soon as possible.

Nutritive value. High in iron and calcium; also contains vitamin A.

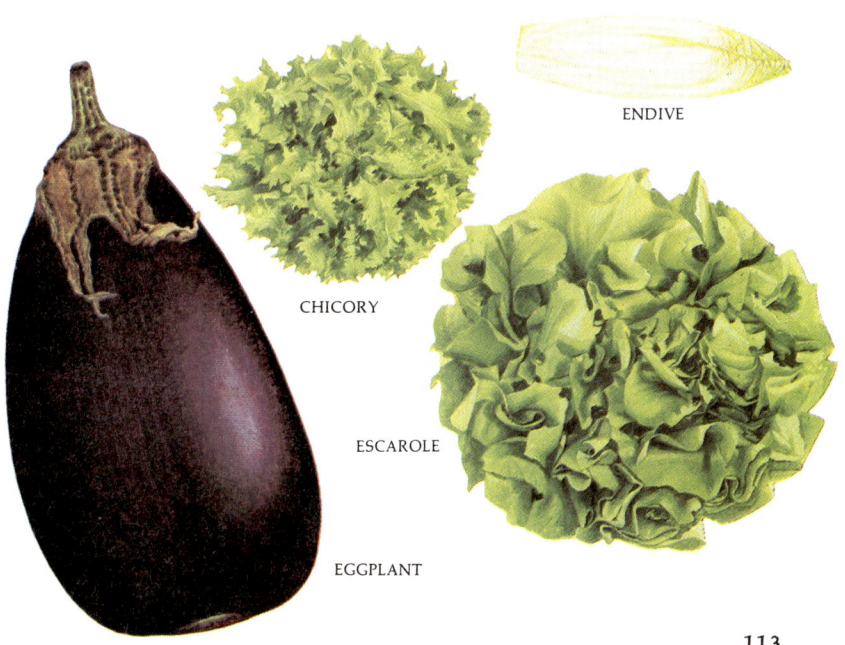

CHICORY

ENDIVE

ESCAROLE

EGGPLANT

Buying Guide
Vegetables

Fennel. A member of the parsley family with a distinct licorice flavor, fennel has been used for centuries in Italian and French cooking. The French treat it as an herb, using the seeds as a spice and the feathery leaves for salads and seasonings or raw as a vegetable, whereas the Italians use it mainly as a vegetable. In Italy and the United States, the variety most commonly grown is *finocchio*, or Florence fennel, whose stalks and bulb can be eaten raw or cooked.

When to buy. October to April; peak in November and December.

What to look for. Well-rounded stalks, white to pale green. Avoid bulbs with brown areas.

How to keep. Store in a plastic bag in the refrigerator.

Nutritive value. Fennel leaves are very high in Vitamin A.

Garlic. This pungent bulb—like onion, a member of the amaryllis family—is one of the oldest and most widespread of cultivated plants. At various times it has been prescribed for every kind of human ailment, and in fact its juice does contain allicin, a natural antibiotic.

With its emphatic flavor and persistent odor, garlic has always evoked strong reactions, both pro and con. It has long been an essential part of southern French and Italian cooking. In the United States, it was not a popular seasoning until well into the 20th century.

When to buy. Available all year.

What to look for. Firm bulbs with unbroken white or purplish skins.

How to keep. Buy one or two bulbs, which will keep for weeks in a cool, dry, well-ventilated place.

Ginger. Grown in tropical regions, this pungent tuber is an essential ingredient of Indian chutneys and many Chinese dishes. It found great favor in 16th-century England, where Queen Elizabeth I is reputed to have "invented" gingerbread men by having ginger-spiced cakes baked in the likenesses of court favorites. Since colonial times, Americans have been similarly addicted to gingerbreads, cookies, and candies. Fresh ginger—peeled and then diced, shredded, or grated—is preferable to the dried kind for flavoring meat and vegetable dishes. It can be found at many greengrocers and Oriental food stores.

When to buy. Available all year.

What to look for. Firm, plump tubers. Newly harvested ginger has a glossy pale-tan skin and greenish flesh, whereas mature ginger has slightly hardened skin and whitish flesh.

How to keep. Ginger will keep in the refrigerator, loosely covered, for two or three months; cut ends might mold but can be trimmed. Peeled ginger may also be stored in dry vermouth and refrigerated.

> ### Growing Your Own
> A sure way to get the freshest possible vegetables for your table is to grow your own. You need not be an experienced gardener or have an acre of land. You can grow many vegetables in a window box. Some of the easiest and most satisfying crops you can start with are lettuce, cucumbers, and tomatoes. If you don't want to bother with seeds, most garden centers carry an attractive supply of seedlings and can give you advice on the growing season in your area. Ask for hardy, disease-resistant plants. If you have no time to clear a sunny garden spot, think about using a section of a flower bed or an unused strip of land along the garage wall. Bear in mind, however, that a small seedling can become the size of a bush by summer.

Horseradish. Sometimes called "German mustard," horseradish is grown chiefly for its sharp-flavored white roots, which contain a volatile oil. The wild variety has been gathered in many parts of the world since ancient times: the Greeks and Romans used it both gastronomically and medicinally, and the Jews have always used it ceremonially as one of the five "bitter herbs" of the Passover seder. In Northern Europe it is usually grated or crushed and added to meat and fish sauce. Freshly grated horseradish can be served as a condiment or added to sauces. It loses some of its sharpness during cooking.

When to buy. Fresh horseradish is available in late fall and early spring, usually before the Jewish Passover festival.

What to look for. Firm, white roots with no soft spots or shriveling.

How to keep. Fresh horseradish will keep in the refrigerator for as long as three months.

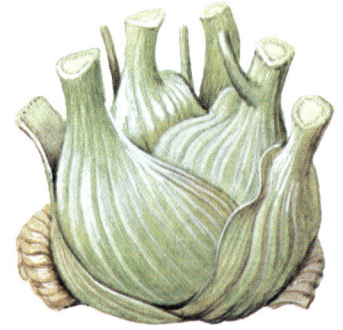
FENNEL

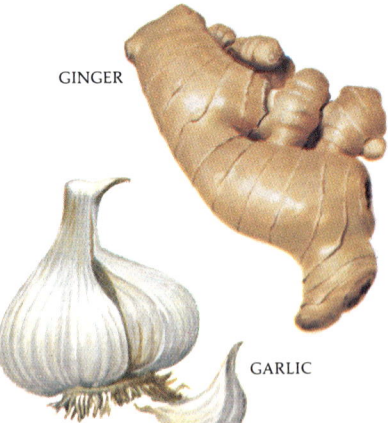
GINGER

GARLIC

FAMILY FOOD GUIDE

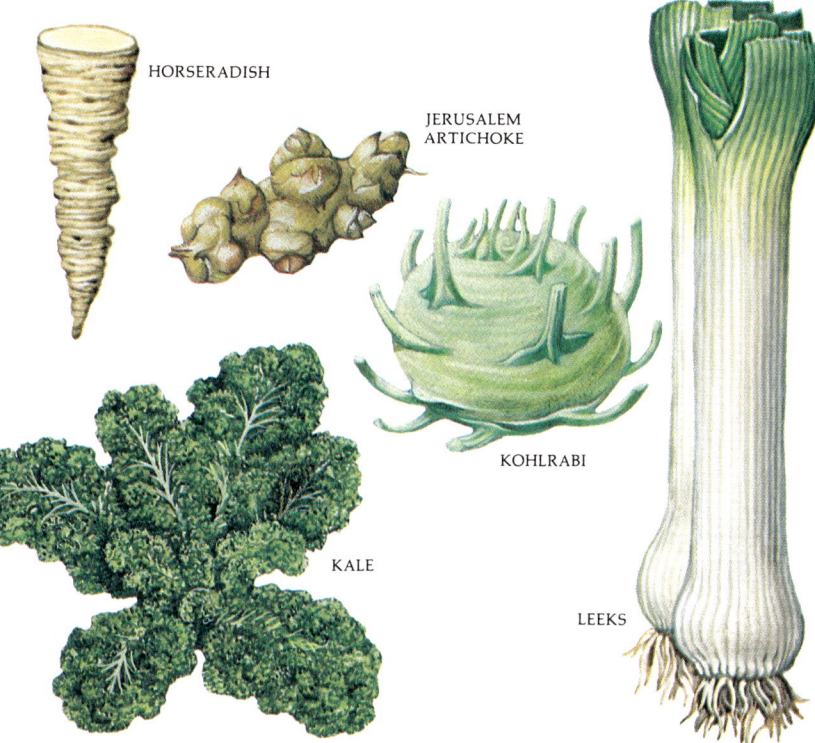

Jerusalem Artichoke. This oddly named plant does not come from Jerusalem but from North America, and it is totally unrelated to the globe artichoke. The tuber of a type of sunflower, it was extensively cultivated by American Indians. In 1605, French explorer Samuel de Champlain found the tubers in an Indian garden on Cape Cod and supposedly gave them their name. The bumpy, elongated tubers, also called "sunchokes," resemble sweet potatoes; they can be cooked in similar ways or sliced raw for salads and garnishes. Boil in their skins and then peel.

When to buy. Mid-November to mid-July.

What to look for. Firm, tan-jacketed tubers with no shriveling.

How to keep. Jerusalem artichokes shrivel quickly when exposed to air; they should be wrapped tightly in plastic and refrigerated.

Nutritive value. These vegetables are not starchy but contain inulin, a type of sugar that can be tolerated by diabetics. Raw, they are a source of calcium, iron, and magnesium.

Kale. Like collards, kale is a non-heading cabbage, impressively rich in nutrients. Because it has heavily crimped leaves, the French call it *chou frisé* ("curly cabbage"). In the United States, kale is most appreciated in the South, where it is often cooked with other greens like turnip tops and collards. Kale is easy to grow and extremely winter hardy.

When to buy. Available all year; peak in late fall and winter.

What to look for. Broad, crimped leaves of dark green to purple, depending on the variety. Kale should be crisp and cold when bought, with no drooping or damaged leaves.

How to keep. Wash, drain well, and refrigerate in the vegetable crisper; use as soon as possible.

Nutritive value. Kale is very rich in vitamin A, calcium, and iron; it also contains vitamin C, B vitamins, phosphorus, and potassium.

Kohlrabi. A bulbous plant with fairly sparse leaves, kohlrabi more closely resembles a turnip than a cabbage and is sometimes called "turnip cabbage." Kohlrabi is not a root vegetable—the bulb is a swelling of the stem just above the ground—but a true cabbage. Since it is grown mainly for its globular stems, the leaves are not always attached when you buy it, but if they are, they can be cooked like other greens. The bulbs have a mild, sweet, turniplike taste.

When to buy. Available in limited amounts May through November, with peak in June and July.

What to look for. Firm, light-green or purple globes about 1 to 3 inches in diameter; larger ones may be woody. The skin should be tender enough to pierce with a fingernail.

How to keep. Refrigerate and use within a few days.

Nutritive value. Contains vitamin C, calcium, and potassium.

Leeks. These hardy vegetables look like scallions of heroic proportions, but they are sweeter and milder than other onions (see separate entry). Their place of origin is unknown, but they appear often in Celtic lore. In Scotland, cock-a-leekie soup, made with chicken and leeks, is a national favorite, but in some countries the leek has been sniffed at as a humble food, "the poor man's asparagus." Leeks were largely ignored in the United States until 1913, when a French chef in New York, Louis Diat, created vichyssoise—an elegant cold potato-and-leek soup which became fashionable and drove up leek prices.

When to buy. Available all year; peak from October to May.

What to look for. The stems should be straight, thick, and well blanched, branching at the tops into dark green leaves. Yellow or wilted tops indicate poor quality.

How to keep. Refrigerate in the vegetable crisper and use within a week. Leeks must be well washed before cooking because soil or sand often lodges between the leaves. Split the leek lengthwise and rinse under cold water.

Buying Guide
Vegetables

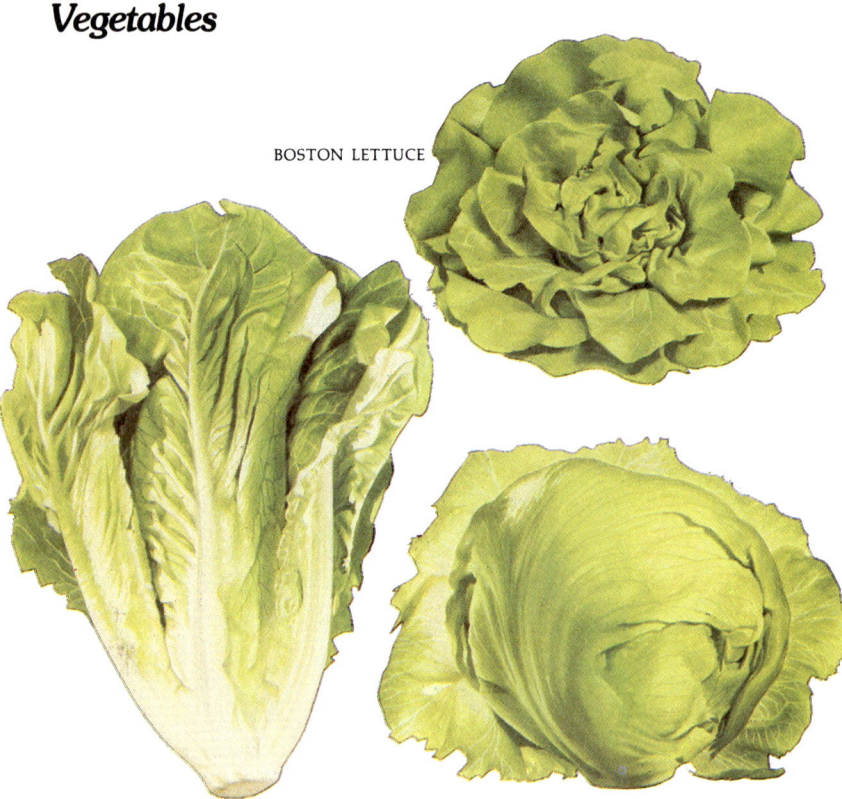

BOSTON LETTUCE

ROMAINE LETTUCE

ICEBERG LETTUCE

Lettuce. The numerous varieties of this salad plant fall into four main groups: crisphead lettuces such as *Iceberg*; the softer butterheads, such as *Boston* and *Bibb*; the long, loose-headed *Romaine* or *Cos*; and the leaf lettuces. Of these, the most popular lettuce is the crisphead Iceberg. Apart from its crunchy texture and ready availability, it has little to recommend it; other lettuces are richer in both flavor and nutrients. The tender, succulent leaf lettuces, which come in many varieties, are favored by gardeners as an easy to grow cool-weather crop.

When to buy. Crispheads are available all year; others, in spring and summer.

What to look for. In crispheads, clean, solid, well-shaped heads with medium-green outer leaves and paler inner leaves. Romaine should be crisp and dark; other varieties are softer but should be clean, bright colored, and fresh, with little or no discoloration and no signs of decay.

How to keep. Before serving, wash lettuces, drain well, and pat dry. Wrap unused portion in damp towel or crisper bag and refrigerate. Crispheads will keep longer than looseheads and leaf lettuces, which should be used within a few days.

Nutritive value. Varies with type. Romaine and loose-leaf varieties have more vitamin A and calcium—and butterheads more iron—than crispheads. All are high in fiber.

Mushrooms. Thousands of species of this edible fungus exist throughout the world. In mushroom-loving countries like France, at least 80 are eaten, but in the United States and Britain, only one—a cultivated form of *Agaricus bisporus*—is grown commercially. (Others may be found,

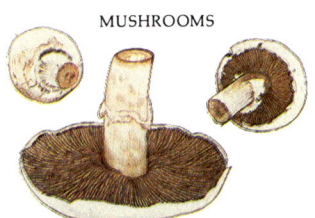

MUSHROOMS

dried or canned, in Oriental groceries and specialty food shops.) The fresh mushrooms in American markets vary only in size and degree of maturity: those with partially to fully opened caps are most strongly flavored; the younger button mushrooms, with closed caps, are milder.

The gathering of wild mushrooms should be left to the experts. Deadliest of the poisonous species is the "death cup," *Amanita phalloides*—the one fed to the Roman emperor Claudius by his wife in order to hasten the succession of her son, Nero.

When to buy. Available all year.

What to look for. Buy clean, creamy-white or light-tan mushrooms; avoid spongy, discolored, or "sweaty" ones. The gills should be pinkish or light tan.

How to keep. Refrigerate and use within a day or two. Wipe mushrooms clean but do not peel or soak.

Mustard Greens. The ubiquitous mustard plant, which grows so freely it scarcely needs cultivation, is usually harvested for its seeds, from which dry and prepared mustard and mustard-seed oil (a spicy cooking oil) are made. One African species, however, has spawned several varieties that are grown especially for their tender, sharp-flavored, highly nutritious leaves, which are harvested before the seeds form. Most popular in the American South, this "leaf mustard" has also found a place in Chinese and Italian cooking. Mustard greens are not always found outside the South but are easily grown in home gardens.

When to buy. Depending on the area, available all year; peak from October to April.

What to look for. Small, crisp, tender leaves, either flat or curly, with no seed stems.

How to keep. Refrigerate and use in a few days.

Nutritive value. High in vitamins A and C, calcium, and iron, as well as other minerals.

FAMILY FOOD GUIDE

Okra. Both of the names by which this curious-looking plant is usually known—"okra" and "gumbo"—come from African words. The plant itself, a relative of the tropical flower hibiscus, was first brought to the United States by African slaves. Young okra pods have a tart, distinctive taste, but the vegetable's most notable characteristic is its sticky consistency, which makes it a useful thickener for the well-known Louisiana gumbo, a stew named for its most essential ingredient.

Okra, which is sometimes called "ladies' fingers," is grown in warm to tropical regions—India, the Middle East, the Caribbean, Africa. In the United States, it is most often used in soups and stews, though it can also be cooked as a vegetable. (If they are steamed quickly, the pods will be crisp-tender and not release their sticky juices.)

When to buy. Available all year; peak from June through August.

What to look for. Bright-colored, tender pods, 2 to 4 inches long, that bend easily. Avoid tough, fibrous, or discolored pods.

How to keep. Refrigerate in a plastic bag; use within a few days.

Nutritive value. Okra is high in calcium; it also contains moderate amounts of potassium and other minerals, as well as B vitamins, A, and C.

Onions. As a cultivated plant, the onion is so ancient and so widespread that its origins are lost in prehistory. An early Turkish legend describes how, after Satan was booted out of heaven, garlic grew on the spot where his left foot touched the earth and onions under his right foot. In the ancient world, onions were usually considered a food for the poor and were shunned by aristocrats, possibly because the bulbs were so abundant and cheap. Much later, in Europe, onions began to acquire respectability: medieval French peasants were often required to give onions as rent to their feudal lords.

The varieties of onions now grown commercially in the United States fall into five main groups: the strong-flavored yellow globe onions, used primarily for cooking (the Spanish onion is a large, mild globe); the Bermuda onions, which are pungent enough for cooking and mild enough for eating raw; the large red Italian onions, whose delicate sweetness makes them popular for salads; the small scallions or green onions, whose immature white bulbs and green tops are used for salads and seasonings. Still another member of the onion family are the even smaller chives, usually sprinkled over food in the same way as fresh herbs. The small globe onions known as boiling or pickling onions are simply immature forms of other varieties. Leeks and shallots are discussed separately.

When to buy. Available all year.

What to look for. Chives and scallions should have fresh, tender green tops, and scallions should have narrow white bulbs and thin skins. Dry or mature onions should be bright, well shaped, and hard, with small necks, crisp papery skins, and no green sprouts.

How to keep. In cool weather, mature onions will keep for weeks in a cool, dry place with good air circulation; they may be refrigerated in hot weather, but should be used before they sprout or soften. Refrigerate scallions and chives in the vegetable crisper and use within a few days. Chop unused portion of an onion or chives, wrap tightly, and freeze.

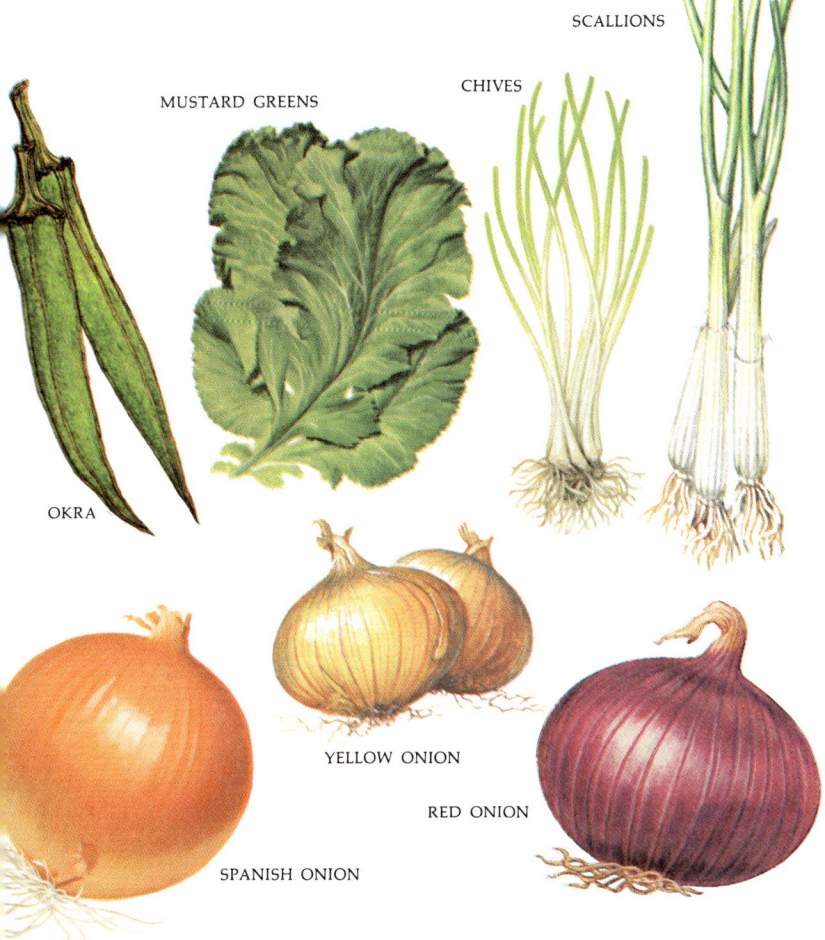

MUSTARD GREENS
CHIVES
SCALLIONS
OKRA
YELLOW ONION
RED ONION
SPANISH ONION

117

Buying Guide
Vegetables

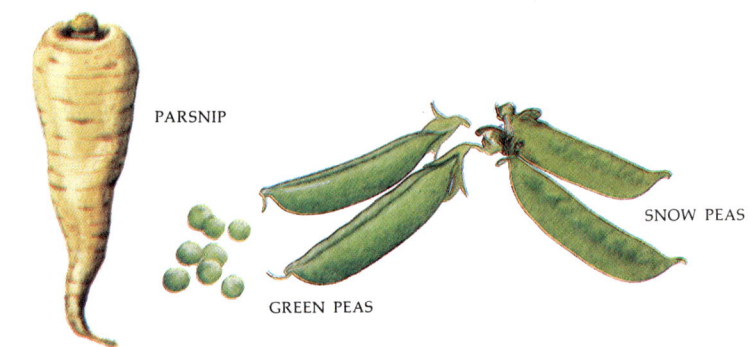

Parsnips. Superficially this vegetable resembles a pallid, overgrown carrot, but it is sweet, nutty, and aromatic. Like Brussels sprouts, parsnips are primarily a winter vegetable; some believe their flavor is at its peak after the first frost.

Parsnips were a staple food in medieval Europe, but by the late 19th century, they had been ousted from favor by the blander-tasting potato. Parsnips are used often to flavor homemade soup. However, the U.S. Department of Agriculture has found parsnips high in toxic chemicals called psoralens that have proved harmful to laboratory animals.

When to buy. October through April, with limited supplies in other months.

What to look for. Firm, smooth, small to medium-sized roots; avoid coarse, flabby, or shriveled ones.

How to keep. Parsnips will keep in the refrigerator wrapped in plastic for at least two weeks.

Nutritive value. High in calcium and potassium.

Peas. Fresh garden peas are becoming a rarity in U.S. markets because few customers want to shell them, preferring to buy them canned or frozen. Unfortunately, those that are available are often large, starchy, and relatively tasteless—a far cry from the tiny, flavorful fresh peas known by their French name of *petits pois*. These were actually developed in Italy during the Renaissance; before that time, most Europeans had eaten dried peas. The English, who imported peas from France, also developed their own varieties of tender garden peas, which were brought to the New World by English settlers.

Besides garden or shell peas, there are two other edible-pod varieties: the small, flat, snow—or sugar—peas often used in Chinese cooking and the plumper sugar snap peas, a new variety that can be either eaten raw or cooked and shelled when mature.

When to buy. Shell peas peak in May and June; snow peas and sugar snap peas, May through September.

What to look for. Smooth, bright pods, well filled but not swollen.

How to keep. Buy peas cold and refrigerate them in their pods; warmth turns their sugar to starch.

Nutritive value. Peas are high in protein, niacin, iron, and phosphorus and supply some calcium, thiamin, and vitamin C.

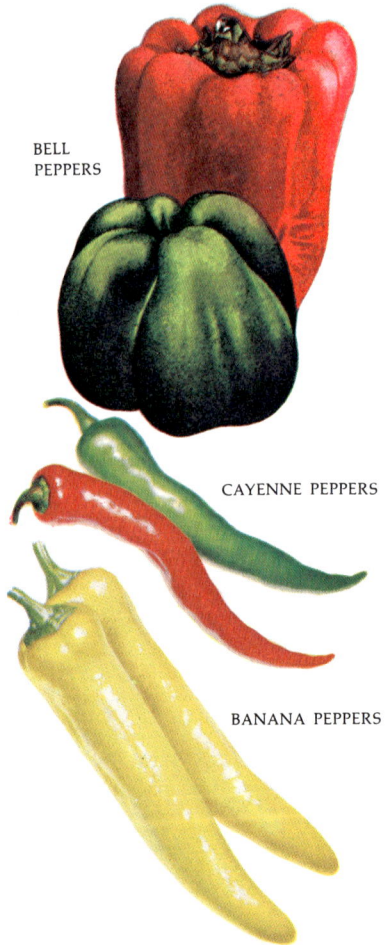

Peppers. Sweet bell peppers and their more explosive cousins, the hot "chili" peppers, are in no way related to the Asian vines that produce peppercorns; peppers are tropical New World plants of the genus *Capsicum*. They were originally misnamed by Christopher Columbus, who was served a dish seasoned with powdered chili by Caribbean Indians and thought it was true pepper.

Capsicums are divided into two groups: the sweet or mild-flavored varieties primarily used as vegetables; and the hot peppers, often called chilies, that are used for sauces and seasonings. Among the many pungent varieties are paprika peppers (the Hungarian seasoning of the same name is not made from these peppers); cayenne peppers; and the fiery Mexican Tabasco peppers, which fuel the well-known sauce of that name. Green bell peppers, which turn bright red when mature, are the type most often found in U.S. markets, but other sweet peppers—such as the long, yellow banana peppers, which can be used for salads or frying—are also available.

When to buy. Sweet peppers are available all year, with slight peak in summer.

What to look for. Peppers should be firm, bright, thick fleshed, and well shaped. Avoid dull, flabby peppers and those with thin skins or soft watery spots.

How to keep. Refrigerate peppers in the vegetable crisper; use within a few days.

Nutritive value. Peppers are an excellent source of vitamin C.

Potatoes. There are several myths about the potato: that it was first cultivated in the Virginia colony, that it was taken to England by Sir Walter Raleigh, and that it achieved instant success in Europe. In fact, potatoes were first cultivated by South American Indians of the high Andes, and taken to England in 1586 by Sir Francis Drake. From there their cultivation spread to Ireland, continental Europe, and finally, in 1719, to the American colonies.

Modern potatoes, the best of which are a far cry from the small, floury originals, fall into three general groups. New potatoes are the tender, thin-skinned ones usually harvested during late winter and early spring; they are used for boiling, creaming, and potato salads. All-purpose potatoes (such as *Katahdin*, *Kennebec*, *Norland*, *Norgold Russet*, *Red Pontiac*, and *White Rose*) can be boiled, mashed, baked, or fried. And the *Idaho*, or *Russet Burbank*, is a popular baking potato.

When to buy. Except for new potatoes, available all year.

What to look for. All potatoes should be firm, clean but not washed, fairly smooth and well shaped, with no sprouts, wilting, or decay. Avoid any with "light burn" (green discolorations which must be cut away). Also avoid those with numerous "eyes," cuts, or bruises.

How to keep. Potatoes should be stored in a cool, dark, well-aired bin rather than in the refrigerator.

Nutritive value. Fresh potatoes, especially those cooked in their skins, provide vitamin C, phosphorus, and potassium. A plain baked potato is only about 145 calories.

Pumpkin. The fabled jack-o-lantern of Halloween is a variety of winter squash. Bees sometimes hybridize pumpkins with other squashes, producing curious anomalies like the green-and-orange "zumkins," but the classic pumpkin is smooth and round, with a hard, ribbed, orange-colored rind. Selection of pumpkins depends on use: for cooking, the small sugar pumpkins, averaging about 7 pounds, are best; for scaring the neighbors' children, varieties like the *Big Max* (100 pounds or more) are unbeatable.

When to buy. September to November; peak in late October.

What to look for. Firm, bright, shapely pumpkins, heavy for their size, with few scars or bruises and no signs of rot.

How to keep. Store in a cool place until ready to use.

Nutritive value. Pumpkins are very high in vitamin A.

Radishes. These crunchy root vegetables come in a variety of shapes and colors—from round to elongated, from white to black. Popular varieties include *Scarlet Globe* and *Cherry Belle* (both globular red radishes), *French Breakfast* (an elongated, white-tipped red radish), *White Icicle* (long and mild tasting), and the Japanese *daikon*, a long, sharp-tasting white radish.

When to buy. Available all year; peak, March through May.

What to look for. Firm, bright radishes of medium size.

How to keep. Remove leafy part of the tops and refrigerate. Use within two weeks.

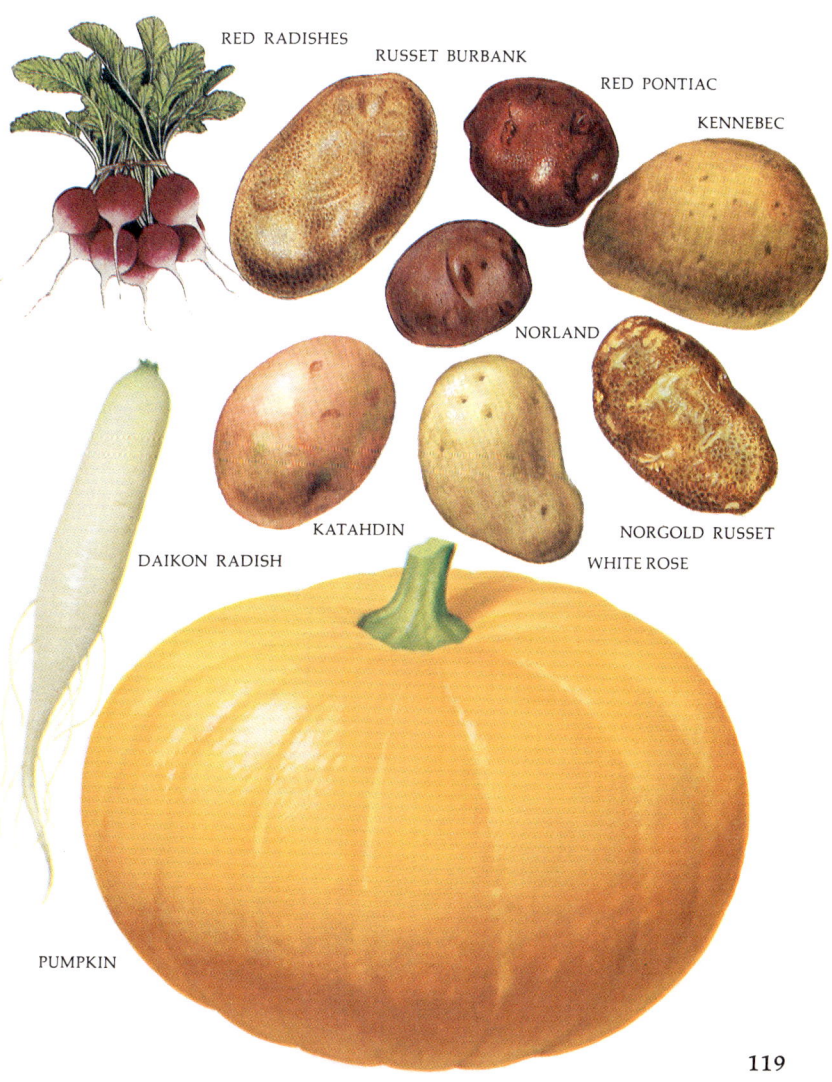

RED RADISHES
RUSSET BURBANK
RED PONTIAC
KENNEBEC
NORLAND
DAIKON RADISH
KATAHDIN
NORGOLD RUSSET
WHITE ROSE
PUMPKIN

Buying Guide
Vegetables

Nutrition Scorecard

This list reflects the overall nutritive value of vegetables, starting at the top with the most nutritious. A food gains points for protein, vitamins A, B_2, B_3, and C, iron and calcium, and complex carbohydrates, and loses points for such substances as fat, cholesterol, and sodium naturally present in the food.

Spinach	2 cups	91
Collard greens	½ cup	90
Sweet potato	1 medium	82
Potato	1 medium	71
Kale	½ cup	71
Winter squash	½ cup	70
Broccoli	½ cup	68
Asparagus	½ cup	67
Brussels sprouts	½ cup	58
Tomato	1 medium	56
Rutabaga	½ cup	54
Carrot	1 medium	48
Green peas, frozen	½ cup	45
Sweet corn	1 ear	41
Cauliflower	½ cup, raw	36
Cabbage, chopped	1 cup, raw	36
Artichoke	½ bud	23
Green beans	½ cup	22
Summer squash	½ cup	22
Turnips	½ cup	21
Bean sprouts	½ cup	18
Eggplant	½ cup	18
Lettuce, Romaine	1 cup	17
Onion, chopped	¼ cup, raw	12
Lettuce, Iceberg	1 cup	11
Mushrooms	½ cup, raw	9
Avocado	½ medium	6
Cucumber	5 slices	6

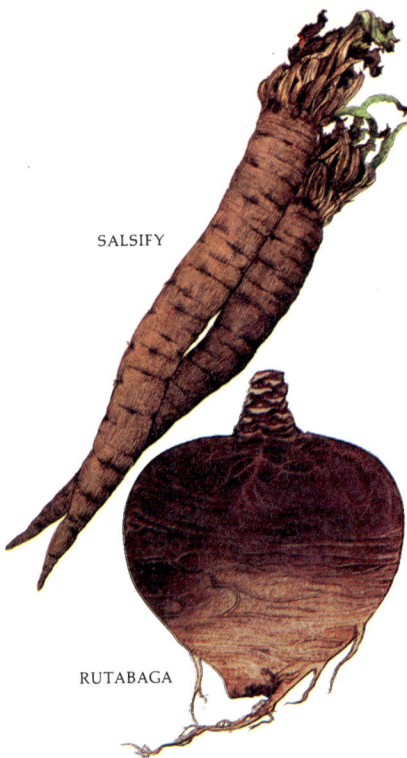

SALSIFY

RUTABAGA

Rutabaga. A relative newcomer to the plant world, this vegetable was first cultivated in Europe in the 17th century. Rutabaga is known by several names—yellow turnip, Swedish turnip, and just plain Swede—but it is larger, coarser, and more emphatically flavored than the turnip, of which it may be a mutant form.

Rutabagas are cool-weather crops, harvested in fall and winter. Like potatoes, they store well for long periods of time, and they are often waxed to prevent moisture loss.

When to buy. The largest supplies are available October to March. They are grown commercially in Canada and the northern United States.

What to look for. Rutabagas are more elongated than turnips, often with purple-tinged tops; most have yellow or orange flesh but some have white. They should be firm and heavy for their size (though size itself does not affect quality), without cuts or bruises.

How to keep. Store in a cool place, and peel before cooking.

Nutritive value. Rutabagas are high in vitamin A; they also contain calcium, potassium, and vitamin C.

Salsify. Just as the parsnip resembles an overgrown carrot, salsify resembles a long, thin parsnip. Like the parsnip, it is one of the few fresh vegetables available in cold weather. It ripens in fall and, in many areas, can be left in the ground all winter; exposure to cold improves its flavor. The root has a mild, sweet taste, which—to some people, at least—suggests that of oysters, hence its other names, "vegetable oyster" and "oyster plant."

When to buy. October and November.

What to look for. Choose young, firm, well-shaped roots with no soft spots.

How to keep. Salsify can be refrigerated in the vegetable crisper for several weeks. If roots are peeled before cooking, they should be dropped into a bowl of water with a little lemon juice or vinegar added to prevent discoloration; or they can also be peeled after cooking.

Shallots. These small bulbs are often confused with both scallions and garlic, and shallots can be considered a variety of onion but they have their own subtle flavor. Their former Latin name, *Allium ascalonicum*, derived in part from the story (probably apocryphal) that shallots were introduced to Europe by crusaders returning from Ascalon in the Holy Land.

Like garlic, shallots grow in tight clusters of six or more little bulbs, sharing a common root system. Delicate in flavor, shallots form an essential component of such classic French sauces as Béarnaise and *beurre blanc* (white butter).

When to buy. October to May; peak in March and April.

What to look for. Shallots should have firm bulbs with a paper-thin reddish skin.

How to keep. Store in a cool, well-ventilated place. They should keep for several months.

FAMILY FOOD GUIDE

Spaghetti Squash. This curious vegetable is not a true squash but an edible gourd with a smooth, pale-green or yellowish rind. Sometimes called "vegetable spaghetti," it is cultivated in the same way as squash. It can be baked or boiled whole; and when the cooked vegetable is cut in half and the seeds are removed, the flesh can be pulled out in spaghettilike strands. It can be served hot, with various seasonings or a spaghetti sauce, or cold in salads.

When to buy. Summer months.

What to look for. Spaghetti squash should have a firm, hard, unblemished rind.

How to keep. Store in a cool, dry place.

Nutritive value. Similar to that of squashes (see page 122).

Spinach. As a cultivated plant, spinach probably originated in or near Persia and was introduced to Spain by the Moors, perhaps about the 11th century. It later became a favorite Lenten vegetable in Europe, since it is ready for harvest in spring. Just when or how spinach came to North America is unknown, but it was being grown in U.S. gardens by the early 19th century.

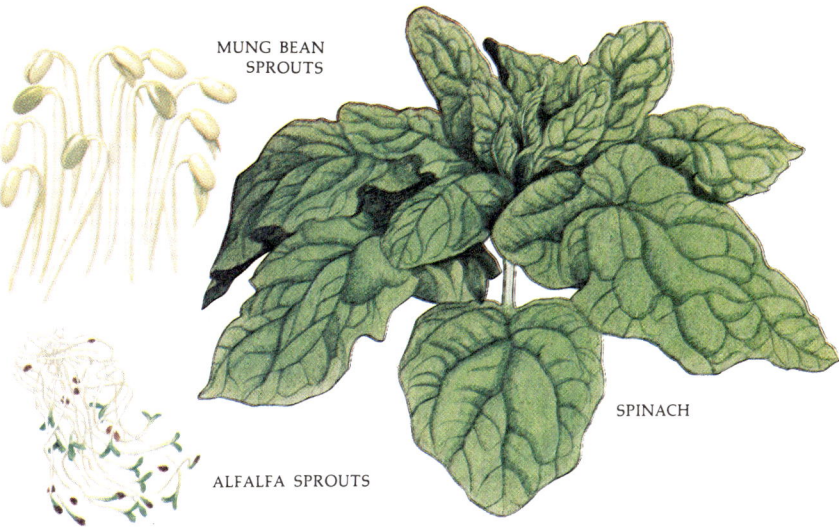

MUNG BEAN SPROUTS

ALFALFA SPROUTS

SPINACH

Spinach can be either smooth leafed or, more commonly, of the crinkle-leafed "Savoy" type; it can also be round seeded or prickly seeded. The prickly seeded varieties, once thought to be the hardiest, are most often grown in the United States, whereas the newer smooth-seeded types—thought by many people to be superior in flavor—are more popular in Europe. Fresh young, tender leaves are delicious in salads or steamed with a little water until just tender.

When to buy. All year, with peak March to June.

What to look for. Fresh, crisp, dark-green leaves that are not wilted, crushed, or bruised. Clipped leaves in bags should feel full and springy.

How to keep. Refrigerate in a plastic bag in the vegetable crisper and use within a few days; wash thoroughly before using.

Nutritive value. Spinach is especially rich in vitamin A and iron and has good supplies of vitamin C, calcium, and other minerals.

Sprouts. The dried seeds of many leguminous plants can be used to grow sprouts, the small, crunchy, delicate shoots that have long been part of Chinese cooking. Packages of alfalfa and mung bean sprouts may be found at many supermarkets, greengrocers, and Oriental food stores. (They are also easy to grow from seed at home; see pages 164-165.)

When to buy. Sprouts are available all year long.

What to look for. Sprouts should be young, very pale, crisp, and short—an inch or two long—with fresh tips. Avoid any with signs of mold.

How to keep. Refrigerate in a tightly closed plastic bag or container and use within a few days.

Nutritive value. Alfalfa sprouts are high in vitamin A; mung bean sprouts contain potassium.

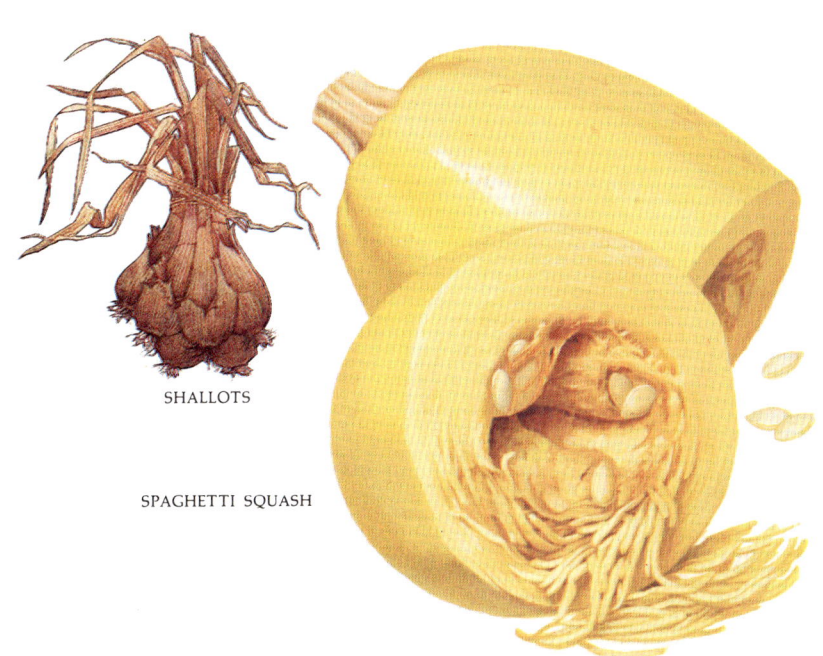

SHALLOTS

SPAGHETTI SQUASH

Buying Guide
Vegetables

Squash. When European explorers first encountered squashes in the Americas, they described the plants as gourds or melons, both of which were familiar species in the Old World. But squashes are, in fact, a specifically New World species; they were probably among the first—and certainly most important—food plants to be cultivated by the Indians of North and South America and the Caribbean.

Squash is generally divided into two types: the quick-growing, tender-skinned "summer" squashes, which are harvested immature; and the larger, slower growing, hard-shelled "winter" squashes, harvested when fully mature. Summer squashes, such as *yellow crooknecks*, *pattypans*, and *zucchini*, are eaten whole. Winter squashes like *Hubbards*, *butternuts*, *acorns*, and *sugar pumpkins* (see entry on Pumpkin) have inedible skins but tastier, more nutritious flesh than summer varieties.

When to buy. Squash is available all year, with hard-shelled varieties most plentiful in fall and winter.

What to look for. Summer squash should be young, tender, and fresh looking, with a glossy skin. Winter varieties should have uniformly hard, thick rinds and be heavy for their size, with no sunken or moldy areas.

How to keep. Summer squashes should be refrigerated and used within a few days; winter squashes will keep for months at cool room temperatures.

Nutritive value. Varieties of winter squash are more nutritious though both types contain vitamins A and C and minerals.

Sweet Potatoes. Yams and sweet potatoes are often confused. Both are edible tubers, but they are from different plant families. Yams probably originated in West Africa, whereas sweet potatoes, like squash, are native New World vegetables. They were called *batatas* (from which comes the English word "potato") by the Caribbean Indians who introduced them to Columbus.

Sweet potatoes come in many varieties but are of two basic types: the dry fleshed, with rather mealy, pale-yellow flesh; and the moist fleshed, with deep-yellow to orange-red flesh (often incorrectly called a yam.)

When to buy. Available all year; peak, September to December.

What to look for. Look for firm tubers with bright, smooth, evenly colored skins. Avoid any tubers with signs of wet, soft decay, dry decay (shriveled and discolored ends), or dry rot (sunken, discolored patches on the sides).

How to keep. Sweet potatoes are far more perishable than white potatoes. Do not refrigerate; but store in a cool, dry place.

Nutritive value. Sweet potatoes are rich in vitamin A and a good source of calcium.

Swiss Chard. A type of beet grown for its leaves rather than its root, Swiss chard is also called the leaf beet. The root, in this case, is inedible, but the leaves can be cooked like spinach and the stalks like celery.

When to buy. April through November, with the peak season from June through October.

What to look for. Large, crisp, dark-green leaves, and firm white stalks. There is also a red variety that resembles rhubarb.

How to keep. Refrigerate chard in a plastic bag in the vegetable crisper, and use within a few days. Wash well before cooking.

Nutritive value. Very high in vitamin A and low in calories.

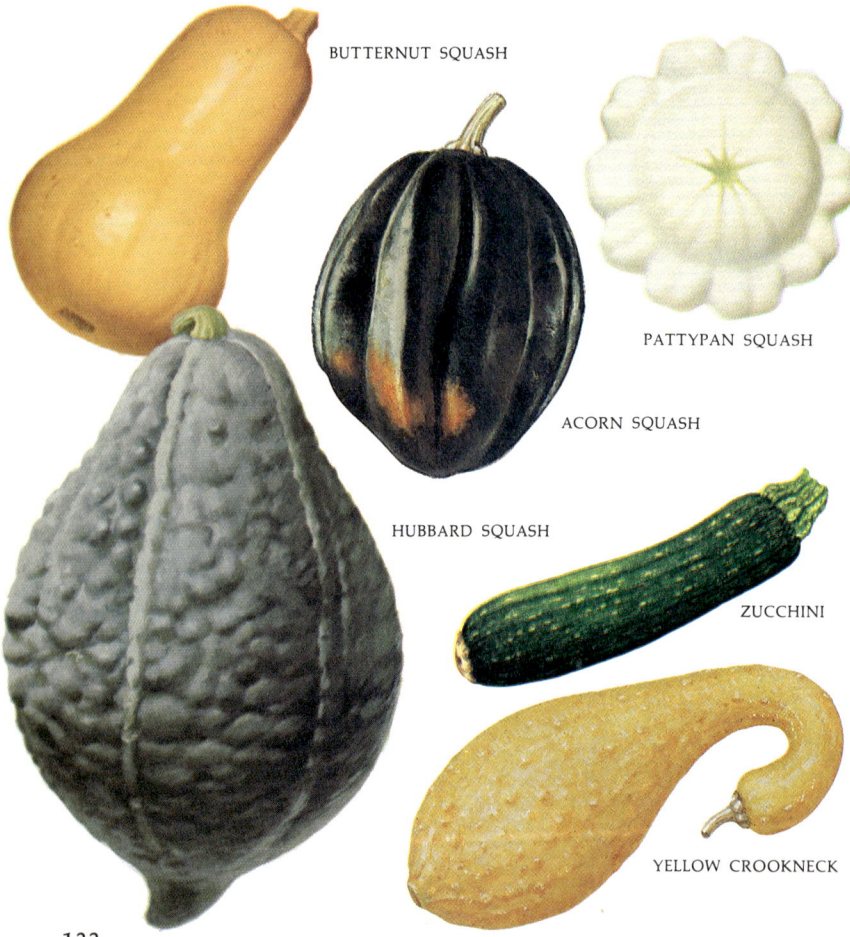

FAMILY FOOD GUIDE

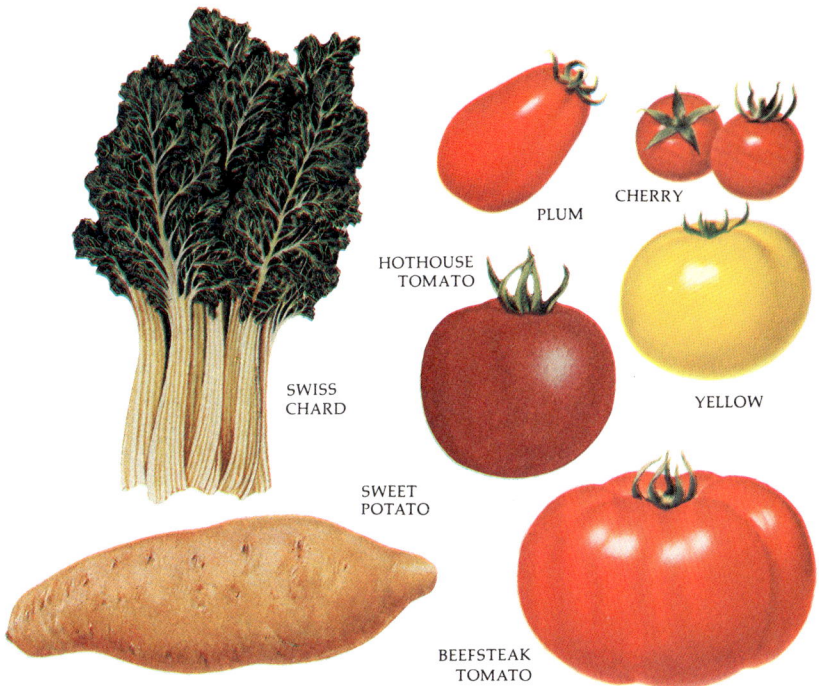

Tomatoes. Today's thick-skinned commercial tomatoes, usually picked green and "ripened" with ethylene gas, have nothing to recommend them beyond the dubious values of the marketplace: ease of shipment and long shelf life. The best tomatoes, as every tomato lover knows, are the succulent, vine-ripened ones bought in season from local farms or grown in home gardens; really ripe tomatoes are much too delicate for long-distance shipment.

The earliest tomatoes, which were gathered wild by Indians of the lower Andes, had small yellow fruits, about the size of today's cherry tomatoes. When they were first imported to Europe in the 16th century, these "golden apples" were grown chiefly as ornamental plants; their fruits were thought to be toxic. Varieties of tomatoes available today include the large, all-purpose *beefsteak* types; the oval *plum* variety, used chiefly for cooking; the small, tasty *cherry* tomatoes, often served in salads; and the large, yellow or orange low-acid tomatoes.

When to buy. For vine-ripened tomatoes, the peak is May to September, depending on the area.

What to look for. Firm, plump fruits with a strong tomato smell (the gas-treated ones are odorless).

How to keep. Commercial tomatoes will not ripen more and must be refrigerated at once to keep from becoming mushy. Slightly underripe homegrown fruits can be ripened in a paper bag or in light—not sunlight. Ripe tomatoes may be refrigerated.

Nutritive value. Tomatoes are a good source of vitamins A and C.

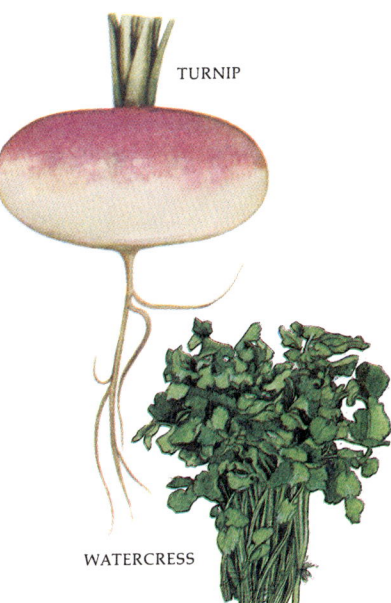

Turnips. Through much of recorded history, the turnip has been dismissed by gastronomes as a food fit only for peasants and livestock. This may have come about because turnips grow so obligingly in meager, sandy soils, and because out-of-season turnips—unlike the crisp young ones—are indeed woody and bitter.

Turnips are found in innumerable varieties, but in the United States the roots are most commonly white fleshed, with purple or green tops. A distinct-tasting vegetable, turnips go well with braised beef or pork roast. Some varieties are bred especially for their leaves, which are far richer in nutrients than the roots.

When to buy. Turnips are available all year long; their peak is from October to March.

What to look for. Firm, smooth, small to medium-sized turnips with few fibrous root ends. Tops, if attached, should be fresh and green.

How to keep. Refrigerated turnips keep for long periods, but remove tops and use as soon as possible.

Nutritive value. Turnip greens are rich in vitamins A and C and calcium.

Watercress. This delicate, round-leafed salad plant is found in every state in the United States, growing freely along the edges of ponds and the banks of gently running streams; it is also cultivated and sold in supermarkets. Since ancient times, cress has been prized for two seemingly contradictory qualities: its taste is sharp and peppery, but it is cooling and refreshing to the mouth.

When to buy. The supply peaks in spring and summer, but it is available throughout the year.

What to look for. Choose bunches of crisp, tender green leaves with no signs of yellowing or wilting.

How to keep. Refrigerate in a tightly closed container or plastic bag and use as soon as possible.

Nutritive value. Watercress is rich in vitamin A.

Buying Guide
Fruits

A fragrant golden peach or a shiny crisp apple is a delicious finale to a meal. Fresh fruit also makes a nutritious, low-calorie breakfast food or snack and often provides dietary fiber. Although the U.S. Department of Agriculture has established grades for fruit based on size, maturity, color, and lack of defects, these standards are voluntary, and you are most likely to find only the two top grades in markets—U.S. Fancy and No. 1. In selecting fruit, keep in mind the tips in this section. Many fruits are shipped underripe over long distances; the tastiest and most economical buys are tree- or vine-ripened fruits during the peak season in your area. Always wash fresh fruit before eating.

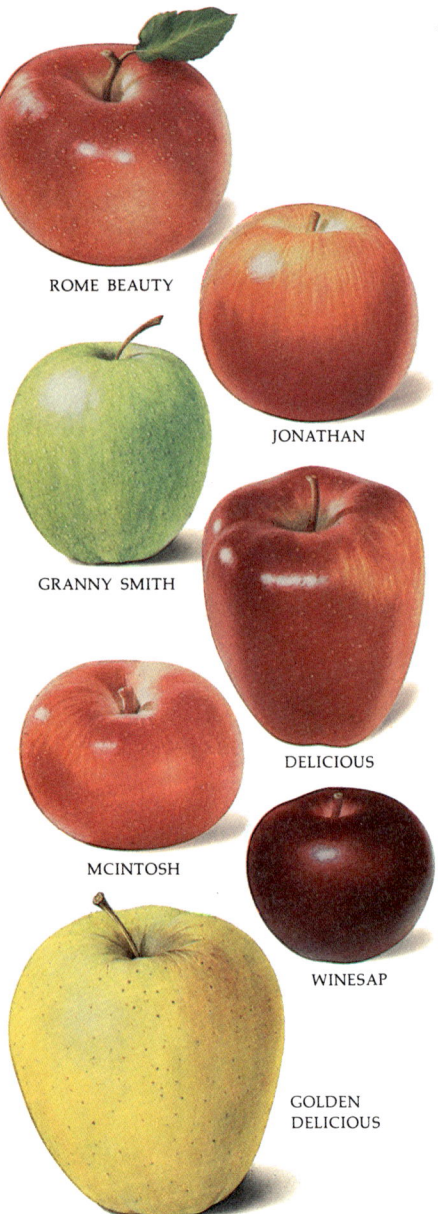

ROME BEAUTY
JONATHAN
GRANNY SMITH
DELICIOUS
MCINTOSH
WINESAP
GOLDEN DELICIOUS

Apples. More than 7,000 varieties of this "king of fruits" have been recorded in the United States alone. Many of today's supermarkets, however, carry only a few of the most profitable kinds. Some of today's most popular varieties originated as mutants, sown accidentally from seed—like the world's top seller, the Delicious, which first appeared uninvited in an Iowa orchard in the 1860s.

The apples shown here are the ones most widely available in markets across the country. The division of apples into "cooking" and "eating" categories is not hard and fast; many "all-purpose" varieties are suitable for both, as indicated below. *Jonathan* apples (peak season, September) are bright red and juicy; they are used for cooking, baking, and eating raw. The *Rome Beauty* (October to March) is also bright red, juicy, and firm. Seldom eaten raw, it is very good for baking, applesauce, pies, and general-purpose cooking. The bright-green, rather tart *Granny Smith* (March to September), mostly imported, is a favorite for eating because of its crisp texture. The brilliant *Red Delicious* (September to May) is an eating apple that keeps well but has a rather neutral flavor; the *Golden Delicious* (September to March) is also an eating apple but can be used for salads and baking. Both *Winesaps* (November to June) and *McIntoshes* (September to April) are excellent all-purpose apples with bright-red skin and juicy flesh. Other excellent all-purpose varieties include *Cortland, Newtown, Northern Spy, Stayman, Gravenstein,* and *Wealthy,* and for cooking, *York* and *Rhode Island Greening.*

When to buy. Generally, apples can be found all year, but lowest availability is July and August. The peak season for individual varieties is mentioned above.

What to look for. Choose mature, firm, crisp apples with stems attached, of good color for the variety; avoid fruit with punctures, shriveling, softness, or brownish bruises. To remove wax coating from apples that have been protected in this way, see page 213.

How to keep. Refrigerate apples or store in a very cool place, but serve at room temperature for best flavor.

Nutritive value. Apples are a good source of fiber.

Apricots. Fresh apricots are delicate fruits with a short season and, once picked, a short life span. Because they are so fragile, only a small proportion of the crop is sold fresh; the rest is dried or canned. Apricots were first cultivated in China about 4,000 years ago; from there they spread to Mesopotamia, to Persia (where they were once called "eggs of the sun"), and eventually to Europe's Mediterranean coast. They may have been introduced to California by the Spanish mission fathers in the 18th century; today the West Coast still supplies most of the U.S. crop.

When to buy. Generally available May to August, with the peak in June and July.

What to look for. Apricots should be picked when mature but still firm. Look for plump, orange-yellow fruits that yield to gentle pressure. Avoid hard, greenish to pale yellow (undermature) fruit and soft, dull, or mushy (overmature) fruit.

How to keep. Refrigerate immediately and use in a few days.

Nutritive value. Apricots are a good source of vitamin A.

FAMILY FOOD GUIDE

Bananas. Botanically, this tropical fruit par excellence is not a fruit at all but a giant herb, the largest on earth. The original wild bananas, native to both Asia and Africa, were (and are) hard, bitter, and full of seeds, whereas today's cultivated varieties are seedless and sterile—new plants are produced from pieces of rootstock. In 1516, cultivated bananas of African stock were brought to the New World island of Hispaniola, and from there banana culture spread with astonishing speed through the Caribbean, Central America, and parts of South America. But the fruit's importance as an export crop had to wait for the advent of refrigeration and specially constructed, steam-powered "banana boats" at the turn of the 20th century. Today bananas are the top-selling fruit in the United States, outranking even homegrown favorites like apples and oranges.

The green or greenish-yellow *plantains* are also called "vegetable" bananas because they are starchy, not sweet, and must be cooked before eating. They are delicious fried, usually as a side dish to meat.

When to buy. Bananas are imported year round from Central and South America.

What to look for. Buy plump, firm, unbruised bananas. Avoid any with dull, grayish skins; they will not ripen properly. If the banana is covered with small brown specks, it is fully ripe. Buy bananas in bunches with the stems intact; they will keep longer. The peel of a plantain is usually greenish and marked with blemishes, which do not affect its quality or taste.

How to keep. Green, or partially green, sweet bananas will ripen, uncovered, at room temperature. Fully ripe ones may be refrigerated for a few days; refrigeration will cause the peel to turn dark brown but will not change the taste of the banana.

Nutritive value. Bananas have potassium, phosphorus, and a high fiber content and are easy to digest.

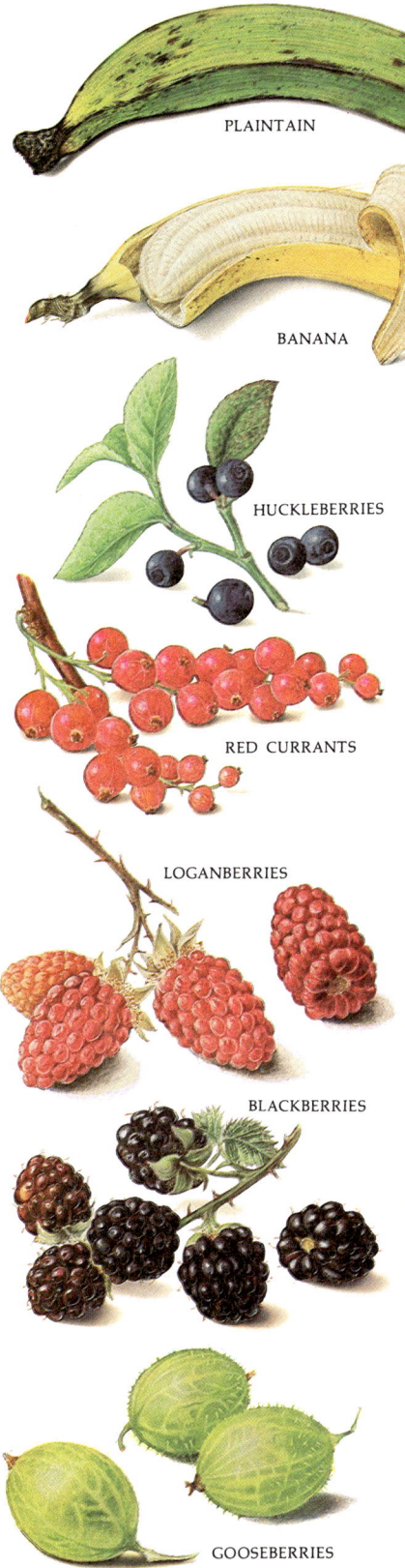

PLAINTAIN

BANANA

APRICOT

HUCKLEBERRIES

RED CURRANTS

LOGANBERRIES

BLACKBERRIES

GOOSEBERRIES

Berries. The berries discussed here are of limited availability; other kinds—blueberries, cranberries, raspberries, and strawberries—are listed separately.

Blackberries (season, May to August), both wild and cultivated, are large, purplish black, and glossy. They can be eaten fresh or used in pies, jams, and jellies, and wine-making. *Currants* (June to August) are glossy, clustered berries with a sweet-tart flavor, used raw and in compotes, jams and jellies, and fruit salads. *Gooseberries* (May to August) are closely related to currants but have translucent, veined skins of green, yellow, red, or white. Used in pies, tarts, and jams, they can be found in some farmers' markets. *Huckleberries* (June to August), gathered wild and sold locally, are sharper tasting and have larger, harder seeds than wild blueberries. Deep blue in color, they are excellent for pies. *Loganberries* (June and July) have a blackberry shape, a raspberry color, and an acid taste. Extremely perishable, they are generally sold canned and are used for pies, jams, and the like.

What to look for. Fresh berries should be plump, firm, and brightly colored. Check the underside of the container—a badly stained carton probably indicates mushy or moldy fruit (mesh plastic cartons will give you a better view).

How to keep. Empty the carton gently onto a plate, discarding any damaged berries. Refrigerate the rest in a flat container (to avoid crushing them). Just before using, wash berries gently in cold water and drain well.

125

Buying Guide
Fruits

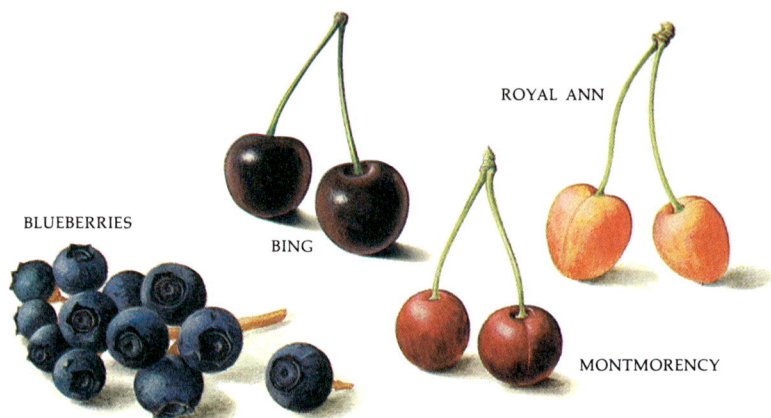

Blueberries. To many people's taste, cultivated blueberries are a poor substitute for the wild form of this native American fruit, with its distinctive, tart-sweet flavor. Cultivated blueberries are larger, blander, sweeter, and far more plentiful than the wild ones, which are found in limited quantities, fresh or canned. Wild blueberries are preferred for pies, but both types have many uses: as a dessert fruit; in cobblers, cakes, tarts, muffins, and pancakes; and for jams, sauces, and jellies.

When to buy. Available May to September, with peak supply in July.

What to look for. Cultivated blueberries are dark blue with a silvery gloss; wild ones are smaller and slightly paler with a lavender tinge. Choose plump berries of uniform size, free of stems and leaves; avoid stained or leaky containers. Remember, there is no waste with blueberries.

How to keep. Always pick over the berries before storing. Blueberries can be refrigerated, covered, for a few days or frozen in sealed freezer bags. Wash gently just before using.

Nutritive value. Blueberries are good sources of vitamins A and C.

Cherries. Since prehistoric times, wild cherries have existed in temperate parts of Asia, Europe, and North America. The early American colonists developed cultivated varieties from the native wild species, as well as importing cultivated cherries from Europe—some of which, in turn, "escaped" and reverted to their original wild forms.

The hundreds of varieties of cherries on the market today may be generally classified in terms of sweetness and color. *Bing* and *Royal Ann* cherries, for example, are both sweet, but Bings have deeply colored juice, whereas the juice of the Royal Ann variety is colorless. Sour cherries—the ones most favored for cooked desserts—are similarly divided: "morellos" have colored juice, and "amarelles" colorless. The popular tart cherry *Montmorency* is light to dark red with red juice.

When to buy. For sweet cherries, May through August with peak in June and July; for fresh sour cherries, late June to mid-August.

What to look for. Plump, bright, glossy cherries with fresh stems and good color for the variety. Examine dark cherries carefully: their deep color can mask signs of decay. Avoid small, hard, immature fruit, for it will not ripen.

How to keep. Discard damaged cherries; refrigerate the rest in a sealed plastic bag and use in a day or two. Wash them just before eating.

Nutritive value. Sour cherries are very high in vitamin A and potassium and contain vitamin C, iron, and calcium.

Cranberries. We have the American Indians of the Northeast to thank for the invention of cranberry sauce; it was they who first cooked the wild berries with honey or maple sugar to accompany meat dishes—a technique they passed on to the English settlers in the 17th century. Today's cranberries, cultivated primarily in Massachusetts and Wisconsin, are larger and more plentiful than their wild ancestors, but their sharp flavor remains much the same.

When to buy. September to December.

What to look for. Cranberries should be firm, plump, and lustrous, medium to blackish red in color. Avoid shriveled or soft berries.

How to keep. Cranberries may be refrigerated for up to a week, or frozen in their original containers.

Dates. These sugary fruits are a boon to desert dwellers, growing in hot, dry regions where most food plants cannot—yet they have their own rather temperamental requirements. Date palms must have a source of underground water, but any moisture in the air will keep the fruit from setting, and temperatures below 70°F will keep it from ripening. The trees themselves can survive in cooler, wetter areas, but their nutritious fruits cannot.

When to buy. Available all year.

What to look for. Fresh (sun-ripened) dates are plump and shiny, with lighter, smoother skins than the dried ones; the latter may contain added sweeteners and preservatives. Fresh dates may be described as "soft," "semi-dry," or "dry," depending on the softness of the ripe fruit.

How to keep. Covered and refrigerated, dates will keep indefinitely.

Nutritive value. Dates are rich in potassium, iron, and other minerals.

Figs. Fresh figs have been a prized delicacy for at least 5,000 years. They were grown in the Hanging Gardens of Babylon, mentioned frequently in the Bible, and exported by the ancient Greeks, who may have introduced their culture to Italy. In the 18th century, Spanish missionaries planted figs at the first mission in San Diego, California; the so-called *Mission* fig is still an important variety in California, which grows 99 percent of the U.S. fig crop.

When to buy. Season for fresh figs, June to mid-November. Dried figs are available all year.

What to look for. Fresh figs are usually pear shaped, with greenish-yellow, purple, or black skins; when ripe, they should be soft but not mushy. Avoid any with broken skins or a sour, fermented smell (an indication of overripeness).

How to keep. Fresh figs should be refrigerated and used, if possible, on the day of purchase.

Grapefruit. The grapefruit is not a hybrid (the product of a deliberate crossbreeding of two species) but a distinct plant species in itself, one of the world's youngest. Grapefruit first appeared sometime during the 18th century in Barbados or Jamaica, probably as a mutant form of a Southeast Asian citrus fruit, the pomelo or Shaddock, which had been brought to Barbados by a trader named Captain Shaddock in 1696. Although similar to the pomelo, the grapefruit is far sweeter and smoother textured, and the young trees yield heavily within five years of planting.

The grapefruit was officially recorded as a species (*Citrus paradisi*) in 1830. By that time the first Florida grove had already been planted, but commercial cultivation did not get under way there until 1890. Today the United States grows 90 percent of the world's crop, principally in Florida and Texas but also in California and Arizona.

When to buy. In general, Florida and Texas grapefruit are available fall through spring, and western grapefruit in summer.

What to look for. Buy firm, heavy, thin-skinned fruits with a springy feel. Avoid puffy or coarse-skinned fruits with pointed stem ends. Russeting, a discoloration of the surface of the rind, does not affect flavor.

How to keep. Refrigerate grapefruit, uncovered, and use within two weeks.

Nutritive value. High in vitamin C; pink and red varieties contain more vitamin A.

> ## Dried Fruits
>
> The practice of drying fruits is centuries old, dating back to biblical times. Today, fruits are dried for commercial sale either in the sun or by various other processes that cause the water to evaporate.
>
> During dehydration, the nutrients (except vitamin C and thiamin) become concentrated in the remaining solids. Thus, dried fruits have more nutrients—and more calories—by weight than fresh fruits. For example, you need 6 to 8 pounds of fresh apricots to equal the amount of nutrients packed into just 1 pound of dried apricots.
>
> Light-colored fruits, such as apples, apricots, peaches, pears, and golden raisins, are treated with sulfur dioxide to prevent discoloration and to help preserve nutrients. Some people think it is harmful to ingest sulfur dioxide, but this has not been proved. Dates, figs, prunes, and raisins are not usually sulfured. The package label will state whether sulfur has been used. Some dried fruits are also treated with potassium sorbate, a preservative that prevents the growth of mold and fungi. All imported dried fruits, and some domestic ones, are fumigated—a process that destroys insects and larvae. By the time the fruit reaches the consumer, however, the gas has dissipated. If you want to be extra sure, open the package and let it stand for a few minutes before using.
>
> Raw, dried fruits are good as snacks; soaked or cooked, they are used in compotes, stuffings, and baked goods.

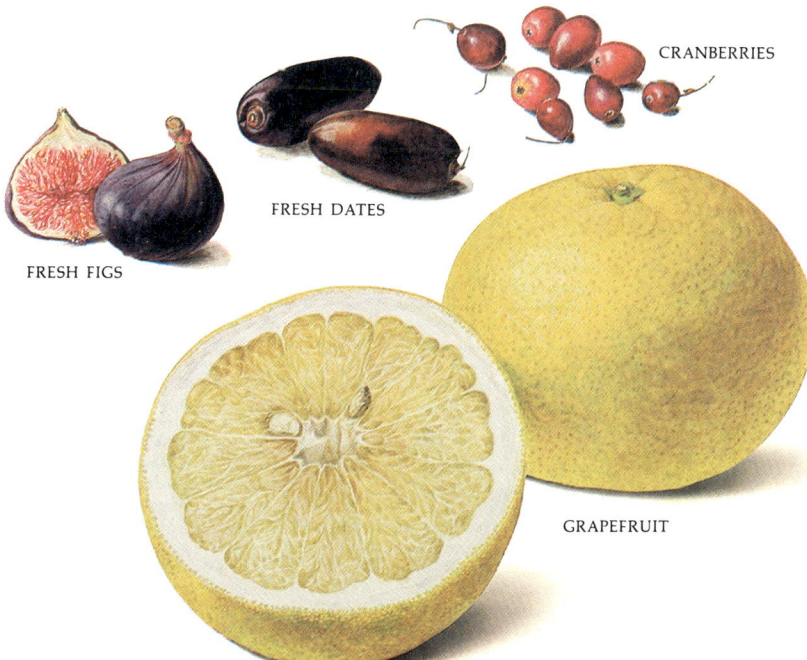

FRESH FIGS

FRESH DATES

CRANBERRIES

GRAPEFRUIT

Buying Guide
Fruits

Grapes. Whether for winemaking or for the table, grapes have always evoked images of luxury and indolence. They are also among the oldest foods of man, having been cultivated for at least 6,000 years.

The Romans may have been the first to grow distinct varieties for winemaking, for eating fresh, and for drying as raisins, but all of the thousands of Old World varieties that exist today are descendants of one species, *Vitis vinifera*, the basic wine grape. The grapes grown commercially in the American West—like the popular green *Thompson Seedless* and the red table grape *Emperor*—are also descendants of this Old World species, but most eastern table grapes derive from native American species or hybrids. The western varieties have adherent skins, but the eastern grape separates easily into skin and pulp. The *Concord*, an eastern grape, is a cross between the European grape and the American "fox grape" (*Vitis labrusca*).

When to buy. Depending on the variety, grapes are available all year, with peak supply July through November.

What to look for. Plump, well-colored grapes, firmly attached to green stems. Avoid wrinkled or leaky grapes.

How to keep. Refrigerate grapes and use them within a week. Wash thoroughly before eating.

Guavas. These small, thin-skinned tropical fruits are usually processed into jams, jellies, preserves, and the well-known guava paste of the Caribbean—a semisolid, gelatinlike dessert—but they can also be eaten fresh. The fruits are round to pear shaped, usually less than 3 inches in diameter, with green or bright-yellow skins; some have a reddish blush. Ripe guavas have a musky, pungent odor. They contain small, hard seeds that can irritate the throat, but some of the newer varieties are relatively free from seeds. Guavas are native to tropical America and are sensitive to frost; they are grown in California and Florida.

When to buy. Available in the fall and January to June.

What to look for. Guavas for eating fresh should yield to slight pressure. Firmer ones may be used for cooking.

How to keep. Refrigerate ripe guavas and use as soon as possible.

Nutritive value. Guavas are extremely rich in vitamin C and also contain minerals.

Kiwi Fruit. An egg-shaped fruit with a fuzzy brown outer skin and sweet green flesh, the odd but appealing kiwi is a native of New Zealand. The fruit was originally (and misleadingly) called the Chinese gooseberry; the name was changed to kiwi for the export market, in honor of the flightless bird that has become the national symbol of New Zealand. Similar in taste and texture to the honeydew melon, the kiwi is now grown commercially in California.

When to buy. Available all year.

What to look for. Kiwi fruits may be bought firm and home ripened at room temperature; when the skins yield to gentle pressure, they are ready to eat. Avoid any with puckered skins.

How to keep. Refrigerate ripe fruits.

Nutritive value. Kiwis are rich in vitamin C.

Kumquats. The smallest of all citrus fruits, kumquats have been cultivated for thousands of years in China and Japan (their name means "golden orange" in Chinese) but were virtually unknown in the West until the mid-19th century, when an English plant collector brought some specimens to Europe.

The kumquats grown in California and Florida are often sold preserved in sweet syrup, to be used for marmalades and garnishes, but fresh ones are delicious for fruit salads or eating out of hand. Kumquats are eaten skin and all—the orange rind is quite sweet but the pulp is tart and juicy.

When to buy. November through February.

What to look for. Fresh kumquats should be bright, firm, unblemished, and heavy for their size.

How to keep. Store at room temperature or refrigerate. Wash thoroughly before eating.

Nutritive value. Kumquats are rich in vitamin A, potassium, and calcium, and provide vitamin C.

Lemons. Seldom are these citrus fruits eaten for themselves—it takes raw courage, after all, to bite down on a raw lemon—yet they remain one of the world's most indispensable foods. Fresh lemon juice is a remarkably versatile flavoring agent, adding piquancy to dressings, fish and meat dishes, vegetables, soufflés, pies, sherbets—the list is nearly endless.

Lemons were known to the ancient Romans, but their culture did not become widespread in the Mediterranean region until the conquering Moors established lemon orchards in Spain and Sicily in the 8th century. Lemon trees thrive in warm, humid, but relatively rainless coastal areas, like the coast of Southern California, which grows about 80 percent of America's commercial lemon crop.

When to buy. Available all year; peak from May through August.

What to look for. Choose plump, heavy, fairly smooth-skinned lemons with a rich yellow color; avoid those with coarse or shriveled skins.

How to keep. Lemons may be refrigerated for several weeks. To get the maximum of juice, bring them to room temperature and apply gentle pressure with a rolling motion before cutting.

Nutritive value. Like other citrus fruits, lemons are high in vitamin C.

Limes. British seamen acquired their famous nickname "limeys" in the 19th century, after lime and other citrus juices were added to their daily rum ration to prevent scurvy, a disease caused by vitamin C deficiency.

Most of the limes marketed today are the bright-green Persian varieties. They are the size of lemons, with strong-flavored, very acid, greenish-yellow pulp. The smaller Florida Key limes—the ones used for the famous pie—have thin, leathery, yellow rinds and green pulp.

When to buy. Available all year, with peak from June to August.

What to look for. Green limes should be heavy, with glossy, fine-textured skin. Avoid any with dull, dry skin, soft spots, or mold.

How to keep. Limes may be refrigerated or kept at room temperature.

Nutritive value. Limes contain vitamin C and potassium.

Mangoes. Mangoes are the most luscious of tropical fruits; but when they are not of fine quality, the flesh can be disagreeably fibrous, with a flavor of turpentine. These highly perishable fruits also vary greatly in size—anywhere from 6 ounces to 4 or 5 pounds—and shape: they can be round, oval, pear or kidney shaped, or even long and thin. The tough skin is usually dull green, with red and yellow areas that broaden as the fruit ripens. Some people have an allergic skin reaction to the fluid beneath the peel and must wear protective gloves when peeling the fruit.

Mangoes have been grown for thousands of years on the Indian subcontinent, and India still produces nearly 80 percent of the world's crop. Mango culture was introduced to Brazil and the West Indies in the 18th century, and to southern Florida in the 19th century.

When to buy. Available all year.

What to look for. Buy firm mangoes with no wilting, grayish discoloration, or black spots.

How to keep. Ripen mangoes at room temperature until very soft, then refrigerate.

Nutritive value. Very high in vitamin A and contains vitamin C, potassium, calcium, and magnesium.

Nutrition Scorecard

This scorecard, like the one for vegetables on page 120, rates fruits as to their nutritive density. The higher the number, the more nutritious the fruit.

Watermelon	10" × 1" slice	68
Cantaloupe	¼ medium	60
Mango	½ medium	52
Orange	1 medium	49
Grapefruit	½ medium	42
Banana	1 medium	36
Honeydew melon	7" × 2" slice	35
Strawberries	½ cup	34
Pear	1 medium	29
Peach	1 medium	26
Tangerine	1 medium	26
Apple	1 medium	23
Blueberries	½ cup	21
Pineapple	½ cup	18
Cherries	½ cup	17

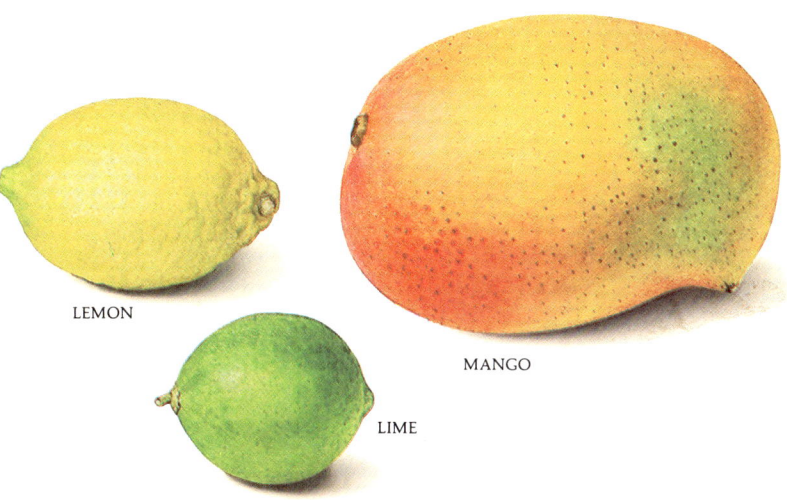

LEMON
MANGO
LIME

Buying Guide
Fruits

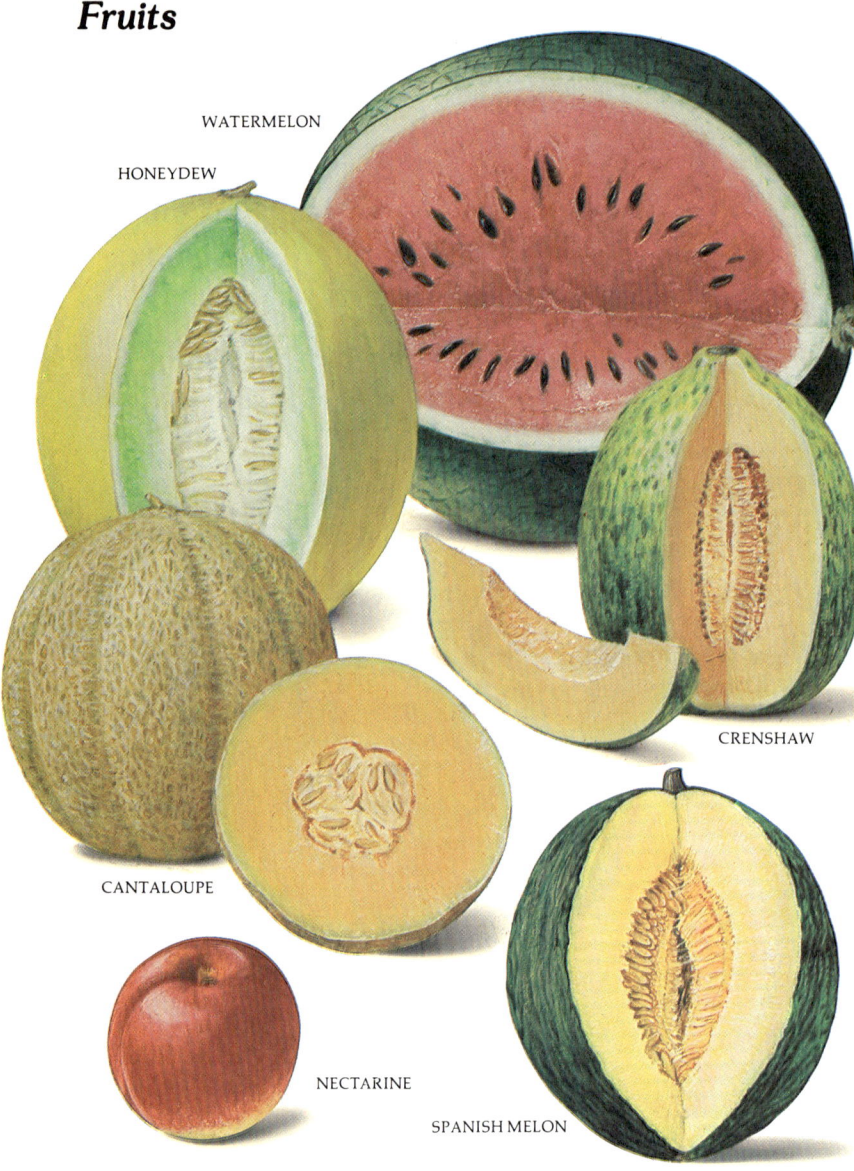

WATERMELON
HONEYDEW
CRENSHAW
CANTALOUPE
NECTARINE
SPANISH MELON

Melons. The individual characteristics of these fruits vary so greatly that there is no one rule for choosing a melon of perfect ripeness. There are, however, some useful clues. *Muskmelons*, or *Cantaloupes* in North American parlance, have rinds with thick, raised netting. Ripe cantaloupes, and the larger, more finely netted *Persian* melons, have yellowish skin under the netting, a pleasant aroma, and a smooth, rounded scar (called a "full slip") at the stem end. *Cranshaws*, or *Crenshaws*, favorites of melon lovers, are rounded at the blossom end and pointed at the stem end. When ripe, the smooth, slightly furrowed rind is a deep golden yellow. They have a pleasant aroma and yield to slight pressure at the blossom end. *Cranshaws* are sometimes confused with *Casabas*, which have deeper furrows but no odor when ripe. *Spanish* melons are dark green with a taste similar to the Cranshaw. *Honeydews*, and the smaller *Honeyballs*, are creamy yellow to white, with a faint aroma and a slight softening at the blossom end. *Watermelons* have a smooth surface and a creamy underside; cut watermelons should be bright and juicy, with dark seeds.

When to buy. Most varieties are available June to October.

What to look for. See above. Characteristics to avoid include excessive hardness or softness, lackluster color, punctures, and sunken or water-soaked areas on the rind.

How to keep. Refrigerate ripe melons and use as soon as possible. Wrap cut melons in plastic so that the aroma will not penetrate other foods.

Nutritive value. Cantaloupes and watermelons have an especially high vitamin A content, as well as vitamin C and potassium.

Nectarines. These small stone fruits are often described as a cross between a peach and a plum, but actually they are smooth-skinned peaches.

Like other peaches, nectarines can be clingstone, freestone, yellow fleshed, or white fleshed, and must be harvested mature if they are to gain their full flavor. The flesh is rich, sweet, and juicy, and is well suited for use in ice cream, pies, and fruit salads in addition to eating fresh.

When to buy. June to September.

What to look for. Buy plump, well-colored fruits (orange-yellow to red) with a slight softening along the seam. Avoid hard, dull, or shriveled fruits, or any with large green areas.

How to keep. Soften at room temperature until ripe, then refrigerate.

Nutritive value. High in vitamin A.

Oranges. These citrus fruits have been cultivated in China, their original habitat, for at least 4,000 years. Like lemons, oranges were brought to the Mediterranean lands by the Moors, where their cultivation flourished. Orange seeds or saplings were carried to the New World by Christopher Columbus, who planted them on the island of Hispaniola in 1493.

The sour or bitter oranges, like the *Seville*, which is used in making marmalade, are probably closest to the original wild fruits. Sweet eating oranges include the western *Navels* (season, November to May), the Florida *Temples* (December to March), the smaller *Mandarins* (November to January), and the imported *Jaffa* oranges (March to May), all of which are easy to peel and section and have an excellent flavor. *Valencia* oranges (March to October) are used for slicing, juicing, and eating whole, whereas the thin-skinned *Hamlins* and *Parson Browns* (October through December) are used mainly for juicing.

What to look for. Buy firm, heavy oranges with fairly smooth skin for the variety; avoid those with soft spots or any that are light, puffy, spongy, or markedly coarse skinned. The orange color is not a reliable indication of ripeness. If coloring has been added to the skin, oranges must be stamped "color added."

How to keep. Refrigerate and use as desired.

Nutritive value. Oranges are rich sources of vitamin C, and contain vitamin A and minerals as well.

Papaya. A native of the Caribbean, the papaya now grows abundantly throughout tropical America. The fruit is usually pear sized and has a central cavity filled with edible, pea-sized black seeds; the sweet, juicy flesh is rather bland, with a slight muskiness and a melonlike texture.

Unripe papayas can be boiled or baked as vegetables, and the leaves, if attached, are often cooked as greens. The juice and leaves of this versatile plant are also the source of an enzyme, papain, which is the active ingredient in commercial meat tenderizers. Like mangoes, papayas secrete a fluid that can often cause an allergic skin reaction in some people. To avoid this, wear rubber gloves while peeling the fruit.

When to buy. Available all year.

What to look for. Choose fruit that is at least half yellow, with smooth, unbroken skin that yields to slight pressure.

How to keep. If necessary, ripen until soft; then refrigerate.

Nutritive value. Papayas are very rich in vitamin A.

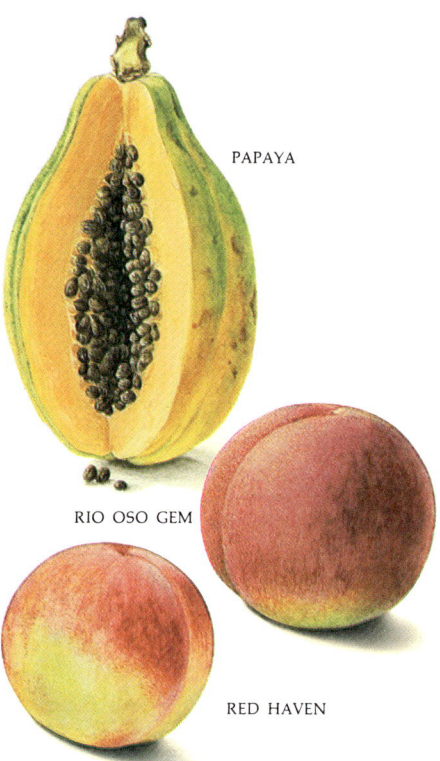

PAPAYA

RIO OSO GEM

RED HAVEN

Peaches. In China, their original habitat, peaches were long venerated as symbols of immortality. Their cultivation spread to Rome, and eventually to the New World.

The many varieties of peaches are divided into two categories: "freestones," with soft juicy flesh that separates readily from the stone, and "clingstones," with firmer flesh that adheres tightly to the stone. Clingstone varieties like the *Red Haven* are generally used for canning; freestones like the *Rio Oso Gem* are eaten fresh or frozen.

When to buy. May through September.

What to look for. Choose mature fruit, fairly firm to slightly soft, with cream to yellow background color and a red blush. Avoid very hard, greenish (immature) peaches, or very soft fruit with bruises or pale-tan spots, which are signs of decay.

How to keep. Ripen at room temperature until soft enough to eat, then refrigerate. Use as soon as possible.

Nutritive value. Peaches are very high in vitamin A.

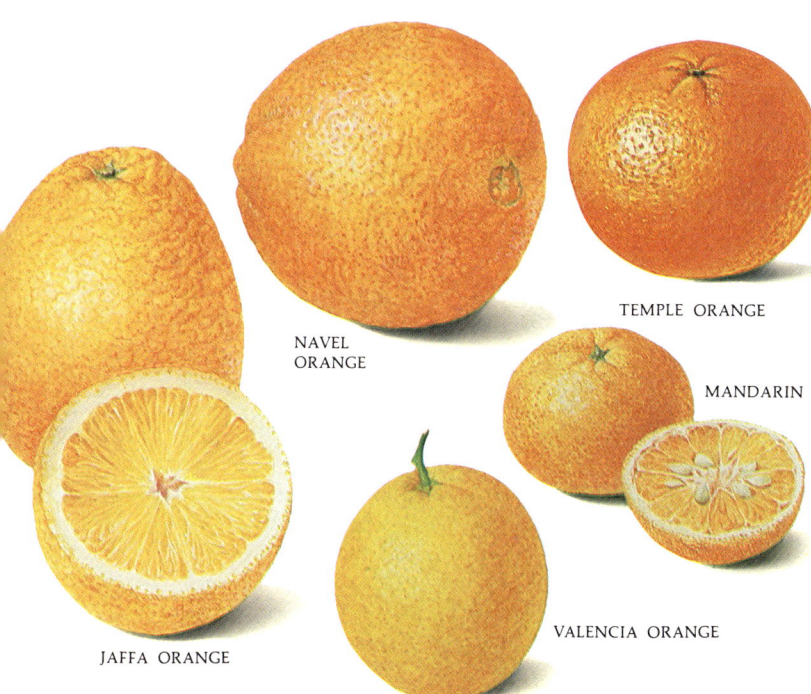

NAVEL ORANGE

TEMPLE ORANGE

MANDARIN

JAFFA ORANGE

VALENCIA ORANGE

Buying Guide
Fruits

Pears. The pear is a delicate, aristocratic, temperate-zone fruit that exists in thousands of varieties—with new ones being constantly produced. Few fruits vary so greatly in color, texture, flavor, size, and shape. Pears are also an exception to the usual rule that tree-ripened fruits are best—they are picked when full grown but still green, and attain their finest texture and flavor (soft on the inside but still firm on the outside) off the tree.

America's most widely grown pear, the *Bartlett*, is bell shaped, with yellow skin and a red blush when ripe. It is excellent for poaching, canning, or eating raw (season, July to mid-October). The yellow-green *Comice*, which also develops a slight red blush, is a soft-fleshed, highly perishable winter pear (season, October to March) of exceptional flavor. The elongated *Bosc*, yellow with russet-brown overtones, is buttery and juicy (season, October to March). Other popular varieties include the large, yellow-green *D'Anjou* and the small, very juicy, granular-textured *Seckel*.

What to look for. Pears should be ripened at room temperature until they yield to slight pressure. Avoid dull, shriveled, or bruised fruit, or any with soft areas near the stem.

How to keep. Refrigerate ripe pears and use as soon as possible.

Nutritive value. Pears contain vitamins A and C.

Persimmons. The very word "persimmon" causes many a mouth to pucker in protest, but in fact these fruits can be very palatable—somewhat astringent, but rich and sweet. The key is ripeness: commercially grown persimmons are picked and marketed unripe because of their extreme perishability; they must be held at room temperature until quite soft for the flavor to develop. Most of the persimmons grown for the U.S. market are an Oriental type—the tomato-shaped, bright-orange fruit known as "kaki."

When to buy. October to January.

What to look for. Buy bright, glossy fruits with stem caps attached. Use soft ones first and ripen firmer ones for later use. Avoid mushy, spotted, or punctured fruits.

How to keep. Refrigerate ripe fruit and use as soon as possible.

Nutritive value. High in vitamins A, C, and minerals.

Pineapple. The first Europeans to encounter the pineapple were the men of Columbus' second voyage, who tasted it on the island of Guadeloupe and were "astonished and delighted" by its succulence. By the late 16th century pineapples were grown in Africa, India, the East Indies, and China.

Pineapples were not planted in Hawaii until 1790, and Hawaiian plantations did not dominate the world market prior to the 20th century because these fruits, which must be ripened on the plant for optimum flavor, spoiled rapidly during shipment. Today, field-ripened pineapples from Hawaii, Mexico, and Central American countries are flown to the continental United States.

When to buy. Available all year, with peak supply April to June.

What to look for. Select plump, heavy fruits with fresh, green crown-leaves, a fragrant aroma, and a very slight separation of the eyes (pips). Avoid fruit with sunken or pointed eyes, dull, discolored, or bruised skin, or brown leaves. An easily removed crown leaf is not a sure indication of ripeness. Though the shell turns yellow with time, pineapples do not ripen after harvest.

How to keep. Refrigerate ripe pineapples; use as soon as possible.

Nutritive value. Pineapples contain vitamins C and A.

Plums. Plums are the most diverse and widely distributed of stone fruits, with varieties suitable to almost any climatic condition; in fact, they are grown on every continent except Antarctica. Prunes are the firm-fleshed variety of plums with a high enough sugar content to permit drying without fermentation around the pit.

Most commercially grown plums are descendants of either European or Japanese varieties. The European plums, oval or round in shape, include all the purple to black varieties (like the *El Dorado*) as well as the smaller, greenish-yellow, richly flavored

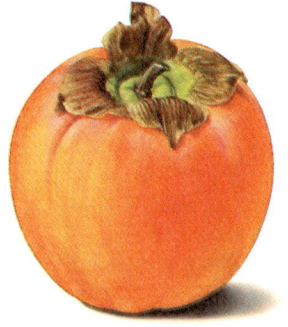
PERSIMMON

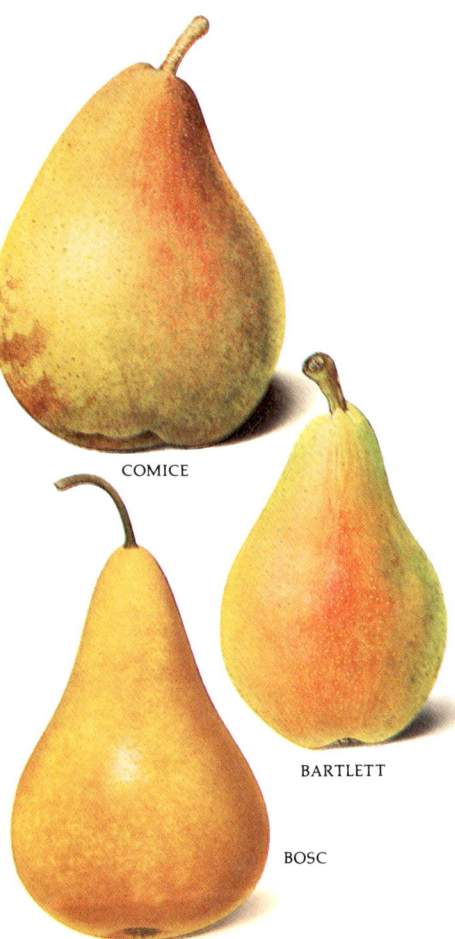
COMICE
BARTLETT
BOSC

Green Gage. The small, bluish-black *Damson* is prized for jams and preserves. The larger, dark-purple *Stanley* is usually eaten as fresh fruit.

The Japanese varieties are larger, with yellow to red skins and juicy flesh—like the crimson *Santa Rosa.* Native American varieties are seldom grown commercially, but they have been extensively hybridized with Japanese plums to increase their hardiness.

When to buy. For prune plums, June to October; for others, late May through September.

What to look for. Buy slightly soft fruits of good color for the variety. Avoid unripe, very hard fruits of dull coloring.

How to keep. Ripen firm fruits at room temperature; refrigerate others and use as soon as possible.

Nutritive value. Plums are a good source of vitamin A.

Pomegranate. An ancient symbol of fertility, this many-seeded fruit is mentioned in the Old Testament and is central to the Greek legend of Persephone, who was condemned to spend half of each year in the kingdom of Hades after she had eaten six forbidden pomegranate seeds.

Pomegranates are exotic-looking fruits about the size of an orange, with thin, tough skins—usually golden to deep red—filled with edible seeds in crimson pulp. (There are, however, a few seedless types.) The flavor ranges from acid to sweet, depending on the variety. Pomegranate juice is used to make grenadine syrup.

When to buy. September to November.

What to look for. Buy bright red or pink fruits with unbroken skins.

How to keep. Refrigerate ripe pomegranates and use within a few days.

Quince. Most people demand sweet fruits and may find fresh quinces inedible, but this was not always so. These yellow fruits, which probably originated in Asia Minor, have been cultivated for more than 4,000 years; at least through medieval times, most Europeans ate them fresh as well as cooking and preserving them.

Quinces were once thought to be a type of pear, and in fact pears are often grown on quince rootstock, but the two fruits cannot be hybridized. Until the late 18th century, marmalade was usually made from quinces: the word "marmalade" derives from *marmelo,* Portuguese for quince.

When to buy. Available end of July to October.

What to look for. Buy firm, smooth, bright-colored quinces with no punctures, bruises, or soft spots.

How to keep. Refrigerate and use them when desired.

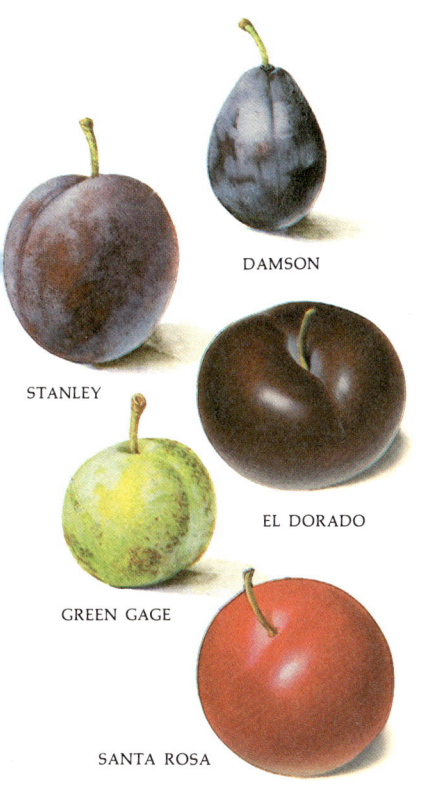
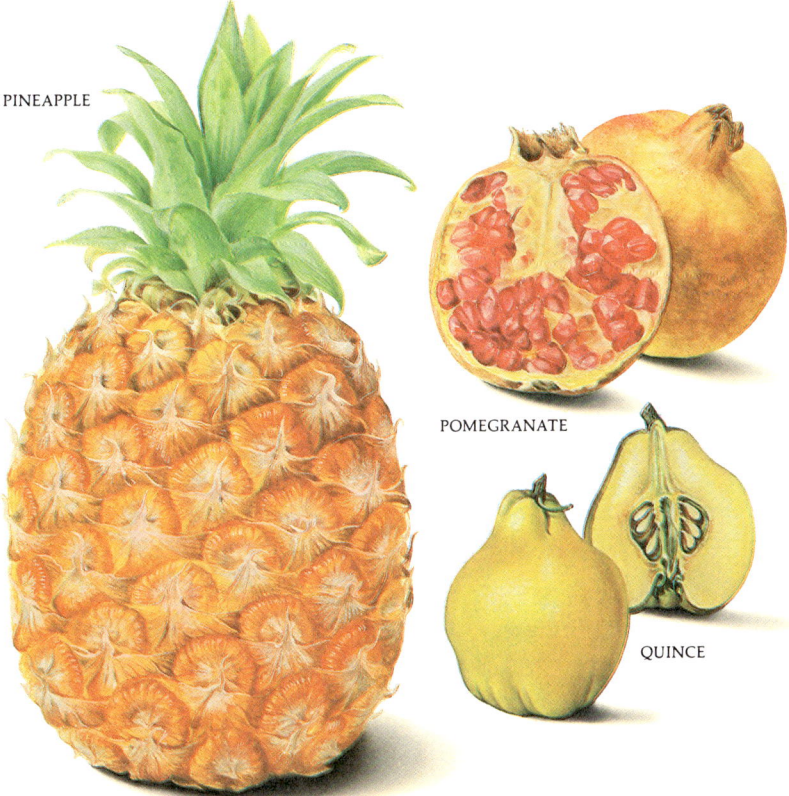

133

Buying Guide
Fruits

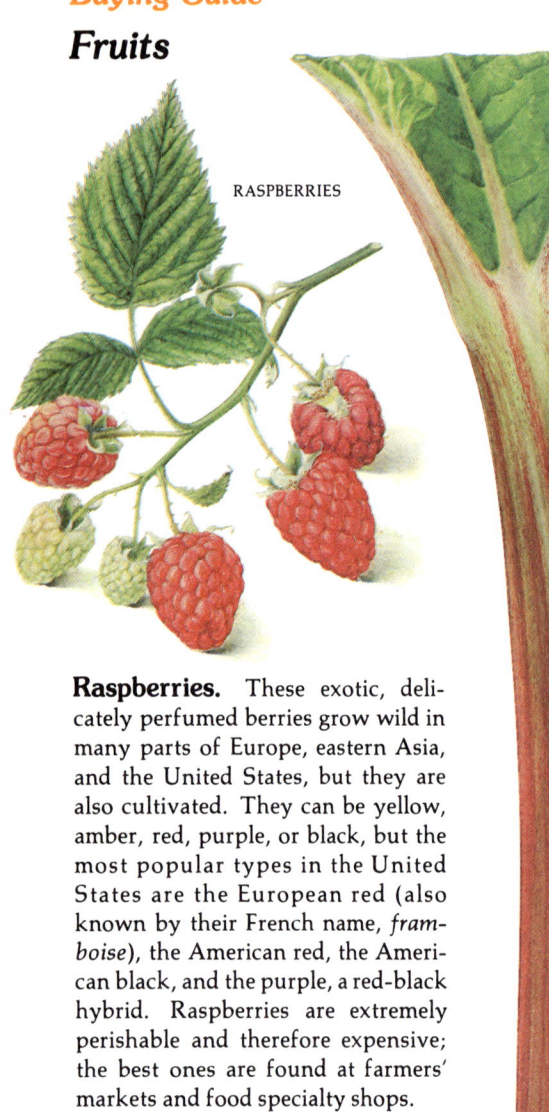

RASPBERRIES

RHUBARB

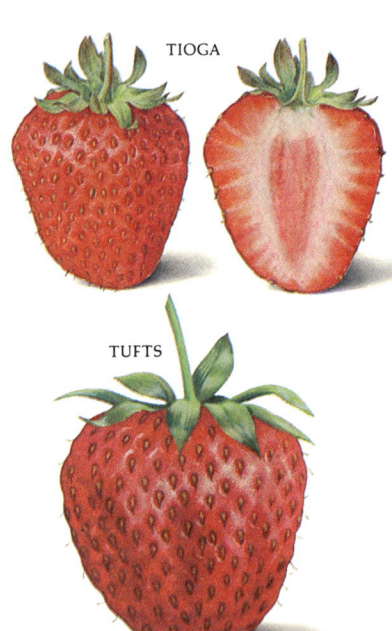

TIOGA

TUFTS

Raspberries. These exotic, delicately perfumed berries grow wild in many parts of Europe, eastern Asia, and the United States, but they are also cultivated. They can be yellow, amber, red, purple, or black, but the most popular types in the United States are the European red (also known by their French name, *framboise*), the American red, the American black, and the purple, a red-black hybrid. Raspberries are extremely perishable and therefore expensive; the best ones are found at farmers' markets and food specialty shops.

When to buy. June to October.

What to look for. Raspberries are always sold hulled. Choose plump berries in dry, unstained containers.

How to keep. Use on day of purchase. Before serving, wash berries very gently, discarding any that are mushy or moldy.

Rhubarb. For thousands of years, rhubarb was grown only for its roots, which were used medicinally as a purgative. Few people thought of using the plant for food until the 17th century, when some misguided English botanists tried cooking and eating the leaves, which contain dangerous amounts of oxalic acid. The pink stalks, however, are edible.

Botanically a vegetable, rhubarb stalks are always used as a fruit. They are especially good for pies but can also be stewed, baked, or used in puddings, sauces, jams, and jellies.

When to buy. February to June, with peak in April and May.

What to look for. Field-grown rhubarb has larger, redder stalks than the hothouse kind and may need peeling. To do this, choose firm, crisp stalks and discard the coarse green leaves.

How to keep. Refrigerate and use as desired.

Nutritive value. Rhubarb is rich in minerals.

Strawberries. As one strawberry lover put it in the early 17th century: "Doubtless God could have made a better berry, but doubtless God never did." Doubtless, too, the writer was speaking of wild strawberries, whose sweet fragrance, flavor, and juiciness are equaled only by their extreme perishability.

Most of today's cultivated strawberries are descendants of two wild species which were accidentally hybridized in the 18th century: the so-called Chilean strawberry, native to the Pacific coasts of both North and South America, and the Virginia strawberry, from North America's East Coast. From this hybrid have come many varieties, suitable for climates as different as those of Florida and the Canadian prairies.

Cultivated strawberries are classified as one crop (those that bear a single crop each season, like the *Tufts* and the *Tioga*) or everbearing (those that bear a succession of crops until frost, like the *Ozark Beauty*).

When to buy. Available all year, with peak April through June.

What to look for. Buy bright, firm berries with green stem caps attached; avoid leaky or moldy berries. In general, very large berries have less flavor than small to medium ones.

How to keep. Refrigerate and use as soon as possible. Wash and hull berries just before eating.

Nutritive value. Strawberries are rich in vitamin C.

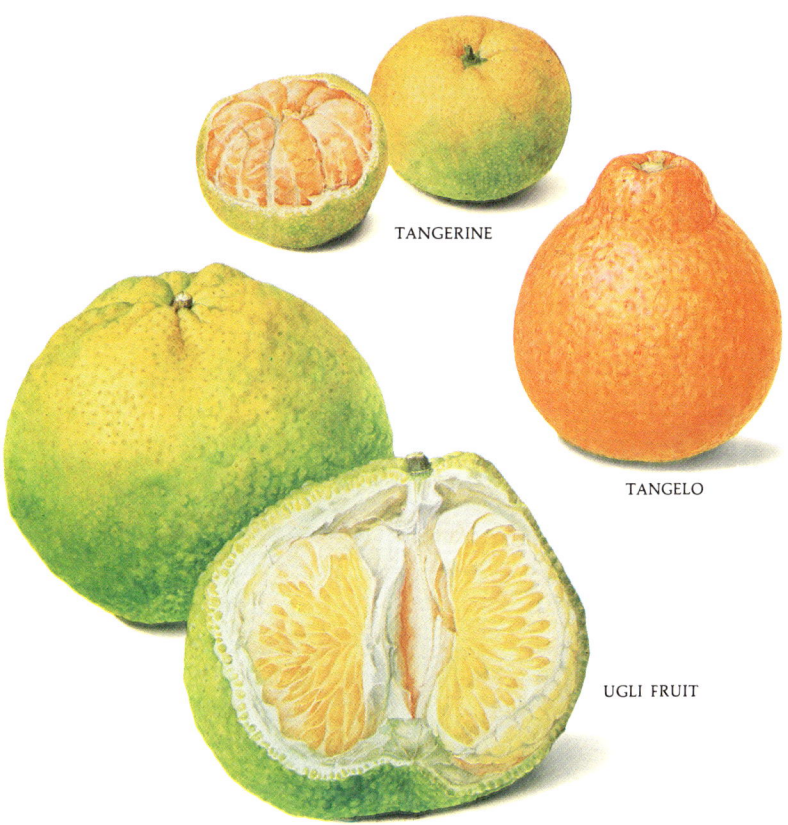

TANGERINE

TANGELO

UGLI FRUIT

Tangelo. A citrus fruit with a rather complex family tree, the tangelo is not one hybrid but a group of hybrids. Tangelos are created by crossing either the Mandarin orange or the tangerine with the grapefruit or the closely related pomelo (see entry for Grapefruit). Whatever the combination, the result is a large, thin-skinned, orangelike fruit that is "necked" (drawn out at the stem end). The flesh is rich and juicy. Tangelos are excellent for juicing, fruit salads, or eating whole.

When to buy. October through January.

What to look for. Tangelos are delicate and easily bruised. Buy firm fruits, heavy for their size, with a minimum of blemishes.

How to keep. Store at room temperature or refrigerate.

Nutritive value. Tangelos contain vitamin C.

Tangerine. Named after the city of Tangier in North Africa, this small, loose-skinned citrus fruit is actually a variety of Mandarin orange—the most important variety. Unlike other Mandarins, which are often canned, tangerines are generally marketed fresh. The juicy segments, which separate readily, are dark orange, with a sweet, delicate flavor. The skin ripens to a deep orange-red.

When to buy. Available all year, with peak in late November through early March.

What to look for. Choose deep-orange to orange-red fruits, heavy for their size, with a bright luster. Loose skin is normal, but avoid fruits with punctures, mold, soft spots, or very pale skins.

How to keep. Refrigerate and use as soon as possible.

Nutritive value. Tangerines contain vitamins C and A.

Ugli Fruit. This coarse-skinned citrus fruit lives up to its billing: it resembles a grapefruit with a bad case of adolescent acne. The skin is thick, knobbly, loose fitting, and altogether unprepossessing, but the flesh is sweet and juicy, with an orangelike flavor and a few seeds.

The origins of this odd fruit are obscure: it may be a grapefruit-tangerine-Seville orange hybrid, or possibly a mutant tangelo. It was first discovered in Jamaica in the early 20th century, and most of the U.S. supply is still imported from that Caribbean island.

When to buy. Usually available December to May.

What to look for. Mature fruit should be orange with light-green blotches. Loose skin is normal, but the fruit should be heavy for its size.

How to keep. Store at room temperature or refrigerate.

Buying Guide
Freshwater Fish

A nutritious food, fish can be more economical to serve than meat. In general, there is less waste with fish, and it takes less time and energy to cook than meat. Shown on these two pages are some of the popular varieties of freshwater fish; for saltwater fish, see pages 138-139. When buying any fish, consider the following information. A fish sold in the form in which it was caught is called a *whole fish*. You will need about ¾ of a pound of whole fish for each person. A *dressed fish* has had the head, tail, fins, entrails, and scales removed; buy ½ pound per serving. *Fillets* are the sides of the fish cut away from the backbone; *steaks* are crosscuts; *portions* are pieces cut from large blocks. When buying fillets, steaks, or portions, allow about ⅓ of a pound per person.

What to look for. Fresh fish should look clean and have a pleasant odor; the flesh should bounce back when poked. The eyes should be clear and bulging; the gills pink or red. If fillets or steaks, they should not have dry, brown edges. If buying frozen fish, be sure it is frozen solid, has little or no odor, and is not discolored.

How to keep. Use fish as soon as possible. If you store fish, wrap it tightly in an air- and moisture-proof wrapping such as aluminum foil. Frozen fish will keep 4 to 6 months.

Nutritive value. Fish contains high-quality protein, many vitamins, minerals, and polyunsaturated fats. The so-called lean fish is less than 2½ percent fat whereas an oily fish contains more than 5 percent fat.

Black Bass. This is a type of sunfish that includes the *largemouth bass*, *redeye bass*, and *smallmouth bass*. In general, the flesh of a black bass is firm, white, and bland to sweet tasting; the skin, however, is unpleasant tasting. Market size for black bass ranges from 1 to 4 pounds.

Buffalofish. Caught in shallow rivers and large lakes primarily in the Plains states, buffalofish are members of the sucker family. The *bigmouth buffalo*, the largest of the species, usually weighs from 3 to 12 pounds but can be as much as 80 pounds. The *smallmouth buffalo* is smaller but generally better tasting than the bigmouth buffalo. Both have lean, firm flesh.

Carp. This fish is found in lakes, streams, and ponds all over the United States. It prefers warm, slow, shallow waters, but it can tolerate unfavorable water conditions. The market size can vary from 2 to 20 pounds. Edible carp flesh is light in color, lean, and firm; it is sold fresh, smoked, and pickled. Carp should be skinned, and the dark part of the flesh should be removed before eating.

Catfish. Found mostly in the southern and central parts of the United States, catfish have firm, moist, white flesh that has a delicate flavor. The *channel catfish*, *white catfish*, and *blue catfish* are very popular. The channel catfish likes clean streams and large lakes; it cannot tolerate polluted waters. It is best when small (3 pounds) but can weigh up to 60 pounds. The blue catfish is considered to be the best-tasting catfish; it prefers fast-moving, clear streams. The white catfish is a coastal species and is often found in brackish waters; it averages 1 pound.

Cisco. A cold-water lake fish, the cisco is found in the Great Lakes and lakes in the northern United States and Canada. The flesh is delicate and white, but oily. It is available fresh and smoked; when cisco is smoked, it is called *smoked chub*.

Crappie. A member of the sunfish family, it is found in lakes and rivers in the central, southern, and northern parts of the United States. Two important types are the *white crappie* and the *black crappie* (*calico crappie*, *calico bass*). Both have lean, tender, white flesh. Black crappies prefer clear waters and weigh 1 to 2 pounds. White crappies like silty waters and weigh under 1 pound.

Freshwater Drum. These fish are caught in large rivers and lakes in the central and eastern parts of the United States from Canada down to the Gulf of Mexico. Although they prefer clear waters, they are generally found in silty waters. Freshwater drum, also known as *sheepshead* and *grunter*, has coarse, lean, white flesh and can weigh 1½ to 5 pounds.

Perch. These fish are found in cool, clean lakes and rivers in the northern and central United States from the east to the west coasts. *Walleye* is the largest member of the perch family. Though usually weighing from 1 to 3 pounds, walleye can grow to be about 20 pounds. *Yellow perch* are smaller. Both perches have lean, white, firm flesh that has a sweet, pleasant taste. Yellow perch is also known as *ringed perch* and *striped perch*.

Pike. These fish are found most often in the Great Lakes area. *Northern pike*, *pickerel*, and *muskellunge* are three types of pike. Pike are bony; the flesh is white, firm, lean, and sweet but dry. Pike can weigh 4 to 10 pounds; muskellunge usually weigh up to 30 pounds. *Pickerel* (young pike) weigh 2 to 3 pounds.

Smelt. This is a very small, oily fish found along the Atlantic and Pacific coasts, in the Great Lakes, and in small lakes in the northeastern United States. About 10 smelts equal one pound. Smelts can be eaten whole, bones and all; their flesh is sweet and delicate. They are available fresh, canned, or smoked.

Temperate Bass. The *white bass* and *yellow bass* (not shown) are temperate basses; they are relatives of and look similar to the striped bass (shown on page 139). Yellow bass are found in lakes and rivers in the central United States; white bass are found in lakes from the Great Lakes down into the southern and southwestern United States. Yellow and white bass weigh ½ to 2 pounds.

Trout. This popular fish is caught in lakes and streams in the northern United States. The flesh varies in color from white to red depending on the diet of the fish and whether it is wild or from a commercial fishery. The taste also depends on the diet as well as the quality of the water that the fish lived in; those taken from fresh, clear water will taste the best. Some trout are anadromous, that is, they migrate between fresh and salt waters. *Brook trout* is considered to be the finest trout. Other trouts are *brown trout* (sea-run version is the *sea trout*), *golden trout*, *rainbow trout* (sea-run version is the *steelhead trout*), and *lake trout* (*togue, mackinaw, gray trout*). Trout is sold fresh or smoked; it weighs 1 to 20 pounds depending on the type.

Whitefish. These fish are caught in the Great Lakes and lakes in the northeastern and northwestern United States. The most available whitefish is the *lake whitefish*. Two others are the *mountain whitefish* (*Rocky Mountain whitefish*) and the *round whitefish* (*Menominee, greyback*). Whitefish weigh 1 to 4 pounds; its flesh is oily but white, flaky, and delicately flavored. It is available fresh and smoked.

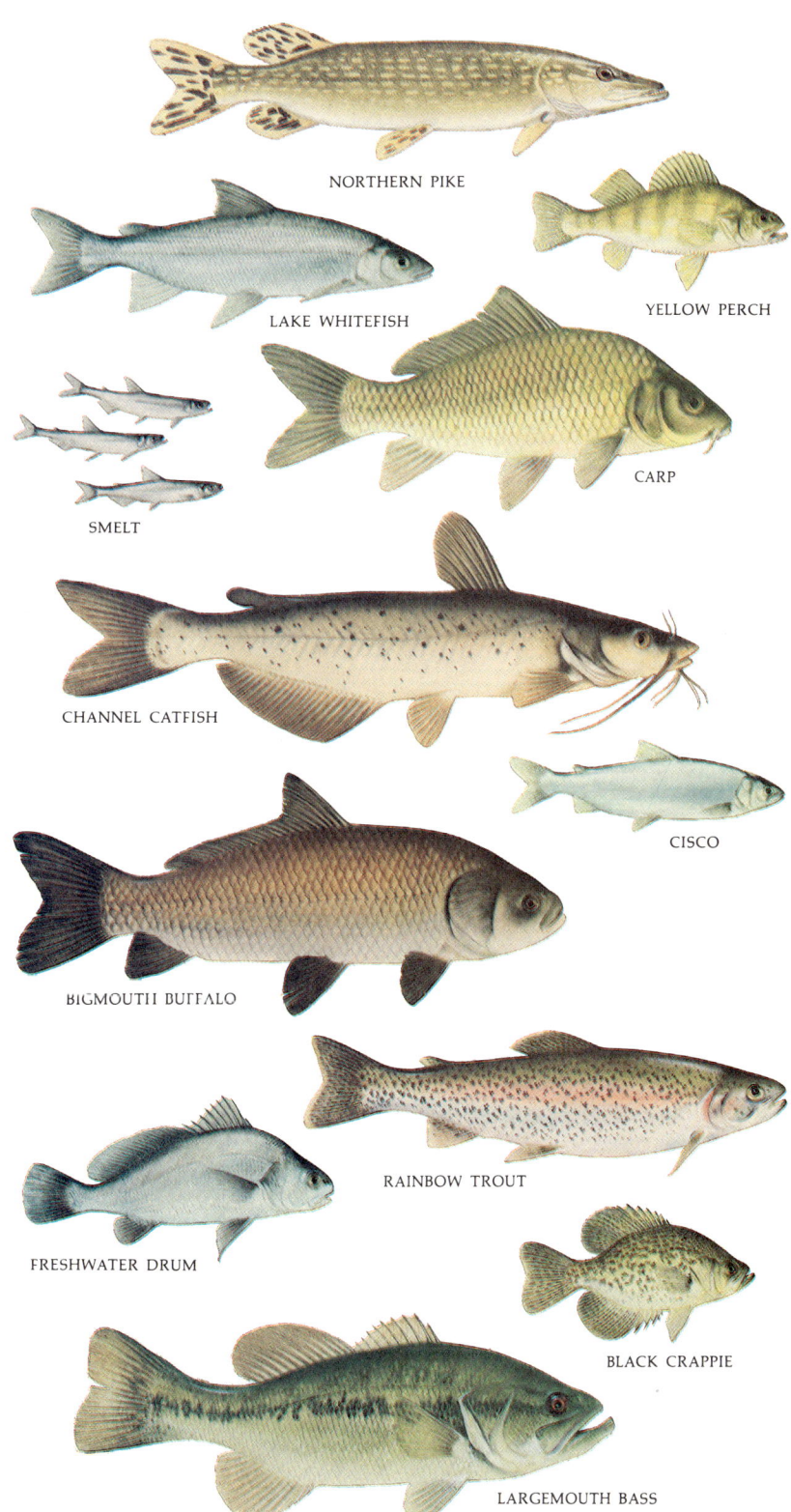

FAMILY FOOD GUIDE

NORTHERN PIKE
LAKE WHITEFISH
YELLOW PERCH
SMELT
CARP
CHANNEL CATFISH
CISCO
BIGMOUTH BUFFALO
RAINBOW TROUT
FRESHWATER DRUM
BLACK CRAPPIE
LARGEMOUTH BASS

Buying Guide
Saltwater Fish

Saltwater fish, like their freshwater cousins, are high in vitamins B_1, B_6, D, niacin, and pantothenic acid and in phosphorus, sulfur, and selenium. In addition, saltwater fish are also good sources of chloride, fluoride, and iodine. Although they contain sodium, the level in the fish (unless it is smoked) is not high enough to exclude saltwater fish from low-salt diets. Some of the more popular saltwater fish are presented on these two pages. Swordfish and tuna, two of the bigger fish, are not illustrated because the average fish market does not sell these fish whole. When buying and storing saltwater fish, follow the same guidelines as given on page 136.

Black Sea Bass. Found in the Atlantic Ocean from Cape Cod to Florida, the black sea bass has a firm, dark, and flaky flesh. It usually weighs 1 to 3 pounds. Large males are called *humpbacks*.

Bluefish. This fish is found in the Atlantic Ocean from Nova Scotia to Florida. Its flesh is soft, dark, and mild tasting; because bluefish are oily, they are more perishable than nonoily fish. The usual market size is 10 to 12 pounds.

Butterfish. A small fish (less than 1 pound), it gets its name from its high fat content. Found in the Atlantic Ocean from Nova Scotia to the Gulf of Mexico, butterfish have white, very tender, good-tasting flesh.

Cod. This is a North Atlantic and North Pacific fish that has lean, white, firm flesh. Usually weighing 4 to 7 pounds, it is sold fresh, smoked, canned, and salted. The *Atlantic cod* is one of the most important. Another member of the cod family is *pollock*. Pollock is sold fresh or smoked, and the market size is usually 4 to 5 pounds.

Flounder. This large family of flatfish includes flukes, halibuts, turbots, and dabs. Flounder flesh is firm, white, and lean and has a delicate taste. Two important flounders are the *summer flounder* and *winter flounder*. Much of the fish sold as *sole* is actually flounder. The winter flounder is often sold as *grey sole* or *lemon sole*. Flounder are caught along most of the eastern coast of the United States.

Haddock. The haddock is a member of the cod family generally weighing 1 to 6 pounds. Haddock flesh is white, firm, and flaky. It is available fresh or in smoked form. Haddock that has been smoked is also known as *finnan haddie*.

Hake. This fish is a member of the cod family. There are several types of hakes, two of which are the *silver hake* and the *red hake*. Hake flesh is a little bit coarser than cod but tastier. The average market size of hake is 1½ pounds.

Halibut. This is a flatfish belonging to the flounder family. Caught in the Atlantic and Pacific oceans, the most popular halibuts are the *Atlantic halibut* and the *Pacific halibut*. All are excellent-eating, white-flesh fish. Halibuts are usually quite large; the Pacific halibut can weigh up to 600 pounds. Very small halibut (those that weigh about 5 pounds) are called *chicken halibut*.

Mackerel. A good-tasting, oily fish, mackerel is caught in the Atlantic and Pacific oceans. Some popular mackerels are the *Atlantic mackerel, cero mackerel, Spanish mackerel*, and the *wahoo*. Mackerel can weigh from 2 to 30 pounds; is sold fresh, smoked, salted, canned, or pickled.

Mullet. Found in both the Atlantic and Pacific oceans, mullet are very rich in iodine. Two important types are *white mullet* and *striped mullet*. Mullet has a mild, nutty flavor. It is available fresh; those high in oil are usually smoked.

Ocean Perch. A North Atlantic fish, ocean perch is also known as *redfish, rosefish, Norway haddock, red perch*, and *sea perch*. Its average weight is 1 pound. Most ocean perch is sold frozen as fillets or in the form of fish sticks.

Porgy. This fish has firm, white flesh and a delicate taste. Some of the most common porgies are the *red porgy, jolthead porgy, white porgy*, and *scup*. Caught in the Atlantic and Pacific oceans, most porgies weigh 1 to 4 pounds; the red porgies can weigh up to 12 pounds. Porgies have small, sharp bones.

Salmon. Found along the Atlantic and Pacific coasts of the United States, salmon live in the sea but migrate into freshwater rivers in order to spawn. The best-known salmon are the *Atlantic salmon, chinook salmon, coho salmon*, and *sockeye salmon*. The taste of the flesh depends on the waters where the fish was caught; the color of the flesh varies according to the type. Chinook flesh is white, Atlantic salmon flesh is white or pink, and sockeye flesh is red. The average market size is 10 pounds; salmon is sold fresh (usually in steak form), smoked, salted, or canned.

Seatrout. These fish are caught along the eastern coast of the United States; they are members of the drum family. The *spotted seatrout* (*speckled trout*) weighs 4 to 10 pounds and has fine, white, delicately flavored meat. Other seatrouts are the *sand seatrout* and *silver seatrout*. Sea trout (two words) is the sea-run version of brown trout (page 137).

FAMILY FOOD GUIDE

Shad. Members of the herring family, two popular shad are the *American shad* and the *hickory shad*. Shad are caught along the eastern coast of the United States, and they range in weight from 1½ to 8 pounds. The flesh is soft but bony; shad is sold fresh, smoked, or pickled.

Snapper. This is a tropical-water fish also caught along the southeastern seaboard of the United States. Among the most common snappers are the *grey snapper* and the *red snapper*. The red snapper weighs 4 to 6 pounds; the grey snapper is usually less than 1 pound. Snapper meat is white and sweet.

Sole. This flatfish is found in European waters. Most of the sole sold in the United States is actually flounder.

Striped Bass. Found in both the Atlantic and Pacific oceans, this fish is a relative of the temperate bass (page 137). South of New Jersey, striped bass is called *rockfish*. Although it can be much larger, striped bass is best when it is 6 to 8 pounds. The taste of the fish is affected by its diet and the quality of the water it lived in.

Swordfish. Found all over the world in temperate and tropical waters, swordfish (not shown) has firm, flaky, good-tasting meat. It is considered an oily fish and can therefore spoil faster than a nonoily fish. Swordfish is available fresh or frozen but usually only in steak form.

Tuna. A member of the mackerel family, tuna (not shown) is caught in both the Atlantic and Pacific oceans. There are many types of tunas, including *albacore tuna*, *blackfin tuna*, *bluefin tuna*, and *yellowfin tuna*. Tuna are very large fish. Most of the tuna caught is canned, and only albacore tuna can be labeled as being "white meat tuna."

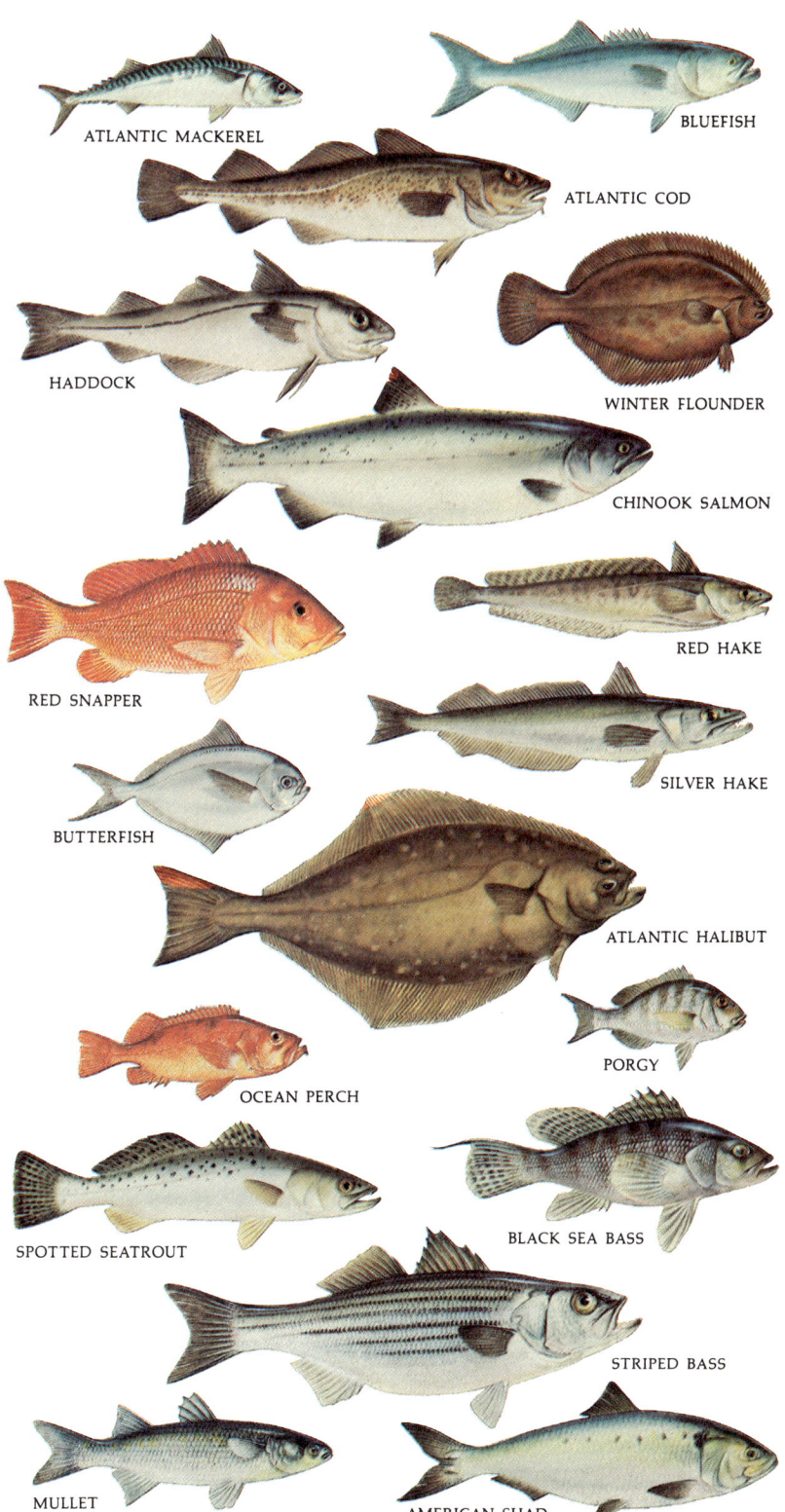

ATLANTIC MACKEREL
BLUEFISH
ATLANTIC COD
HADDOCK
WINTER FLOUNDER
CHINOOK SALMON
RED HAKE
RED SNAPPER
SILVER HAKE
BUTTERFISH
ATLANTIC HALIBUT
PORGY
OCEAN PERCH
SPOTTED SEATROUT
BLACK SEA BASS
STRIPED BASS
MULLET
AMERICAN SHAD

Buying Guide
Shellfish

Some of the most popular of all the seafoods are included in this group known as crustaceans and mollusks but more commonly referred to as shellfish. Of the shellfish discussed on these two pages, crabs, crayfish, lobsters, and shrimps are crustaceans; all of the others are mollusks.

Note: Clams, oysters, and mussels get their food by filtering microscopic particles from the water that passes through their bodies. As a result, these shellfish can become toxic from polluted waters. Those grown in commercial beds are screened and inspected for wholesomeness before going to market. If gathering the shellfish yourself, check with the local authorities as to the cleanliness of the water and bed.

How to keep. All crustaceans and mollusks are highly perishable, taste best when freshly caught, and should be used as soon as possible. If purchased fresh, store in the coldest part of the refrigerator; if frozen, keep in the freezer until ready to thaw and use. Some shellfish—crabs, lobsters, clams, mussels, and oysters—can be purchased live. For information on **What to look for,** see the individual entries.

Nutritive value. Crustaceans and mollusks are good sources of high-quality proteins and polyunsaturated fats. They are also good sources of many vitamins (thiamin, riboflavin, niacin, B_6, B_{12}, and pantothenic acid) and minerals (calcium, zinc, copper, fluoride, and phosphorus). All of them (except crayfish) are especially high in iodine; all but oysters and soft-shell clams are too high in sodium to be recommended for low-salt diets. Shellfish have as much cholesterol as meat and milk products; however, some egg products and cuts of beef have even more cholesterol than fish and shellfish. All shellfish are easily digested.

Abalone. This mollusk (not shown) is found in many parts of the world, including the waters off the California coast. *Red abalone* has a reddish shell about 6 inches wide. Abalone meat is white and is usually cut into steaks or fillets. It is available fresh (in California) or canned; buy ¼ pound per person.

Clams. The most popular East Coast clams are the *hard-shell clam (quahog)* and *soft-shell clam (steamer)*. Hard-shell clams are named according to their size—the *Little Neck clam* is about 1½ inches across and the *cherrystone clam* is about 2 inches across. Any hard-shell clam over 2 inches wide is called a *chowder clam* and is used in chowders. Some West Coast clams are the *Pismo, goeduck,* and *littleneck* (one word). *Razor clams* are found on both coasts. Clams are sold live and shucked (flesh removed from the shell). Shucked clams can be fresh, frozen, smoked, or canned. Buy 16 to 20 clams per serving. If buying live clams, the shells must be closed or, if open, they must close when you tap on them. If buying fresh-shucked clams, the meat should be plump and surrounded with clear liquid with no signs of shell. Never refreeze thawed clams.

Crab. The most common crab, the *blue crab*, is found along the East Coast, primarily in the Chesapeake area. The *stone crab* is caught off the Florida coast. Two Pacific crabs are the *Dungeness crab* and the *king crab*. King crab is very large (10 pounds average) and is found off the coast of Alaska. A *soft-shell crab* is any crab that has molted its shell; most often, the soft-shell crabs sold in markets are blue crabs. Crab is sold live, fresh, frozen, or canned. If buying live crabs, choose those that move their legs, feel heavy in proportion to their size, and have a fresh, ammonia-free odor. Buy a 1-pound hard-shell crab per serving; buy 2 soft-shell crabs per serving. If buying shelled crabmeat, figure ¼ pound per person.

Crayfish. These freshwater crustaceans can be found in all parts of the United States, especially the South. They are similar to lobsters in appearance and taste but are generally much smaller. Crayfish can be as small as 1 inch, but the preferred eating size is about 6 inches. Buy about 10 crayfish per serving.

Lobster. The most common lobster in the United States is the *American lobster*, many of which are caught off the coast of Maine. The shell is dark green or blue but turns red when cooked. Another popular lobster is the *spiny lobster*, which is also called *crawfish* and *rock lobster*. Spiny lobsters do not have claws; most of the meat comes from the tail. Lobster is sold frozen and live. When buying live lobster, pick active ones with both their claws. Buy 1 lobster (about 1½ pounds) per serving.

Mussels. These mollusks are found on both coasts of the United States; *blue mussels* are the most common type. When buying live mussels, select those with tightly closed shells; if slightly open, the shells should not move from side to side. Mussels are also sold shucked, fresh, or frozen. Figure on 18 to 24 small or 12 large mussels per serving.

Octopus. This mollusk is caught in the Atlantic and Pacific oceans. The two most common types are the *Atlantic octopus* and the *Pacific octopus*. Octopus is usually cut up and then sold fresh. It can also be purchased frozen, canned, salted, pickled, or smoked. Buy about ¼ pound of octopus per person.

FAMILY FOOD GUIDE

Oysters. Found along both the Atlantic and Pacific coasts of the United States, their taste, size, shape, and color will depend on the oyster bed. Some popular oysters are the *New Orleans oyster*, *Blue Point oyster*, and *Cape Cod oyster*. If buying live oysters, choose those with tightly closed shells or open shells that close when you tap on them. Oysters are also sold shucked, fresh, frozen, canned, or smoked. Buy about 12 medium-sized oysters per serving.

Scallops. The *bay scallop* (shell measures about 3 inches across) is considered to be more tender and tastier than the sea scallop; bay scallops are caught in inlets and bays from Cape Cod to Cape Hatteras. *Sea scallops* are larger (5-inch-wide shell) than bay scallops and are found in the waters from Labrador to New Jersey. Scallops are usually sold as shucked meat, which should be creamy in color. Buy ⅓ pound per person.

Shrimp. The main supply of shrimp for the United States comes from the South Atlantic, the Gulf of Mexico, and Alaska. There are many types of shrimp, varying in color and size. Shrimp are available fresh, frozen, smoked, dried, or canned. Fresh shrimp should be firm and smell fresh, with no ammonia odor. They are sold according to the count per pound; for example, 10 to 15 shrimps per pound. The count will vary according to the size of the shrimp. In general, 2 pounds of uncooked shrimp in the shell equals 1 pound after shelling and deveining. Buy ½ pound of shrimp per serving.

Squid. Although these mollusks can vary in size from 1 inch to 6 feet, the average market size is 3 inches. The flesh is firm and lean and becomes yellow when cooked. Figure about ¼ pound of squid per person. Squid is available fresh, frozen, salted, pickled, dried, or canned.

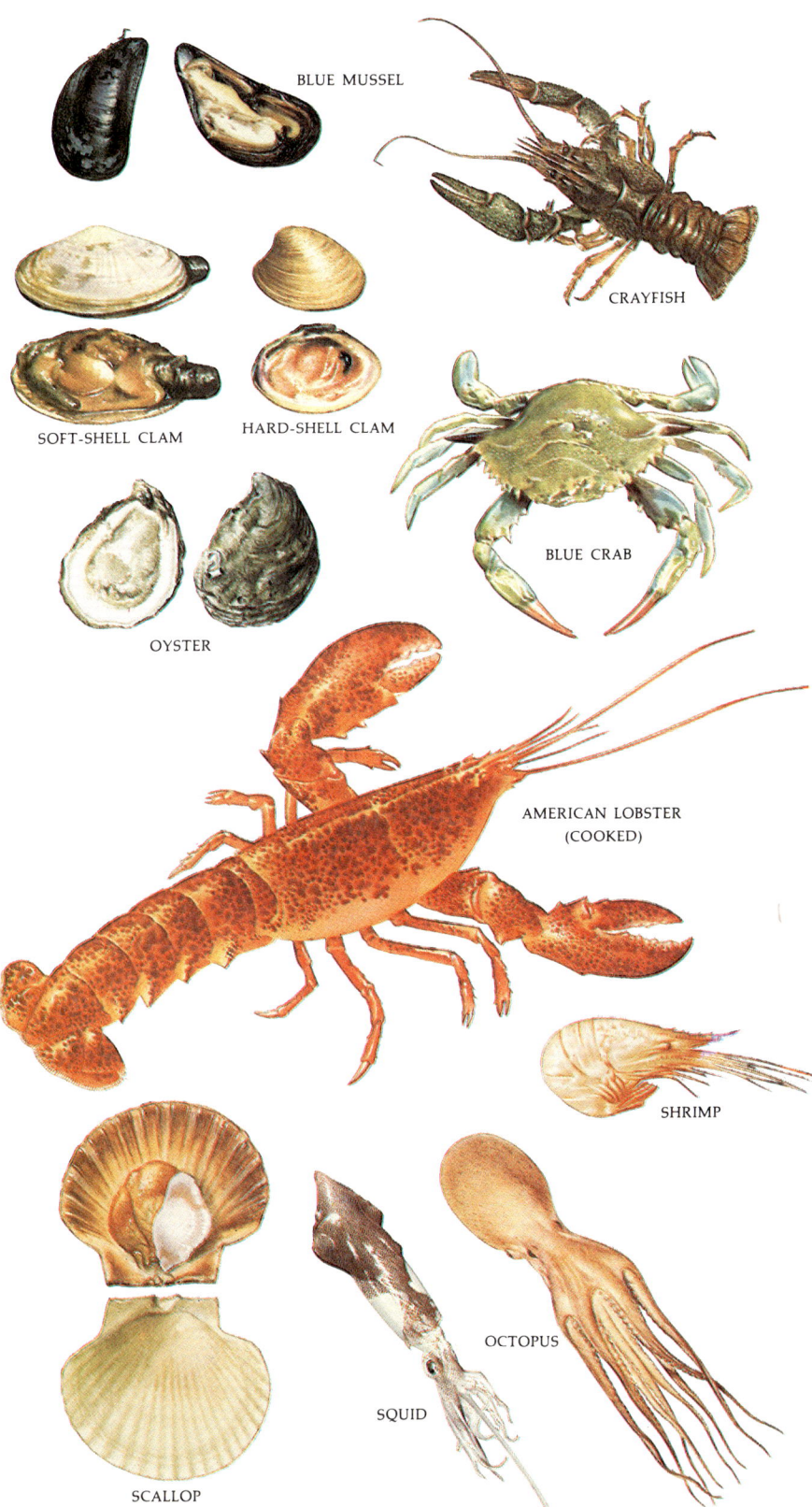

Buying Guide
Beef

All beef sold in the United States must be inspected for wholesomeness by federal or state authorities; most is graded for quality by the U.S. Department of Agriculture. Usually, only USDA Choice or Good grades are sold in markets; the top grade, USDA Prime, as well as the lower grades, are rarely available to the shopper. Most of the tender steaks can be broiled or fried; tougher cuts of beef should be cooked in moist heat, that is, braised or stewed. Not all cuts are illustrated.

What to look for. Cuts from the least used muscles, such as in the rib, short loin, and sirloin sections, are usually the most tender.

How to keep. Wrap loosely in paper to keep surfaces dry and refrigerate. Avoid packaged meat with accumulated liquid. For storage times and tips on freezing, see pages 204-209.

Nutritive value. Meats are good sources of high-quality proteins, vitamin B_{12} and niacin, and many minerals such as iron, phosphorus, sulfur, potassium, chloride, sodium, and magnesium.

Rib
Rib roast. Taken from the top of the rib, this tender cut has both fat and bone. It can be cut into *rib steaks*.

Rib eye roast. This boneless roast, also called *Delmonico roast*, is the eye muscle from the center of the rib. It can be cut into *rib eye steaks*.

Short Loin
Loin tenderloin roast. Cut from the top back part of the short loin, tenderloin is boneless, tender, good tasting, and has little fat. Also called *filet mignon*, it can be cut into steaks.

Loin porterhouse steak. A tasty steak cut from the top back part of the short loin, it contains a back and finger bone and the tenderloin.

Loin T-bone steak. This is a steak cut from the top middle of the short loin. It is similar to a porterhouse steak but with less tenderloin.

Loin top loin steak. This steak, from the top of the short loin, has a backbone. It is also called *shell steak* or *club steak*.

Sirloin
Sirloin steaks. When cut from the top front part of the sirloin, the steak is called a *loin pinbone sirloin steak*. It contains some tenderloin and parts of the back and hipbones. The *loin flat bone sirloin steak* is from the top center of the sirloin; it has some tenderloin and a long, flat hipbone. The *loin wedge bone sirloin steak*, from the top back of the sirloin, has parts of the back and hipbones. Any of the sirloin steaks can also be boneless.

Tip roast. This is a lean, boneless roast cut from the bottom of the sirloin or round sections.

Chuck
Chuck blade roast. A tasty piece of meat from the top back of the chuck, this can be cut into *chuck blade steaks*. The closer the cut is to the rib (called "first cut"), the more tender it is. Better grade roasts can be oven roasted. First-cut blade steaks can be broiled or fried; braise other cuts.

Chuck eye roast (boneless). This cut is the center, meaty portion of blade chuck. It has some fat and can be roasted or braised. It can also be cut into *chuck eye steaks* that can be broiled, fried, or braised.

Chuck arm pot roast. A flavorful, tough cut with a round arm bone, it should be cooked with moist heat.

Chuck shoulder pot roast (boneless). This cut is from the front top section of the chuck. Better grades can be oven roasted; cook lower grades in moist heat. Chuck shoulder can be cut into *chuck shoulder steaks* that are good braised.

Chuck short ribs. These small, rectangular cuts have bone, meat, and fat; braise or cook in liquid.

Short Plate
Plate skirt steak. This boneless cut is flavorful but not tender. It can be braised, broiled, or fried. It is also called *diaphragm*.

Flank
Flank steak. Often called *London broil*, this boneless, oval cut of meat has very little fat and is not very tender. Better grades can be broiled.

Brisket and Fore Shank
Brisket. Not a very tender piece of meat, brisket should be cooked with moist heat. There are two cuts: *point half boneless (thick cut)* and *flat half boneless (thin cut)*. Corned beef is usually made from brisket.

Shank crosscuts. These are cut perpendicular to the shank bone. Cook crosscuts in liquids, as in soups.

Round
Round rump roast. Cut from the top of the round, this roast contains some bone, fat, and the top round, bottom round, and eye of round muscles. Round rump is usually sold boned and rolled. Cook Good and lower grades in moist heat; better grades can be roasted.

Round roasts. These are cut from the center of the round as a *round top round roast, round bottom round roast,* or *round eye of round roast*. Each is boneless with a surface layer of fat. Choice grade of top and eye of round roasts can be oven roasted; cook others with moist heat. Bottom round roasts can be braised or roasted. Round roasts can be cut into *round steaks*. Better grades of top and eye of round steaks can be broiled or fried; cook others with moist heat.

Round heel of round. This boneless, wedge-shaped piece, from the bottom of the round, is not tender and should be cooked with moist heat.

FAMILY FOOD GUIDE

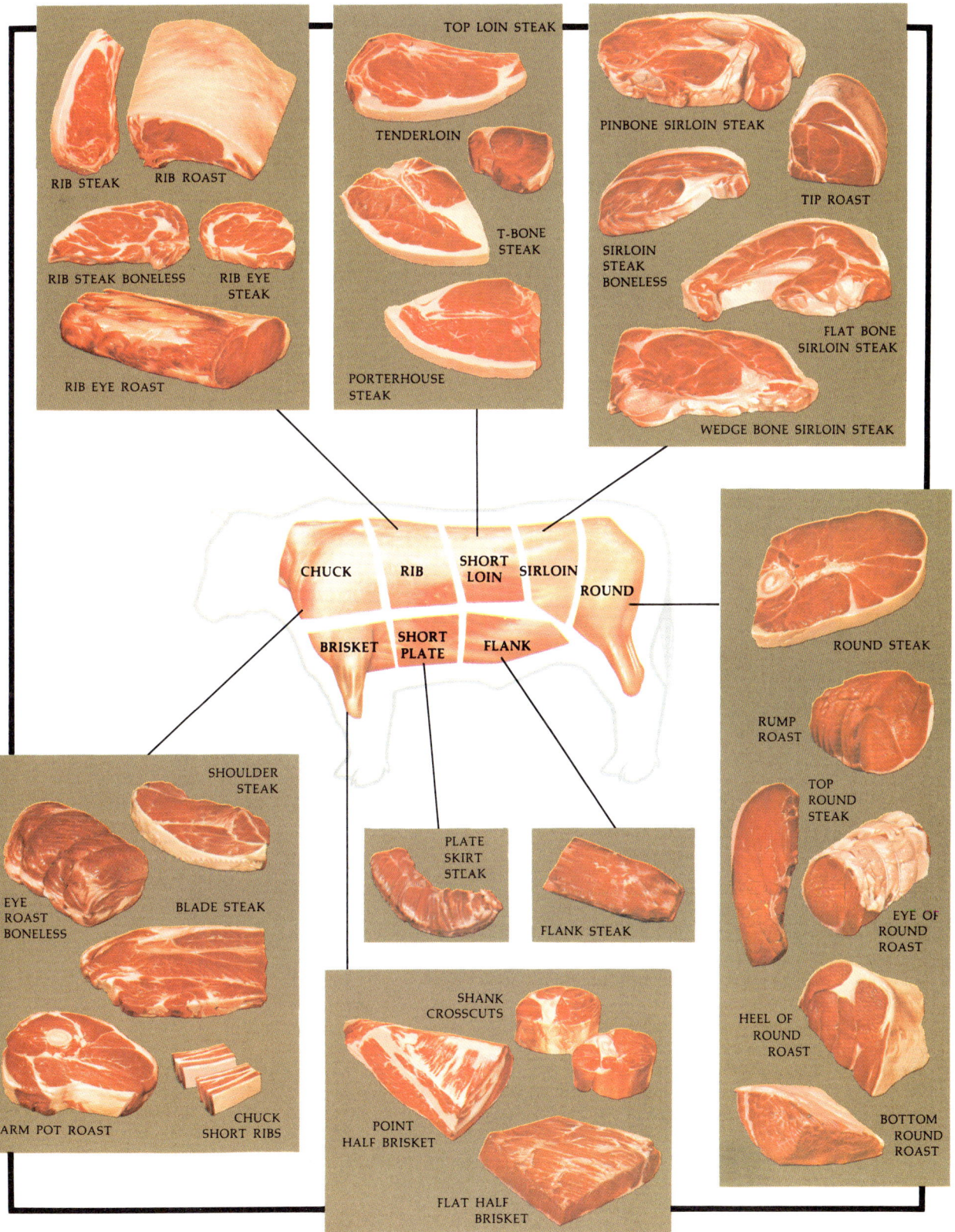

143

Buying Guide
Veal

Veal is the meat of young beef. The most tender veal comes from calves that are under three months old, have been fed a milk diet with little or no roughage, and weigh 150 to 250 pounds. However, most veal sold in this country is from older, heavier calves that have eaten foods other than milk. This veal is darker and less expensive than the milk-fed veal. Like beef, veal is inspected for wholesomeness before it can be sold; it is graded by the U.S. Department of Agriculture or an independent agent. USDA Choice and Good are the grades sold in most stores; USDA Prime, the topmost grade, is rarely available to consumers. Not all cuts are illustrated. For example, ground veal and veal cubes are not shown on the next page. Like beef, ground and cube meat can be cut from more than one section of the animal, and the taste, tenderness, and fat content of the meat will depend on the section it was cut from. For **Nutritive value** of meat and **How to keep** it, see page 142. In general, since veal has less fat than beef, its cholesterol level is lower than that of beef. Because of its low fat content it needs to be cooked slowly. Veal roasts can either be oven roasted or braised; steaks and chops are good fried or braised.

What to look for. Veal flesh should be smooth, moist looking, and pale pink to pink in color. The bones, if any, should be soft, small, and reddish; there should be little fat covering.

Shoulder
Shoulder arm roast. This roast is cut from the lower part of the shoulder section of the animal. It contains several bones and is also called *shoulder roast* and *round bone roast*. Shoulder arm roast can also be cut into *shoulder arm steaks*. These steaks are also referred to as *round bone steaks* and *shoulder steaks*.

Shoulder roast (boneless). Cut from the lower or top back part of the shoulder section, this roast is boned, rolled, and tied. Boneless shoulder roast is also known as *rolled veal shoulder* and *rolled roast*.

Shoulder blade roast. Cut from the top back part of the shoulder, this roast contains the blade bone, backbone, and ribs. It is also called *shoulder roast* and *blade roast*. Shoulder blade roast can be cut into *shoulder blade steaks*, which are also known as *shoulder steaks* or *shoulder veal chops*.

Rib
Rib chops. These are cut from the rib section of the young calf. They contain several bones; the primary muscle in the chop is the rib eye. Loin end rib chops are better than those cut from the shoulder end. Rib chops are also called *veal chops*. Another cut from the rib section of veal is the *rib roast*. This roast is usually about seven ribs wide and should be oven roasted.

Sirloin
Leg sirloin steaks. These steaks come from the sirloin of the animal. Each steak contains some backbone and hipbone. They are also called *sirloin steaks* and *sirloin veal chops*. A *leg sirloin roast* is made up of leg sirloin steaks and is also referred to as *sirloin roast*. Leg sirloin roasts also come boned, rolled, and tied. Veal sirloin roasts should be oven roasted.

Cubed steaks. These are square or rectangular, boneless pieces of meat usually cut from the leg section (sirloin or round). The cubed texture is produced by a machine and is a way of tenderizing the meat.

Round
Leg round roast. This is a conical piece of meat cut from the center portion of the round. It contains the leg bone and the top, bottom, and eye muscles; it is also called *leg roast* and *leg of veal*. The roast can be cut into *leg round steaks*; these are sometimes referred to as *veal scallopini* and *veal steaks*.

Leg rump roast. Cut from the top of the round, this wedge-shaped roast has some bone and fat and the three round muscles—the top round, bottom round, and eye of round. It is also sold as *rump roast* and *rump of veal*. Roast or braise this cut of veal.

Cutlets. These are thin slices of boneless veal cut from the leg. They are very lean pieces of meat and can be braised or fried.

Loin
Loin roast. Cut from the loin section of a young calf, loin roast contains the backbone, a T-shaped bone, and the top loin and tenderloin muscles. The roast can be sliced into *loin chops*, which look like rib chops except that rib chops do not have the tenderloin muscle. Those loin chops cut from the rib end of the loin are smaller than those cut from the sirloin end. Veal loin chops are also sold boneless, with the tenderloin removed; in this form they are known as *veal loin top loin chops*.

Breast
Breast. This cut of meat is from the breast section and has ribs and layers of fat and lean meat. It can also be bought boneless and then stuffed. Breast of veal can be either braised or roasted.

Shank
Shank. Cut from the shank of the animal, this piece contains the leg bone. Veal shank is also available sliced and known as *shank crosscuts*. Shank and shank crosscuts should be braised or cooked in liquid.

FAMILY FOOD GUIDE

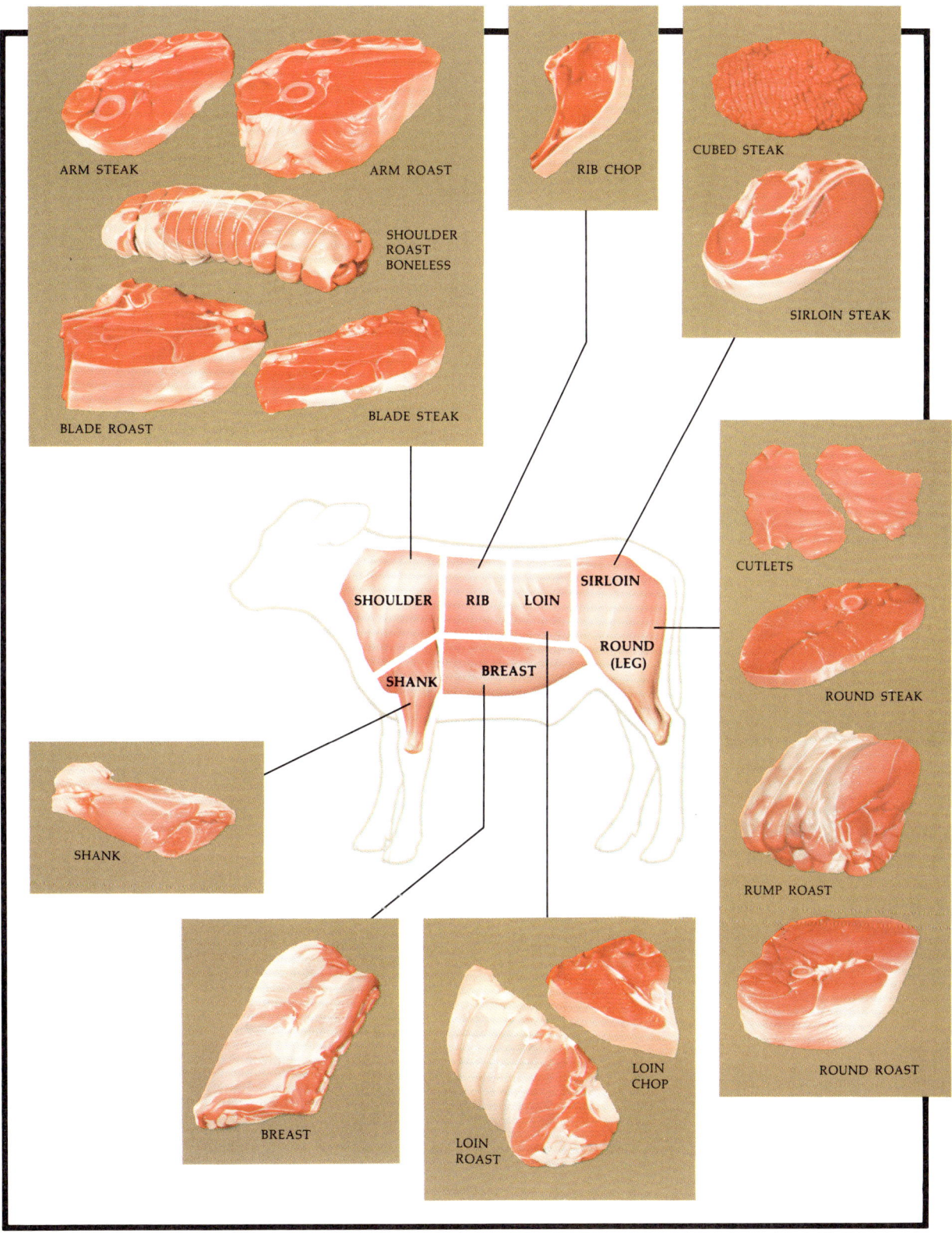

145

Buying Guide
Lamb

Most lamb sold in markets is from animals that are four to eight months old; when this young, the meat is tender and delicate in flavor. Older lambs, especially those over a year old (yearling and mutton), have tougher, stronger-tasting meat. Lamb is inspected for wholesomeness and can be graded for quality. USDA Prime is the best grade, but usually only USDA Choice or Good is sold in stores. In general, the cuts from the least-used muscles of the animal (rib and loin sections) are the most tender but not necessarily the tastiest. The more tender chops can be broiled, fried, or oven roasted; the more tender roasts can be oven roasted. However, tougher chops or roasts should be cooked with moist heat. For information on the **Nutritive value** of meat and **How to keep** it, see page 142.

What to look for. Young lamb should be firm, lean, and light pink in color; the fat should be white and the bones streaked with red. Older lamb will be darker, drier, fattier, and will have less red in the bones.

Rib
Rib roast. The most tender of all the lamb roasts, it is cut from the rib section and contains the backbone, rib bones, and the rib eye muscle; this roast is also called *rack roast* and *hotel rack*. It can be cut into *rib chops*. Also called *rack lamb chops*, the chops cut from the loin end are tastier and more tender but smaller than those cut from the shoulder end.

Loin
Loin chops. Cut from the loin section of the animal, loin chops are very tender. They contain a T-shaped bone, part of the backbone, the eye muscle, and the tenderloin. There is some fat along the outer surface.

Boneless double loin roast. This is the loin from both sides of the animal. It contains the top loin and tenderloin muscles and is boned and rolled. It can be cut into *boneless double loin chops*, also called *English chops*.

Leg
Lamb leg whole. This lamb roast includes the sirloin, the leg, and the hind shank sections of the animal. It weighs 5 to 9 pounds and is very meaty, with a moderate amount of fat. A *French style lamb leg whole* is one in which meat has been removed to expose 1 inch of the shank bone.

Lamb leg sirloin half. This is a small, bony, tender roast from the sirloin and the top of the leg.

Lamb leg shank half. This is meatier than the sirloin half of the leg. Cut from the lower half of the leg, it weighs 3 to 5 pounds and includes the hind shank as well. It is a very meaty roast that has some fat. When meat is removed to expose about 1 inch of the shank bone, it is known as a *Frenched lamb leg*.

Lamb leg American style roast. This is the same cut as the Frenched lamb leg except that the shank bone is removed and the meat is tucked back.

Sirloin
Sirloin roast. Cut from the sirloin section, this is a small roast that can serve three or four people. It can be cut into *sirloin chops*, which are also called *lamb sirloin steaks*. Both the roast and chops contain backbone and hipbone. Chops cut from the loin end are tastier and more tender than those from the leg end of the sirloin.

Hind Shank
Hind shank. This is a cut from the lower part of the back leg that is good when it is braised or cooked in liquid (stewed). It contains a good deal of bone.

Shoulder
Shoulder square cut whole. This is a square-shaped roast that contains blade, arm, and rib bones. It is fatty and will be easier to carve if the shoulder bone is cracked by the butcher. It is also known as *shoulder block* and *shoulder roast*.

Boneless shoulder roast. This roast, cut from the arm and blade sections of the lamb, is boneless, and the meat is rolled and tied. It is tender and juicy but contains a good deal of fat. It is also called *boneless shoulder netted* and *rolled shoulder roast*.

Shoulder blade chops. These are larger and meatier than loin or rib chops, but the meat is not as tender nor as delicately flavored. The more desirable blade chops are from the rib end of the shoulder; these have thinner blade bones than chops from the neck end of the shoulder. They are also called *shoulder blocks*, *blade cut chops*, and *shoulder lamb chops*. They can be sold boneless.

Shoulder arm chops. Cut from the lower part of the shoulder, these chops contain rib bones and a round arm bone. The meat is less flavorful than that of blade chops. Arm chops are also known as *shoulder blocks*, *lamb round bone chops*, *arm cut chops*, and *shoulder chops*.

Fore Shank
Fore shank. This cut from the foreleg is bony but very tasty. Fore shank is usually braised or stewed; it is also known as *lamb trotter*.

Breast
Breast. This is a very bony, fatty cut that is large enough to serve two people. It can be boned and rolled, or boned and then stuffed. Braise or roast breast of lamb.

Spareribs. These are sections of the breast that can be roasted, braised, or barbecued. Spareribs can be cut into smaller portions called *riblets*, which can be cooked in the same ways as spareribs.

FAMILY FOOD GUIDE

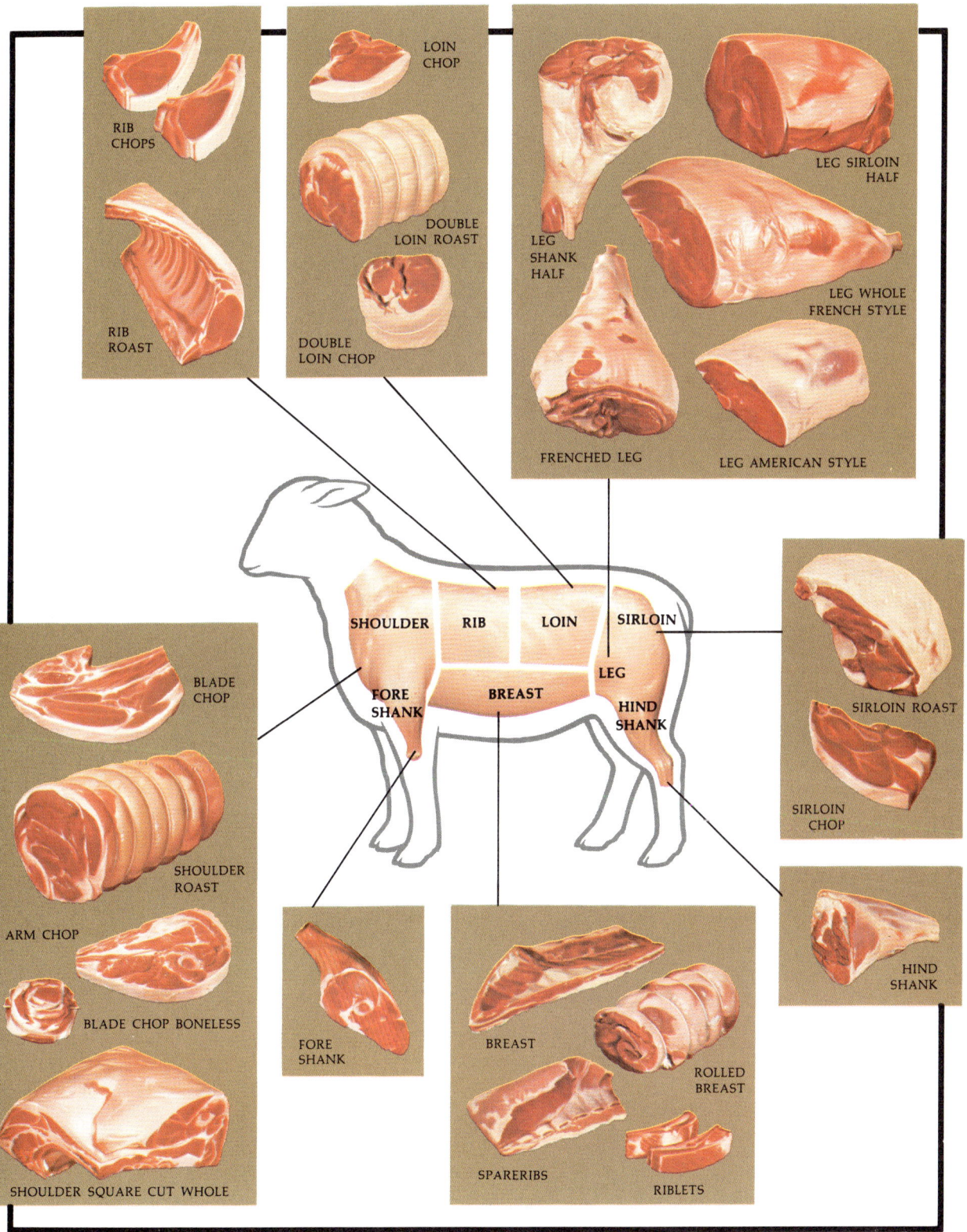

Buying Guide
Pork

Of all the pork sold in the United States, less than half is sold as fresh meat; the rest is cured, smoked, pickled, or processed. The federal grades for pork are No. 1 (the best), No. 2, and No. 3. For full flavor and because pork is susceptible to the parasite trichina, it should be cooked to an internal temperature of 170 degrees. Risk of trichinosis is also reduced if pork is kept frozen at 0 degrees for 20 days. Cured or "fully cooked" pork does not need additional cooking for health safety. Many curing solutions, however, contain sodium nitrite or sodium nitrate, additives whose safety is a matter of controversy. Some cured and smoked hams are labeled "water added"; this means that up to 10 percent of the curing solution remains in the meat. Any of the chops or steaks can be braised or fried; the more tender ones can be broiled. Fresh pork roasts are usually oven roasted or cooked in liquid; the cured and smoked roasts can be oven roasted. Pork is a very good source of thiamin (vitamin B_1); for more on the **Nutritive value** of meat and **How to keep** it, see page 142.

What to look for. Young, lean cuts are best. The meat should be pinkish-gray and have white fat; the bones should have a red tinge.

Boston Shoulder
Shoulder blade (Boston) roast. Cut from the top of the shoulder, this roast is fatty and contains the blade bone. It is also called *pork butt*, *Boston shoulder*, and *butt roast* and comes fresh or cured and smoked. It can be cut into *shoulder blade steaks*, which are also called *pork loin 7-rib cut*. A shoulder-blade roast can be boned and tied or put into a bag and called *shoulder blade roast boneless*.

Smoked shoulder roll. This is the boneless eye muscle of the shoulder blade roast in a cured and smoked form. It is also called *smoked shoulder butt*, *cottage butt*, and *daisy ham*.

Loin
Loin blade roast. Cut from the front of the loin, this bony roast is also called *loin 7-* or *5-rib roast* and *rib end roast*. It can be sliced into *loin blade chops* that are also known as *pork chops end cut*.

Loin center loin roast. This roast from the center of the loin contains the tenderloin and rib eye muscles, fat, and rib and T-shaped bones. It is also called *center cut* and *pork roast*.

Loin chops. These contain the eye muscle, tenderloin, backbone, and T-shaped bones; they are also called *center loin chops*.

Loin butterfly chops. These thick, boneless chops from the eye muscle are cut nearly in half and spread open.

Loin rib chops. From the center of the loin, these chops have eye muscle, fat, backbone, and often a rib bone. They are also called *rib cut chops*.

Loin top loin chops. These chops have top loin muscles and some backbone and fat; they are also called *center cut loin chops*.

Loin sirloin roast. A bony roast that contains the eye of loin and some tenderloin. Also called *hipbone roast*, it can be cut into *loin sirloin chops*.

Loin top loin roast boneless (double). Two roasts tied together, this is also called *boneless loin roast*.

Loin tenderloin whole. This is the tenderloin muscle from the center of the loin. It is also called *pork tender*.

Loin back ribs. These contain rib bones with layers of meat between. Also known as *country backbones*, they can be roasted, braised, broiled, barbecued, or cooked in liquid.

Leg
Leg (ham). When the cut is the whole leg boned, skinned, and tied or put into a net bag, it is called *leg (ham) boneless*, or *rolled ham*. Two bone-in hams are the *leg (ham) shank portion* and *leg (ham) rump portion*. The rump portion is from the upper leg and is meatier than the shank portion (lower leg). Ham rump is also called *ham butt end* and *ham sirloin end*. Fresh hams can be roasted or cooked in liquid; cured and smoked hams can be roasted. Center sections of cured and smoked whole hams can be cut into *ham center slices* and roasted, broiled, or fried.

Pig's Feet
Pig's feet. Also called *trotters*, pig's feet can be bought fresh, smoked, or pickled. They are often used in stews, soups, and sauces.

Spareribs and Bacon
Spareribs. Cut from the side of the pig, these bony pieces can be roasted, broiled, stewed, or barbecued.

Slab bacon. This is a boneless, fat and lean piece that is cured and smoked; it is also available as sliced bacon. *Salt pork* is slab bacon that is salt cured but not smoked; it is used in soups and stews.

Picnic Shoulder
Shoulder arm picnic. This is a roast having the shoulder muscle, bones, and some fat. It is also known as *picnic* and *picnic shoulder*, and is sold fresh or cured and smoked. It can be sliced into *shoulder arm steaks* that are also known as *picnic steaks*. Braise or fry the steaks.

Shoulder arm roast. This meaty part of the shoulder arm picnic contains the arm bone.

Hocks. These oval, 3-inch-thick cuts contain shank bones, meat, and fat. Also called *shank*, they are good braised or cooked in liquid and are sold fresh or cured and smoked.

Jowl
Jowl. This is meat from the cheek of the animal and is used like bacon.

FAMILY FOOD GUIDE

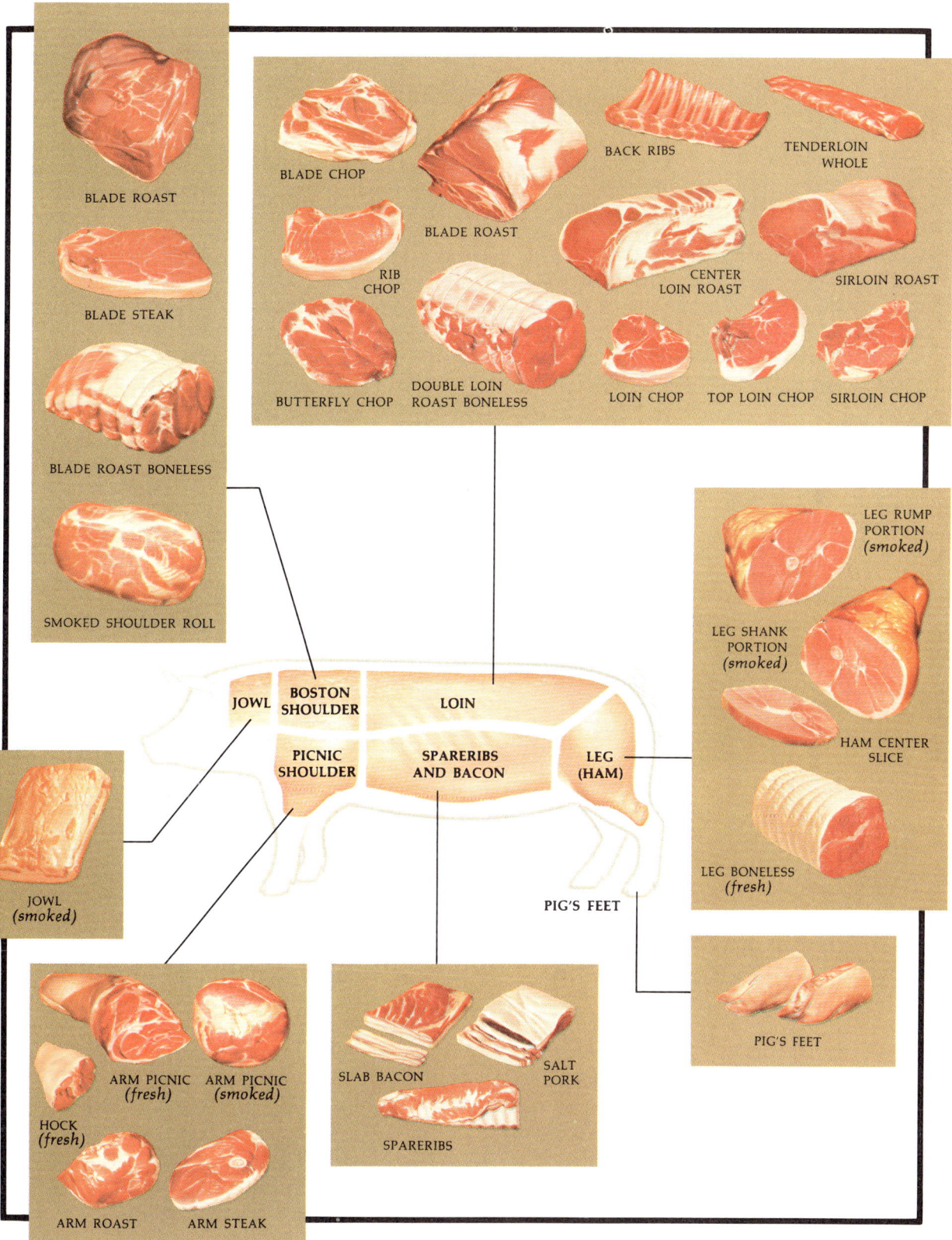

Buying Guide
Variety Meats

Variety meats are those edible parts of the animal left after it has been cut into the more popular cuts of meat. The variety meats found most often in the stores are discussed here. For each serving, buy about ¼ pound of brains, heart, kidneys, liver, sweetbreads, and tongue. If tripe, buy ½ pound per person; if oxtails, buy 1 pound per serving.

What to look for. See individual entries.

How to keep. Wrap and refrigerate fresh variety meats. Cook brains, liver, and tripe the same day as purchased; cook the others in two days.

Nutritive value. All variety meats are nutritious and are a good source of molybdenum. Kidneys are a good source of vitamin B_{12}, folic acid, pantothenic acid, and biotin. Liver is the most nutritious variety meat and is a good source of vitamins B_1, B_2, B_6, B_{12}, niacin, A, D, and E, folic acid, pantothenic acid, biotin, iron, zinc, and copper. Liver, however, accumulates residues of the chemicals given to the animal, and for this reason some sources suggest that you eat the livers of young animals, such as calves, and that you limit it to once a week.

Brains. Of all the variety meats, brains have the most delicate flavor and texture; veal brains in particular are the most desirable. Pork brains and beef brains are stronger in taste than veal or lamb brains. Lamb brains, however, are not as readily available as the others. Brains are especially good sautéed. Before cooking, soak brains for 1 to 2 hours in cold water with lemon and salt to remove any traces of blood.

What to look for. Fresh brains should be pale pink, plump, have a clean odor, and be free of blood clots and stains.

Heart. This is a very tough muscle, but one that is tasty and the least expensive of all the variety meats. Veal heart and beef heart are most readily available. Beef heart is the largest, contains the most fat, and requires the most cooking; lamb heart is the smallest and most tender. Pork heart is in between lamb and veal for both tenderness and taste. Heart is best prepared by slow cooking in liquid. (Poultry hearts are usually cut up and used in gravies and sauces.)

What to look for. Heart should be plump, bright red, and have a fresh smell.

Kidney. The most delicately flavored of all the kidneys are those of veal and lamb. Beef kidney is the strongest tasting; pork kidney is milder than beef. These are most often cooked slowly in a liquid, as in braising and stewing. Beef kidneys are used in the popular English dish beef and kidney pie. Veal and lamb kidneys are best broiled, sautéed, or used in stews or pies.

What to look for. Beef and veal kidneys are lumpy; lamb and pork kidneys are smooth and kidney-bean shaped. Kidneys should smell fresh and clean and should be shiny and slightly firm.

Liver. This organ is the most popular variety meat. The two kinds most available are calves' liver and beef liver. Calves' liver is considered to be the best tasting of the animal livers; beef has the strongest flavor. Sauté or broil calves' liver and lamb liver, but cook beef liver and pork liver slowly. Poultry livers are usually cut up and sautéed or used in pâté.

What to look for. Fresh liver should be moist and shiny with no objectionable odor.

Oxtails. These are tails of young steers; they are very tasty and should be cooked with moist heat. Oxtails are usually used in stews or soups

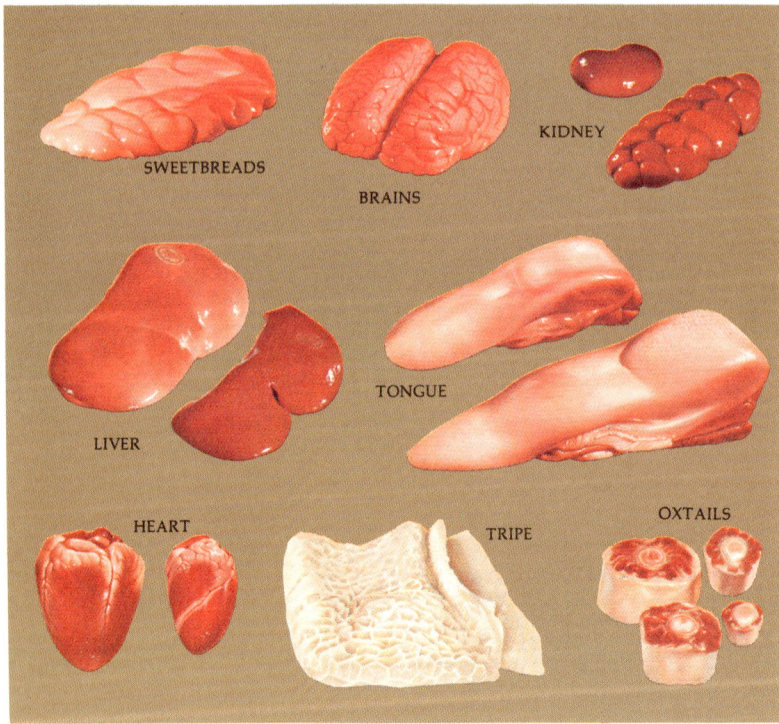

Sausages

and, although they are bony, have a good deal of meat on the bones.

What to look for. Fresh oxtails should have red flesh and a pleasant smell.

Sweetbreads. These are the thymus glands of young animals, usually calves. Sweetbreads are generally sold as a set, the pair being the throat sweetbread and the heart sweetbread (the larger of the two). They are usually sautéed or braised. Before cooking, sweetbreads should be soaked for 1 to 2 hours in cold water to remove traces of blood.

What to look for. Sweetbreads are not readily available and may have to be specially ordered. They should be creamy in color (the whiter they are, the better), plump, shiny, and have a clean smell.

Tongue. The largest and tastiest fresh tongue is beef tongue. Beef tongue can also be purchased cured, smoked, canned, corned, or pickled. Use moist heat to cook tongue. (Cured tongue can be kept refrigerated up to 8 days. Fresh tongue can be frozen for about 4 to 6 months; cured tongue does not freeze well.) Veal, lamb, or pork tongues are usually sold as processed meats that are canned, ground, or pickled.

What to look for. Fresh tongue should be pink to gray and free of blemishes.

Tripe. This variety meat is the lining of the inner stomach of beef. There are two types of tripe—plain and honeycomb. Honeycomb tripe is the more desirable of the two; both are soft, chewy, and bland tasting. Fresh tripe must be partially cooked before buying, but it will need more cooking in moist heat, after which it is usually braised or added to stews or soup.

What to look for. Tripe is not always available and may have to be specially ordered. Choose tripe that is thick, white, and has a fresh smell.

A sausage is chopped or ground meat that is flavored with seasonings and stuffed into a casing that is usually edible. Most sausages are made of pork or pork in combination with another meat, usually beef. Whatever the meat, most often the less lean, lower grades of meats and variety meats are used. One large group of sausages is referred to as luncheon meats—processed meats that are usually sliced or spread and served cold in a sandwich. Some sausages can be served cold; others must be cooked before eating (see individual entries). The package label usually specifies if the product has to be cooked; if in doubt, ask the butcher. In general, sausages are high in sodium and saturated fats. Many of the ready-to-eat types contain chemical additives whose safety is being studied. If the sausage is cured or smoked (see page 148), it most likely contains sodium nitrite and/or sodium nitrate, two additives that some claim are linked to certain types of cancer. To be sure you know what you are buying, always read the package label for a listing of ingredients.

Fresh Sausage. This type of sausage requires thorough cooking. *Italian sausage*, *bratwurst*, and many breakfast sausages are fresh sausages. Some fresh sausages such as *Bauernwurst* are smoked, but they must still be cooked because the smoking process does not cook them enough.

How to keep. Wrap, refrigerate, and use in a few days. Keep frozen sausages for up to 2 months.

Cooked Sausages. For the most part, these sausages are ready-to-eat. Many of the liver sausages, or *liverwursts*, are in this category.

How to keep. Refrigerate and use within a week. They do not freeze well.

Cooked Smoked Sausages. The most popular cooked smoked sausages are frankfurters and bolognas. Although frankfurters can be eaten cold, they taste better heated. Under the U.S. Department of Agriculture's standards of composition (page 194), frankfurters and bolognas can contain only skeletal meat and up to 30 percent fat, 10 percent water, and 2 percent corn syrup. Frankfurters or bolognas with by-products (variety meats) must comply with the above percentages, contain at least 15 percent skeletal meat, and each by-product must be in the list of ingredients. If the frankfurters or bolognas with by-products also contain nonmeat binders, there can be only up to 3½ percent binders, and they too must be in the list of ingredients.

How to keep. Refrigerate and use in one week; they do not freeze well.

Semidry and Dry Sausages. These are smoked, dried, and ready to eat. The drying period for the semidry (summer) sausages is less than that for the dry sausages. *Cervelat*, *Genoa salami*, *hard salami*, *pepperoni*, and *mortadella* are in this group.

How to keep. Although they can be unrefrigerated for a few days, they keep better if refrigerated. Use in 2 weeks.

Luncheon Meat Loaves. There is much variety within this type. Besides meat, some luncheon meat loaves contain nonmeat products like olives, pimientos, or pickles. Some of them are *olive loaf*, *headcheese*, *Dutch loaf*, *luncheon meat*, *chopped ham*, and *souse*.

How to keep. Refrigerate and use within a few days of purchase or of opening if it is a prepackaged type.

Buying Guide
Poultry

The U.S. Department of Agriculture grades for poultry are A, B, and C; Grade A is the best. The age of the bird (see the individual entries) is a good indicator of its tenderness—the younger the bird, the more tender it will be. After preparing poultry, wash your hands, all utensils, and work surfaces to get rid of any traces of salmonella, a food-poisoning bacteria commonly found in poultry. Cooking poultry to an internal temperature of 165 degrees destroys salmonella. When buying chicken or turkey, buy ¾ to 1 pound of meat with the bones or ½ pound of boneless meat per person. With Rock Cornish game hens, a small hen (about 1¼ pounds) will serve one person; a larger hen (1½ to 2 pounds) will serve two. If buying duck, figure on 1½ pounds of meat with the bones or ½ duck per person. If buying goose, buy about 1 pound per serving. If serving several people, purchase a few small geese rather than one large one.

What to look for. All poultry should be plump, well formed, and have a fresh odor. The skin should be soft, not too thick, and lack pinfeathers. The skin color is determined by the breed as well as the diet. A frozen bird should not have any frozen liquid with it.

How to keep. Loosely wrap and keep refrigerated for up to 2 days or freeze right away for longer periods (see pages 204-209).

Nutritive value. Poultry is easily digested and is a good source of high-quality protein, sulfur, phosphorus, selenium, and copper. Except for goose and duck, poultry is low in fat; much of the fat in duck and goose can be drained off in cooking if the skin is pricked in a few places. Any poultry will be lower in fat if cooked without its skin.

Chicken. The three most common types of chicken sold are the broiler-fryer, roaster, and the hen. A *broiler-fryer* is an 8- to 9-week-old chicken that weighs up to 4 pounds. Whole broiler-fryers are usually roasted; when cut into pieces, the meat can be broiled, roasted, or braised but is especially good sautéed and served with or cooked in a sauce. Because it is suited to so many cooking methods a broiler-fryer is also referred to as an *all-purpose chicken*. Roaster chickens are 4 to 8 months old and weigh 3½ to 6½ pounds. They are slightly tastier and meatier than broiler-fryers, but they also have a bit more fat. Roasters are perfect for roasting; they can also be barbecued. Older, heavier chickens are hens, and are also referred to as *fowl, stewing chicken,* or *bro-hen*. They are about 10 months old, weigh up to 8 pounds, and are fattier and tougher than either a roaster or a broiler-fryer. Hens should be braised or stewed; they are also very good for making soups, stocks, and chicken salad.

Capon. The *capon* is a male desexed chicken that is about 7 months old and weighs 5 to 8 pounds. Neutering makes the bird docile which, in combination with its diet, produces a chicken that is meatier than a roaster but has the flavor and tenderness of a young broiler-fryer. Capons have a good deal of white meat on their breasts; this is one of the reasons that capons make the best type of roasting chicken. They are suitable for a dinner party because one capon will usually serve 6 to 8 people. You might have to order in advance.

Rock Cornish Game Hen. A cross between two strains of chickens, this is a very small bird (1 to 2 pounds), but it has a proportionately high amount of white breast-meat. Whole Rock Cornish game hens are delicious when roasted and stuffed with a wild rice stuffing.

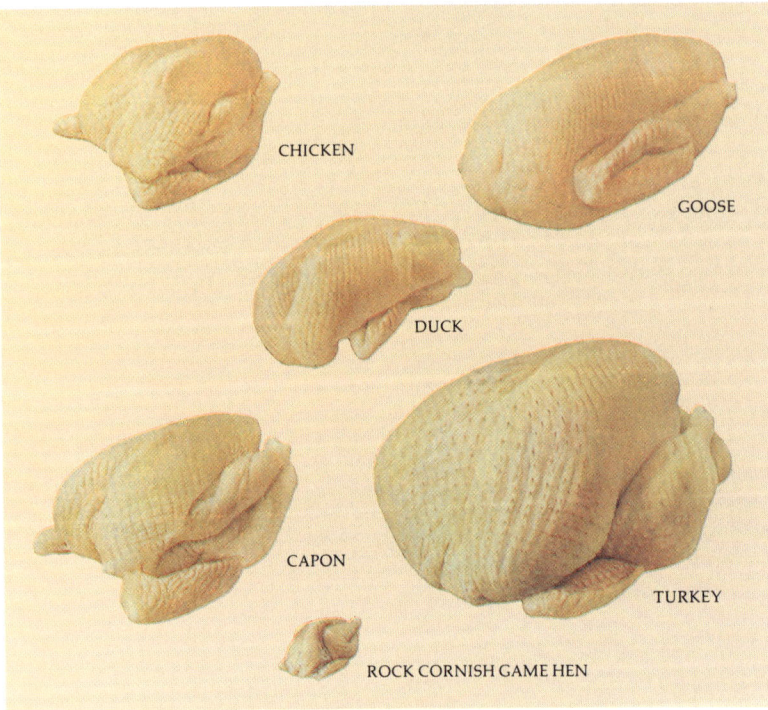

FAMILY FOOD GUIDE

Eggs

Turkey. Although they can grow larger, most of the turkeys sold today are young and weigh about 20 pounds or less. If the turkey has a pointed breast, it is probably a *tom* (male) and it will tend to be slightly less tender than would a *hen* (female) turkey of the same weight. Young turkeys can be oven roasted. Older, heavier *yearling turkeys* can also be roasted, but they are very good when they are used in soups, stews, or as meat for salads. Turkeys are also sold as parts, such as legs, breasts, thighs, or wings, some of which are also available boneless. The larger pieces can be roasted; the smaller ones, however, are best when cooked in liquid. Also available are whole, boneless turkeys and ground turkey meat.

Duck. Most of the ducks sold are *ducklings* (young ducks), 7 to 12 weeks old and weighing 3 to 5½ pounds. Duck meat is very fatty. Duckling is excellent when roasted. Older, heavier ducks are good when braised in sauerkraut or red cabbage. Most duck is sold frozen, either as a whole duck or as duck halves or parts. You might have to order duck in advance of the day you need it.

Goose. Although often considered a gourmet food to be eaten mostly at Christmas time, frozen goose is available all year round and, from late spring to Christmas, goose can be had fresh. When cooked, goose has a slightly gamy, sweet-tasting meat that is also tender and juicy. Geese can weigh up to 18 pounds, but most weigh 5 to 9 pounds and can be called *goslings*. Goslings weigh under 9 pounds and are very tender; they are the best geese to buy. Like duck, goose is very fatty. Goslings are best when roasted. Older geese, which are less tender but fattier than young geese, should be braised and are very tasty when cooked with chestnuts and sausage or fruit stuffing. You might have to order goose in advance.

Eggs are inspected and graded by government agencies. The two top grades, AA and A, are most often available in the stores, and sometimes also Grade B. No matter what their grade or shell color, all eggs are equally nutritious. The primary difference between eggs is their appearance (see below). A Grade AA egg has a firm, high yolk centered in a clear, thick albumen (white). A Grade A egg has a thinner albumen than a Grade AA egg, and the yolk is not as high nor as centered. A Grade B egg is still flatter, runnier, and with an off-center yolk. Blood spots and cloudy whites are safe to eat; they indicate that the egg is very fresh. The white, ropelike part, or chalaza, which holds the yolk to the albumen, is also edible. Eggs are also classified according to their size (weight): Jumbo, Extra Large, Large, Medium, Small, and Pee Wee. Most often only Extra Large, Large, and Medium are in the stores. The minimum weight per dozen eggs must be 30 ounces for Jumbo, 27 ounces for Extra Large, 24 ounces for Large, 21 ounces for Medium, 18 ounces for Small, and 15 ounces for Pee Wee.

What to look for. Buy only clean, unbroken eggs. If you break one, use it the same day and be sure to cook it thoroughly. Cracked eggs can harbor salmonella, a bacteria that is destroyed in cooking.

How to keep. Refrigerate in the carton and use within two weeks. Eggs stored pointed end down will keep longer (see pages 204, 207).

Nutritive value. An egg contains high-quality protein (all eight essential amino acids), sodium, chloride, sulfur, iron, pantothenic acid, and vitamins A and B_{12}; the yolk contains biotin and vitamin D. Eggs, however, are high in cholesterol.

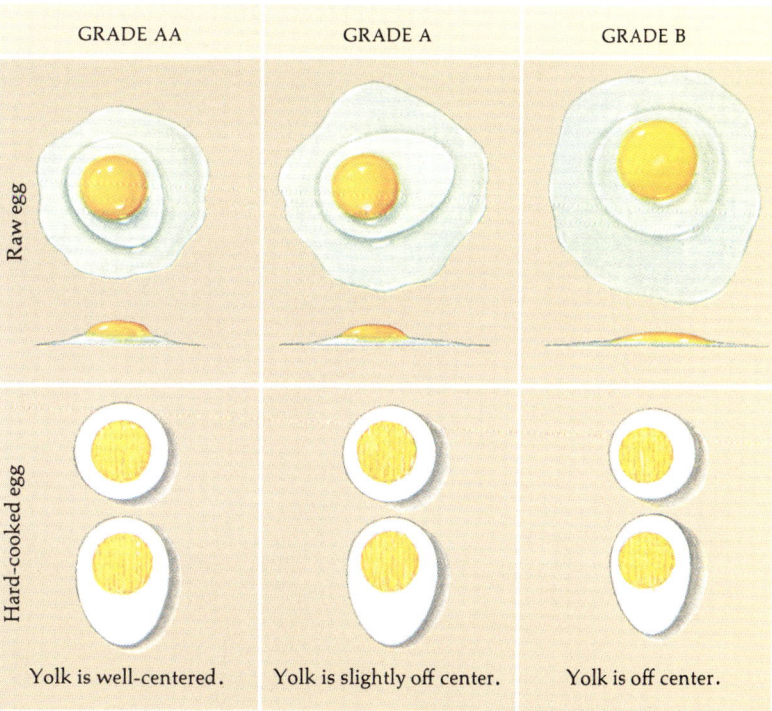

Buying Guide
Milk Products

Milk products include sweet and sour creams, butter, yogurt, some frozen desserts, and cheese (see opposite page). Almost all are made from cow's milk. Fresh milk is sold in waxed cartons or glass and plastic bottles. Nonfat dry milk, available in packets or boxes, has about half the calories of fresh milk. Goat's milk is easier to digest than cow's milk and has more protein and calcium. For those who are allergic to regular milk, there is soy milk, made from soybeans and sold fresh, canned, or powdered

All Grade A milk products are *pasteurized*, a process that kills bacteria with heat. The process also destroys some nutrients and changes the flavor of the milk. Most milk is also *homogenized*, a process that prevents the cream from separating and rising to the top.

Nonfat dry milk with a U.S. Extra Grade shield from the U.S. Department of Agriculture means it has passed strict quality-control inspections. Sweet butter with a U.S. Grade AA, also called U.S. 93 Score, is the best quality butter, with U.S. Grade A not far behind. U.S. Grade B butter may be made from sour cream instead of sweet.

What to look for. For the freshest product, always choose the one with the latest date (see dating, page 197).

How to keep. Store dairy products in the refrigerator or freezer. Milk, butter, some types of cream, and yogurt may be frozen. Use fresh milk within a week of purchase. Do not pour unused milk from a pitcher back into the carton but refrigerate separately.

Nutritive value. Milk products are an excellent source of high-quality protein, calcium, and riboflavin. They are a good source of vitamins A, D (when fortified), and B_{12}, plus phosphorus, potassium, sodium, magnesium, chloride, and sulfur. Milk products also contain sugar and saturated fat.

Whole Milk. Whole milk is at least 3.25 percent milk fat, two-thirds of which is saturated; 8.25 percent is nonfat milk solids (protein and carbohydrates); and the remaining 88.5 percent is water. Most fluid milk sold is homogenized, pasteurized, and fortified with vitamins A and D. Other milks are also sometimes available for those with special tastes. Bottled *raw milk* is not pasteurized and may contain harmful bacteria. *Certified raw milk* is usually safer to drink because dairies must comply with strict sanitary codes. Call your state department of health (food and agriculture division) for information about local certified dairies. *Evaporated milk* is sold in cans. It is thick because 60 percent of the water has been removed. Canned *condensed milk* is evaporated milk sweetened with at least 40 percent sugar.

Low-Fat Milk. Similar in taste to whole milk and its nutritive equivalent, low-fat milk has between .5 and 2 percent milk fat and at least 8.25 percent nonfat milk solids. Also called *2 percent*, *1 percent*, or *99 percent fat free*, this milk is usually fortified with vitamins A and D. Low-fat milk can be made at home by mixing equal amounts of whole milk and skim milk.

Skim Milk. Also called *nonfat milk*, skim milk has less than .5 percent milk fat and at least 8.25 nonfat milk solids. Usually fortified with vitamins A and D, it has the same nutritive value as whole milk without the saturated fat and calories. Adding a teaspoon of instant nonfat dry milk to a glass of skim milk will improve its flavor and nutritive value.

Acidophilus Milk. Usually made from skim or low-fat milk, this milk (similar to diluted yogurt) is cultured with acidophilus bacteria for easier digestion. It is usually pasteurized, homogenized, and fortified with vitamins A and D. It has the same nutritive value as regular milk. Its effectiveness in relieving digestive problems is now being studied.

Buttermilk. Old-fashioned buttermilk, unavailable commercially, is the liquid remaining after butter is churned. Today, buttermilk is made from pasteurized skim or partially skim milk that is cultured with a harmless bacteria to make it thicker and more tart. It has about the same nutritive value and low-fat content as skim milk. Salt is added to retard spoilage and improve flavor.

Sweet Creams. All creams are pasteurized and are at least 18 percent milk fat. Some may contain dry or skim milk, emulsifiers, stabilizers, or flavorings. *Light cream* has between 18 and 30 percent milk fat; *heavy cream* has at least 36 percent milk fat; and *half-and-half* (a mixture of milk and cream, homogenized) is at least 10.5 to 18 percent milk fat. *Imitation creams*, including *coffee whiteners*, may be made with animal fats, vegetable fats, sweeteners, chemical additives, or artificial coloring and flavorings. A nondairy creamer does not mean it is nonfat. Some vegetable oils, such as coconut and palm, have more saturated fat than regular cream.

Sour Cream. Old-fashioned sour cream was sweet cream allowed to sour. Modern sour cream is pasteurized and homogenized light cream that is cultured with bacteria and may contain nonfat dry milk, enzymes, or

FAMILY FOOD GUIDE

Cheese

chemical additives. Sour cream contains at least 18 percent milk fat.

Butter. Made from milk or cream or a mixture of both, butter must be at least 80 percent milk fat. Salt and coloring may be added. *Salted butter* may be made from either sweet or soured cream.

Yogurt. Although there is no proof that it will enable you to become a centenarian, yogurt has all the nutritive value of milk, is easier to digest and, some experts believe, is beneficial to the digestive tract. Yogurt may be made from whole, low-fat, or nonfat milk that is cultured with a harmless bacteria. If the label does not say low fat, then the yogurt is made with whole milk, and will thus have more fat and calories. The label will also say if the milk has been pasteurized. Yogurt is sold plain or flavored. It may have fruit, sugar, nonfat milk solids, chemical additives, or imitation flavorings added. Flavored low-fat yogurt may have even more calories than whole-milk yogurt because of added sugar. Check the label or buy plain low-fat yogurt and add your own fruit, jam, or nuts.

Frozen Desserts. These include *ice cream, frozen custard, frozen yogurt, ice milk, sherbet*, and *ices.* Ice cream is made from cream, milk, and sugar. Flavorings and stabilizers may be added. Regular ice cream is at least 10 percent milk fat. Richer ice cream is 16 percent milk fat. Frozen custard, also called *French ice cream,* contains egg yolks. Frozen yogurt has less fat but more sugar than ice cream. They have about the same amount of calories. Ice milk is between 2 and 7 percent milk fat and is made with milk, sugar, stabilizers, and flavorings. Sherbet is at least 1 to 2 percent milk fat and is made with milk, fruit or fruit juice, stabilizers, and twice as much sugar as ice cream. Ices have no milk solids or fat.

Cheese is usually made from the milk of cows, goats, or ewes. The milk is heated with an enzyme, rennin, to separate the curds from the liquid whey. The curds are collected and pressed and may be salted or cured. Curing (also called aging or ripening) develops the flavor and texture of the cheese by keeping it for a certain time at controlled temperature and humidity levels. Some cheeses acquire a protective skin, or rind, during curing; others are dipped in wax. The longer a cheese is cured the harder the texture and the stronger the flavor. There are four basic types of cheeses: *very hard, hard* or *firm, semisoft,* and *soft.* Hard cheeses keep the longest; semisoft are soft but not runny; soft cheeses are the most perishable. Some cheeses voluntarily carry a U.S. Department of Agriculture grading. Grades AA and A are the best. Others may carry a USDA Quality Approved shield, which guarantees the wholesomeness of the cheese.

What to look for. When buying cheese, look for cut surfaces that are moist, not dry or cracked. Brown discoloration should not mar blue cheeses. Soft cheeses should not have an ammonia smell.

How to keep. Refrigerate cheeses in foil or plastic wrap. Ripened cheeses may be kept for a few weeks; unripened cheeses, such as ricotta, should be used in a few days. Serve cheese at room temperature, except unripened cheeses, which should be served cold.

Nutritive value. Since cheese is made from milk, it is similar to it in nutritive value. However, many cheeses are high in sodium and fat content. Contrary to popular belief, cheese made from partly skim milk is not always low fat because extra cream may be added to it. Moreover, some part-skim cheeses (for example, Jarlsberg) are as fatty as whole-milk cheeses that are high in water (soft cheeses such as Brie); the more water a cheese contains, the lower its overall percentage of fat.

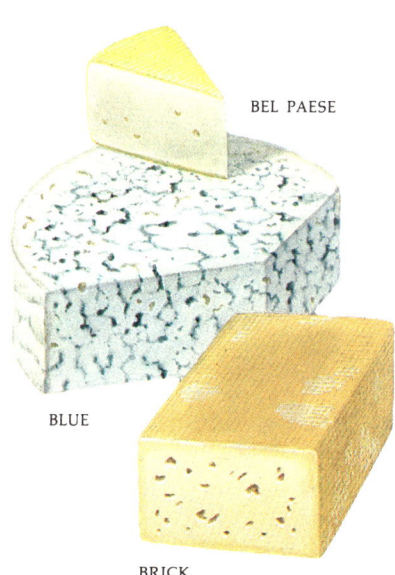

BEL PAESE

BLUE

BRICK

Bel Paese. An Italian table cheese whose name means "beautiful country," this semisoft creamy cheese is mild to robust in flavor. Its gray or brownish surface is sometimes coated with yellow wax. Imported Bel Paese has a map of Italy on the wrapper. It is sold in small wheels or wedges.

Blue. Spelled *bleu* on those imported from France, this tangy cheese is made by injecting a harmless mold into the cheese that causes blue-green veins to form. Blue cheese is aged from 2 to 6 months and has a semisoft, crumbly texture. It is made from cow's or goat's milk; *Roquefort* is made exclusively from ewe's milk.

Brick. Originally made in Wisconsin, this semisoft cheese takes its

Buying Guide
Cheese

name from its rectangular shape. Brick has a sweet, pungent taste, somewhere between Cheddar and Limburger. Made from cow's milk and aged 2 to 4 months, brick can be sliced without crumbling. Its interior is dotted with small holes.

Brie. Made in France since the 8th century, this pale-yellow, creamy cheese is ripe when the edible, white crust is tinged with brown, and the cheese yields slightly to the touch. Made from cow's milk, Brie ranges in flavor from mild to pungent. Since it is very perishable, buy only the amount needed. Avoid any with an ammonia smell. Brie is sold in whole wheels and pie-shaped wedges.

Caciocavallo. This pear-shaped cheese, known in Italy as "cheese on horseback," derives its name from the fact that a pair of caciocavallos resembles a pair of saddlebags. Usually made from cow's milk but also from a mixture of cow's and ewe's milk, this firm, ivory cheese has a golden rind and is similar to provolone in flavor. It is sold whole with a cord attached or cut into pieces.

Camembert. Supposedly named by Napoleon after the hamlet where it was first made, this soft, slightly tangy French cheese has a creamy-yellow interior with an edible, thin white or gray-white crust. It is made from cow's milk. A ripe Camembert will be plump and yield slightly to the touch. If its rind is hard, it is overripe. Avoid any with an ammonia smell. Camembert is sold whole in small round boxes and in wedges.

Cheddar. Named for the English village where it originated, Cheddar is a hard, cow's-milk cheese whose color ranges from white to a deep yellow-orange, which comes from annatto-seed dye. The color, however, does not affect the taste. Avoid any that are very dry or cracked. *Mild Cheddar* is aged from 2 to 3 months; *mellow* is aged for more than 4 months; and *sharp Cheddar* is aged 6 to 12 months. The best Cheddars are aged for more than a year. The top-ranked American Cheddars are made in New York and Vermont.

Colby. First made in Colby, Wisconsin, this variation of Cheddar is softer, moister, and milder and ranges in color from white to yellow-orange. It does not keep as well as Cheddar. Made from cow's milk and aged 1 to 3 months, Colby is sold whole in a cylindrical shape or as cut pieces.

Cottage Cheese. Made from skim cow's milk or nonfat dry-milk solids, the soft, white-curd cottage cheese varies from bland to tangy. Usually some cream is added. When the cream makes the cheese 4 percent or more fat, it must be called *creamed cottage cheese*. Low-fat cottage cheese is made with skim cream. *Pot cheese* is drier than cottage cheese and is made without cream and salt. *Farmer cheese* is cottage cheese pressed into a rectangle. When the container is stamped with the date, always buy the freshest one available.

Cream Cheese. Made with cream from cow's milk, this soft, unripened white cheese originated in the United States. It has a smooth, firm consistency, often aided by gum arabic, an emulsifier. Usually sold in 3- to 8-ounce foil-wrapped packages, it is also whipped and packaged in containers. Cream cheese has many uses, from the popular cream cheese and jelly sandwich to cheesecake.

Edam. A Dutch cheese since the Middle Ages, this round, semifirm cheese is made from partly skim cow's milk and is coated with red wax. Small holes dot the interior, which varies in color from pale yellow to orange. A mild cheese, Edam has a nutlike flavor and is sometimes salty. It is similar to Gouda but is firmer and has less fat. It is also sold in pieces.

Feta. Called a pickled cheese because it is cured and stored in brine, this moist, crumbly cheese is sharp tasting and salty. Traditionally made in Greece from ewe's milk, feta is now also made from goat's milk and in the United States from cow's milk. The best is aged from 4 to 6 weeks. Store feta in milk to prevent drying.

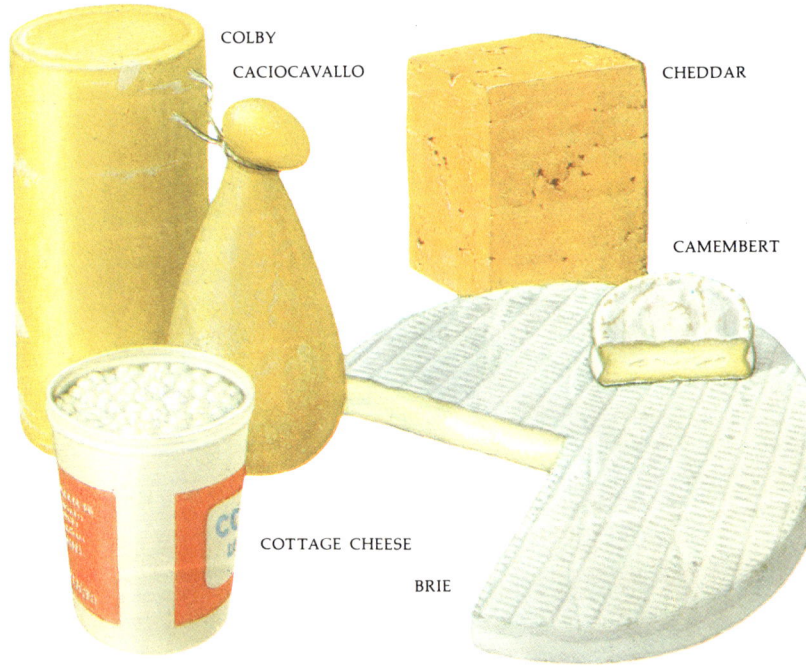

COLBY
CACIOCAVALLO
CHEDDAR
CAMEMBERT
COTTAGE CHEESE
BRIE

Fontina. Named after Mont Fontin, which overlooks the Piedmont region in northern Italy, Fontina was first made only in Italy. Now Scandinavian and American versions are widely available. *Italian Fontina* is firm, pale yellow with a dark-gold rind, and ranges from bland to strong tasting, depending on its age. It sometimes has a few holes in it. *Scandinavian Fontina* is softer and milder. *American Fontina* is bright yellow with a red covering and is bland when compared with the other two.

Gjetost. A Scandinavian favorite, gjetost is said to have been the cheese carried by seafaring Vikings. Made from the whey of goat's milk or a mixture of whey from cow's and goat's milk, unripened gjetost is a golden-brown paste with a sweet flavor. It is most uncheeselike, and newcomers to it usually learn to like it after several servings. It is often sold in small, foil-wrapped rectangles.

Gorgonzola. One of the most pungent of the blue cheeses, the spicy *Italian Gorgonzola* is made from cow's or goat's milk or a mixture of both. It has a creamy-white interior marbled with blue-green veins. Aged Gorgonzola is drier and more crumbly than younger ones. Gorgonzola is moister than Stilton and Roquefort. It is also now made in Wisconsin and Michigan.

Gouda. A Dutch table cheese named after the town where farmers marketed their cheeses, the mild-tasting Gouda is semisoft or firm, depending on its age, and ranges from creamy-yellow to yellow-orange in color. Irregular holes are scattered throughout. Gouda may have a red or yellow wax covering over its round and flattened shape. Made from cow's milk (whole or part skim), it is similar to Edam but has more fat. The round *Baby Goudas* weigh a pound or less.

Gruyère. Made from cow's milk on both the French and Swiss sides of the Alps, this firm cheese is similar to Swiss but is creamier, sharper, and has smaller holes. It has a sweet, nut-like flavor. Aged 3 to 10 or more months, the light-yellow Gruyère is too old if it has a sandy texture or if there are cracks in its brown rind. It is different from processed Swiss Gruyère sold in foil packages.

Processed Cheese

This is a mixture of shredded cheeses pasteurized (heated) together. Pasteurization not only kills any bacteria in the cheese but also stops the cheese from ripening further, keeps the flavor and texture uniform, and increases its shelf life. The mixture is then poured into molds to solidify before being packaged for sale. Emulsifiers and stabilizers are usually added for consistency, and the cheese is sometimes artificially colored. Of the three types of processed cheeses, *pasteurized process cheese*, such as American cheese slices, contains the most cheese. *Pasteurized process cheese food* is about half cheese and half water mixed with another dairy product. *Pasteurized process cheese spread* has the most water and is the most spreadable. *Cold-pack*, or *club cheese*, is processed cheese that has not been heated and may be sweetened.

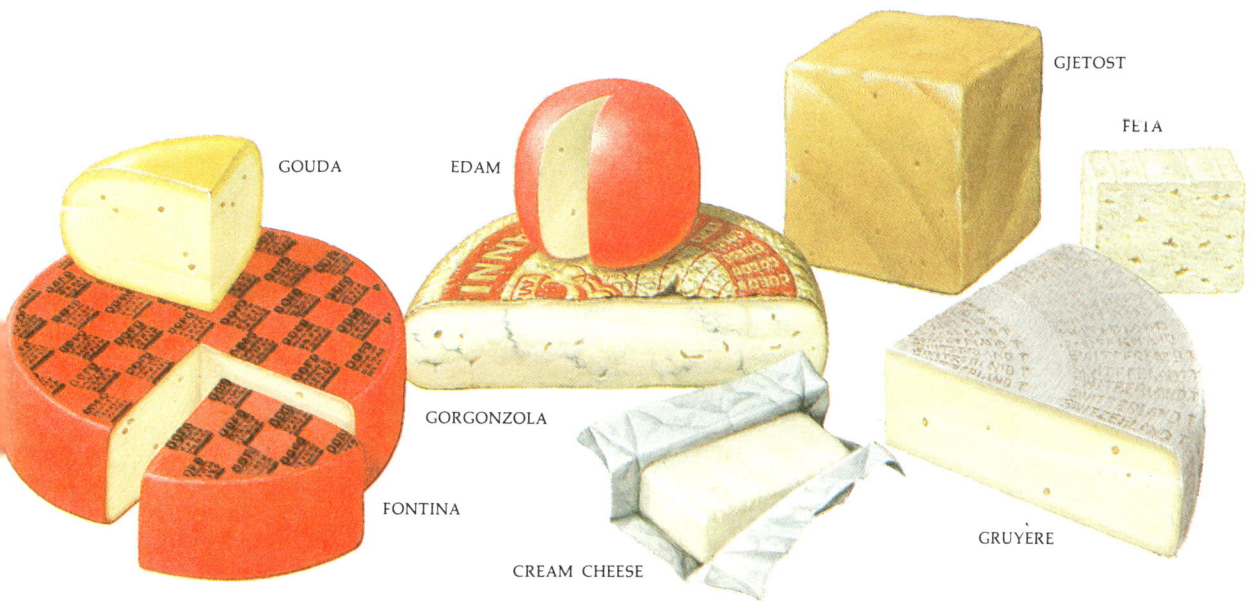

Buying Guide
Cheese

Jarlsberg. A Norwegian cheese that is twin to Swiss Emmentaler, Jarlsberg is sweeter and more delicate in flavor. Like Swiss Emmentaler, it is made from cow's milk and has large holes in its firm yellow interior. It is sold in wedges cut from a large wheel that is covered with a yellow wax rind.

Liederkranz. Named after a New York singing group that raved about its taste, Liederkranz is a soft, surface-ripened, strong-smelling cow's-milk cheese that is milder than Limburger. As it ages, its color changes to honey while its edible rind turns from yellow to brown. Made principally in Ohio, Liederkranz is usually foil-wrapped and dated, indicating ripeness.

Limburger. Known as the king of the smelly cheeses, this pungent, soft Belgian cheese has a reddish-yellow rind and a creamy-white interior. Some experts say its strong flavor comes from its harmless surface-ripening bacteria. Limburger is usually sold in small rectangles.

Monterey. Also called *Jack cheese*, or *Monterey Jack*, this semisoft cheese varies in flavor from bland when aged 2 to 3 weeks to very sharp when aged 6 months or more. Young Monterey is similar to Gouda, whereas ripened Monterey is closer to Cheddar. When made from low-fat milk, Monterey is a hard cheese best suited for grating. It is sometimes called *Dry Monterey* or *Dry Jack*.

Mozzarella. Originally made in Italy only from buffalo's milk, mozzarella is now also made from cow's milk. When freshly made, unripened mozzarella is soft, white, and mild. Most mozzarella is factory made and has a rubbery consistency that makes it good for cooking, such as a topping for pizzas or lasagnas. It is usually sold in small, round chunks or shredded. Some mozzarella is smoked.

Muenster. American-made Muenster is yellow with a thin, orange rind. It is milder than the original Muenster made by monks in France and another type made in Germany. Muenster is made from cow's milk and is similar to brick. Its interior is dotted with tiny holes. Muenster is sold round, in wedges, or sliced.

Parmesan. Parmesan is the popular name for a group of very hard Italian cheeses known in Italy as *Grana*. *Parmigiano* and *Reggiano* belong to this group and are named after their places of manufacture, Parma and Reggio, respectively. Sometimes Reggiano is known as *Reggiano Parmesan* or, like the others of the Grana group, as simply, Parmesan. Made from cow's milk and aged at least a year or more, this sweet-tasting cheese is used both as a table cheese and for grating. Older Parmesan is golden-yellow, whereas a younger type, *Grana Padano*, is paler and not as strong tasting. American-made Parmesan is not as flavorful as that made in Italy. It is sold in wedges and grated.

Port Salut. Still made by Trappist monks in France according to their secret formula, Port Salut was named for the abbey to which the monks returned after the French Revolution—Port of Salvation. Port Salut manufactured elsewhere is similar but not identical. Made from cow's milk, Port Salut is a semisoft, yellow cheese covered with an orange rind. A mild cheese similar to Gouda in taste, it nonetheless has an aroma not unlike a mild Limburger. Bland or rubbery Port Salut is not top quality.

Provolone. Sold in a variety of shapes—including sausage, pearlike, and wedge—this firm, smooth, Italian table cheese made from cow's milk has a white-yellow interior and a light-brown or gold glossy rind. Its flavor ranges from mild when aged just 2 months (*provolone dolce*) to piquant and biting when aged 4 to 6 months (*provolone piccante*). Still older provolone is good for grating. Some provolones are smoked.

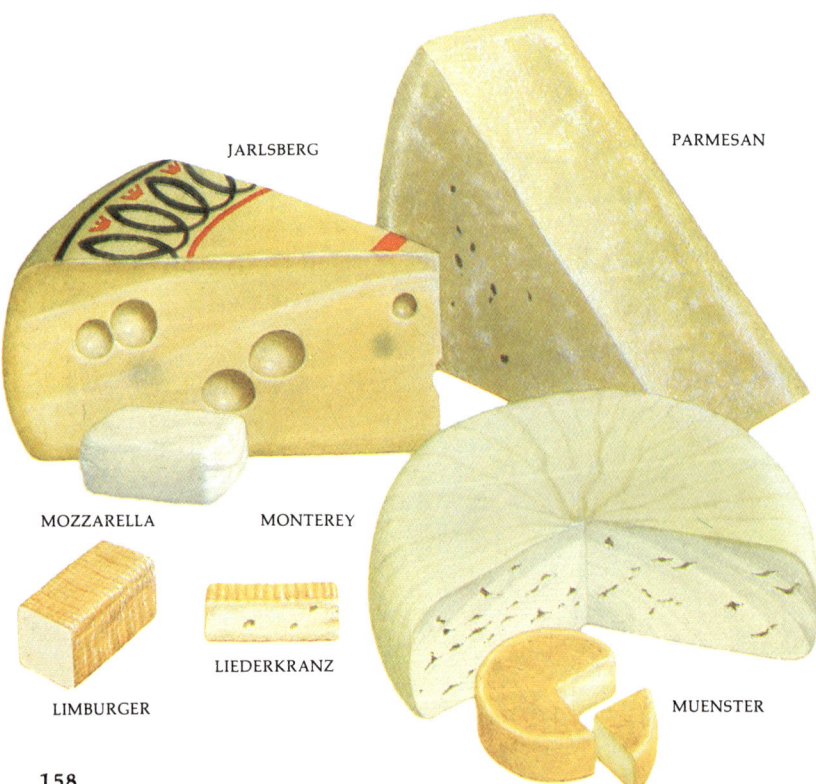

158

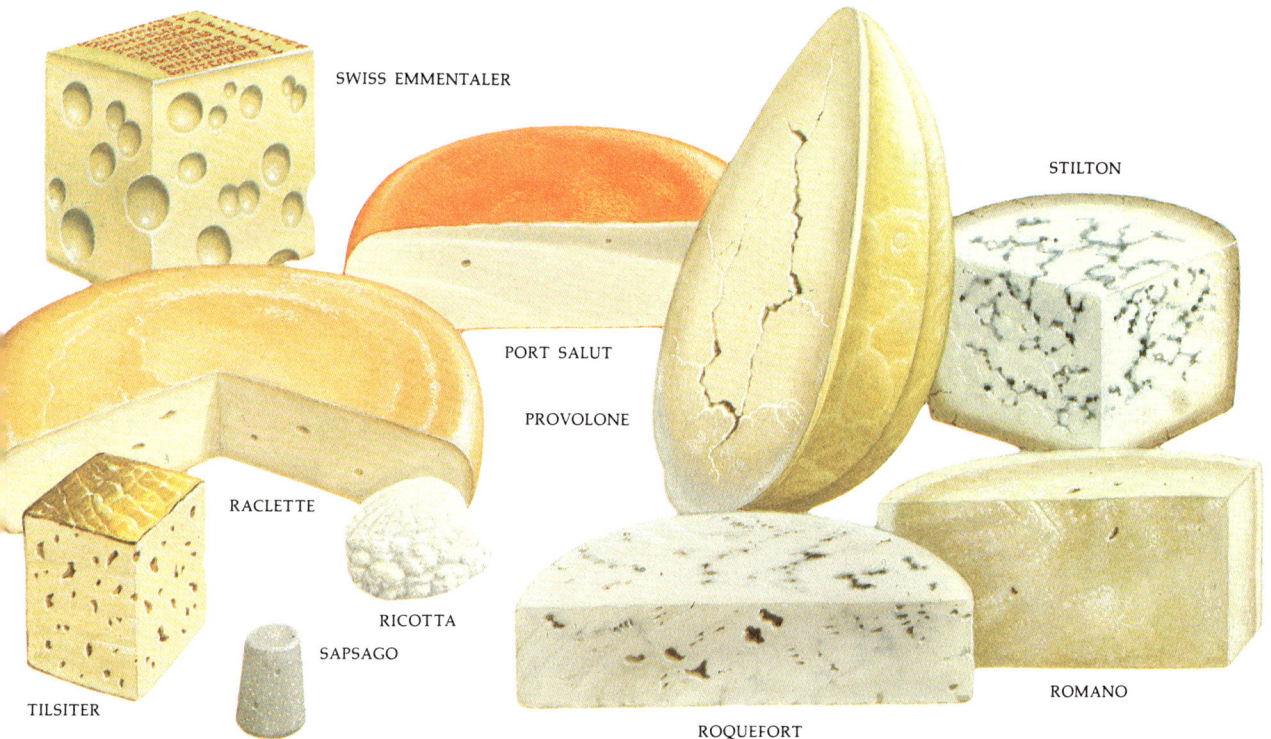

Raclette. A cow's-milk cheese, raclette is mild and nutty tasting. It has a brown rind and a yellow-amber interior that is marked with small, irregular holes. Raclette was first used as a melting cheese in a Swiss specialty dish from which it takes its name.

Ricotta. Similar to cottage cheese, white and moist soft-curd ricotta is made from whole or partly skim cow's milk or from cow's whey with milk added. Sweet and nutlike in flavor, unripened ricotta is sold in containers stamped with a date for freshness. Buy the freshest one since ricotta spoils easily. Avoid any with yellow discoloring. Dry ricotta is pressed into rectangles similar to farmer cheese and can be sliced.

Romano. This very hard, granular cheese is made in Italy from ewe's milk and is called *Pecorino Romano*. In the United States, it is made from cow's milk and is called *Vacchino Romano*. When aged for less than a year, Romano may be used as a table cheese. The older Romanos are best for grating purposes.

Roquefort. Made from the milk of ewes and aged in special limestone caves, Roquefort is unique in flavor among the blue cheeses. Best when it is creamy rather than crumbly, French Roquefort is sold foil wrapped with the image of a sheep stamped on it. Only cheese from the Roquefort area in France may use that packaging and the Roquefort name.

Sapsago. A very hard granular cheese used for grating, the pungent, herblike *Swiss sapsago* is made from skim cow's milk to which a powder ground from special clover leaves is added. This gives sapsago its sharp, herbal flavor and aroma and its greenish color. It is sold in cone shapes.

Stilton. Milder than Roquefort or Gorgonzola, this English blue cheese is creamy white and marbled with blue-green veins of mold. Made from cow's milk and aged 4 to 6 months, Stilton tends to dry out, so keep it wrapped in a damp cloth.

Swiss Emmentaler. Characterized by its large holes caused by expanding gases during fermentation, the original Swiss cheese is called Emmentaler after the river valley in central Switzerland where it was first made. Swiss Emmentaler is a firm, cow's-milk cheese, ripened from 5 to 10 months, with a mild, sweet, and nutlike flavor. Its color is light yellow. The rind of Emmentaler is stamped many times with the name "Switzerland." Swiss cheese made in the United States or from other countries cannot use the name "Emmentaler" and is thus called simply *Swiss cheese*.

Tilsiter. Popularly called *Tilsit*, this cow's-milk cheese was first made by Dutch settlers in East Prussia and is now made in Germany, Switzerland, and other countries. It is a mild table cheese similar to brick and is characterized by the many cracks in its white to yellow, semisoft interior.

Buying Guide
Legumes

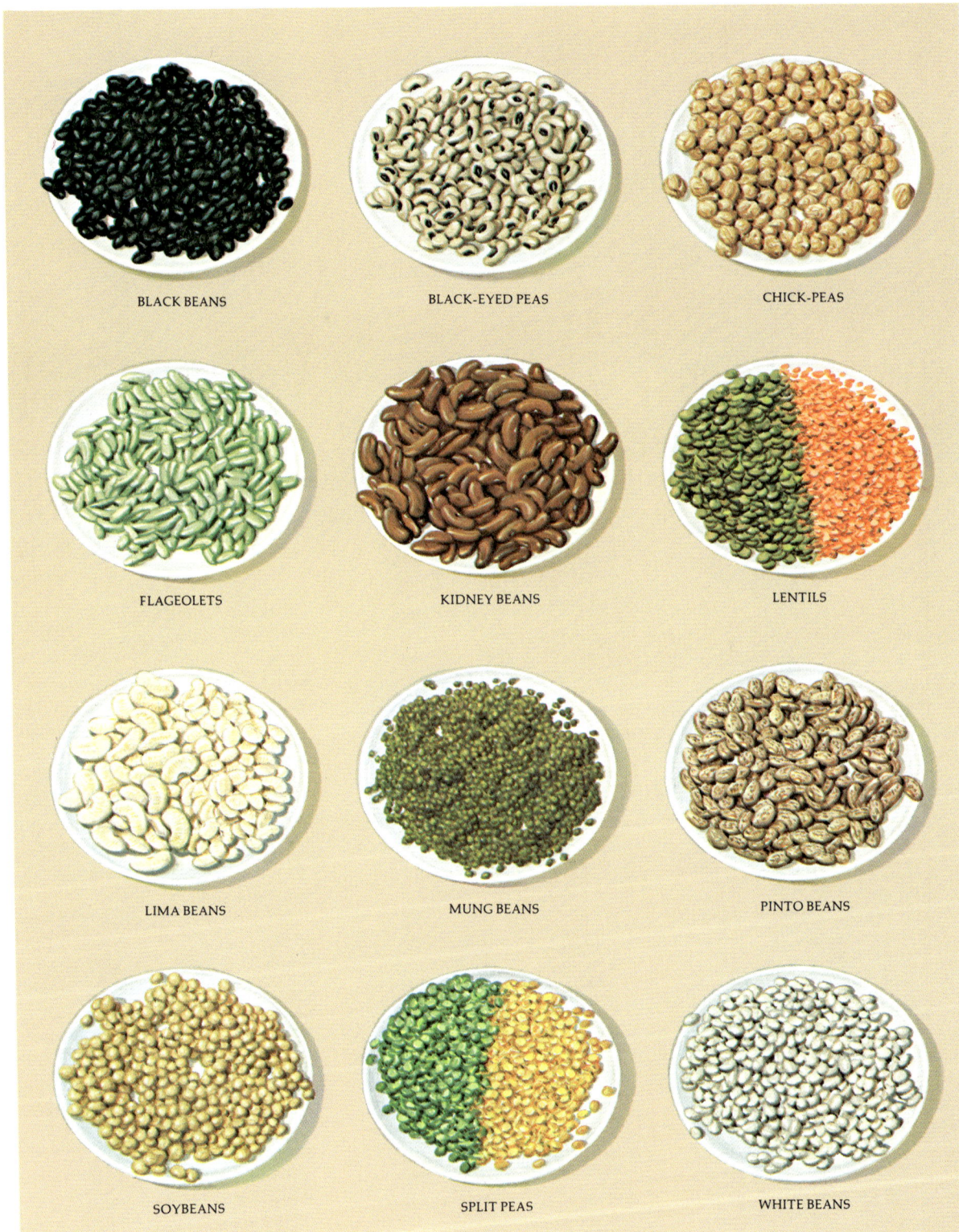

Legumes are the dried seeds of certain plants such as peas, beans, and lentils. Long a part of the diets in the Middle East, India, Asia, and Central and South America, legumes have recently gained greater popularity in Europe and the United States because of their low cost, high nutritive value, and versatility in cooking.

Available all year, legumes are usually sold in clear plastic bags or see-through boxes that carry a federal grade. For example, the top grades are U.S. No. 1 for peas, lentils, and black-eyed peas; U.S. No. 1 Choice Handpicked or Handpicked for pinto beans and white beans; and U.S. Extra No. 1 for lima beans. Lesser quality legumes are not usually sold to consumers. Legumes can also be purchased loose by the pound. Precooked frozen or canned legumes, such as baked beans, usually cost more than dried legumes. For example, 2 cups of dried legumes (1 pound) generally yield 6 cups of cooked beans whereas 3½ pounds of canned beans are needed to equal the same amount.

What to look for. Look for beans or peas with a bright, uniform color that are about the same size and that lack visible defects such as cracked seed coats, foreign matter, and pinholes made by insects.

How to keep. Store legumes in tightly covered containers in a dry, cool place. Use within 6 to 9 months. Do not mix legumes purchased at widely different times because the older ones will be drier and therefore require longer cooking.

Nutritive value. Very high in protein, legumes also provide iron, thiamin, riboflavin, niacin, potassium, phosphorus, fiber, and complex carbohydrates. Legumes do not contain cholesterol and are low in sodium and saturated fat.

Black Beans. These popular South and Central American beans are shiny black on the outside and cream colored on the inside. Also known as *turtle beans*, black beans are smaller in size than kidney beans. They are the main ingredient in the renowned black bean soup of the American South; the national dish of Brazil, *feijoada completa* (a stew of meat, greens such as kale or collards, onions, black beans, rice, meat, and sometimes banana); and the traditional black beans and rice dish of Puerto Rico and Cuba. Their flavor is enhanced by adding lemon juice, garlic, or cumin.

Black-Eyed Peas. Also called *cowpeas*, these oval, creamy-white legumes with their distinctive black spot on one side are actually beans. Originally brought to America from Africa by slave traders, black-eyed peas have been a standard ingredient in Southern cuisine, particularly in soul food. According to a New Year's Day custom in and around South Carolina, eating black-eyed peas mixed with rice and perhaps some ham or bacon (a dish called hoppin' John; recipe on page 263) will bring you good luck in the coming year. Black-eyed peas make a tasty dish mixed with tomatoes and onion.

Broad Beans. Nicknamed *horse beans* because of their large size, these beans (not shown) are also known as *Windsor beans*, *English beans*, and *fava beans* (from the botanical name *Vicia faba*). These oversized beans range in color from white to beige to brown. Broad beans are usually available fresh, dried, or canned. Some people think that broad beans have a bitter taste. Eating broad beans or inhaling their pollen may cause favism, a form of anemia that afflicts people of the eastern Mediterranean region, who have a genetic tendency to develop the disease.

Chick-Peas. When the French occupied Sicily during the Middle Ages, the Sicilians determined a person's French or Sicilian origins by asking him to pronounce the Italian word for chick-peas, *ceci* ("tchay-tchee"). If the person failed to pronounce it correctly, he was judged to be French and killed. The Spanish call chick-peas *garbanzos*. Their botanical name, *Cicer arietinum*, refers to the fact that they are shaped like the head of a ram—*aries*. In ancient times, the nut-flavored chick-peas were paired with bacon to make a version of pork and beans; today, navy beans are used. Chick-peas are available whole or split. They are used in salads, casseroles, soups, and as a separate vegetable. When pureed with spices and other ingredients, these legumes make up the well-known Middle Eastern specialties *hummus* (Arabic for chick-peas) and *falafel*. When made into soup with pasta added and topped with Parmesan cheese, the result is an Italian dish called "thunder and lightning." Chick-peas and chick-pea flour are dietary staples in India and throughout the Middle East.

Flageolets. These small, French-imported kidney-shaped beans come in two varieties, green or white. The green ones have a more delicate flavor. They may be available in specialty food shops and can be purchased dried, fresh, or canned. Flageolets are a good complement to meat, especially lamb, and are an ingredient of the French *cassoulet*, a stew of sausage, pork, lamb, or game.

Kidney Beans. These large, dark-red beans are perhaps the most ver-

Buying Guide
Legumes

satile and popular of all the legumes. They figure in the cuisines of such diverse regions as New England, the South, the Southwest, and of Mexico. The Pilgrims supposedly learned to cook kidney beans and corn together in bear grease from the Narraganset Indians, who called the dish *misickquatash*. Today, this type of succotash is still a favorite in New England—minus the bear grease, of course. In New Orleans a dish of red beans and rice is still the traditional noonday meal on Mondays. Many popular Central American dishes are made with kidney beans, notably chili, tamales, and *frijoles refritos*, "refried beans" (see also pinto beans). Kidney beans are grown in the United States in New York State, Michigan, and California.

Lentils. Biblical experts believe that the "mess of pottage" for which Esau sold his birthright was a bowl of lentils, possibly in combination with lamb and herbs. Long scoffed at as the poor man's meat, lentils have the most protein of all the legumes except soybeans. Lentils need no advance preparation and are ready to eat after about 45 minutes of cooking. The length of cooking time depends on how old and therefore how dried the lentils are. Lentils and split peas (see separate entry) are the only legumes that do not require soaking before being cooked. Most of the lentils available in this country are brown or brown-green but are called green lentils. A red variety may also be found. Grown in Washington State and in Idaho, lentils are used mainly in soups or pureed and made into patties. Lentils are a popular food in the Middle East, in countries along the Mediterranean, and Asia and North Africa.

Lima Beans. There are two main types of lima beans: small, known as *baby lima beans*, and large, called *Fordhooks*. Choose baby limas when possible because the large ones shed

Preparation Tips

Although legumes are easy to prepare, you may find the following hints helpful.
- Legumes should first be rinsed and any foreign matter and damaged beans removed.
- All legumes—except split peas and lentils—must be soaked before cooking. Soak overnight or for 6 to 8 hours, or bring to a slow boil, simmer 2 minutes, and soak (covered) 1 hour away from heat.
- Split peas and lentils will cook in 45 to 50 minutes; others take 2 to 3 hours after soaking.
- Remember to allow room for legumes to expand. One cup of dry legumes will yield 2 to 3 cups of cooked beans or peas.
- Legumes should always be simmered; rapid boiling breaks them apart.
- Add 1 tablespoon of vegetable oil or other fat to the pot to reduce the amount of foam that develops during cooking.
- Keep the lid of the pot partially open to prevent the beans from boiling over the sides.
- Do not add salt or acid substances such as lemon, tomatoes, or vinegar until the legumes are nearly cooked, since these ingredients will impair the softening of the beans.

their skins during cooking. *Calico beans* are limas with purple markings on them. Lima beans, sometimes referred to as *butter beans*, are grown in California and are also available fresh or frozen. Baby lima beans can be served as a separate vegetable or in a casserole, whereas large limas are preferred in soups.

Mung Beans. Best known for their use as sprouts (see pages 164-165), these small, round beans can also be served as a vegetable or added to soups and casseroles. Mung beans, which can be green, golden, yellow, or black, are usually available whole, split, or skinless. They are native to India, where they are ground into flour. Split peas can often be substituted in recipes calling for mung beans.

Pinto Beans. Related to kidney beans, these beige-colored, speckled legumes are the basis of many chili recipes and *frijoles refritos*, "refried beans). Refried beans are not actually refried. In Spanish the prefix *re* can mean "well" or "thoroughly." Thus, *refritos* means "well-fried," not fried again. Black beans or kidney beans may be used instead of pintos in *frijoles refritos*. Pinto beans are grown in North Dakota, Colorado, and Idaho and turn reddish-brown after cooking. Thick, hot brews of pinto beans and beef were often relished at chuck wagons and campfires in the Old West. *Pink beans* are similar to pinto beans, but have a smoother, brownish-red skin.

Soybeans. These small, round beans, about the size of peas, have been providing protein to the peoples of the Orient for more than two millennia, and in recent times, to those of the Western world as well. Introduced to the United States in the early 19th century, soybeans were first used as animal fodder. Today, the United States not only grows more soybeans than any other bean but also produces most of the world's supply. Soybeans, which can be yellow, green, brown, black, or mottled, are one of the few known vegetable sources of protein that contain nearly as many essential amino acids as do animal foods. Despite its high protein rating, soy is lower in one of the essential amino acids than animal protein and must be supplemented with animal-protein foods such as milk or cheese. Still, soybean protein is the highest quality vegetable protein and the reason soybeans are a good substitute for meat. One cup of cooked soybeans contains nearly 20 grams of protein. Soybeans are also a good source of B vitamins, vitamin A, potassium, calcium, phosphorus, and some iron. They are the basis of many other products, described below. A recent study, however, has shown that some of these soy products, such as soy flour, may interfere with the absorption of iron from vegetable sources.

Split Peas. Green or yellow split peas are specially grown whole peas that are dried, have their skins removed, and are then split in half. Some people think the green ones are tastier than the yellow. Both make excellent purees and can be used anytime as substitutes for whole peas.

The Versatile Soybean

Soybeans are an extremely useful food source. Some soy-based products now available include:

Soy sauce. Natural soy sauce is sold in this country as *tamari*, made from whole soybeans that are fermented from six months to one year. Tamari does not contain additives. Most but not all of the soy sauces sold on the supermarket shelves contain added ingredients such as caramel coloring, corn syrup, salt, and sodium benzoate as a preservative. The list of ingredients on each product will tell you what it contains. Tamari and other soy sauces all have a high sodium content.

Soy sprouts. Soybean sprouts are a good source of vitamin C. Buy them already sprouted or sprout your own (see pages 164-165). It is a good idea to cook soy sprouts by sautéing lightly before adding them to salads or other dishes; the body cannot assimilate the protein from raw soybeans.

Soy "nuts." Widely available in supermarkets, soy "nuts" are made from deep-fried whole soybeans. They are sold salted and unsalted and are very similar to peanuts but contain more protein. *Roasted soybeans* have even more protein than soy "nuts."

Soy flakes. These are dry-roasted soybeans that have been run through a roller miller, which flattens the beans before cutting them into flakes. They cook faster than whole soybeans.

Miso. This is a soybean paste made by fermenting soybeans, rice, salt, water, and other ingredients. It can be used as a base for bouillon, a stock for soups or stews, and instead of soy sauce in sauces and dips.

Soy milk. Soy milk contains about as much protein as cow's milk but it is lower in fat. Soy milk is available in ready-to-use, dry, concentrated forms. You can substitute it for whole milk or use half soy milk and half skim milk.

Soy flour. Made from ground dried soybeans, soy flour is best used with other flours to enrich baked goods with protein. Since it contains no gluten, the substance that causes yeast breads to rise, soy flour must be used with other flours when baking bread. Store soy flour in a cool, dry place to keep it from turning rancid.

Soy oil. Unlike other soy products, soybean oil has no protein. However, it is rich in polyunsaturated fatty acids (discussed on page 21). With its mild flavor, it can be used both as a cooking and a salad oil. Store in the refrigerator after opening.

Textured vegetable protein. Made from soy flour or soy concentrate into tiny granules, this soy product can be added to main dishes to extend their protein content or used as analogs—look-alike substitutes for meat, fish, chicken, and other foods.

Tofu. This white, bland cheeselike soy product has been a source of protein in the Orient for more than a thousand years and has been rapidly gaining popularity elsewhere because of its nutritive value, versatility, and low cost. It contains no cholesterol and little saturated fat and provides calcium, vitamin E, iron, and phosphorus. It may be used in place of soft cheeses in many dishes, by itself, crumbled into soups and salads, and also added to spicy main dishes and desserts.

Tofu comes in firm, regular, and sometimes soft cakes; the firm ones have the most soy content, and therefore more nutritive value, the least water, and hold their shape the best. Look for tofu in your local produce market or specialty store.

Tofu should be refrigerated and will keep about a week after purchase. If it is to be used within 24 hours of purchase, drain and store without water; this will help preserve tofu's delicate flavor. Otherwise, drain and add fresh water every day until it is ready to be served. For firmer tofu, drain a few hours before serving.

Buying Guide
Legumes

Unlike most other legumes, split peas do not need to be soaked before cooking. The most familiar dishes made with green split peas are split-pea soup and the English pease pudding.

White Beans. There are several varieties of white beans, all of which can generally be used interchangeably in soups, stews, and casseroles. Some of the most popular are *marrow* or *marrowfat beans, Great Northern beans, cannellini beans, navy* or *Yankee beans,* and *pea beans.* Marrow beans are the roundest and largest of the white beans and have a less delicate taste than Great Northerns. They are grown in the eastern part of the United States. Great Northerns are raised in Nebraska, Wyoming, and Idaho. They were often used by New Yorkers to make homebaked beans (called New York baked beans) instead of the navy beans used by Bostonians. Great Northerns do not hold their shape as well as pea or navy beans.

Cannellini beans are a bit larger and plumper than navy beans and are more kidney shaped than round. They are used in many Italian dishes. They are sometimes referred to as *Italian white beans.*

Navy or Yankee beans are the most widely used white beans since they are traditionally made into baked beans. Navy beans are so called because the U.S. Navy served them so often, sometimes even at breakfast. Although grown in Michigan, navy beans are nicknamed Yankee beans because they are used for the famous Boston baked beans. Since the strict New England Puritans were forbidden to cook on the Sabbath, they fixed enough navy beans to last from Saturday supper to Sunday lunch. This rich brown brew of beans, molasses, and salt pork is still a custom on Saturday nights in many parts of New England. (Pinto or kidney beans may be substituted for white beans.) Navy beans are also known for their part in the famed Senate bean soup served daily in the Congressional dining rooms. Many canning manufacturers use navy beans in their pork and bean mixtures.

Pea beans are the smallest white beans. They are oval and hold their shape in cooking. They are often used for Boston baked beans. In fact, some growers do not differentiate between navy and pea beans.

Whole Peas. Available in green or yellow varieties, these versatile legumes can be used as a separate vegetable dish or in soups, casseroles, puddings, or purees. Whole peas that are dried are produced in Idaho and Washington State.

Is It True What They Say About Beans?

Throughout the ages, bean eating has been associated with flatulence—expelling digestive gas. The gas, which is mainly nitrogen and carbon dioxide, is produced when bacteria in the intestines break down complex carbohydrates in the beans. While there is no known antigas remedy, the following are rumored to help: adding a teaspoon of baking soda (but this destroys thiamin in the legumes) or a pinch of ginger to the beans during the cooking, or chewing on peppermint. A proven way, however, is to eat beans in small quantities. One expert has offered a flatulence rating for beans from the most to the least gas-producing: soybeans, pink beans, black beans, pinto beans, California small white beans, Great Northern beans, baby lima beans, chick peas, large lima beans, and black-eyed peas.

Sprouting Your Own See[ds]

Every seed that is suitable for sprou[t]ing is a miniature storehouse of n[u]trients. Not all sprouts are equa[lly] nutritious. Many provide vitamin[s C] and A as well as some B vitamins, b[ut] they are not the miracle food, as so[me] claim. However, sprouts are low [in] calories and are easier to digest th[an] the beans themselves.

Sprouts can be purchased fresh [or] canned, but they are easily ho[me] grown from almost all dried peas a[nd] beans as well as some grains and se[eds] (see table opposite). Be sure to b[uy] the beans and seeds from a superm[ar]ket, specialty store, or a mail-or[der] supplier; stores vary in their sto[ck.] Use only edible seeds; never spr[out] seeds sold for gardening because t[hey] have been treated with fungicides t[hat] are poisonous.

Homegrown sprouts are more e[co]nomical than store-bought ones [. On] the average, ¼ cup dried peas or be[ans] yields at least 1 cup of sprouts) a[nd] more nutritious (some of the vitam[ins] and minerals are lost during stora[ge).] Keep sprouts refrigerated in an [air]tight plastic bag or container. For b[est] flavor and highest food value, [use] sprouts within 2 to 3 days. A[dd] sprouts to salads, soups, cassero[les,] or stir-fry as vegetables; gree[n] sprouts are especially good in sal[ads] or on sandwiches.

You do not need any special equ[ip]ment to grow sprouts at home. J[ust] follow the directions outlined h[ere] and consult the table for sprout[ing] times. Some sprouts, such as alfa[lfa] may be harvested at seed len[gth] (when the sprout is the same siz[e as] the seed) or they can be allowe[d to] grow longer. Use a jar or tray la[rge] enough to hold your sprout c[rop,] which may be four times greater t[han] the amount of seeds used. Alw[ays] drain rinse water thoroughly, s[ince] et seeds will sour and eventually ot. Many seeds will shed their husks uring sprouting. The remaining usks can be washed away in the final nsing. It is a matter of taste, but emember that the husks contain vimins. However, many sprouts are etter tasting and more tender withut their husks. Grain sprouts—alfala, wheat, barley—can be exposed to ght (a window sill is good) on the st day so they become green (with hlorophyll).

SEED	DRY MEASURE	YIELD	SPROUTING TIME	SPROUT LENGTH	EAT RAW OR COOK?
Alfalfa	¼ cup	½ to 4 cups	1 to 2 days 4 to 6 days	⅛ inch or 1 to 2 inches, greened	both
Barley	¼ cup	½ cup	3 to 5 days	seed length	cook
Chick-pea	¼ cup	nearly 1 cup	3 to 5 days	¾ to 1 inch	both
Lentil	½ cup	1 to 2 cups	3 to 4 days	¼ to ½	both
Mung Bean	¼ cup	1 to 2 cups	3 to 8 days	⅓ to 3 inches	both
Soybean	¼ cup	nearly 1 cup	3 to 6 days	½ to 1 inch	both
Wheat	¼ cup	1 cup	2 to 3 days 4 to 7 days	¼ inch or 1 inch, greened	both

ar Method

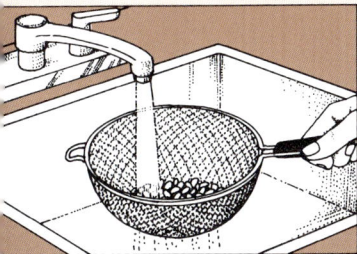

The jar method generally works best r mung or soybeans. (Small seeds, such alfalfa and barley, can be sprouted in a ay.) Measure out desired amount of eans or seeds (see table above). Discard y that are cracked or discolored, and nse the remainder in a sieve or strainer.

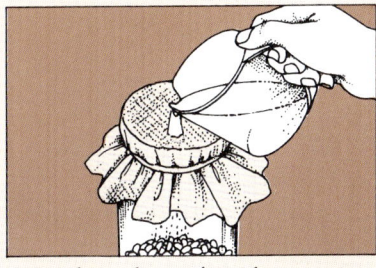

2. Put the seeds in a clean glass container, such as a canning jar, and secure a layer of cheesecloth over the top with a rubberband. Add 1 cup of lukewarm tap water (or 4 times the amount of seeds) and soak, unrefrigerated, with jar standing upright, for 8 hours or overnight.

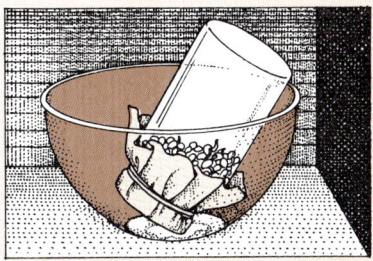

3. Thoroughly drain the remaining water through the cheesecloth and shake the jar to spread the seeds over the inner surface. Invert the jar and place at an angle in a large bowl or pot so still more water can drain out. Keep in a dark place, such as a kitchen cabinet or a closet.

Tray Method

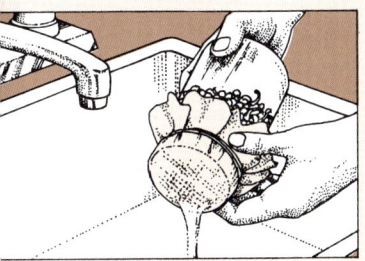

Rinse seeds twice daily—morning and ening—by running cold water into the , swirling it around, and pouring it out rough the cheesecloth. Remove any oldy seeds. Seeds should remain moist t not wet. Chick-peas and soybeans ed 4 to 6 rinsings a day.

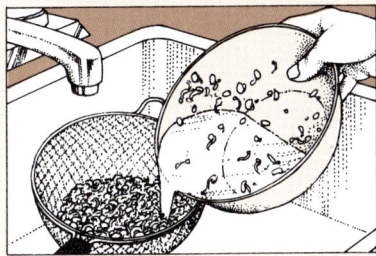

5. After sprouts reach desired length, place in a bowl and cover with water. Pour off some of the water and any loose husks. Drain the sprouts in a sieve or strainer. Husks that cling to the bowl can be washed away. Repeat this process if necessary. Refrigerate sprouts.

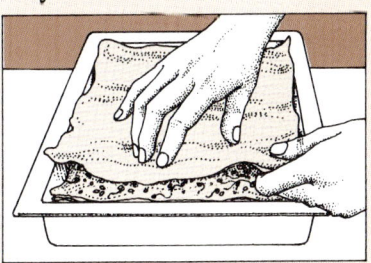

1. Follow steps 1 and 2 above. Then line a shallow tray with a layer of moist cheesecloth and spread the soaked seeds over it. Cover with another layer of moist cheesecloth. Sprinkle occasionally with water to keep the seeds moist. Place seeds in light on last day so the tiny leaves turn green.

Buying Guide
Nuts and Seeds

Nearly all nuts are dried tree fruits—called kernels or nutmeat—inside hard shells. Seeds are the embryo and food supply of new plants. They are graded by the U.S. Department of Agriculture. U.S. No. 1 is the finest grade; second grade includes U.S. No. 2, U.S. Commercial, and U.S. No. 1 Mixed. Popularly, "nuts" is a broad term that includes seeds such as cashews and Brazil nuts, and legumes such as peanuts.

What to look for. Nuts and seeds are sold shelled and unshelled and are available all year (except for chestnuts). Look for shells without cracks, holes, or mold. If the nuts rattle in their shells when shaken, it means they are shriveled or stale. When buying shelled nuts, choose plump ones of uniform size and color; avoid those that are soft, rubbery, or shriveled. Shelled nuts are sold whole, halved, in pieces, chopped, slivered, or ground. They may be plain, roasted (fried in reheated oil), toasted (dry roasted in the oven), blanched (outer skin of kernel removed by hot water), salted, smoked, sugared, spiced, or packaged raw with preservatives. Nuts in vacuum-packed jars or cans usually stay fresh longer than ones in bags. Unshelled nuts cost less, but about half the weight is shells; 1 pound unshelled nuts yields 1 to 2 cups nutmeat depending on the nuts.

How to keep. Nuts can be stored for a few months in a cool, dry place, but will keep longer if refrigerated. Nuts may also be frozen.

Nutritive value. Nuts and seeds are 10 to 25 percent protein, high in polyunsaturated fat, and a good source of iron, calcium, potassium, phosphorus, thiamin, riboflavin, vitamin E, and fiber. Seeds are very high in protein, iron, potassium, and phosphorus.

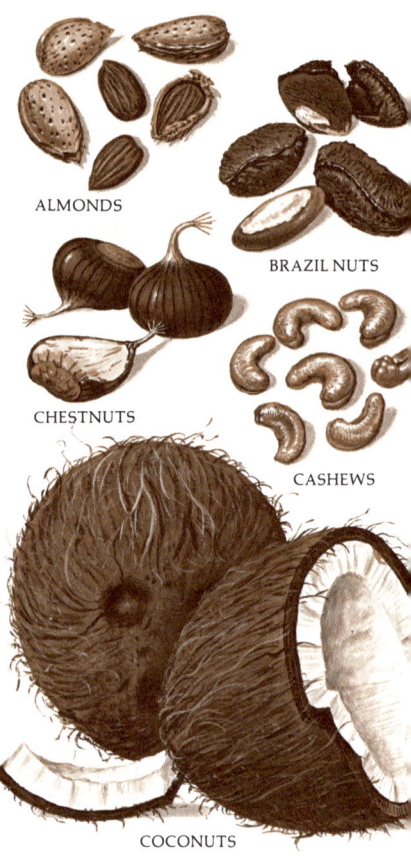

ALMONDS

BRAZIL NUTS

CHESTNUTS

CASHEWS

COCONUTS

Almonds. These are small, oval, flat nuts in easy-to-crack, light-brown shells. The white nutmeat has a delicate flavor. There are two types of almonds: bitter and sweet. Bitter almonds are used commercially for almond-based products such as almond extract. Sweet almonds can be eaten raw or cooked. Almonds are available whole, shelled or unshelled, ground, slivered, chopped, blanched, plain, roasted, salted, sugared, or smoked.

Brazil Nuts. These large, three-sided nuts have hard, dark-brown shells. The nutmeat is white, firm, and oily. They turn rancid sooner than other nuts because of their high oil content. They are available shelled and unshelled, whole, sliced (called chips), chopped, salted, or unsalted.

Cashews. These kidney-shaped nuts are the only ones sold without their shells because the shells are toxic. Cashews are usually available roasted and salted.

Chestnuts. Unlike most other nuts, the hard, shiny-brown, shelled chestnuts have less fat, more starch, and fewer calories. They are the only nuts served as a vegetable. Chestnuts are available fresh, roasted, canned, or dried. Although they can be eaten raw, most people prefer them cooked.

Coconuts. White coconut meat can be eaten raw or dried, or it can be grated and squeezed into a rich, fatty "milk." Buy heavy coconuts that are full of liquid (shake them to make sure). Avoid those with wet or moldy "eyes" (the three circles at one end). Unopened coconuts will keep at room temperature for about two months. Coconuts are high in calories and saturated fats.

Filberts or Hazelnuts. These brown-shelled nuts are actually fruits of the same bush that differ only in their shape. To distinguish between the two, hazelnuts are shorter and rounder than filberts. They have the sweetest meats of all the nuts and are used mainly in desserts and candies. They are available shelled and unshelled, whole, chopped, or ground.

Macadamias. Also called *Queensland nuts* since they are native to Australia, macadamias have honey-brown shells that are very difficult to crack. The crisp, creamy-white nutmeat has a slightly sweet flavor. They are usually sold roasted and salted and can be served as cocktail or dessert nuts.

Peanuts. Botanically classified as underground peas of the legume family, peanuts are also called *ground*

FAMILY FOOD GUIDE

peas, *ground nuts*, and *goobers*. Of the two varieties, the small, round *Spanish peanuts* are used for candy, peanut butter, and peanut oil. The larger, oval-shaped *Virginia peanuts* are used whole. Peanuts are sold shelled, unshelled, plain, roasted, dry roasted, salted, or blanched. About half of the U.S. peanut crop is made into peanut butter.

Pecans. The soft nutmeat of pecans is twin lobed and wrapped in thin, shiny, light-brown shells. They are available shelled, unshelled, whole, halved, chopped, dry roasted, plain, or salted.

Pine Nuts. Also called *Indian nuts*, *piñons*, *pignolias*, and *pinocchios*, these sweet-flavored, high-protein nuts vary in size (⅓ to 2 inches), shape (cylindrical to round), and color (white to pale yellow). Pine nuts are mostly sold shelled and blanched.

Pistachios. These green nuts have ivory-beige shells that split open upon maturity. Those with red shells have been colored with vegetable dye, and those with white shells have been coated with salt. Most are sold unshelled, roasted, and salted.

Walnuts. The two types of walnuts are *black* and *English*. Black walnuts have a strong flavor, and their dark-brown shells are difficult to open. The more popular *English*, or *Persian walnuts* (grown in California), are white on the inside and golden tan to amber on the outside. Their light-brown shells are easy to open. English walnuts can be eaten raw or cooked and are sold unshelled, shelled, whole, chopped, or ground.

Pumpkin Seeds. These thin-shelled seeds are sold shelled, unshelled, fresh, and dried. They can be eaten raw (shell and all), toasted, or salted. Keep them refrigerated.

Sesame Seeds. Also called by their African name *benne*, these tiny beige or brown seeds are sold whole and are eaten raw or toasted. The term "'open sesame''' is based on the ease with which the seeds pop out of their hulls.

Sunflower Seeds. These high-protein seeds can be eaten raw, toasted, or cooked. They are available shelled, unshelled, plain, or salted. To prevent discoloration when cooking with the seeds, use a small amount of one of the following: vinegar, lemon juice, orange juice, brown sugar, baking soda, or molasses. Refrigerate the seeds to retard spoilage.

Peanut Butter

A sandwich made with 2 tablespoons of peanut butter on enriched white bread or whole-wheat bread is a very nutritious lunch—and an economical one as well. It supplies 20 percent of the recommended daily protein intake for an adult, as well as 30 percent niacin, 10 percent iron, 6 percent calcium, 18 percent magnesium, 17 percent phosphorus, and 7 percent zinc. Peanut butter is about 50 percent fat, most of which is unsaturated.

All peanut butter must, by federal regulation, be at least 90 percent peanuts. The remaining 10 percent is limited to salt, sugar, and hydrogenated fat or oil (to prevent the natural oil in peanuts from rising to the top). No artificial colors, flavorings, or chemical preservatives can be added to peanut butter, but these are permitted in peanut spreads. Chunky peanut butter has small bits of peanuts added and is outsold 3 to 1 by the smooth variety.

Look for peanut butter that is light brown and avoid any that is grayish or uneven in color. When you open the jar, it should not have a musty or chemical odor.

Peanut butter can also be easily made at home by grinding unsalted peanuts in your blender or food processor. You may need to add a tablespoon of oil per ½ pound of peanuts for smoother blending. The natural peanut oil that rises to the top can be stirred back in. Refrigerating homemade peanut butter will prevent it from separating.

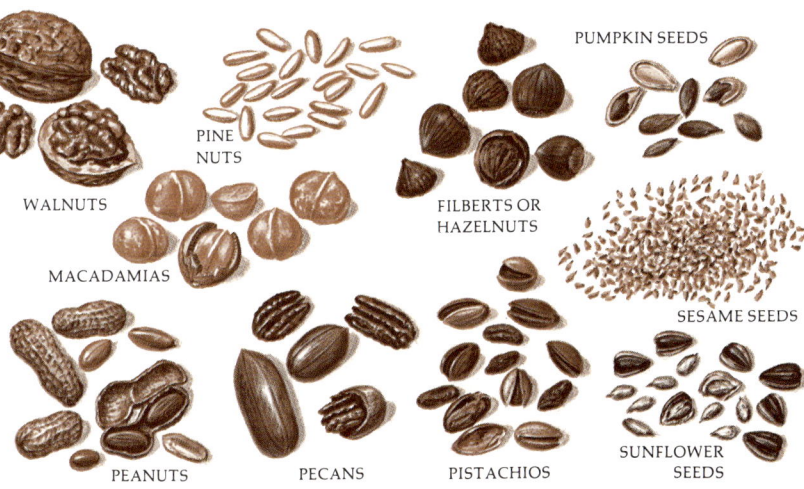

Buying Guide
Grains and Grain Products

Grains are the seeds of food grasses and other plants and include barley, corn, millet, oats, rice, rye, the hybrid triticale, and wheat. Buckwheat, usually grouped with grains, is actually a botanical relative of rhubarb. Grains were the first cultivated food. Once man learned to plant crops he could give up the nomadic way of life and settle down to farming. Usually, the locally grown grain became the staple food of the area—rice in the Far East, oats in Scotland, wheat in the United States. Grains can be eaten whole, such as brown rice, or processed into cereals or flour for a multitude of other food products.

How to keep. Store grains and grain products in an airtight container—preferably a glass jar with a tight lid—in a cool, dry place. To prevent whole grains and whole-grain products, such as whole-wheat flour, from turning rancid, keep at room temperature for no more than two weeks or refrigerate for longer use. **What to look for** and specific storage information are mentioned in individual entries.

Nutritive value. Grains are very low in fat, sugar, and sodium and high in starch and fiber. The nutrient content will depend on whether the grain is highly milled or not and also on whether the product has been enriched or fortified. Most are a good source of niacin, thiamin, riboflavin, B_6, phosphorus, magnesium, copper, chromium, manganese, selenium, and molybdenum.

Barley
In ancient times, before wheat and rye were used to make raised yeast breads, barley was the chief grain for baking flat breads. The Bible tells that Jesus fed 5,000 people with 5 loaves of bread made from barley. Centuries later, the Scottish poet Robert Burns personified Sir John Barleycorn as the king of grain. Barley was celebrated not only for its role in breadmaking but also because malted barley is the basis of beer and whiskey. Today, a large part of the world's barley crop is fermented into alcohol.

In Scotland, where barley is widely grown, it is commonly eaten as a breakfast cereal and as Scotch broth, a mutton-based barley soup. When barley is boiled with lemon peel and strained, it becomes barley water, an old-fashioned broth for the sick.

Whole barley. Also called *Scotch barley*, *pot barley*, and *hulled barley*, whole barley is often sold in specialty food stores. This brown barley is nuttier and chewier than pearled barley and must be soaked before cooking.

Pearled barley. The only type usually found in supermarkets, pearled barley is polished white after the hull and bran are removed. It is sold in fine, medium, and coarse grinds and can be used in soups and casseroles.

Malted barley. The main ingredient in beer and malt whiskey, malted barley is made by sprouting and pulverizing the grain into a powder before processing it into alcohol. There is little nutritive value in malt liquors. *Extract of malt*, which retains the nutrients of the grain, is also produced from malted barley. When combined with powdered milk, it becomes malted milk.

Buckwheat
Although used as a grain, the strong-flavored buckwheat is botanically a fruit. Buckwheat seeds, produced from flowers, consist only of a kernel (called a groat) inside a shell. It is a good source of protein, thiamin, riboflavin, potassium, iron, and is low in calories. Groats are used for breakfast cereal, puddings, and stuffings. Roasted groats are called *kasha*, which is a traditional Eastern European food. Buckwheat is also the source of a dark, strong-tasting honey.

Corn
Now also a vegetable, corn was first thought of only as a grain. Grain products such as grits and cornmeal are made with *field corn*, which has more starch and less sugar than *sweet corn*, the variety eaten as corn on the cob. Both kinds of corn are raised in two varieties: yellow and white. The two are nutritionally similar, but yellow corn is richer in vitamin A.

Hominy. The American Indian word for hulled and dried corn, hominy is sold dried (it must be soaked before cooking) or canned (precooked). Hominy has neither the bran nor the germ of the whole corn kernel.

Grits. Also called *hominy grits* or *corn grits*, grits are ground hominy and are sold in fine, medium, and coarse grinds. Grits have larger granules than cornmeal. Cooked grits are a traditional dish in the South.

Cornmeal. Made from dried kernels, cornmeal can be stone-ground or ground by steel rollers. It is sold in fine, medium, or coarse grinds. The most commonly available is steel-rolled, a process that removes the germ and the bran from the kernels, thus lengthening the storage time of the meal. This is called *degermed cornmeal*. Stone-ground cornmeal is often labeled "old-fashioned." *Bolted cornmeal* has only a portion of the bran removed. *Enriched cornmeal* has riboflavin, niacin, thiamin, and iron added according to government standards.

Keep cornmeal in an airtight container in a cool, dark place. If old-fashioned cornmeal is freshly ground, it should be used within 2 weeks of purchase. If not fresh, it should be refrigerated or it may turn rancid.

Cornmeal is used to make many traditional American specialties, including cornbread, spoon bread, johnnycakes (or journey cakes), hasty pudding, hush puppies, and hoecakes. Cornmeal is also the basis of Italian polenta and Central American tortillas.

Cornstarch. A common thickener used in cooking, cornstarch is made from the starch in the endosperm of the corn kernel.

Popcorn. A gift from the Indians at the first Thanksgiving, popcorn remains a favorite American snack. Popcorn kernels are larger than other corn kernels, and when they are heated, the moisture trapped within bursts the kernels open. If the kernels do not pop, it usually means they are dried out. Soak them for a few days in a little warm water and stir occasionally. Try popping them again after the water is absorbed.

The two types available are *yellow* or *white*. White popcorn has slightly smaller kernels and some people think they are more tender and tastier. Store kernels in a cool place in an airtight container. They will keep for about a year.

Popcorn is low in calories (only 25 calories in 1 unbuttered cup), high in fiber, and not without nutritive value. It has a little protein, phosphorus, iron, riboflavin, and niacin.

Millet

A yellow, bland, and nutritious grain, millet is available in specialty food stores in the United States. It is sold *whole* and *cracked* and usually without its tough, inedible hull. Used in cakes, cookies, bread puddings, and as a substitute for rice, millet has nearly as much protein as wheat. Since millet swells greatly in cooking, a small amount will yield a large portion. Millet is a dietary staple in the Orient, India, and Africa.

Oats

First thought of as just useless weeds crowding out other grains, oats have more protein than any other grain plus ample amounts of calcium, iron, phosphorus, and potassium. Although long a dietary staple in Scotland and Ireland, oats were used as animal feed in America until the middle of the 19th century when Ferdinand Schumacher, a German immigrant, developed the first quick-cooking hot oat cereal. However, 90 percent of the American oat crop is still used to feed livestock. Unlike wheat and rye, oats do not have gluten—a

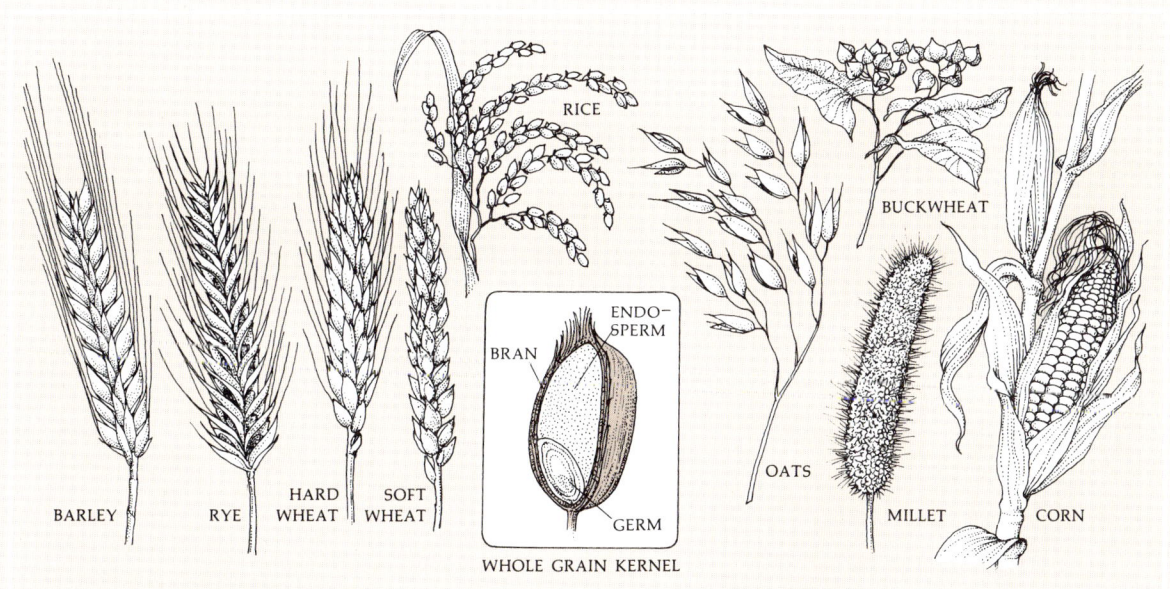

What Is a Whole Grain?

Most of us never see grain growing in the field—what we buy has been processed to one degree or another. Shown above are stalks of some staple grains and the flowering buckwheat; at center is a representation of a kernel of whole grain. Every kernel consists of the bran, germ, and endosperm inside an inedible husk, or hull. The bran forms the protective inner covering and is a source of dietary fiber. The germ is the embryo of a new plant and a source of protein, vitamins, and minerals; it also contains polyunsaturated fats. The endosperm supplies most of the protein and carbohydrates primarily as starch.

Buying Guide
Grains and Grain Products

protein that interacts with yeast and causes dough to rise. Oats contain fiber and polyunsaturated fats because the bran and germ are not removed in processing. Refrigerate oat products to prevent the fats from becoming rancid, or keep in a cool place for not more than 3 weeks.

Whole oats. Called *groats*, whole oats consist of the bran, germ, and endosperm of the whole grain with the outer hull removed. Whole oats are softer than wheat grains and can be crushed at home. They are available in specialty food stores.

Rolled oats. The most common form of oats, rolled oats are so-called because the whole groats are steamed and then flattened between rollers before being made into flakes. Rolled oats are popularly called *oatmeal*. They are available in three thicknesses, and the thicker the flake, the longer the oats will take to cook. *Scotch* or *steel-cut oats* are the thickest, and are sometimes called *Scotch* or *Irish oatmeal*. *Table-cut* or *regular old-fashioned oats*, sold in specialty stores, are nuttier and chewier than quick-cooking oats but are otherwise the same. *Quick-cooking* or *instant oats* are the thinnest flakes. Some think they have a raw taste compared with other oats. Do not confuse instant oats with *instant oatmeal*, which may be packaged with sugar.

Rice

A grain that grows in water, rice is one of the two most important foods in the world. The other is wheat. Although the West considers rice as an accompaniment to a main dish or a substitute for potato or bread, rice is central to Eastern cuisine and is prized for its simplicity and nourishment.

Rice was first grown in the United States in South Carolina. It was so profitable that it came to be known as "Carolina gold." During the American Revolution, however, when the British occupied Charleston, all the rice was sent to England, including the seeds for the following year's planting. Thomas Jefferson remedied the situation by smuggling rice kernels out of Italy while on diplomatic business there in 1787.

Rice is mainly a source of carbohydrates, but it also provides protein, calcium, iron, phosphorus, potassium, niacin, and riboflavin. Brown rice and enriched, or converted, white rice have similar nutritive values, but brown rice has more fiber.

Both white and brown rice are available in long-, short-, or medium-length grains, and are sold packaged or loose in bins or sacks. When cooked, *long-grain rice* kernels are lighter, fluffier, and firmer than short-grain rice and do not cling together. Therefore, long-grain rice is used with poultry, seafood, and meat and for cold salads, pilafs, curries, and Chinese and Japanese dishes.

Medium and *short-grain rice* are plump, oval grains, moister than long grains, and cling together when cooked. This cohesiveness makes them good for porridge, croquettes, and desserts. Long and medium grains are usually identified as such.

Rice purchased loose should be rinsed in cold water before cooking. Packaged rice does not need to be washed unless the rice is whitened with talc and glucose, in which case the directions will say so. Most rice, however, is not coated with whiteners. Washing enriched rice will reduce its nutritive value by about 15 percent because the water-soluble vitamins may be washed away.

One-half cup of raw rice will yield 1½ cups cooked rice. An average serving of cooked rice is ⅓ to ½ cup per person. The best way to prevent rice from turning soggy is *not* to stir it while it is cooking.

White rice should be kept in an airtight container in a cool, dry place. If a glass jar is used, store in a dark place. Brown rice should be refrigerated if not used within a month of purchase to delay its turning rancid.

Brown rice. Brown rice retains both the bran and the germ of the rice kernel. It has a nutlike flavor and a chewy texture. It needs to be cooked in more water than white rice and takes longer to cook.

White rice. When both the bran and the germ are removed by milling and polishing the rice kernels, only the white, starchy endosperm is left. Most white rice is enriched with some of the nutrients lost during milling, namely thiamin, iron, and niacin. Riboflavin is not replaced because it turns the raw rice yellow. Rice that is enriched will say so on the label.

Converted (parboiled) rice. This is brown rice that is steamed and pressurized before being milled and polished into white rice. The steam pressure forces the nutrients from the bran and germ into the endosperm before the bran and germ are removed. Packaged rice dinners usually use this type of white rice.

Quick-cooking (instant) rice. This is precooked white rice that has been dehydrated before packaging. It is usually lower in minerals than other kinds of rice.

Wild rice. Not rice at all, but the seeds of a tall aquatic grass, wild rice is expensive because it is scarce and difficult to grow commercially. Ninety percent of all wild rice grows on or near the Chippewa White Earth Reservation in the Great Lakes region of the United States. Only the Indians are permitted to gather it, and their ancient methods are still used. As Waverley Root, noted food historian, describes it, "They harvest it as they always have, from canoes which glide almost invisibly through the water among the tall plants. They bend the stalks over the canoes, smack them with a stick, and the grain drops into the canoe—or more exactly, about 10 percent of it does. The other 90 percent falls into the water, where . . . it reseeds the stand and feeds fish and wild ducks."

Wild rice, which is gray-brown,

should be washed before cooking to remove any foreign particles. Wild rice has twice the protein of white rice and less calories. It is sometimes sold packaged with long grain white rice.

Rye

Popular in Scandinavia and Eastern Europe, rye is similar to wheat in nutritive value. But since it is low in gluten (the protein necessary to make yeast bread rise), it is frequently combined with wheat when baking bread. Rye is also fermented to make whiskey.

Unlike other grains, rye is susceptible to ergot, a poisonous fungus. Chemical preservatives are therefore often added to rye bread to prevent ergot's growth. Use opened packages of rye bread that do not have preservatives within a few days of purchase.

Whole and cracked rye grains. Available in specialty stores, whole and cracked rye kernels can be cooked as cereal, combined with cracked wheat or oats, or ground into flour for home use. *Rye grits* have more nutritive value than hominy grits.

Sorghum

Related to millet and a dietary staple in Africa and Asia, sorghum can be used as you would rice, as a porridge, or in soups, or popped like popcorn. A sweet syrup is produced from some varieties. Sorghum may be difficult to find in the United States.

Triticale

Pronounced "triticaylee," this hardy hybrid of wheat and rye is generally available in specialty stores as grain or flour. Triticale flour combines the gluten of both rye and wheat, producing a bread dough more delicate than either parent grain.

Wheat

Grown throughout the world, wheat was one of the first grains ever cultivated by man.

Although there are many varieties of wheat, they all fall into two categories: those high in gluten, called *hard wheats* (or *bread wheats*), and those with little gluten, called *soft wheats* (or *pastry wheats*). Hard and soft wheats are grown in colder climates where they are planted in spring (known as *spring wheats*) or in warmer climates where they are planted in the fall (known as *winter wheats*). The farther north the wheat is planted the more protein it will have. The most common varieties of wheat are as follows: *hard red spring wheat*—these kernels are short, thick, and hard with large amounts of gluten. They make the best flour for bread; *hard red winter wheat*—these kernels are longer and thinner than the spring wheat kernels, with varying amounts of gluten, depending on where they are grown. Most of the wheat grown in the United States is this type. It is widely used for bread and other baked goods. *Soft red winter wheat*—these kernels are long and chubby with less gluten and more starch than hard wheats. This wheat is used for pastry flour. *Durum wheat*—these kernels are amber and pointed. They are ground into flour for whole-wheat pasta and semolina (see page 173) for regular pasta. Wheat is available whole, cracked, or ground into flour.

Whole-wheat grains. Whole-wheat grains, also called *wheat berries*, are usually sold in specialty food stores. Check the label on the sack or barrel to be sure it specifies that the kernels are for human consumption. Do not purchase whole kernels intended for planting because they are coated with toxic chemicals. Whole-wheat grains can be cooked as porridge or used as a side dish instead of rice.

Cracked wheat. These are whole-wheat kernels that have been broken or crushed into smaller pieces for faster cooking. Cracked wheat can be used instead of whole-wheat grains or bulgur in recipes, but it will cook faster than whole-wheat grains and slower than bulgur.

Bulgur. Also known as *wheat pilaf, burghul,* and *parboiled wheat,* bulgur is similar to cracked wheat but has been partially cooked and dried before being cracked. Sometimes the bran, the dark-brown covering, is removed, so check to see, if possible. Interchangeable with cracked wheat, bulgur has a slightly nuttier taste and cooks faster. It is usually sold in three grinds: coarse, medium, and fine. Bulgur is used as cereal, in soups, salads, and casseroles. A staple grain in Eastern Europe and the Middle East, bulgur is the main ingredient in tabouli, a Middle Eastern salad (see recipe, page 259).

Bran. This is the coarse, dark-brown outer layers of a grain. Wheat bran is well-known for its high fiber content. (Fiber is discussed on pages 18-19.) Bran is separated from the wheat kernels when they are milled into white flour. Bran adds texture, sweetness, nuttiness, and color to cereals and baked goods such as bread, muffins, and cookies.

Wheat germ. Actually the embryo from which a new wheat plant can grow, the germ contains most of the vitamins and minerals of the wheat grain and much of the protein. Wheat germ is rich in vitamin E. It also contains polyunsaturated fats, which can cause the wheat germ to turn rancid if not refrigerated. The germ is extracted from the kernels when the wheat is milled into white flour. This increases the shelf life of the flour. Wheat germ is sold both raw and toasted and can be eaten as cereal, added to bread, salads, or casseroles; sprinkle on top of yogurt or vegetables for added crunch.

Farina. Farina wheat is commonly used as a breakfast cereal, though there are other uses for it. Farina's bran and germ are removed. *Enriched farina* has iron, thiamin, riboflavin, and niacin added to it according to government standards.

Buying Guide
Grains and Grain Products

Cereals — Breakfast in a Box

Before the day of ready-to-eat dry cereals packaged in colorful cartons, breakfast cereals were the stick-to-the-ribs variety such as hot oatmeal and porridge. These whole-grain cereals were usually cooked on the stove for many hours and served with hot syrup, butter, cream, or sugar.

Today, whole grains for ready-to-eat cereals are first steamed, dried, pressurized, and toasted. Then they are rolled, flaked, shredded, puffed, sugared, colored, flavored, or fortified, resulting in a bewildering array of breakfast cereals, each with its healthful benefits proclaimed on the package.

The best buys are usually cereals that are not highly processed and that have the least amount of sugar, salt, artificial flavoring, artificial coloring, and preservatives. Always check the list of ingredients on the package to see what has been added. (For information on how to read labels, see pages 196-198.)

Here are some of the terms you will probably encounter in trying to make sense of cerealmakers' claims.

Fortified cereals. These are cereals to which manufacturers have added nutrients whether or not they are present in the cereal grains themselves, such as vitamin D. Fortified and enriched cereals are not the same (see enriched, below). Both hot and cold cereals may be fortified.

Manufacturers may add as many nutrients as they wish, or none at all. However, if the manufacturer adds any nutrient, or makes a nutritional claim, he must provide a nutritional label on the package. If 50 percent or more of the Recommended Dietary Allowances for any nutrient is added to a cereal, the cereal must be labeled a *dietary supplement*. The more a cereal is fortified, the more a manufacturer will usually charge for it.

Some nutrition experts are leery of people depending overly much on a single food that supplies 100 percent of the Recommended Dietary Allowances of a nutrient. It would be unwise to conclude that if you meet your vitamin and mineral needs by eating a breakfast cereal that supplies 100 percent of the RDA for these vitamins that you can forget about your choices of food for the rest of the day. Remember that no food fills all of your nutrient needs, even when it is highly fortified. Don't put all of your nutrient eggs in a single basket.

Enriched cereals. These are cereals to which nutrients destroyed during processing are added in amounts set by the government. The amounts may be higher than those found naturally in the grains. However, some nutrients lost in milling are not replaced. Trace minerals are not replaced; nor is fiber, unless the cereal is made with bran. Both hot and cold cereals may be enriched.

Ready-to-eat cereals. These dry cereals may be single grain or a combination of two or more. They are sold plain, flavored, colored, sugared, with or without fruit, and come in a variety of sizes and shapes. Ready-to-eat cereals are often fortified and/or enriched.

Nearly all ready-to-eat cereals contain sugar. Many are 40 percent sugar but some are less than 10 percent sugar. Many cereals specify on the label how much sugar there is in a 1-ounce serving. One way to cut back on sugar is to buy unsweetened cereals. If you insist on extra sweetening and do not want to use fruit, you can add your own sugar. Since the price of sugar in presweetened cereals is about 6 times that of sugar, you will save money.

"Natural" cereals. For the most part, these are cereals to which no artificial or synthetic ingredients have been added and which have been only minimally processed. However, since the use and meaning of the term "natural" are not regulated by any federal agency involved with labeling, be sure to check the list of ingredients to see how much sugar or sweeteners and fat is in each serving. If the cereal is enriched, the label must so state. Both hot and cold "natural" cereals are sold.

Hot cereals. Also called *cooked cereals*, these require cooking before being served, such as oatmeal. Hot cereals do not necessarily have more nutritive value than cold ones. For example, unenriched farina has very little nutritive value. Enriched oatmeal, though, is nutritious. Many hot cereals are enriched or fortified, so check the label. Check also for added sugar, perservatives, and other ingredients.

Quick cereals. These cereals take less time to prepare than hot cereals because the grains are cut thinner and smaller. Otherwise they are just as nutritious as hot cereals.

Instant cereals. These precooked cereals require only the addition of boiling water before being served. Sometimes sugar or other ingredients and preservatives are added.

Flours

Almost all the wheat produced today for human consumption is ground into flour for making breads, cookies, cakes, pastries, and pasta. Wheat flour can be either whole wheat, which is brown and includes the bran and germ of the grain, or white wheat flour, which is white because the bran and germ have been removed in processing. Most white flour is enriched and/or bleached (see below). Only flours made from wheat and rye have more than a trace of gluten, the protein needed to make yeast bread rise. (For a step-by-step guide to baking yeast bread, see pages 270-272.) Bakers sometimes mix nonwheat flours, such as oat or soy flour, with wheat flour for variety in taste, texture, and nutritive value. Nonwheat flours can also be used for other baked goods.

What to look for. The terms "wheat flour" and "wheat bread" printed on packages mean only that wheat is the grain that has been used, not any other grain, such as rye or corn. If you want whole-wheat flour or whole-wheat bread, be sure the package or the label says "whole wheat" or "100 percent whole wheat."

How to keep. Flour should be stored in a cool, dry place in a tightly closed container. If a clear glass jar is used, it should be kept in a dark place. White flour will stay fresh longer than whole wheat. Refrigerate or freeze whole-wheat flour if not used within two or three weeks of purchase to prevent it from turning rancid.

Wheat Flours

All-purpose flour. A blend of finely ground hard and soft wheats, this white flour is suitable for baking breads and pastries. (The blend varies, however, from one region of the country to another. For example, in the South, where quick breads are popular, the texture of all-purpose flour is closer to cake flour; in the North, however, where more yeast breads are usually baked, more hard wheat goes into the flour to provide additional gluten.) Although all-purpose flour has the bran and germ removed, government regulations mandate that all-purpose flour be enriched with certain nutrients. All-purpose flour may be bleached or unbleached or have barley flour added to replace needed enzymes lost in milling. It can be used to make breads, cakes, cookies, and pastries.

Bleached flour. This is flour that has been chemically treated to age it and/or make it whiter. Aged flour produces better baking results. Bleaching prolongs the shelf life of flour, but it also destroys the vitamin E content. Unbleached flour is creamier in color and has a better taste, according to some.

Cake flour. With a silky and soft consistency, this low-gluten flour is made from uniformly and finely ground bleached soft wheat and is used mainly in making cakes and pastries.

Enriched flour. This is white flour to which certain nutrients have been added in accordance with government regulations to replace nutrients lost in milling. Iron and three B vitamins—thiamin, riboflavin, and niacin—are added. The amount of B vitamins added to enriched flour is usually higher than in the natural wheat grain. However, neither bran nor the following vitamins and minerals are replaced: vitamin B_6, pantothenic acid, folacin, vitamin E, choline, calcium, phosphorus, potassium, magnesium, sodium, chromium, manganese, cobalt, copper, zinc, selenium, and molybdenum.

Gluten flour. High in protein and low in starch, this flour is made by washing the starch from wheat flour and then drying out and grinding the remains. When gluten flour is combined with the correct proportion of low-gluten flours, it becomes a substitute for all-purpose flour and can be used to make yeast breads. Gluten flour is a common ingredient in breakfast cereals.

Instant flour. Manufactured to dissolve quickly in liquids, this flour does not lump when used in making sauces and gravies; in addition, it does not need to be sifted before it is used. Except for making pie dough, instant flour should not be used as a substitute for baking with all-purpose flour.

Self-rising flour. Leavens, such as baking powder, and salt are added to bleached all-purpose flour by the miller to make self-rising flour as a convenience to the home baker. Since leavens lose their potency over a period of time, this flour should be used within 1 to 2 months of purchase. Available as self-rising all-purpose flour or self-rising cake flour, it is not recommended for baking yeast breads. Self-rising flour is used in commercially prepared mixes for biscuits, cakes, and pancakes.

Semolina. Finely ground from durum wheat, semolina is used commercially to make pasta. (For homemade pasta, use whole-wheat or unbleached all-purpose flour.) Semolina has a natural yellow color. It is also used to make the grains for *couscous*, a North African dish. Couscous is sold in some specialty stores.

Whole-wheat flour. Ground from the whole-wheat kernel, this brown flour has the bran, germ, and endosperm of the whole grain. It contains fiber and more vitamins and minerals than enriched white flour. *Stone-ground whole-wheat flour* is simply ground between stone wheels rather than steel rollers. It is coarser and heavier than steel ground, and some prefer the nutty taste. Sometimes

Buying Guide
Flours

whole-wheat flour is called *Graham flour*, after Sylvester Graham, proponent of whole-wheat flour and for whom the Graham cracker is named. When some of the coarser bran flakes are sifted out, the result is *whole-wheat pastry flour*, which produces a lighter-texture product. Whole-wheat pastry flour should not be used for making yeast bread because it is low in gluten.

Other Flours

Barley flour. Low in gluten, barley flour should be combined with wheat flour for breadmaking. This flour produces products with a cakelike consistency and sweetness and is thus generally used for pastries.

Buckwheat flour. Two types of buckwheat flour are made: *dark* (from unhulled groats) and *light* (from hulled groats). Buckwheat flour is used mostly for pancakes and blinis, and for a Japanese commercial fast-food noodle called *soba*.

Oat flour. Because it contains an antioxident that delays fat from turning rancid, oat flour mixed with whole-wheat flour will prolong the freshness of whole-wheat bread. Oat flour should be combined with wheat flour to make yeast breads.

Rice flour. Made from finely ground brown or polished white rice, this flour is used in baked products as a thickener and in baby cereals. Rice flour is more easily digested than wheat flour. Brown rice flour is sold in specialty food stores.

Rye flour. With its low gluten content, rye flour makes a heavy, low-rising bread with a rich flavor. It is thus frequently mixed with wheat flour—which has more gluten—to make a lighter, higher loaf. Rye flour ranges from light to dark grades. Light rye flour has been "bolted," or sifted, to remove some of the bran. Dark rye flour is unbolted and coarser and is sometimes called *pumpernickel flour*. Commercially baked pumpernickel bread may be prepared with dark rye flour or a mixture of rye and wheat flours or it may be darkened with molasses or caramel coloring.

Soy flour. Ground from whole, dried soybeans, this flour is high in protein and fat. Three types of soy flour are marketed: *low fat*, *defatted*, and *full fat*. (See The Versatile Soybean, page 163.)

Triticale flour. Although higher in protein than wheat flour, this sweet-tasting hybrid of wheat and rye is low in gluten. Therefore, it should be mixed with wheat flour for breadmaking. Triticale flour is usually sold in specialty food stores.

Bread—White vs Whole Wheat

The argument over white bread versus whole wheat goes back to the time of the Roman Empire. In those days, wheat was ground between two stones to produce a coarse, dark flour with bits of stone and chaff in it. According to one observer, Roman bread was "so heavy that it would sink in water." Lighter bread was made by regrinding and resifting the flour and the addition of milk and chalk—all of which also made it whiter as well. Because all this meant more work, white bread was expensive and only wealthy Romans could afford to buy it. Not until the 1870s, when mechanized roller mills could mass produce white flour, did white bread become everyman's food.

Today the debate is not about cost but about nutrition. Whole-wheat bread contains the fiber of the bran, vitamin E of the germ, and all the other vitamins and minerals found naturally in the wheat kernel. If the whole-wheat flour is stone-ground, some claim it is even more nutritious because the millstones do not get as hot as steel rollers and therefore more nutrients are preserved.

This would seem to tilt the scales toward whole wheat. However, white bread is enriched, in compliance with government regulations, with four nutrients—thiamin, niacin, riboflavin (all B vitamins), and iron. Calcium and vitamin D may also be added. Moreover, the amount of B vitamins are increased to levels greater than those found naturally in wheat. But fiber, vitamin E, and 22 other nutrients lost in milling are not replaced. Also, white bread stays fresh longer than whole wheat because it lacks wheat germ, whose fat content turns the bread rancid with time.

Another factor that enters into the argument is that whole-wheat bread contains phytic acid, which interferes with the body's ability to absorb calcium and iron. But according to nutritionist Jean Mayer, much of the phytic acid is destroyed during leavening. Moreover, phytic acid is not a serious problem if a balanced diet is followed.

When all these points are taken into account, whole-wheat bread is generally considered slightly more nutritious than white bread.

Pasta and Noodles

A well-known food of Italy, pasta also includes the dumplings and noodles of both Europe and the Far East. Most Italian-style pasta is made from semolina, a flour ground from durum wheat, and water. Other pastas are made with eggs (or egg solids) and different flours. The word *macaroni* is sometimes used as a general term for pasta as well as being a type of pasta itself, such as elbow macaroni. Pasta should be cooked until it is al dente, or firm to the bite, not soft or mushy. Adding a teaspoon of vegetable oil to the cooking water will help prevent pasta from sticking together when drained.

What to look for. Most pasta is yellow-white in color. Avoid any that is gray or too powdery. Light brown pasta is made with whole-wheat flour and tastes slightly nutty. Other pasta is made with bleached or unbleached flour. (Flours are discussed on pages 173-174.) Green pasta (*pasta verde*) is made with spinach or other green vegetable puree added to the flour, and red pasta with tomato or other red vegetable puree. Colored pasta tastes about the same as regular pasta. For those who wish to avoid artificial colors, be sure that the pasta label says vegetable coloring. Fresh pasta, sold in its doughy form before it is dried, can often be purchased in specialty food stores or in an Italian neighborhood.

How to keep. Keep boxed pasta in a cool, dry place. If pasta is transferred to a glass jar, do not keep it in the light for more than a few weeks. Refrigerate fresh pasta in a sealed bag or container or freeze for not more than two weeks.

Nutritive value. Very high in carbohydrates, pasta is low in fat (spaghetti is less than 1 percent fat) and contains some protein, calcium, potassium, and phosphorus. Pasta made with enriched flour has thiamin, riboflavin, niacin, and iron. Whole-wheat pasta, egg, and colored pasta are slightly more nutritious than regular pasta.

Italian Pasta

Although legend says that the Venetian explorer Marco Polo brought back pasta from China to Italy in 1295, records show that Romans were eating ravioli and fettucine at least a decade earlier. In Italy a meal is usually not considered complete unless it is preceded by a small pasta course.

Almost all pasta is made from semolina flour mixed with water. The dough is pressed through a variety of metal designs into hundreds of different shapes. Pasta can be grouped according to its uses: those that can be stuffed, such as *ravioli*, *agnolotti*, *cannelloni*, and *manicotti*; those that are flat, such as *lasagna* and *tagliatelle*; those that are "strings," such as *spaghetti* and the spiral-shaped *fusilli*; and those in a variety of special shapes, such as *farfalle* ("butterflies" or "bows") and *stellini* ("little stars"). Some pasta, such as *fettucine* and *tortellini*, has eggs added to the dough, and in Italy this type of pasta is called *pasta all'uovo*.

The most popular pasta, of course, is spaghetti. It is also the most versatile and can be bought in a variety of widths. Use very thin spaghetti, such as *vermicelli* ("little worms"), with seafood sauces, and the wider spaghetti, such as *linguine* ("little tongues"), with tomato sauces. Meat sauces can be served with pasta that is short, curled, or ridged—such as shells or spirals—so that the bits of meat will be trapped in the pasta's twists and curls.

European Noodles

The origin of the word *noodle* is rooted in the European words for dumpling—in German it is *nudeln*; in the Bavarian part of Germany it is *knödl*; and in Austria it is *knödel*. Dumplings preceded the development of the noodle and were made by tossing bits of uncooked dough into soups and stews. Variations of this custom spread throughout Europe. It is the Germans, however, who are credited with being the first to add eggs to the dough and shape it into the now familiar flat noodle. Noodles with a deep yellow color have a higher egg content than those that are pale yellow. Two favorites of the European region are a noodle pudding that is baked with raisins and cheese and *spätzle* ("little sparrows"), which are small unfilled dumplings served as a side dish with veal or cabbage or mixed with vegetables.

Oriental Noodles

Most Oriental noodles are long and thin, to symbolize long life. They are usually sold in specialty food stores, and some supermarkets or in bundles by weight in Oriental food shops. In Oriental neighborhoods, most of the noodles available in the stores are made from rice flour. They have a distinctive flavor and include *rice sticks*, *rice noodles*, and the thread-thin *rice vermicelli*. But there are noodles made from many other ingredients, too. One type of noodle is made with eggs and/or wheat flour and is called *egg noodles* or *wheat noodles*. *Cellophane noodles* (also called *transparent noodles*, *bean threads*, *pea starch noodles*, or *vermicelli*), are made from mung-bean flour and become translucent and slippery after they are cooked. They readily absorb the flavors of other ingredients. Other noodles are made from soybean, buckwheat, or seaweed flours. *Wonton* wrappers are the Chinese version of the European dumpling and Italy's ravioli.

Buying Guide
Herbs and Spices

Herbs are the leaves, stems, flowers, or roots, and sometimes seeds of plants and shrubs that are used for seasoning, fragrance, or as medicine; spices—used for the same purposes—come from the roots, bark, fruit, or berries of perennial plants such as cinnamon, nutmeg, and pepper and cannot be easily grown at home. The aroma and flavor of herbs and spices come from the essential oils that are released when they are crushed, ground, or chopped. Featured below are 11 herbs that are often sold fresh in markets but which are also easy to grow in the garden, or indoors in a flower pot. All except parsley and chives also appear in the chart on the next two pages. Herbs and spices are a calorie-free way of flavoring foods while limiting the use of salt. When substituting dried herbs for fresh, use one-third to one-half of the amount called for in the recipe. A common mixture of herbs is a *bouquet garni*, usually parsley, thyme, and bay leaf, tied in cheesecloth. It is used to flavor soups or stews and is removed before serving.

What to look for. Fresh herbs often have better flavor than those that are dried, packaged, and sold in stores. Whole herbs and spices stay potent longer than if they are ground, powdered, or crumbled.

How to keep. Store dried herbs and spices in airtight jars away from heat and sunlight. To preserve most fresh herbs, dry out or freeze in plastic bags or jars with screw-top lids. Herbs that freeze well are parsley, chives, tarragon, dill, summer savory, sweet marjoram. Replace dried herbs and spices when color or aroma has faded or changed.

Basil. The word basil comes from the Greek *basilikon*, meaning "kingly." There are several varieties of this pungent herb. The most common is *sweet basil*, which grows about 18 inches high and has small white flowers and pairs of veined, green oval leaves. *Bush basil*, another variety, is a good indoor plant because it is short. An annual, basil seeds can be sown outdoors after the last frost; if grown indoors, seeds can be started anytime. Pick basil before the flowers open. The leaves may be preserved by drying, freezing, or storing in olive oil. Though leaves may turn black when preserved, the flavor remains.

Chervil. A member of the parsley family, chervil's lacy leaves resemble parsley but are a lighter green in color. Chervil tastes slightly like anise and is highly prized in French cooking. An annual, with spreading, delicate foliage and white flowers, chervil is a good indoor plant because it grows to a height of 2 feet or less and needs only moderate light. If grown outdoors, sow seeds in early spring; for a steady supply, sow thereafter every few weeks. Pinch back flower buds to encourage new leaf growth. Harvest before flowers open.

Chives. The smallest member of the onion family (see page 117), chives grow from tiny underground bulbs in grasslike clumps. Chives have a mild onion flavor that adds zest to foods such as omelets and salads. They are often used in *bouquets garnis*. The thin, tubular, bright-green leaves grow to about 10 inches. Fluffy, round, lavender flowers bloom in the summer. A hardy perennial that thrives without much attention, chives may quickly outgrow their pot or crowd out neighboring plants. Propagate by root division or from seed. Because chives lose their color and good taste when dried, use fresh or freeze.

Dill. Once thought to ward off witches and cure hiccoughs, today dill is a widely cultivated culinary herb. It grows 2 to 4 feet high and has light-green, feathery leaves and yellow flower clusters. The plant is used in two forms—dillweed, the leaves of the plant, and as dill seed, from the flowers. Dill is an annual that likes full sun and well-drained soil. If left undisturbed, plants will usually reseed themselves in the fall. Dillweed is most flavorful when the flowers are in bloom; gather seeds when ripe.

Marjoram. Sweet marjoram (*Origanum Majorana*) and oregano (*Origanum vulgare*) are often mistaken for each other. (Oregano is actually another species of marjoram.) A member of the mint family that grows as an annual in the North and as a perennial in the South, sweet marjoram is a low-spreading plant with small, oval, gray-green leaves that are soft to touch. The white, pink, or purplish flowers grow in dense clumps resembling knots, from which the herb's nickname, *knotted marjoram*, is derived. Sweet marjoram can be grown from seeds or cuttings.

Mint. The two most popular members of the large mint family are *spearmint* and *peppermint*. The characteristic coolness of mint comes from the menthol-containing oil in the plant's leaves and stems. Both are perennials that spread rapidly. Peppermint has dark-green leaves on purplish stems with violet flowers. Spearmint has pointed, deeply veined, crinkled leaves with purple or pink flowers. Both can be propagated by root division or stem cuttings. Pick leaves at any time to use fresh; to preserve them, pick when flowering begins. Dried mint makes a tasty tea.

Oregano. Botanically, oregano is wild marjoram, or pot marjoram, and is thus often confused with its cousin, sweet marjoram (see above). To add to the confusion, some commercially sold dried "oregano" is a species of a different plant from Mexico. Oregano, or *wild marjoram*, is a sprawling perennial that grows about 2 feet high, topped with fragrant purple, pink, or white flowers. Oregano is better suited to outdoor gardens because of its spreading root system. It can be grown from seeds or by root division or cuttings. Pick leaves just after buds appear for fullest flavor.

Parsley. There are many varieties of parsley, but the two most popular types are curly and flat. The bright-green curly parsley has crinkled leaves that grow in small tufts. The more piquant flat-leaf parsley, often called *Italian parsley*, has scalloped-edged leaves. A biennial grown as an annual, parsley is so slow to germinate that legend says the seed makes 7 round trips to the devil before sprouting. Parsley should be picked before it blooms because after flowering the leaves become bitter. Frozen parsley makes an excellent flavoring for soups and stews but is usually too limp to be used as a garnish. The stems, too, are rich in flavor.

Rosemary. A perennial rich in both legend and fragrance, rosemary has pale-blue flowers and deep-green, pinelike needles that perfume the air with their spicy, resinous aroma. In mild climates, rosemary grows as high as 6 feet. According to a story, the blue flowers got their color from the Virgin Mary's sky-blue cloak, which she laid on a rosemary bush to dry. Although rosemary can be grown from seed, the plant will develop faster from cuttings.

Savory. Sometimes called the "bean herb" because its spicy, peppery flavor enhances dried beans and lentils, savory is cultivated in two varieties: *winter* and *summer*. The more popular summer savory is an annual about 18 inches high with small, narrow, shiny green leaves and tiny white or lavender flowers. Winter savory is a hardy, woody perennial with narrow, glossy, dark-green pointed leaves that are stiffer than those of summer savory. Both can be grown from seed; winter savory can also be grown from cuttings.

Thyme. A low-growing, shrublike perennial, common thyme has tiny, oval, gray-green leaves that are highly pungent. Oil of thyme is used for many products, including perfumes and cough drops. Lilac-color flowers grow in small clusters along the stem. *Wild thyme*, another variety, makes a good ground cover. Keep the plant well pruned for a bushy look, and harvest when the first flowers open. Thyme can be propagated by cuttings, root division, or from seed.

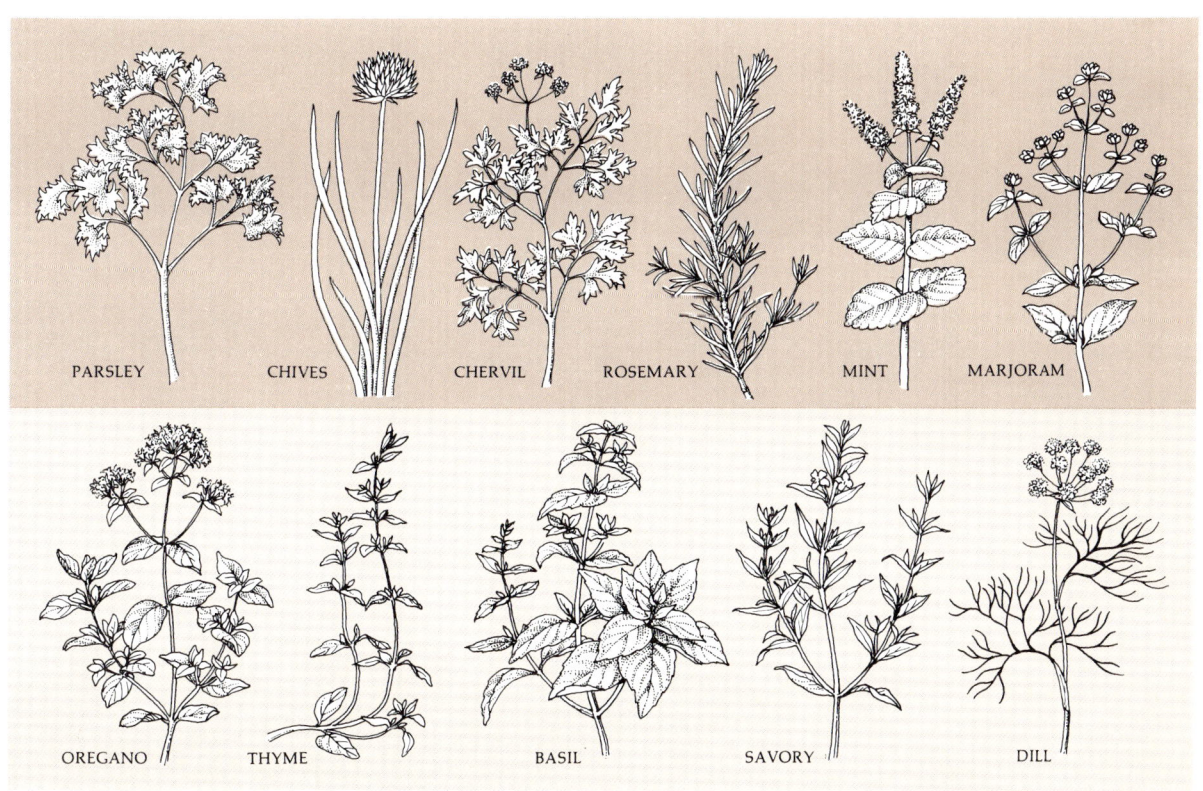

Buying Guide
Herbs and Spices

The following chart includes many familiar and some less familiar herbs and spices and a wide choice of dishes that are made more delicious by their use. Some combinations, such as basil and tomatoes, are standard, whereas others, such as fennel and baked fish, may be less common. Herbs and spices can also take the place of salt if you are on a restricted diet or simply wish to reduce sodium intake. Experiment

SPICES	SOUPS	MAIN DISHES
Allspice	beef, split pea, potato, tomato, vegetable	beef or lamb stew, boiled ham, pot roast
Basil	dried bean, fish chowder, gazpacho, minestrone, potato, tomato, vegetable	sautéed chicken, baked fish, omelet, spaghetti sauces
Bay Leaf	dried bean, bouillabaisse, chicken, fish chowder, minestrone, oxtail, Scotch broth	beef or lamb stew, corned beef, boiled chicken, poached fish, pot roast, veal roast
Caraway	dried bean, borscht, cabbage	cabbage rolls, scrambled eggs, lamb stew, roast pork, sauerbraten, Welsh rabbit
Chervil	spinach, tomato, vichyssoise	beef with béarnaise sauce, omelet, veal roast
Cinnamon	cold fruit	baked ham, lamb roast, sauerbraten
Cloves	beef-vegetable, onion, pea, potato, tomato	corned beef, roast chicken, chili, baked ham, meat loaf, tongue
Coriander	black bean, clam broth, lentil, pea	game, pork, sausage
Cumin	black bean, eggplant, squash	bean-rice dishes, baked chicken, beef hash, chili, enchiladas, meatballs, meat loaf, shrimp curry
Dill	dried bean, borscht, chicken, fish chowder, tomato, vegetable	bean-rice dishes, boiled beef, creamed chicken, roast chicken, broiled fish
Fennel	borscht	braised duck, baked fish, pizza, Italian sausage, spaghetti sauces
Ginger	eggplant, Indian vegetable, zucchini	baked chicken, broiled fish, Chinese pepper steak, Swedish meatballs
Marjoram	fish chowder, minestrone, onion, potato	stewed beef, roast chicken, baked fish, sausage, spaghetti sauces
Mint	cold cucumber, split pea	lamb stew, roast lamb
Nutmeg	fish chowder, pumpkin, vichyssoise	French toast, quiches, Swedish meatballs
Oregano	dried bean, fish chowder, minestrone, onion, tomato, vegetable	stewed beef, chicken cacciatore, lasagna, meat loaf, roast pork, spaghetti sauces, roast turkey
Rosemary	vegetable	roast chicken, lamb, or pork, spaghetti sauces, stuffing for poultry, broiled swordfish
Sage	corn, turkey, vegetable	sautéed chicken, roast pork, pork sausage
Savory	fish chowder, lentil	stewed beef, chicken or meat pies, meat loaf, omelet, roast pork
Tarragon	chicken, fish chowder, lentil-tomato, mushroom	beef with béarnaise sauce, chicken in cream sauce, omelet, spaghetti sauces
Thyme	chicken, lentil, onion, vegetable	stewed beef, lamb, or pork, broiled fish

FAMILY FOOD GUIDE

with a variety to discover which combinations you prefer. Because these flavorings are so versatile, you are limited only by your imagination and taste preference. Some dishes, such as chili, require a substantial quantity of one spice, but usually just a small amount will have an impact on flavor. If using whole herbs or spices in cooking, it is preferable to remove them before serving.

SALADS	VEGETABLES	DESSERTS	OTHER
pear	carrots, spinach, squash	spice cake, stewed fruit, mince pie, pumpkin pie	cider, eggnog, fruit punch
chicken, cucumber, egg, mixed green, potato, seafood, tomato	green beans, peas, ratatouille, broiled tomatoes, tomato sauce	none	corn bread, tomato juice
none	dried beans, eggplant, lentils	none	cheese balls
pickled beets, coleslaw, cucumber, potato, tuna fish	green beans, Brussels sprouts, stewed onions, sauerkraut	none	biscuits, yeast breads, liqueur (kümmel)
cucumber, guacamole	mushrooms	none	tartar sauce
Waldorf	baked beans, carrots, sweet potatoes, squash	applesauce, apple pie, cherry pie, cobblers	eggnog, hot chocolate, tea
apricot, pear, plum	baked beans, carrots, sweet potatoes, spinach	fruit cake, spice cake, cooked fruit, pumpkin pie	cider, punch, tea
cucumber and yogurt	beets	cooked apples, gingerbread	yeast breads, chutney
chicken	kidney beans	none	chick-pea appetizer, spiced rice
coleslaw, cucumber, mixed green, potato, seafood	green beans, carrots, peas, potatoes, ratatouille, zucchini	none	tomato juice, yeast breads
mixed green, raw vegetable platter	carrots, potatoes	none	fennel, date and lemon chutney
fruit cup	baked beans, glazed carrots, sweet potatoes	spiced cooked fruit, broiled grapefruit, orange slices, pumpkin pie	chutney, mincemeat
asparagus, chicken, mixed green, seafood, vegetable	eggplant, peas, spinach, tomato dishes, zucchini	mixed fruit	yeast breads
fruit, tabouli, Waldorf	stuffed artichokes, peas	applesauce, pineapple	fruit juice, tea
none	green beans, carrots, sweet potatoes, spinach, squash	applesauce, egg custard, rice pudding, pumpkin pie	eggnog, hot cider, milk shake
three-bean, mixed green, seafood	corn, eggplant, mushrooms, onions, stewed tomatoes, zucchini	none	tomato juice
mixed green	lima beans, boiled potatoes, tomatoes	none	corn bread, yeast breads
chicken, turkey	lima beans, onions, potatoes, tomatoes	none	biscuits, corn bread
bean, mixed green	dried beans, green beans, lentils, tomatoes	none	herbal yeast breads
chicken, mixed green, seafood, sliced tomatoes	lima beans, mushrooms, spinach, tomatoes	none	tomato or vegetable juice
mixed green	mushrooms, onions, potatoes, spinach, tomatoes	none	corn bread, creole sauce

Gathering Foods from the Wild

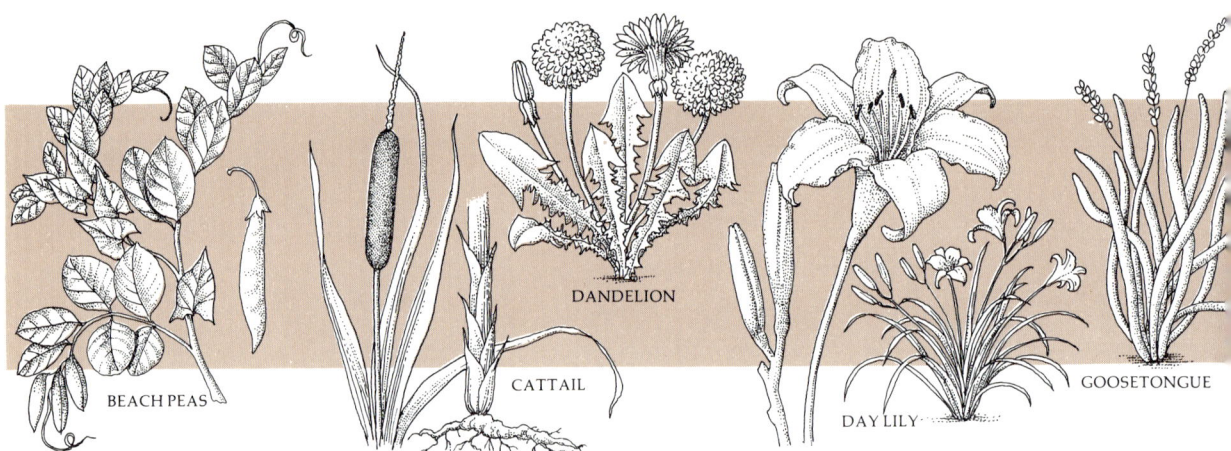

Gathering edible plants in the field, marsh, desert, or along the seashore is a very satisfying activity. These gifts of nature can be as tasty as what you buy at the market or grow in your garden. One way to get started on this fascinating hobby is to invite a friend who is familiar with edible plants to accompany you on your first expedition. Until you feel confident about identifying plants, take along a reference book with clear pictures and descriptions. *Never eat anything you cannot identify. Don't take chances; some plants are similar in appearance, but one may be poisonous and make you ill whereas another is safe to eat. Also, know which part of the plant you want to eat and when it is edible.*

The pictures and descriptions on these two pages include only the most common plants with wide distribution across the United States. When gathering wild foods, be sure to cut off only what you plan to use. Some plants with edible roots should be picked sparingly, to save the plant for another year's growth.

Beach Peas (*Lathyrus maritimus*). These low-to-the-ground vines grow along the beaches or on lake shores. The blue-green leaflets, which are oval in shape, either alternate or grow in pairs on stems that end in curly tendrils. Look for arrowhead-shaped leaf at base of leaf stalk. The pink to purple flowers resemble sweet-pea blossoms; the pea pods look like garden peas, only smaller. The young, inch-long pods can be sautéed or stir-fried. Shell mature peas and cook in little water until tender. The leaf buds can be used raw in salad. *Found from Maine to New Jersey, on the shores of the Great Lakes, and from California to Alaska; gather from May to October, depending on what part of the plant you want to use.*

Cattail (*Typha latifolia*). Long, swordlike leaves and tall, straight stems topped with flower spikes that resemble torches are characteristics of the swamp cattail. (Be sure that the water where the cattails grow is not polluted.) The spikes are made up of hundreds of tiny, green flower heads that turn dark brown as they mature. In spring, the young stalks can be easily pulled up. Slice the tender, white part of the stalk and add raw to salads, or steam pieces in a little water for about 15 minutes. Young green flower heads can be eaten like corn on the cob. Remove the husk and boil in a small amount of water for about 5 minutes. *Found throughout the United States; gather flower heads in early summer.*

Dandelion (*Taraxacum officinale*). A common garden weed, the dandelion grows from 2 to 10 inches tall. The dark-green, oblong, toothed leaves are thickly clustered at the base of the plant, and the leafless, hollow stems that originate from the center are topped with yellow flower heads.

Collect leaves in early spring, as they become increasingly bitter. Wash leaves thoroughly and use in salad or steam as a vegetable. Buds, too, may be added raw to salads. Very young dandelion blossoms can be dipped in batter and deep-fried. *Found throughout the United States; gather in spring.*

Day Lily (*Hemerocallis fulva*). The showy orange or yellow blossoms sit atop branching stalks that grow from 2 to 4 feet tall. The long, tapered leaves grow in a cluster at the base.

The young stalks that appear in spring can be cooked like asparagus. Pick buds when fully formed and steam in a small amount of water for about 5 minutes (caution: some people may experience diarrhea from eating the buds). Flowers can be dipped in batter and fried. The unpeeled tubers are delicious eaten raw or cooked for about 15 minutes in little water. *Found from Maine, south to Missouri, Tennessee, and North Carolina; gather stalks in April; buds and blossoms in July and August; tubers in early spring and late fall.*

FAMILY FOOD GUIDE

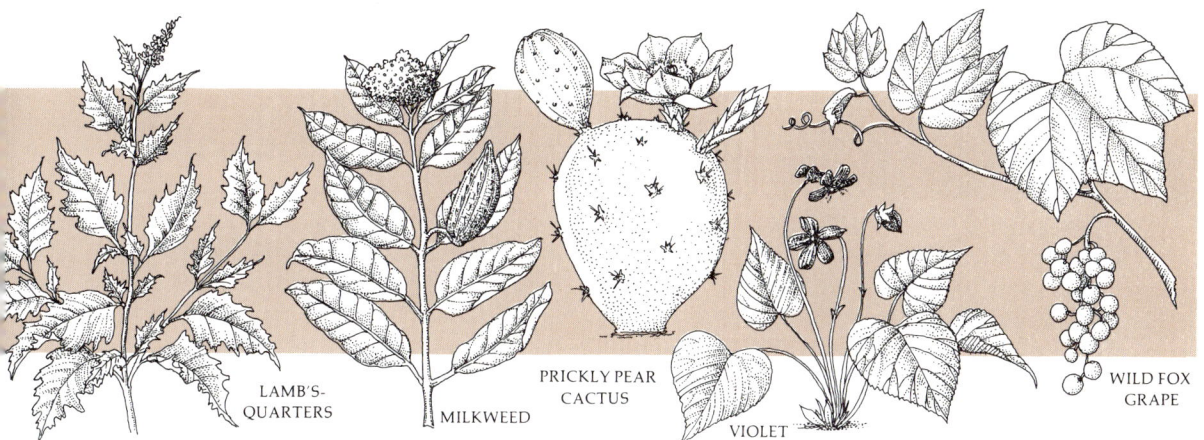

LAMB'S-QUARTERS MILKWEED PRICKLY PEAR CACTUS VIOLET WILD FOX GRAPE

Goosetongue (*Plantago oliganthos*). Also called *seaside plantain*, goosetongue is found along the shore. It grows 4 to 6 inches high and has long, narrow, fleshy leaves. The flower spikes grow on separate stalks, and are oval shaped and brown.

The leaves are sweet and tender into early July but tend to get bitter later on. Goosetongue leaves can be used raw in a salad or cooked for about 20 minutes in a little water. *Found along the shore from Maine to New Jersey and Alaska to California; gather from June to September but best in June and early July.*

Lamb's-Quarters (*Chenopodium album*). This tall, multibranched plant, also called *pigweed*, is a relative of spinach. The green leaves are spade shaped with jagged or toothed edges and are dusted with whitish particles. Leaves are arranged alternately on the tall green stem, which reaches from 2 to 4 feet in height.

Pick tender leaves in spring. Steam the leaves for several minutes in water that clings from washing. Like spinach, they reduce in bulk during cooking. Young leaves can be also added raw to salads. *Found throughout the United States in rich soil; gather leaves in spring or early summer.*

Milkweed (*Asclepias syriaca*). This sturdy meadow plant has large broad oval leaves with a stiff midrib. They are connected to the hollow main stalk by short stems. The plant oozes a sticky white substance when cut. The clusters of fragrant, star-shaped flowers range in color from lavender to pink and purple. After the flowers die, the plant produces pointed pods which, when ripe, open and scatter their seeds.

The unopened flowers make a delicious cooked vegetable somewhat like broccoli. When seed pods are 1 inch long, boil in a small amount of water first and add to soups or stews. *Found from Maine to the Carolinas and west to Kansas; gather buds when formed, pods after flowering.*

Prickly Pear Cactus (*Opuntia ficus-indica*). Like most cacti the prickly pear does not have leaves. The flat, oval-shaped joints are really stems of the plant. Each one is covered by tiny bristles. This cactus grows in clumps up to 5 feet in height. The flowers have yellow petals and bloom from April to July, depending on the rainfall. The fruit, called tuna, can be red, purple, or even yellow.

Peel the tuna and eat raw or make into jam or candy. The stems are also edible. Use only young parts. Remove bristles with thick garden gloves and a knife or scrub brush. Peel, slice, dip in cornmeal or flour, and fry. *Found in Texas, Arizona, and New Mexico; gather when fruit is ripe—stems anytime.*

Violet (*Viola soraria*). This spring-blooming plant, which prefers a shady setting, grows approximately 8 inches tall and has dark-green, heart-shaped leaves with serrated edges. The deep-blue or purple flowers, with lighter centers, each grow on a separate stem.

Gather the leaves after the plant has flowered. Use in a salad, along with the flowers, for a wild food rich in vitamins A and C. Cut up leaves and cook for 15 minutes in a small amount of water; season to taste. *Found from Maine to Georgia, west to Wyoming and southward; gather leaves and blossoms in spring.*

Wild Fox Grape (*Vitis labrusca*). Wild grape vines are usually found in wooded areas. These vines, which grow up to 60 feet, climb along tree trunks or entwine themselves in bushes. The green leaves are deeply lobed with fuzzy undersides. The flowers consist of small green clusters from which the deep-red to deep-purple fruit evolves.

Grape leaves must first be boiled briefly to be palatable for making stuffed grape leaves. The ripe fruit can be eaten raw, or made into jam and jelly. It is not good for winemaking. *Found from Maine to Florida and west to New Mexico; gather leaves in June when they are most tender, and the fruit in September and October when it is ripe.*

Beverages: What's Good for You

All beverages have one basic purpose: to help supply the body's need for water, the most essential of all nutrients. The average person needs about 2.5 quarts of water a day to replace natural fluid loss (see page 50). We get some of this replacement water from the foods we eat. All foods contain water: many vegetables such as asparagus, cucumbers, and radishes are more than 90 percent water; most fruits are over 80 percent water; fish usually fall in the 50 to 60 percent category; and, surprisingly, even spaghetti and macaroni are about 65 percent water. However, most of the water we consume comes from fluids: milk (see page 154) and coffee, tea, and other beverages discussed on the following pages.

Therefore, it is important for us to find out what we actually get from beverages in addition to water, and how to get the best value for our beverage dollar. Does the beverage contain nutrients or little else other than calories? What percent is sugar or alcohol? Are natural or artificial flavors and colors used? How do drugs like caffeine and alcohol affect us? And, finally, in this age of industrial chemicals and pesticides, how do we know if our tap or well water is safe to drink? The challenge facing the consumer is to make an informed, intelligent choice.

Water

For millennia a draft of cool, clear water has been the perfect antidote to thirst. Now, however, questions are being raised about the quality of this basic resource.

Generally, the supplies of drinking water in American cities are among the world's safest, largely because the tap water from the municipal systems has been extensively purified through filtration, chlorination, and other means to remove infectious organisms. But even though waterborne bacterial diseases have mostly been brought under control by these methods, some old problems remain—and new problems have arisen. There is the question of flavor, for one thing. At its best, purified tap water tastes the way water should—clean and refreshing; at its worst, it can be murky and unpleasant, with a pronounced aftertaste of chlorine or sulfur.

Perhaps more crucial than the problem of taste, however, is the question of quality. Rivers and streams are our major sources of water; ground water accounts for about one-quarter of the supply. The use of pesticides, herbicides, industrial chemicals, and other potentially toxic materials means that some of these chemicals may be making their way into our water supply—through storm runoff, industrial dumping, and seepage from poorly maintained waste dumps.

Another recently discovered hazard comes from the very substance used to disinfect our water supplies. Chlorine is known to combine with other organic matter in water to form compounds called trihalomethanes, or THMs, which are strongly suspected of being carcinogenic. THMs have been found not only in surface water (rivers, lakes, and reservoirs) but also in ground water, the vast subterranean supply that was long thought to be naturally protected from pollution. In 1978 the Environmental Protection Agency set maximum allowable levels for THMs and certain pesticides in public water supplies, but many other contaminants are as yet unregulated, partly because they are so numerous and partly because not enough is known about their potential hazards.

Apart from questions of quality and taste, tap water varies considerably in its natural mineral content. Some minerals found in water are calcium, selenium, and zinc. In a broad sense, everything except distilled water is mineral water. So-called "hard" water has a much higher mineral content than "soft" water, which can be either naturally soft or treated to remove part of its mineral content. (Bear in mind that water softeners add sodium to water.)

Both types of water, hard and soft, have advantages and disadvantages: hard water is tastier for drinking; soft water is better for bathing, dishwashing, and cleaning. Hard water can cause mineral buildup on pipes and plumbing fixtures, but soft water can leach out harmful substances such as lead and asbestos if your system contains these materials. (If your water is soft, let it run from the cold tap for a few minutes before using it, and don't cook with water from the hot tap, which may have picked up an off flavor from the water heater.)

Bottled Water

The growing public concern over pollutants in our water supplies has, in part, resulted in a glut of bottled waters on the market. Many people have turned to bottled water for drinking and cooking. In

1980 alone, 370 million gallons of domestic and imported waters were sold in the United States. But is bottled water better than tap water? Not necessarily. It varies considerably in quality, flavor, mineral content and, of course, price.

The taste of bottled water depends on many factors: mineral composition, alkalinity, and the degree of effervescence, for example. Some waters are light and refreshing; others can be explosively bubbly, with a strong aftertaste. You may need to sample several brands to find one you like.

In general, the best quality bottled water is *"natural" spring water* or *"natural" mineral water* from a protected spring or other pure source. It can be still (without carbonation) or naturally effervescent. To comply with federal labeling regulations, "natural" spring water must come from a true spring (some waters list the source on the label); no processing is allowed, although carbon dioxide can be added to make the water effervescent. "Natural" mineral water may contain only those minerals already present at the source; it too is usually from a spring.

Plain *spring water*, on the other hand, may be filtered to remove impurities, and plain *mineral water* can be processed water with minerals removed or added. They can be sparkling or still, depending on the source. *Bottled* or *purified drinking water*, often sold in large, "bulk" containers, is usually purified well or tap water, with or without spring water added.

Club soda and *seltzer* are typically tap water that is carbonated and are usually considered soft drinks (pages 185-186). They have the advantage of usually costing less than sparkling spring waters.

Distilled water, more often used in machinery or in laboratory experiments than for drinking, has been vaporized and condensed to remove all minerals; it has a flat taste.

Spring-type water is purified water with certain minerals replaced. Although the Food and Drug Administration has imposed safety standards on both domestic and imported bottled water, mineral waters have so far been exempted. Many bottlers do not specify the source or the mineral content on the label. Careful buyers should choose among the established brands that list both source and mineral content (some waters have high concentrations of sodium).

Bottled waters are packaged either in glass bottles or plastic containers; the lighter and cheaper plastic containers, some people think, have an adverse ef-

Water—What You Can Do About It

There are a number of ways you can check on the quality of the water you drink.

If you suspect that your drinking water may be polluted, there are several things you can do. First, get in touch with the company that supplies your water. If you live in a sizable town or city, this may be a municipal water department or a public water corporation. Most places monitor their water supplies; ask the supplier about the frequency of testing and whether or not the test results show the presence and quantity of specific pollutants such as THMs, toxic waste, heavy metals, as well as bacteria.

If you are not satisfied with the response, contact the county health department. It may test your water for other pollutants besides bacteria. If it doesn't, and you wish to pursue the matter, you can get in touch with a private laboratory. Look in the yellow pages of your telephone directory under "Laboratory, testing." Make sure it is state certified and find out the cost. If it is expensive, perhaps a group of neighbors would share the cost since you are all probably drinking water from the same source.

If your water is supplied by your own well, go directly to your local health department or county health officer, or try the nearest department of environmental protection. Then take the steps listed above.

You can also get in touch with your local congressman or community action groups such as the League of Women Voters Education Fund, 1730 M Street, N.W., Washington, D.C. 20036. Although the problem of contaminated water is complex and widespread, it is not unsolvable.

Beverages: What's Good for You

Water

fect on taste. To retain maximum flavor, always keep the bottle tightly closed and chilled, and serve water over ice made from the bottled water itself, not from tap water.

Juices

Fruit and vegetable juices, like milk, are more than just thirst quenchers; they contain important nutrients. Tomato juice, for example, is rich in vitamins A and C, carrot juice in vitamin A, prune juice in iron, and citrus juices—especially the all-time favorite, orange juice—in vitamin C.

Today, nearly all commercial fruit juices sold in bottles or cartons, including those found in speciality food stores, are pasteurized to prevent fermentation and spoilage. (This process, besides killing bacteria, prevents the growth of yeasts that would otherwise convert the fruit sugars to alcohol.) Many commercial juices, notably apple and grape, are also filtered to remove plant minerals, fibers, and other particles. Supermarkets always stock this thin, clarified juice because it looks better on the shelf, but many also offer the heavier-bodied, unfiltered variety.

Pasteurization destroys some nutrients, and filtered juices tend to be less flavorful than unfiltered ones. To get maximum taste, freshness, and nutritional content from juice, the best way is still the old way: make your own. Citrus fruits are easy enough to squeeze with a hand juicer, but for most fruits and vegetables, you may wish to buy a heavy-duty juice extractor. For a refreshing drink, you can thin any juice with water if you want to cut back on sugar and calories. All fresh-squeezed juices deteriorate in quality and should be used at once, or refrigerated and used within a day.

Packaging—What it Means

The fruit juice you buy in bottles or cartons can be either full strength (the liquid pressed directly from fruit) or reconstituted (made from concentrate and water); check the label, which should also list any added preservatives or sugar. Nonpasteurized, full-strength juices are sometimes available in areas where the fruits are grown; like homemade fresh-squeezed juices, they are highly perishable. Bottled juice is, of course, bulkier and usually more expen-

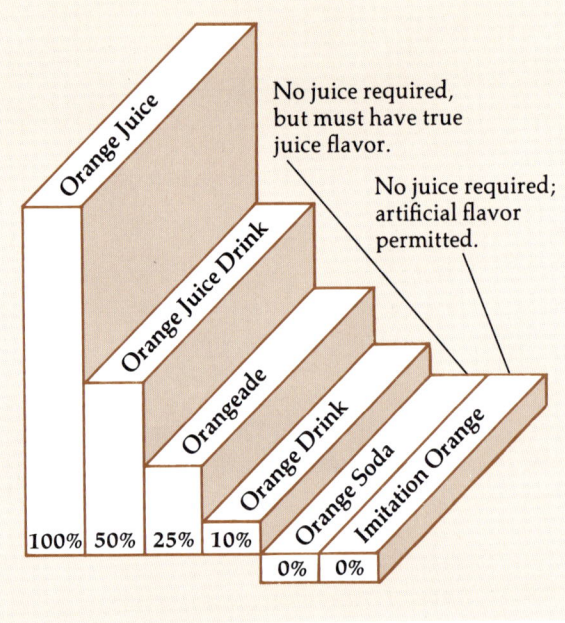

sive than frozen concentrate. Canned fruit juices generally rank lower in flavor than fresh or frozen. As for the nutritive value of canned juices, it depends on whether the juice is fortified or not. If you buy canned juice, avoid cans with lead soldered seams because the acids in the juice can leach out some of the lead. However, more cans are being made with electrically welded side seams, which eliminates the use of lead solder. Frozen concentrate is always packaged in seamless aluminum or fiber containers.

Orange Juice, Real and Otherwise

Of all juices, orange juice is by far the most popular among Americans. A 4-ounce glass provides 100 percent of the Recommended Dietary Allowance for vitamin C, in addition to other nutrients. However, the amount of vitamin C varies somewhat according to packaging and storage. Fresh-squeezed and concentrate score highest in both vitamin content and flavor, provided the concentrate isn't allowed to become thawed too long before being reconstituted. (The liquid in fresh-squeezed orange juice is superior in taste and nutritional quality to reconstituted juice.) And concentrate is usually cheaper than the reconstituted orange juice sold in cartons.

Unfortunately, the very popularity of orange juice has spawned a flood of factory-made substitutes and watered-down orange drinks. Although these substitutes are fortified with nutrients, they are likely to contain added sugar, artificial color, and artificial flavorings. As for the various "drinks," "-ades," etc., not only do they contain sugar and other additives but the fruit-juice content can be as low as 10 percent (see chart). Products labeled "orange soda" and "imitation orange" are soft drinks and need not contain any juice at all—although fruit soda is required to have a "true fruit flavor."

You should also know what the words "nectar," "cocktail," or "punch" mean on a label. In broad terms, fruit nectar must contain between 25 to 40 percent of fruit puree, pulp, juice, or concentrate; a cocktail such as cranberry cocktail must contain at least 25 percent juice, whereas a fruit punch does not need to have any juice at all. Even some frozen juice concentrates, notably grape juice, contain added sugar and vitamins; check the label for content. Also, avoid concentrates in sticky containers—a sign that the contents may have thawed during storage. Finally, remember that some juices—particularly lemon and lime—are highly acidic; excessive quantities can damage tooth enamel.

Soft Drinks

In 1980, the average rate of soft-drink consumption was 39 gallons per person per year, and climbing (see chart). Judging by the sales figures, today's Americans prefer soft drinks to almost any other beverage. Most sweet soda pop is calorie rich and nutrient poor, and contains additives such as caffeine, artificial color, artificial flavorings, and sugar or synthetic sweeteners. Overconsumption of soft drinks tends to promote poor nutritional habits by replacing more healthful foods and beverages in the diet with empty calories. Today, soft drinks, led by the colas, are unquestionably the nation's most popular thirst quenchers, accounting for more than a third of every dollar spent on beverages. There is very little nutritional return for those dollars spent.

What accounts for our national obsession with these sweet, fizzy fluids? The answer seems to be twofold: advertising and availability. We are bombarded with alluring promotions that equate soft-drink consumption with youth, energy, sex appeal, sociability, and all-around good living. And wherever we go, we find soft drinks in enormous quantity: they dominate the vending machines and fill entire aisles in the nation's supermarkets.

Just What Is a Soft Drink?

Although sweetened soft drinks were originally sold as patent medicines in the late 19th century, they were soon being touted as refreshing, nonintoxicating substitutes for alcohol—hence the term "soft," as opposed to "hard," drinks. Technically, a soft drink is any beverage made with artificially carbonated or noncarbonated water and/or sweeteners, edible acids, and natural or artificial flavorings, such as the cola and pepper drinks, root beer, and ginger ale, fruit-flavored sodas, cream soda, tonic water, club soda, and seltzer. (The noncarbonated imitation fruit drinks often sold in powdered form are also considered soft drinks.) Of all soft drinks the nondiet, fruit-flavored sodas have the highest proportion of both artificial colorings and sugar (see calorie chart); the nondiet cola and pepper drinks are high in sugar but may contain as much as 32 to 65 milligrams of caffeine per 12-ounce serving—more than the average cup of black tea (see caffeine feature on pages 188-189). The popular "diet" soft drinks contain everything the others do plus saccharin, a sweetener of questionable safety.

If an average 12-ounce can of nondiet soda has 9 teaspoons of sugar, then its diet counterpart must contain no more than half that amount. Of course, it can always contain even less. However, many diet sodas are higher in sodium than regular sodas. The least controversial of all soft drinks appear to be club

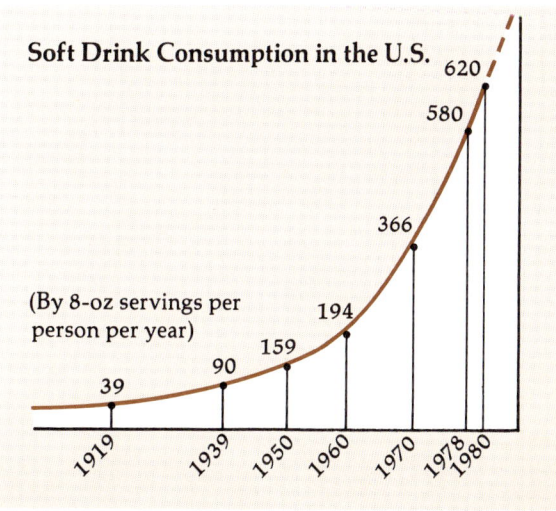

Soft Drink Consumption in the U.S.
(By 8-oz servings per person per year)
39 — 1919
90 — 1939
159 — 1950
194 — 1960
366 — 1970
580 — 1978
620 — 1980

Beverages: What's Good for You
Soft Drinks

soda and seltzer, both of which are essentially filtered water that is charged with carbon dioxide. (Club soda has added minerals and mineral salts, including variable amounts of sodium; seltzer, on the other hand, may contain minerals and is usually lower in sodium.) Neither drink has any calories.

Soft Drinks and Children

The overwhelming popularity of soft drinks among the young makes it imperative for us to understand their effects on the body. One recent study reports that soft drinks are consumed by three-fifths of all American teenage boys, half the teenage girls, and half of all children in the 2-to 11-year-old age group. Even more surprising, the study reported that two-fifths of the children between 1 and 2 years old drink soft drinks, averaging 9 ounces per day! The champion guzzlers, however, are boys 15 to 18 years old; the average daily intake of users in this group is 22 ounces per day. (Soft-drink consumption showed a gradual decline among adults; half of those under 35 but only a third of those over 35 reported using them.)

Many of the most popular soft drinks contain both sugar and caffeine, two substances many parents are already concerned about. Some children who are very heavy users of such soft drinks can become dependent on the "kick" provided by the caffeine, like their parents may be on coffee or tea. Others may exhibit "hyped-up" behavior if they consume very large doses of caffeine. It is important to remember that because of their smaller size, young children get a greater concentration of these substances per pound of body weight than adults do.

For a quick check on how much caffeine your child may be consuming, you can take the following test. Multiply the number of servings by the number of milligrams of caffeine in each serving and then total the results. For soda with caffeine, multiply the number of servings by 40; iced tea, 30; chocolate milk, 6; chocolate candy bar, 20; cocoa, 10. A total score up to 50 milligrams is equivalent to 2 cups of instant coffee for an adult; from 51 to 100 milligrams equals 4 cups of coffee; from 101 to 150, 6 cups, and so on. Of course, all the figures are approximate because the caffeine content varies by brand.

Even in soft drinks without caffeine, the high sugar content unaccompanied by other nutrients is hardly a nutritional plus. Most soft drinks are also very expensive when you take into account the fact that they contain so few nutrients. Moreover, the safety of saccharin in diet sodas is also open to question. Thus there are many reasons why a goodly number of parents feel it is only wise to limit their children's intake of soft drinks and to stock them only occasionally in the house. In their place, the old standbys milk, fruit juice, and water are better choices.

Coffee

More than a thousand years ago, the crushed fruit of the coffee tree is thought to have been used as a food by certain nomadic peoples in Africa, where the plant originated. By the 15th century, however, the Arabians had discovered that the seeds within the fruit—the coffee beans—could be dried, roasted, and ground to make a stimulating, aromatic drink. And by the late 17th century the use of coffee had spread throughout the Islamic world into most of Europe and to the American colonies, where the brew quickly supplanted tea as the beverage of choice, especially among patriots.

Since that time, coffee consumption in the United States has had its ups and downs. The current trend is downward for several reasons: the zooming popularity of soft drinks, the increases in coffee prices in the mid-1970s, and Americans' growing concern about the possible health hazards of caffeine (pages 188-189). Yet despite this decline, coffee is still one of America's most popular beverages: the industry itself estimates that 56 percent of all Americans over the age of 10 drink coffee, averaging about three cups a day.

Most of the world's commercial coffees come from two species, the Arabian (*Coffea arabica*) and the African (*Coffea canephora*, popularly known as Robusta). The best commercial coffees, including all those grown in Central and South America, come from varieties of the Arabian strain, but the quality varies considerably, depending on the growing conditions. The finest beans, such as the famed Colombian, are mountain grown. Brazil, which produces about half the world's coffee, grows beans of a generally lower quality of *arabica*. Robusta coffee is hardier and can be grown in more climates than *arabica*, but it tends to be harsher and consequently lower priced than the Arabian. Robusta coffee is generally mixed with superior blends or used to make instant coffee; the processing tempers the bitter flavor somewhat.

Green (unroasted) coffee has virtually no flavor. After roasting the next step in coffee processing is grinding, which brings out the aromatic oil, or caffeol, and gives coffee its distinctive taste and aroma. Once coffee is ground, however, the caffeol is quickly released, which means that the shorter the time lapse between grinding and brewing, the better the coffee will be.

Buying, Storing, and Brewing Coffee

If you are an avid coffee gourmet, you may want to buy your favorite blend of coffee beans from a food shop that stocks exotic varieties like Java, Jamaica and, of course, high-grade Colombian. Not all of us, however, have access to a gourmet shop or wish to pay the usually higher prices. Fortunately, there are several alternatives.

You can buy bean coffee in many supermarkets, and have it ground to order by the store; or you can grind it at home, as needed, with a hand grinder or electric minigrinder. Another alternative is to buy a reliable brand of ground coffee in a vacuum-sealed can. Once opened, store the can in the freezer—the best place to keep all ground coffee in order to maintain optimum flavor. (Some people prefer to store coffee in the refrigerator.) Finally, there are the instant coffees, both freeze dried and regular. Both are cheaper (per cup) than ground or bean coffee, and most contain much less caffeine, but they are undeniably inferior in flavor, and most are made from low-grade beans. Of the two, freeze-dried instant has the better flavor because it is not heated during processing.

Decaffeinated Coffee and Coffee Substitutes

Many health-conscious people have turned to decaffeinated coffee, but there are some questions about the safety of the decaffeinating process itself. In the United States, most coffee is decaffeinated with chemical solvents, one of which (trichloroethylene) was banned as a suspected carcinogen in 1975; the solvent now used, methylene chloride, is being tested for safety by the National Toxicology Program. For those who prefer to avoid chemical solvents until their safety is fully established, many specialty shops carry decaffeinated coffee made by a method that uses no chemical solvents: the Swiss pure-water process, a steam process.

Although the consumption of coffee substitutes has declined since the advent of decaffeinated coffee, several are still on the market. Most of them are made from roasted grains like whole wheat, bran, barley, and rye, with added flavorings such as chicory, carob, molasses, and even artificial coffee flavor. They are wanting in the true coffee taste, not to mention the caffeine "kick." Also available are true coffees blended with "extenders" such as grain or chicory and flavorings like cinnamon and chocolate; they contain less caffeine, but they may cost more than regular coffee.

Tea

Americans have never been as devoted to tea as their British cousins, though the popularity of this aromatic hot beverage is gradually rising. On the plus side, tea has the following in its favor: except for certain blends found in specialty food stores, it is cheaper; its caffeine content is, on the average, less than half that of coffee; and it comes in an almost infinite variety of flavors. On the minus side, tea contains other methylxanthines besides caffeine, some of which may also have stimulant qualities.

All true tea comes from the leaves of one shrub, *Camellia sinensis*, which originated in China. Tea leaves are divided into three basic types: *black tea*, which is fermented before drying; the greenish-brown *oolong*, which is semifermented; and unfermented *green tea*. Other labels refer to the area of origin (Darjeeling, Lapsang, etc.) or the grade of the leaves (the finest tea, orange pekoe, comes from the younger leaves near the growing tip, whereas souchong leaves are picked farther down the stem). The most desirable leaves—the youngest leaves—also have the most caffeine.

Most of the tea consumed in the United States is black tea, whose full, rich flavor usually appeals to coffee drinkers. Green tea—the kind often served in Oriental restaurants—is thinner and more astringent. Oolong can usually be found in gourmet shops, and many stores stock blends containing two or more types, often with added flavorings like spices, flower buds, or orange rind. In addition, you

Beverages: What's Good for You
Tea

can buy blended teas with names like Earl Grey and Irish Breakfast Tea.

Buying and Brewing Tea

More than half the tea sold in the United States comes in tea bags; unfortunately the confinement of the bag keeps the leaves from opening fully in water and releasing their maximum flavor. Although tea bags are far superior to instant, powdered teas—the best choice by far is loose tea. In general, loose tea is also the cheapest, especially when bought in bulk. To get the freshest leaves, which should have a resilient feel and a strong tea aroma, buy loose tea in a metal canister rather than in a cardboard box or from open bins. Store it in a cool, dry place.

Brewed tea is only as tasty as the water you steep it in. First, pour some boiling water from the kettle into the teapot to warm it. Swirl it around, pour it out, and add the tea (a spoonful per cup, plus one for the pot). Cover it immediately with boiling water. Don't steep for more than 3 to 5 minutes before straining into cups; if brewed longer, the tea will develop a bitter taste from the release of tannin. (Double-strength brewed tea makes a delicious iced tea.) Since teas contain tannins, which can irritate the digestive tract, some people prefer to add milk because milk neutralizes tannins.

Herb Teas

These infusions, sometimes called "tisanes," aren't teas at all but drinks made with herbs. There are nearly 400 herbs and spices that are used by manufacturers of herb teas. Some, like chamomile, linden, and peppermint, are generally safe when taken in moderation, and have a pleasant refreshing flavor. Others, however, contain potent chemical compounds which can be toxic in concentrated doses. Many of these compounds have not been tested for safety. (Sassafras tea, for instance, was banned from the market in 1976 because it contains safrole, a proven animal carcinogen.) Herb teas must be approached with caution. People who suffer from

Caffeine—How It Works

We are accustomed to hearing that tea is "bracing," that coffee has a "kick," that cocoa "picks you up," or that colas are full of "pep." And for once, it's quite true—all these beverages have powerful stimulative effects.

Caffeine and the related substances theophylline (found naturally in tea) and theobromine (occurring naturally in cocoa and other chocolate products) belong to a group of drugs called methylxanthines, or xanthines, of which caffeine is the most potent. All xanthines are central nervous system stimulants, and as such they can have both beneficial and harmful effects. In a sense, the adverse effects of these drugs are extensions of the beneficial ones: just as caffeine in moderation can increase mental alertness and seem to lessen fatigue, too much of it can constrict the blood vessels of the brain, speed up the heart, cause an irregular heartbeat, and also bring on symptoms ranging from restlessness and irritability to twitching muscles and headache.

The methylxanthines are widely used in both prescription and over-the-counter remedies. Caffeine, because it constricts the cranial blood vessels, is found in many headache preparations and other pain relievers (both prescription and nonprescription), and in over-the-counter "alertness" tablets and cold/allergy remedies. Methylxanthines, which stimulate the heart and help regulate the respiratory system, are used in treating asthma, congestive heart failure, and other conditions.

But medically supervised use of these stimulants is one thing; frequent or heavy self-administered doses are, obviously, quite another. The list of documented or suspected side effects of heavy caffeine use is long and getting longer. Scientific studies of adult coffee drinkers have shown that heavy use (1,000 milligrams per day, or about 8 cups) can produce classic anxiety symptoms—dizziness, nervous irritability, tremulousness, insomnia, headaches, and disturbances in the heart rate and rhythm. Heavy caffeine intake can also lead to dependency, increased tolerance, and even withdrawal symptoms—much like heavy use of alcohol or other mood-changing drugs. One of the most common withdrawal symptoms is a headache, which may come on 18 hours after quitting caffeine. Painkillers containing caffeine will get rid of the headache but plain aspirin will not.

ragweed allergy should avoid teas made from flowers such as chamomile, yarrow, and others. Don't buy herb teas unless you are informed about the properties of their ingredients, and use them in moderation. To find out what you are getting, consult the label. If, however, the package does not have a list of ingredients, you will have to contact the manufacturer at the address given on the label.

Cocoa

The word "cocoa" is a corruption of "cacao," the name of the tropical New World tree whose beans are made into chocolate and cocoa. Confectionary and cooking chocolate is made from cocoa nibs, the fermented, roasted, and crushed seeds of the plant, which have a high cocoa-butter content. In beverage chocolate, or cocoa, much of this fat is pressed out before the nibs are pulverized into powder. (In the United States, the fat content of beverage cocoa is regulated by law: a minimum of 22 percent for "breakfast" cocoa, 10 to 22 percent for plain cocoa, and less than 10 percent for low-fat cocoa.)

Hot cocoa is usually prepared with equal amounts of powdered plain cocoa and sugar, plus hot milk, and a little water. This type of cocoa will not mix with cold milk as the instant cocoa mixes do. The mixes, however, contain artificial flavorings and as much as 80 percent sugar; the "complete" mixes also contain powdered milk, so that all you need to do is add boiling water. Many instant mixes are made with "Dutch Process" cocoa, which is not an import from Holland—it is simply cocoa treated with alkali to reduce acidity and enhance flavor.

Children, of course, love cocoa, but those who are allergic to chocolate should avoid drinking it because chocolate is one of the major ingredients of cocoa. Cocoa also contains the stimulants theobromine and a trace of caffeine, as well as tannin. One possible cocoa substitute is powdered carob, made from the pods of the evergreen carob tree. Carob contains

(There have been a few studies on "caffeineism" in children, and similar symptoms have been noted in those who consume large quantities of caffeine-containing soft drinks, cocoa, and chocolate.)

Besides the symptoms already mentioned, high caffeine intake has been associated with diuresis (excessive urination), gastrointestinal problems, and adverse changes in blood-sugar metabolism. Recent studies indicate that caffeine may increase the risk of developing fibrocystic (benign) breast disease and pancreatic cancer. However, not all scientists agree with the conclusions.

The effects of coffee consumption on the unborn fetus are also being studied. In 1980 the Food and Drug Administration issued a warning advising pregnant women to avoid or use sparingly all products containing caffeine because a study had shown that large levels of caffeine produced birth defects in rats. However, more recent studies, at Boston University and at Harvard, found that coffee drinking had no ill effects on the newborn. But these results are not considered conclusive by a number of scientists because the population samples tested were too small for accurate results. The current FDA stand on caffeine during pregnancy is that it is neither safe nor unsafe.

Over the years, researchers have also explored the possible role of caffeine in heart attacks, ulcers, and cancers of the stomach, bladder, and urinary tract, but here too the results so far have been inconclusive.

Although moderate caffeine consumption is thought to be safe for healthy adults who do not have a family history of diabetes, hypertension, or coronary heart diseases, apart from pregnant women and nursing mothers, the caffeine content of many products consumed by children is cause for concern (see Soft Drinks and Cocoa). Children who regularly consume colas and chocolate bars can ingest as much caffeine as adult coffee drinkers, and their growing bodies may be far more susceptible to its effects. Concerned parents should read labels carefully (especially on soft drinks, some of which contain caffeine and some of which do not) so that they can control their children's intake of this powerful stimulant. Further studies are necessary if caffeine is to be removed from the GRAS (Generally Recognized As Safe) list of additives.

Beverages: What's Good for You

Cocoa

tannin but no stimulants, and is probably less allergenic than chocolate products. However, for those who truly enjoy the sweet taste of chocolate, carob may seem like a weak substitute.

Alcoholic Beverages

All alcoholic beverages, including beer, wine, and distilled liquors, have the same active ingredient: ethyl alcohol, a potent mood-changing drug. Alcohol is absorbed rapidly by the tissues and acts as a depressant, or anesthetic, on the central nervous system. In moderation, it produces a pleasant sense of relaxation or euphoria—which explains why many people drink—but larger doses impair judgment and muscular coordination, and still larger ones can lead to total loss of physical control, unconsciousness, and even death.

Although many people feel that beer and wine are healthful additions to the diet, their nutritive value is questionable. In small amounts, wine can stimulate the appetite and increase the absorption of minerals from food taken with it, but it contains few nutrients of its own. (As for beer, most of its nutrients remain in the grain from which it is brewed, not in the beverage itself.) In general, although alcoholic beverages contain some nutrients, their overall effect on nutrition is decidedly negative. Alcohol itself is extremely high in calories (see chart)—more than 7 per gram, as opposed to the 4 per gram in carbohydrate. These "empty" calories make up a good part of the daily caloric intake of heavy drinkers, replacing many essential nutrients. (Alcohol actually increases the body's need for B vitamins, which are used to metabolize it, but at the same time it impairs the body's ability to utilize these and other nutrients, as well as depleting its store of water-soluble vitamins and minerals.)

Approximately 65 percent of Americans over 18 drink alcoholic beverages, but estimates of the number of alcoholics vary widely, from a low of about 5,750,000 to one high estimate of 18 million; the most common figure, however, is about 10 million. Because alcoholism is so extensive a health problem—one too large and complex to be dealt with here—it is tempting to assume that only complete abstainers can live healthy lives, but this is not necessarily so. There is some evidence (albeit inconclusive) that moderate drinking may be harmless and possibly even beneficial for otherwise healthy people. (A "moderate" dose would be one or at most two drinks, for a large person, a day, each one consisting of 12 ounces of beer, 5 ounces of wine, or 1.5 ounces of distilled liquor.) This does not mean, of course, that moderate drinking is a panacea, or suitable for everyone—far from it. For many people—including recovering and recovered alcoholics, those who object to alcohol on moral or religious grounds, those who take drugs that interact adversely with alcohol, and those with other health problems—alcohol in any form is out of the question.

Alcohol/Drug Interactions

Alcohol and other drugs can have complex interactions, with effects ranging from merely unpleasant to lethal. Of the 100 most frequently prescribed drugs, more than half contain ingredients that react adversely with alcohol—especially those drugs which, like alcohol itself, act as central nervous system (CNS) depressants. (Narcotics, barbiturates, "minor" tranquilizers, sedative-hypnotics, prescription painkillers, and over-the-counter antihistamines belong in this category, as do some major tranquilizers and sedatives.) Furthermore, a drug does not have to be taken *with* a drink in order to produce ill effects; as long as the drug is in the system, the potential for harm is there.

If you take prescribed drugs, here are some things the FDA advises you can do to avoid unpleasant alcohol-drug interactions.

• Be honest with your physician when discussing the amount you drink. Knowledge of present and past drinking habits is important in determining how much of certain drugs you should take.

• Be sure to report any changes in your drinking habits. Some people who are chronic alcohol users, whose drug dosage has been adjusted to the metabolic state of their liver, could upset the balance by giving up drinking without having their drug dosage adjusted accordingly.

• Ask your physician about possible alcohol interactions with the drugs prescribed for you.

• Check your prescription drug container for any warnings the pharmacist has attached.

• Read the labels on over-the-counter drug products. Know what's in the product and what side effects you might experience.

Alcoholic Beverages

	Serving	Calories
Distilled Liquors		
liqueurs *(cordials)*		
anisette	1 cordial glass, 1 oz.	75
apricot brandy	1 cordial glass, 1 oz.	65
benedictine	1 cordial glass, 1 oz.	70
creme de menthe	1 cordial glass, 1 oz.	67
curacao	1 cordial glass, 1 oz.	55
brandy, Calif.	1 brandy glass, 1 oz.	73
brandy, cognac	1 brandy pony, 1 oz.	73
cider, fermented	6 oz.	71
gin, rum, vodka, whiskey *(rye/scotch)*		
80-proof	1 jigger, 1½ oz.	104
86-proof	1 jigger, 1½ oz.	112
90-proof	1 jigger, 1½ oz.	118
94-proof	1 jigger, 1½ oz.	124
100-proof	1 jigger, 1½ oz.	133
Wines		
champagne, domestic	1 wine glass, 4 oz.	85
dessert *(18.8% alcohol by vol.)*	1 wine glass, 3½ oz.	137
Madeira	1 wine glass, 3½ oz.	105
muscatel/port	1 wine glass, 3½ oz.	158
red, Calif.	1 wine glass, 3½ oz.	85
sauterne, Calif.	1 wine glass, 3½ oz.	85
Wines		
sherry, dry, domestic table *(12.2% alcohol by vol.)*	1 wine glass, 2 oz.	85
	1 wine glass, 3½ oz.	85
vermouth, dry	1 wine glass, 3½ oz.	105
vermouth, sweet	1 wine glass, 3½ oz.	167
Malt Liquors *(American)*		
ale, mild	8 oz.	100
ale, mild	12 oz.	148
beer, denser liquid	8 oz.	114
beer	12 oz.	65-175
Cocktails		
daiquiri	1 cocktail	125
eggnog *(Christmas)*	4 oz. punch cup	335
gin rickey	8 oz.	150
highball	8 oz.	165
manhattan	1 cocktail	165
martini	1 cocktail	140
mint julep	10 oz.	212
old-fashioned	4 oz.	180
planters punch	4 oz.	175
rum sour	4 oz.	165
tom collins	10 oz.	180
whiskey sour	1 cocktail	138

- When in doubt, don't take a drink while on medication.

Alcohol and Other Health Problems

There are few, if any, organs of the body that alcohol doesn't affect in some way. The liver, which is the only organ that can metabolize alcohol, bears the brunt of overindulgence, with effects ranging from "fatty liver" (accumulated fat deposits) to alcoholic hepatitis and, finally, the degenerative and often fatal condition known as cirrhosis, sometimes accompanied by liver cancer. Heavy drinkers, especially those who also smoke, have a higher than normal risk of contracting other cancers as well. The heart is affected by alcohol in seemingly contradictory ways. There is some evidence that alcohol in moderation may have a protective effect on the coronary arteries, but this is counteracted by the damage it is known to do to the heart muscle. Heavy drinkers are prone to cardiac arrythmia, high blood pressure, congestive heart failure, and other potentially fatal cardiovascular conditions.

Heavy drinking in pregnancy is believed to carry a risk of multiple birth defects known collectively as "fetal alcohol syndrome." In July 1981 the U.S. Surgeon General's office cautioned pregnant women to avoid alcohol altogether. In men, prolonged heavy drinking is associated with lowered testosterone levels, impotence, and infertility. Alcohol also exacerbates existing health problems such as gout, ulcers, and low blood sugar, and it plays a major role in accident and crime statistics. Drinking is a factor in half the traffic accidents and more than half the violent crimes committed in the United States each year. All in all, it seems beyond dispute that alcohol, though pleasurable and relaxing in moderation, is a potentially toxic drug that should be used with extreme care.

Market Basket / A Guide to Shopping

Buying food wisely and preparing balanced, appetizing meals can save money and provide you and the members of your family with good nutrition. When buying food, various factors come into play; many of these are discussed here and on the following pages.

Knowing good nutrition. It is important for everyone to know what good nutrition means. The section of this book called Necessary Nutrients (pages 10-50) gives a concise introduction to carbohydrates, fats, proteins, vitamins, and minerals and the amounts of these nutrients needed by people to maintain good health. By eating a variety of foods from the Basic Four Food Groups (discussed on pages 96-105), you can fulfill your vitamin and mineral requirements and establish a sound nutrition program.

Planning meals and shopping trips. Planning meals can help in several ways. Weekly menus make it easier to see how you can fulfill the recommended number of servings from each of the Basic Four. They also enable you to make up a shopping list, a tool that is very useful when it comes to saving time and money. You can save even more time by grouping the items on the list according to the way they are displayed in the store. Another benefit of a shopping list is that it discourages haphazard or impulse buying—often a wasteful expense.

While planning the weekly menus, read the food ads in the local newspapers to see what is on sale or at a good price, and try to take advantage of these "specials" as much as possible. Since a family's likes and dislikes probably dictate the menus to a large extent, and if some of the favorites are not as nutritious as you would like them to be, compensate by adding more nutritious foods to the same meal. Remain flexible and, wherever necessary, be ready to substitute one food for another in case it is not available or is too costly. This applies especially to fresh fruits and vegetables.

To broaden your scope of ideas for meals, start building up your cookbook collection and recipe file and refer to these when planning the menus. Also, consider using or getting ideas from published, planned menus like the ones shown on pages 278-279 or given in magazines and newspapers.

Know what you are buying. Learn how to recognize good foods by using the Buying Guide (pages 108-179). Know what the food standards and grades mean and use them to your advantage (pages 194-195). Read the labels on food packages to know what is in the foods (pages 196-198); understand what the claims on the labels mean. Here are a few:

Enriched generally means that some of the nutrients that were lost during the processing of the food were put back into the food. For example, white flour is enriched with B vitamins.

Fortified usually means that nutrients that were never in the food are put into it during processing. For example, cereals are fortified with vitamin D.

Dietary supplement is a food, such as a highly fortified "cereal," that supplies more than 50 percent of the U.S. Recommended Daily Allowances of vitamins and minerals.

Imitation food is one that is not so nutritious as the food it is intended to resemble. For example, imitation eggs can be used like real eggs but are not so nutritious as real eggs.

Low calorie means that the food contains no more than 40 calories per serving.

Reduced calorie means that the food has at least one-third fewer calories than a similar food. The label must state what food it is being compared to calorie-wise.

Sugar free means that the food does not contain sucrose (table sugar). It can, however, contain fructose, sorbitol, mannitol, corn syrup, honey, molasses—all of which supply calories.

A term to be especially wary of is "natural." It is used liberally in food advertising, and the tendency is for the price of the food to increase with the use of the term. Although not officially defined and regulated as to its use, the Federal Trade Commission has proposed that "natural" should mean that the food does not contain any artificial or synthetic ingredients. In addition, the food can be no more than minimally processed, such as occurs in washing, peeling, grinding, baking, roasting, aging, homogenization, or canning. For example, foods that contain sugar are not "natural" because sugar is more than minimally processed. Foods labeled "natural" are usually no better nor more natural than similar foods not bearing the word "natural." Two other terms to approach with caution are "no artificial ingredients" and "no preservatives."

Shopping wisely. Since food accounts for a large part of every family's budget, the cost of food is of prime importance to every shopper. Instead of knowing just the price of the package, find out what the price per unit is and use it to compare costs between similar items of different sizes. If there is a unit-price label on the package or on the store shelf, the price per unit of weight, volume, or area will be indicated. If there is no unit-price label, calculate the price per unit by dividing the cost by the weight, volume, or measure. For example, a 16-ounce can of beans costing 64 cents costs 4 cents per ounce.

A more useful cost to establish is the cost per serving. This is done by dividing the price of the package by the number of servings. Many times, the number of servings is given on the label. If not, rely on your experience to make an educated guess as to the number of servings. When calculating for meats and fresh produce, subtract waste from the weight before determining the number of servings. If the package has a nutrition label, you can even determine how much the food costs per gram of protein (page 198).

When comparing costs, consider the store brands and the generic, no-name brands of foods; both are usually less expensive than the big-name brands. Although all three are equally nutritious, the generic foods tend to be lower in quality; that is, their appearance or uniformity is not so perfect as it could be, or they were picked before or after their peak of maturity.

Still another way to save money is to use the cents-off coupons and the refund offers. Most often they can be applied to only the big-name brands which, even at the reduced cost, can sometimes be more expensive than the store or generic brands.

When the price is right and if you have the storage space, consider buying in quantity; many times it will save you money in the long run. Learn how to cut meats and poultry and save even more money—the largest pieces are usually less expensive than chops or parts.

Sometimes, however, what appears to be a bargain is no bargain at all. Do not waste your time and money buying foods that you know your family definitely will not eat. Another waste is to buy spoiled foods. When buying fresh food, avoid those that do not look fresh or that have an off odor. When buying canned foods, never buy any cans that are leaking, bulging, or badly damaged or discolored; the contents could be contaminated with *Clostridium botulinum*, a bacteria that causes botulism, an often fatal food poisoning. If you are buying bottled foods, do not buy bottles with lids that are loose or appear to have been removed and replaced. When buying frozen foods, avoid packages that are soft, damaged, or stained. When buying cereals, flours, or other similar foods, do not buy any if the packaging is torn, cut, or open; bugs or other foreign matter may have entered.

Evaluating the stores. Compare them for quality, price, convenience, range of foods, and cleanliness. Also rate them as to how they handle food—the proper handling of food is very important to its safety and quality. Consider all types of stores, not just the supermarkets. Investigate what the vegetable stand, meat store, health food store, or cheese shop have to offer. If there is a food-buying club or food cooperative in your area, you may want to find out if being a member would help you. In these organizations, the members join together to buy food at wholesale prices and pass the savings on to other members. The range of food available, however, is usually limited.

Where To Go for Help

If you are dissatisfied with the taste or appearance of a commercially packaged food, contact its manufacturer. If you wish to report the sanitary conditions of a store (or restaurant) get in touch with the local health authorities. If you have an inquiry as to the safety, labeling, or wholesomeness of a food, the following list will help you direct your message to the proper agency.

• For food products containing meat or poultry, contact the Food Safety and Inspection Service, U.S. Department of Agriculture, Washington, D.C. 20250

• For food products not containing meat or poultry, contact the U.S. Food and Drug Administration, Rockville, Maryland 20857

• For foods produced and sold within the boundaries of a single state, contact the state or local health department or a similar law enforcement agency.

• For fish and fish products, contact the U.S. Department of Commerce, Washington, D.C. 20230

• For suspected false advertising, contact the Federal Trade Commission, Washington, D.C. 20580

Market Basket
Food Standards

There are many laws pertaining to the safety, quality, composition, fill of container, and representation of foods. Two major areas of regulation are the labeling of foods (pages 196-198) and the additives that can be put into our foods (pages 199-201). Other areas where regulations exist are discussed on these two pages: standards of identity, composition, and minimum quality and fill of container; the grading and inspection of foods.

Standards of identity are set up by the U.S. Food and Drug Administration (FDA). They stipulate what ingredients must be in a food in order for it to be labeled as that particular food. Certain optional ingredients are also allowed. Most of the standards have been revised in recent years to require that all optional ingredients be listed on the label. Mandatory ingredients, however, need not be listed.

The purpose of standards of identity is to let the consumer know that when he buys a certain standardized food, such as mayonnaise or ketchup, it will be like the food he has become familiar with. Standards of identity exist for about 300 foods. Some types of foods that have standards of identity are:

cacao products	cereal flour and related goods
bakery goods	macaroni and noodle products
milk products	cheese and cheese products
margarine	food flavorings and dressings
frozen desserts	canned fruits and fruit juices
sweeteners	jellies and preserves
fruit butters	canned and frozen fish
nut products	egg and egg products
vegetable juices	canned and frozen vegetables

Even though it may not be required, many companies voluntarily list all the ingredients of a standardized food. If they do not list the ingredients and you want to know what is in the standardized food, you can write to the manufacturer of the food and ask for the information, or you can look it up in Title 21 of the Code of Federal Regulations (available in many libraries or from the U.S. Government Printing Office, Washington D.C. 20402).

The Food and Drug Administration has set up mandatory minimum *standards of quality* for many canned fruits and vegetables. These standards may pertain to the color and tenderness of the food and allowable freedom from defects. If the food is below standard in quality, this must be stated on the label. The actual substandard element (for example, excessive peel, excessively broken) is required to be noted on the label. The FDA minimum standard of quality for a fruit or vegetable is the minimum standard established by a USDA grade standard. This is comparable to that of a USDA Grade C for many foods (see next page). Below-standard foods are rarely seen in stores.

Standards of fill of container, set up by the FDA, dictate the minimum quantity of food that must be contained in a package. Their purpose is to prevent deceptive packaging practices, such as the addition of undue amounts of air or water.

For processed meat or poultry foods, there are also *standards of composition* the foods must meet in order to qualify for sale. Set up by the U.S. Department of Agriculture, these standards define the minimum amounts of meat or poultry that must go into the product; however, a manufacturer can always add more meat or poultry to the food. Listed below are just some of the foods that come under this regulation and the minimum percentages of uncooked meat or poultry that must be in the foods. Notice that the percentages differ between meat and poultry for the same types of foods. (For information on other foods, contact your local branch of the Department of Agriculture.) Also helpful to know is that if a product is called "meat and noodles" or "meat and rice," there must be more meat than noodles or rice. Conversely, if a product is labeled "noodles and meat" or "rice and meat," it can have more noodles or rice than meat.

Meat	Poultry
Baby food, high meat dinner: 26%	Baby food, high poultry dinner: 18¼%
Baby food, meat and broth: 61%	Baby food, poultry with broth: 43%
Chile con carne: 40%	Poultry chile: 28%
Chile con carne with beans: 25%	Poultry chile with beans: 17%
Meat with vegetables: 50%	Poultry with vegetables: 15%
Meat casserole: 25%	Poultry casserole: 18%
Meat loaf: 65%	Poultry meat loaf: 65%
Meat pie: 25%	Poultry pie: 14%
Meat ravioli: 10%	Poultry ravioli: 2%
Meat soup, condensed type: 10%	Poultry soup, condensed type: 4%
Meat soup, ready-to-eat type: 5%	Poultry soup, ready-to-eat type: 2%
Meat stew: 25%	Poultry stew: 12%
Meat tamale: 25%	Poultry tamale: 6%

Food Grades and Inspection Stamps

The most common grading system used in this country is the one set up by the U.S. Department of Agriculture. It has developed standards for more than 300 types of foods; private companies voluntarily contract with the government for a federal grader to come and grade their foods. If a food has been graded by a USDA grader, it can carry a USDA shield denoting its quality. Some companies, however, choose to set up and use their own standards and grades.

Listed below is a sampling of foods and the *USDA grades* that apply to those foods. The highest grades are at the top of the columns; foods in these categories tend to be the most expensive. Shown below the list are several of the USDA grade shields found on these foods. Lack of a grade shield, however, does not mean that the food was not graded.

The standards for the USDA grades will vary with the type of food. The higher the grade, the more desirable the food is in such things as taste, texture, or uniformity. With some foods, such as eggs and vegetables or fruits, grade is based primarily on appearance. As a general rule, when buying any food, choose the grade that is best suited to your purpose. For example, if making a stew, where the appearance of the vegetables is not critical, you may want to buy the less expensive, lower grade vegetables.

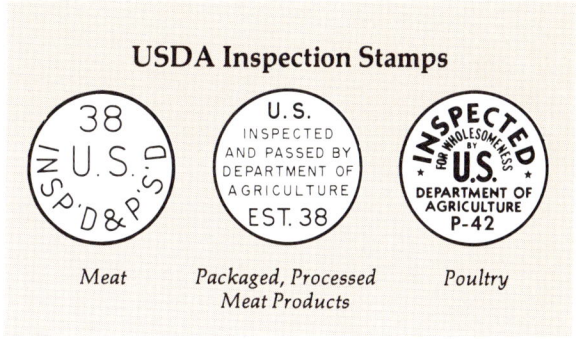

Grade-shield stamps should not be confused with *inspection stamps*. Inspection stamps indicate that the food is wholesome and was slaughtered, packed, or processed under sanitary conditions. Although other food can carry an inspection stamp, three types of food must be inspected, and there is an inspection stamp for each one (see above). Since the meat and poultry stamps are applied to the carcass or bulk package, they might not be visible on cuts packed for retail sale. Sometimes an inspection verification is included on a grade shield, such as is the case with the Grade AA shield for butter shown below.

Food Grades and Inspection Stamps

Beef; Veal; Lamb	Pork	Poultry	Eggs	Milk	Instant Nonfat Dry Milk	Butter; Cheddar Cheese	Cottage Cheese; Process Cheese	Fresh Fruits and Vegetables	Canned and Frozen Fruits and Vegetables
Prime	No. 1	A	AA	A	Extra Grade	AA	Quality Approved	Fancy	A or Fancy
Choice	No. 2	B	A			A		No. 1	B
Good	No. 3	C	B					No. 2	C

USDA Grade Shields

Beef; Veal; Lamb — Pork — Poultry — Eggs — Butter; Cheddar Cheese — Cottage Cheese; Process Cheese

Market Basket
Food Labels

An extremely important part of wise food shopping is reading and understanding the information given on the food labels. By doing so you can compare foods for quality, price, ingredients, and nutritive values and buy the ones that suit your needs.

The type and amount of information on a food label depend on the kind of food and the existing regulations. As of this writing, all food labels must have the name of the food, the net quantity, and the name and address of the manufacturer, packer, or distributor, should the consumer want to contact him. If the food is sold in different forms (for example, green beans can be sold whole or cut), the label must specify what form is in the container. If there is a picture of the food as well, it must accurately depict the food inside the package. The net quantity is given as a weight or a count, whichever is more appropriate to the food. If the food is packed in a liquid, the net weight includes the liquid (the weight of the food without the liquid is the drained weight).

Most labels, however, have more information than just the name, weight, and source of the food. Any food that does not have a standard of identity (see page 194) must list the ingredients in descending order of their predominance by weight. Although this way of listing is helpful, it does not tell you the actual amounts of the ingredients. In addition, food colorings, flavorings, and spices do not have to be specifically identified. With flavorings and colorings, all that has to be stated is whether they are natural or artificial. Spices, no matter how many different ones are used, can be accounted for by using a single word—"spices."

It is to every consumer's benefit to understand and use the list of ingredients on a food label. By reading the list, you get some idea of what the food tastes like, what you are paying for, and you can judge for yourself how "natural" or how additive- or preservative-free the food is. In addition, you may be able to avoid those foods that contain substances or additives that you want to avoid or are allergic to. While reading the lists of ingredients, be especially concerned with how much sugar, salt (sodium), and fats there are in the foods. Most nutritionists recommend that you limit your intake of these three ingredients. The problem, though, is that most processed foods contain them (especially sugars and salts) and that each can be listed in several different ways, as demonstrated by the lists at left. Notice that the fats have been grouped into saturated and unsaturated fats. On the next page is a comparison of the lists of ingredients for two soups.

Whenever a nutrient is added or a nutritional or dietary claim has been made, the food is required to show a nutrition label (see page 198) that lists the calories and the quantity of protein, fats, carbohydrates, and seven specific nutrients that are in one serving of that food. Some manufacturers give more than just the minimum required information.

Sugars, Salts, and Fats

Sugars and Other Sweeteners

beet sugar	fructose	mannitol
brown sugar	galactose	maple sugar
cane sugar	glucose	molasses
corn sugar	honey	sorbitol
corn syrup	invert sugar	sucrose
dextrin	lactose	turbinado sugar
dextrose	maltose	white sugar

Ingredients with Sodium

baking powder or baking soda
plain or flavored salt
self-rising flour
any compound with "sodium" in its name, such as:
    anhydrous disodium phosphate
    dioctyl sodium sulfosuccinate
    disodium dihydrogen pyrophosphate
    disodium guanylate
    disodium inosinate
    monosodium glutamate (MSG)
    sodium alginate
    sodium carboxymethyl cellulose
    sodium chloride (salt)
    sodium propionate
    sodium sulfite
    trisodium citrate

Saturated Fats	**Unsaturated Fats**
animal fats	corn oil
butter	cottonseed oil
coconut oil	olive oil
hydrogenated shortening	peanut oil
palm oil	safflower oil
sour cream	soybean oil
sweet cream	
whole milk	
whole-milk cheese	

Lists of Ingredients

Choosing a product on the merits of its ingredients is not a simple job, as this example illustrates.

Soup No. 1 is condensed, and when reconstituted, costs just over 2 cents an ounce. Soup No. 2 is ready-to-eat and costs just under 3 cents an ounce.

According to the two lists of ingredients, Soup No. 2 seems heartier than Soup No. 1, but it has neither beef stock nor beef fat, as does Soup No. 1. Beef fat, however, is a saturated fat, whereas the fats in Soup No. 2 (soybean and olive oils) are unsaturated. Although water is the first ingredient in Soup No. 2, the amount might be equal to or less than the total amount of water in Soup No. 1 when it is eaten—in addition to the water added for the reconstitution of Soup No. 1, its fifth ingredient is water. Salt is in a relatively middle spot in both soups, but Soup No. 1 also has monosodium glutamate (MSG).

Soup No. 1 Ingredients. Beef stock, carrots, potatoes, tomatoes, water, celery, peas, enriched spaghettini, green beans, pea beans, zucchini, salt, beef fat, potato starch, cabbage, yeast extract and hydrolyzed plant protein, spinach, rutabaga, monosodium glutamate, enzyme-modified Cheddar cheese, and natural flavoring.

Soup No. 2 Ingredients. Water, red kidney beans, Great Northern beans, green lima beans, green peas, carrots, potatoes, celery, cabbage, green beans, tomato paste, chick-peas, macaroni product, salt, soybean oil, dehydrated onions, olive oil, dehydrated garlic, natural flavorings, and spices.

With the advent of computerized checkout systems, many labels have the *universal price-code symbol* imprinted on them. This symbol is a pattern formed by numbers and lines of varying weights and lengths that, when passed over the machine, identifies the product to the computer. The computer then registers the price of the food and updates the inventory of the stock of that item. The customer in turn receives a register tape on which all the items are printed out with their names and prices. Because the prices are stored in the computer, the main worry among consumers is that the stores, hoping to cut costs and work loads, will do away with the practice of pricing individual packages. This would make it difficult, if not impossible, for the consumer to compare prices while shopping.

Other various symbols can also appear on a food label. An "R" means that the name adjoining it is a registered trademark; the letter "C" means that the label has been copyrighted. A "K" or a "U" inside a circle signifies that the food was prepared according to kosher standards. "Pareve," a Yiddish term, assures the consumer that neither milk nor meat was used in the preparation of the food. Two other markings that can appear on a label are a grade shield and an inspection stamp; for information on what these mean, see page 195.

Many foods also carry a date. There are two types of *dating systems*—coded and open. Coded dates are numbers and letters that, because they are part of a code, can be read only by those who understand the code. These coded dates are often used by supermarkets for rotating their stock. The code system can also indicate a plant location or a lot number that can serve to identify suspicious lots that may have to be recalled. Open dating, on the other hand, is an easily understood statement of a date that indicates the age of the product to the consumer. The date is accompanied by an explanation of what it means, such as "use by this date" or "not to be sold after" this date. If you are unsure of what the date means, ask the store manager. Although a date can appear on any type of food, they are most often found on perishable foods such as dairy products, baked goods, and meats.

In general, to get the freshest food, buy the package with the latest date. Poor handling or storage, however, can greatly diminish the freshness of a food. It can even happen that because the food was mishandled, a food with a future date on it can be less fresh, or "older," than the same type of food with an expired date on it. Unfortunately, there is no way for the consumer to know just how a food has been handled in shipping and storage.

Market Basket
Nutrition Labels

A nutrition label is not a separate designation but a part of the label on a package of food. According to regulations of the U.S. Food and Drug Administration, any food to which a nutrient has been added, or any food for which a nutritional claim (such as fortified or enriched) has been made must have a nutrition label. As a consumer you should read nutrition labels and use the information on them to evaluate and compare the nutritive values of foods and to help you select the foods you want.

To begin with, a nutrition label (see below) must tell first the size of a serving and how many servings there are in the package. In general, a serving size is the amount of that particular food that an average adult male, engaged in light physical activity, would be expected to consume as part of a meal. The nutrition label must then list, on a per serving basis, the amount of calories, protein, carbohydrate, fat, and the percentage of the U.S. Recommended Daily Allowances (US-RDAs) of protein, vitamins A and C, thiamin, riboflavin, niacin, calcium, and iron. For most nutrients, the USRDA is the highest RDA for that nutrient of all the age and sex categories (the present RDAs are based on those of 1974). For example, the RDA for iron is the 1974 one for female adults because that is the highest RDA for iron of all the age and sex categories. In addition, quantitative information on the sodium, cholesterol, or fatty-acid content of the food may also be given on the nutrition label.

The listing of any other nutrition information is voluntary. Many manufacturers will give nutrition information on foods that do not require a nutrition label. Some will voluntarily list the amount of sodium or give a breakdown of the types of carbohydrates (sugar, starch, and fiber) and their amounts per serving (see left).

You can use the information on a nutrition label to calculate the price per serving, the cost of each gram of protein, and the percentage of calories supplied by fat. If there is a carbohydrate breakdown, you can also determine the percentage of calories supplied by sugar or starch; fiber does not supply any calories. Use the formulas at left to do the calculations. The numbers in the examples at left are from a 16-ounce box of cereal that cost $1.39.

Formulas

Price per serving

$$\frac{\text{price}}{\text{number of servings}}$$

Example: $\frac{\$1.39}{16} = \$.0868$

Price of each gram of protein

$$\frac{\text{price per serving}}{\text{grams of protein per serving}}$$

Example: $\frac{\$.0868}{4} = \$.0217$

Percent of calories from fat

$$\frac{\text{grams of fat per serving} \times 9^*}{\text{calories per serving}} \times 100$$

Example: $\frac{1 \text{ gr} \times 9}{70 \text{ cal}} \times 100 = 12.85\%$

Percent of calories from sugar or starch

$$\frac{\text{grams of sugar (starch) per serving} \times 4^*}{\text{calories per serving}} \times 100$$

Example: $\frac{5 \text{ gr} \times 4}{70 \text{ cal}} \times 100 = 28.57\%$

*Each gram of fat supplies 9 calories; each gram of sugar or starch supplies 4 calories. Use last formula to calculate percent of calories from sugar or starch.

Nutrition Information Per Serving		Carbohydrate Information	
Serving size:	1 oz	Starch and related carbohydrates	7 gr
Servings per package:	16	Sucrose and other sugars	5 gr
Calories	70	Dietary fiber	9 gr
Protein	4 gr	Total carbohydrates	21 gr
Carbohydrates	21 gr		
Fat	1 gr		
Sodium	320 mg		

Nutrition Information Per Serving
Serving Size: 1 oz.
(about ½ cup cooked)

Servings per container:	16
Calories	100
Protein	2 grams
Carbohydrate	22 grams
Fat	0 grams

Percentage of U.S. Recommended Daily Allowance (U.S. RDA)

Protein	2
Vitamin A	*
Vitamin C	*
Thiamine	8
Riboflavin	*
Niacin	6
Calcium	*
Iron	4

*Contains less than 2% of U.S. RDA of these nutrients.
Ingredients: Long grain rice enriched with niacin, iron (ferric orthophosphate), thiamine (thiamine mononitrate).

Carolina Rice, Riviana Foods Inc.

Additives to Foods

Additives to foods are those natural or synthetic substances in processed foods which are intended to maintain or improve them. Today, much of our food is processed—that is, it has undergone one or more procedures that change it from its natural state. Milk, frozen cheesecake, and even butchered meat are all processed foods. Additives are regulated by the U.S. Food and Drug Administration as three different categories—color additives, food additives, or as an additive "Generally Recognized As Safe" (the so-called GRAS List).

There are many different types of additives, each with a specific purpose. *Anticaking agents* absorb moisture and prevent finely powdered or crystallized substances from caking or lumping. *Antioxidants* delay or prevent foods from turning rancid or changing in taste, odor, and appearance. *Colors*, either natural or artificial, impart a characteristic or appetizing color to foods, or intensify the color. *Emulsifiers* help distribute particles evenly in liquids and prevent them from separating into layers. They also affect texture, volume, and consistency of foods. *Flavors* (either natural or artificial) increase or alter the natural flavor of foods, restore flavors lost in processing, or mask unpleasant flavors. *Flavor enhancers* modify or supplement the original taste or aroma of foods without giving off a flavor or aroma of their own. *Humectants* help foods retain their moisture. *Leavening agents* influence the results of cooking foods, such as the texture or volume. *Maturing* or *bleaching agents* and *dough conditioners* improve the baking qualities of foods and accelerate the aging process of certain ingredients so that they are at the preferred stage for processing. *Nutrients* enrich or fortify foods (see page 192). A *pH control agent* maintains or changes the acidity or alkalinity of foods, thereby affecting their taste, texture, and safety. *Preservatives* prevent foods from spoiling from infectious microorganisms such as molds, fungi, or bacteria and extend the shelf life. *Stabilizers*, *thickeners*, and *texturizers* stabilize emulsions and affect the texture and body of foods. *Sweeteners* make the taste or aroma of foods more pleasant and appealing. A *nutritive sweetener* is metabolized by the body and produces energy. A *non-nutritive sweetener* does not produce energy (or yield calories) in significant amounts.

Given below and on the next two pages is a chart of some of the additives used in foods today. Some, such as mannitol, sorbitol, saccharin, BHA, BHT, sodium nitrite, sodium nitrate, caffeine, and several of the artificial colors are controversial but may be used at present levels until further studies are completed. (By law, food processors must add sodium ascorbate to bacon to block the formation of cancer-causing nitrosamines formed from nitrates.)

ADDITIVE	TYPE	FOODS WHERE FOUND
acetic acid	pH control	candies, sauces, dressings, relishes
acetone peroxide	maturing and bleaching agent	flours, breads, rolls
adipic acid	pH control	beverage or gelatin bases, bottled drinks
ammonium alginate	stabilizer, thickener, texturizer	dessert-type dairy products, confections
annatto extract	natural color (yellow-red)	found in many foods
aspartame	nutritive sweetener	cereals, chewing gum, dry beverage or dessert mixes
baking powder (calcium phosphate, sodium aluminum sulfate, sodium bicarbonate)	leavening agent	quick breads, cake-type baked goods
baking soda (sodium bicarbonate)	leavening agent	quick breads, cake-type baked goods
benzoic acid	preservative	fruit products, acidic foods, margarine
beta carotene	nutrient, natural, artificial color (yellow)	found in many foods
butylated hydroxyanisole (BHA); butylated hydroxytoluene (BHT)	antioxidants	bakery products, cereals, snacks, fats, oils
caffeine	flavor enhancer	baked goods, desserts, candies, colas, other soft drinks
calcium alginate	stabilizer, thickener, texturizer	dessert-type dairy products, confections

Market Basket
Additives to Foods

ADDITIVE	TYPE	FOODS WHERE FOUND
calcium lactate	pH control	olives, cheeses, frozen desserts, beverages, fruits, vegetables
calcium silicate	anticaking agent	table salt, baking powder, powdered foods
caramel	natural color (brown)	found in many foods
carrageenan	emulsifier, stabilizer, thickener, texturizer	chocolate milk, canned milk drinks, whipped toppings, frozen desserts, puddings, syrups, jellies
carrot oil	natural color (orange)	found in many foods
cellulose derivatives	stabilizers, thickeners, texturizer	breads, ice cream, confections, diet foods
citric acid	preservative, antioxidant, pH control	acidic foods, fruits, snacks, cereals, instant potatoes, fruit products, candies, beverages, frozen desserts
cochineal extract	natural color (red)	found in many foods
corn syrup, corn-syrup solids	nutritive sweeteners	cereals, baked goods, candies, processed foods and meats
dehydrated beets	natural color (dark red)	found in many foods
dextrose	nutritive sweetener	cereals, baked goods, candies, processed foods and meats
diglycerides, monoglycerides	emulsifiers	baked goods, peanut butter, cereals
disodium guanylate	flavor enhancer	canned vegetables
disodium inosinate	flavor enhancer	canned vegetables
disodium phosphate	emulsifier, pH control	cheeses, drinks, sauces, cereals
ethylenediaminetetraacetate (EDTA; calcium disodium)	stabilizer	dressings, sauces, margarine
FD&C blue No. 1 or 2; FD&C red No. 3 or 40; FD&C yellow No. 5 or 6; FD&C green No. 3	artificial colors	found in many foods
fructose	nutritive sweetener	cereals, baked goods, candies, processed foods and meats
fruit juices, vegetable juices	natural colors	found in many foods
fumaric acid	pH control	dry desserts, confections, powdered drinks
furcelleran	stabilizer, thickener, texturizer	frozen desserts, puddings, syrups
gelatin	stabilizer, thickener, texturizer	dry dessert mixes, yogurt, ice cream, cheese spreads, beverages
glucose	nutritive sweetener	cereals, baked foods, candies, processed foods and meats
glycerin, glycerol monostearate	humectants	flaked coconut, marshmallow
heptylparaben	preservative	beverages
hydrogen peroxide	maturing and bleaching agent, dough conditioner	flours, breads, rolls
hydrolyzed vegetable protein (HVP)	flavor enhancer	processed meats, gravy mixes, sauce mixes, fabricated foods
invert sugar	nutritive sweetener	cereals, baked goods, candies, processed foods and meats
lactic acid	preservative, pH control	olives, cheeses, frozen desserts, beverages
lecithin	emulsifier	margarine, dressings, chocolate, frozen desserts, baked goods
mannitol	nutritive sweetener, anticaking agent, stabilizer, thickener, texturizer	candies, chewing gum, confections, baked goods, jams, jellies
methylparaben	preservative	beverages, pastries, dressings, relishes
modified food starch	stabilizer, thickener, texturizer	sauces, soups, pie fillings, canned meats

FAMILY FOOD GUIDE

ADDITIVE	TYPE	FOODS WHERE FOUND
monosodium glutamate (MSG)	flavor enhancer	Oriental foods, soups, foods with animal protein
paprika, paprika oleoresin	natural flavors, natural colors (red-orange)	found in many foods
phosphates	pH control	fruit products, beverages, ices, sherbet, soft drinks, oils, baked goods
phosphoric acid	pH control	fruit products, beverages, ices, sherbet, soft drinks, oils, baked goods
polysorbate 60, 65, or 80	emulsifiers	gelatin, puddings, dressings, baked goods, nondairy creams, ice cream
potassium alginate	stabilizer, thickener, texturizer	dessert-type dairy products, confections
potassium bromate	maturing and bleaching agent, dough conditioner	breads
propionic acid (calcium, potassium, or sodium propionate)	preservative	breads, baked goods
propylene glycol	stabilizer, thickener, texturizer, humectant	baked goods, frozen desserts, dairy products, confections
propyl gallate	antioxidant	cereals, snacks, pastries
propylparaben	preservative	beverages, pastries, dressings, relishes
quinine	natural flavoring	carbonated beverages
saccharin	non-nutritive sweetener	special dietary foods, beverages
saffron	natural flavor, natural color (orange)	found in many foods
salt (sodium chloride)	natural flavor, preservative	found in many foods
silicon dioxide	anticaking agent	table salt, baking powder, powdered foods
sodium acetate	pH control	candies, sauces, dressings, relishes
sodium alginate	stabilizer, thickener, texturizer	dessert-type dairy products, confections
sodium benzoate	preservative	fruit products, acidic foods, margarine
sodium citrate	pH control	fruit products, beverages, frozen desserts
sodium diacetate	preservative	baked goods
sodium nitrate, sodium nitrite	preservatives	cured meats, fish, and poultry
sodium stearoyl lactylate	maturing and bleaching agent, dough conditioner, emulsifier	baked goods, pancakes, puddings
sodium stearyl fumarate	maturing and bleaching agent, dough conditioner	yeast-leavened breads, instant potatoes, processed cereals
sorbic acid (calcium, potassium, or sodium sorbate)	preservative	cheeses, syrups, cakes, beverages, mayonnaise, fruit products, margarine
sorbitol	humectant, non-nutritive sweetener	chewing gum, confections, baked goods
spices	natural flavors	found in many foods
sugar (sucrose)	nutritive sweetener	cereals, candies, processed foods
tartaric acid	pH control	dairy desserts, baked goods, beverages
tertiary butylhydroquinone (TBHQ)	antioxidant	snacks, fats, oils
turmeric, turmeric oleoresin	natural flavors, natural colors (yellow)	found in many foods
vegetable gums (acacia, carob bean gum, guar gum, gum ghatti tragacanth gum)	stabilizers, thickeners, texturizer	chewing gum, sauces, desserts, dressings, syrups, beverages, fabricated foods, cheeses, baked goods
yeast	leavening agent, nutrient	breads, baked goods
yeast-malt sprout extract	flavor enhancer	gravies, sauces
yellow prussiate of soda	anticaking agent	salt

Keeping Foods Fresh / On the Shelf

Storing foods in the cupboard or pantry has one major advantage—it is an inexpensive way to keep foods for a long period of time. Many staples can be stored this way as long as certain conditions are met.

Most important of all, keep all foods away from the stove or any other heat source. Use cabinets or shelves above and near your stove for cooking utensils rather than for food supplies.

Choose an area that is dry and cool, preferably where the temperature does not get above 70 degrees. Shelves near the ceiling or in garages are usually not good storage areas because in summer the temperature can get extremely high. It is advisable to store foods away from light, which may destroy nutrients and hasten deterioration.

Dry Foods. Select packages with no cuts or openings, and sizes that will be used up quickly. To protect against dust, moisture, and insects, transfer larger quantities to a large, wide-mouth jar with a screw-on top. Coffee cans or canisters, too, can be used, as long as the tops have a tight seal.

Bottled Foods. Always check the label on bottled foods to find out if they can be stored without refrigeration until opened.

Canned Foods. Most food experts suggest that you keep canned foods for about a year—or less. Although the food in the cans may be safely eaten well past the time restriction, the taste and color can change. For example, acid foods such as tomatoes can pick up a metallic taste. Cherries may lose their color, and onions can turn an unappetizing tan. The nutritive quality of the food, too, can be affected. Some vitamin loss is sure to occur with passing time. For example, the vitamin C loss is about 10 percent when canned fruits and vegetables are stored for a year at 65 degrees. But if the storage temperature is as high as 80 degrees, the vitamin loss can reach 25 percent—and possibly more.

Canned goods are a bargain only if they are properly cared for after you get them home. Here are some tips on how to handle canned foods.

• Always buy cans that are in good shape. A dent along the seams or on the rim can eventually cause a leak.

• Check cans for bulges or leaks. Never open a leaky can or one with a popped lid; return it, and alert the store manager. If you opened a can that appeared normal, but the contents bubbled or spurted, dispose of them in a safe manner without tasting—the contents may harbor toxins that can cause fatal food poisoning.

• Rotate your stock and move the oldest cans to the front of the shelf so that they will be used up first. Write dates on the labels or on the bottoms of the cans with a marker if you wish to keep track of the dates of purchase.

• Always read the storage information on the label. A few types of container foods such as canned hams may have to be refrigerated even if unopened.

• Wipe the top of the can with a damp cloth. Any dust that has collected will mix with the food during opening.

• Although it is safe to leave an unused portion of food in the can if refrigerated, it is better to store leftover food in glass or plastic containers. The metal can impart an off flavor to foods.

Food	Recommended Storage Time	Handling Hints
Staples		
Baking powder	1 year	Keep dry and very tightly covered.
Baking soda	2 years +	Keep dry and covered.
Bouillon cubes	1 year	Keep dry and tightly covered.
Bread	5 days	Refrigerate in hot weather.
Breadcrumbs, dried	6 months	Keep dry and covered.
Cereals		
ready-to-eat, unopened	6-12 months or expiration date	
ready-to-eat, opened	2-3 months	Refold package liner tightly after opening.
cereal to be cooked	6 months	Keep dry and tightly closed.
Cornmeal	12 months	Keep tightly closed.

FAMILY FOOD GUIDE

Food	Recommended Storage Time	Handling Hints
Cornstarch	18 months	Keep tightly closed.
Flour		
white	2 years +	Keep in airtight container
whole wheat	6-8 months	Keep refrigerated. Store in moisture-proof airtight container.
Gelatin, all types	18 months	Keep in original container.
Grits	12 months	Keep in covered, airtight container.
Honey	12 months	If crystals form, warm jar in pan of hot water.
Jams, jellies	12 months	Refrigerate after opening.
Milk, dry		
nonfat, unopened	12 months	
nonfat, opened	6 months	Keep in airtight container.
Pasta	2 years +	
Rice		
white	2 years +	Keep tightly closed.
brown or rice mixes	4-6 months	Keep tightly closed.
Salad dressings		
bottled, unopened	10-12 months	
bottled, opened	3 months	Refrigerate after opening.
made from mix	2 weeks	Refrigerate prepared dressing.
Salad oils		
unopened	6 months	
opened	3 months	Refrigerate large quantities for longer storage.
Shortenings, solid	8 months	Do not refrigerate.
Sugar		
white	2 years +	Cover tightly.
brown	6 months	Refrigerate in airtight container.
Syrups	12 months	Refrigerate after opening.
Vinegar	2 years +	
Canned Foods		
Unopened canned goods	1 year	Keep cool and dry.
Dried Foods		
fruits	1 year	Seal in plastic bags inside glass or metal container in a dry, cool, dark place.
Spices, Herbs, Condiments		
Catsup, chili sauce		
unopened	12 months	
opened	6 months	Refrigerate after opening.
Mustard, prepared		
unopened	2 years	
opened	6-8 months	Refrigerate after opening.
Spices and herbs	6-12 months	Keep in airtight containers away from light and heat.
Others		
Nuts in shell	6 months	Refrigerate after opening. Freeze for longer storage. Unsalted and blanched nuts keep longer than salted.
Peanut butter	6-9 months	
Peas and beans, dried	12 months	Keep in airtight container in cool, dry place.
Vegetables, fresh		Store in ventilated containers
onions	6-7 months	–in cool, dry, dark place.
potatoes, white	4-9 months	–in cool, moist, dark place.

Keeping Foods Fresh
In the Refrigerator

Of all the ways to preserve food, mechanized household refrigeration is a fairly newfangled idea. Before 1923, when the Frigidaire company came out with the first self-contained refrigerator that merely needed to be plugged into an electrical outlet, keeping foods cold in the house was a messy job. Almost daily, blocks of ice had to be delivered to the kitchen door, carried dripping across the floor, and deposited in the tin storage compartment of the so-called ice box. On hot summer days the ice melted, and much of the food spoiled anyway. Today, the refrigerator is the most used appliance in American homes, and fewer than 1 percent of households are without at least one refrigerator.

The refrigerator is most handy for keeping perishable foods. Think of it as a transitory storage place and check the contents frequently. Throw out any foods that have dried or spoiled.

To keep perishable foods safe for eating, be sure the temperature in your refrigerator is between 34 and 40 degrees F. You can check the temperature with a special refrigerator thermometer or a standard indoor-outdoor thermometer. Take several readings at different levels. If the temperature is near 32 degrees, some of the foods will develop ice crystals or freeze; above 45 degrees, bacteria will multiply so rapidly that the foods will spoil much more quickly.

In most frostless or self-defrosting refrigerators, the temperature usually remains fairly even throughout the compartment, including the storage shelves on the door. In a standard type refrigerator, however, the temperature tends to be colder near the freezer and warmer in the door storage area. Also, opening the door frequently on hot, humid days will raise the temperature inside the refrigerator.

Refrigerate foods that need to be kept cold, such as dairy products, eggs, meat, poultry, fish, produce, as soon as you unpack your grocery bags. Nutrient loss and spoilage will take place rapidly if foods are kept at room temperature for more than two or three hours. Suggested storage times for fresh foods are discussed in the Buying Guide to fruits, vegetables, fish, meats, poultry, eggs, milk and milk products, and cheeses, which appears on pages 108-159. However, here are some general pointers to keep in mind about refrigerator storage.

Fruits and Vegetables. Most refrigerators are equipped with a hydrator, or crisper drawer, which provides both cold and moderate humidity for keeping fruits and vegetables fresh. If your refrigerator lacks this feature, you can store your produce in unsealed plastic bags. In general, do not wash fruits and vegetables before storing because any additional moisture hastens rotting.

Eggs. Before storing in the refrigerator, check all eggs for any cracks. Cracked eggs should never be used, even in cooking. Store the eggs with the larger end up and the pointed end down to keep the yolk centered. Since eggs have porous shells, they will quickly lose moisture and absorb refrigerator odors. For this reason, it is best to store them in the original carton or in a covered container.

Oils. If you buy large quantities of oil for salads and cooking, store the opened container of oil in the refrigerator. Although fats turn rancid more quickly at room temperature, you can keep a small quantity in your cupboard for daily use. Some oils may become cloudy or solidify when refrigerated, but this is not harmful. They will become clear and liquid when warmed to room temperature.

Meat, Poultry, Fish. Store meats at once in the coldest part of the refrigerator or in a special meat keeper if you have one. Unrefrigerated meat will begin to spoil rapidly because of bacterial growth and the production of toxins. Prepackaged meat, poultry, and fish can usually be left in the original packaging. However, if there is any blood, repackage the meat. Use within the time recommended in the storage chart, and rinse food under running cold water before cooking to remove surface bacteria. Handle fish carefully, since bruised fish spoils more quickly; wipe fish with a damp cloth before cooking.

Leftovers. Using leftovers can be economical and save hours of work in the kitchen, but only if they are properly handled.

When you have some food left over from lunch or dinner that you plan to use for another meal, refrigerate it promptly—even if the food is still slightly warm. Though the temperature in your refrigerator compartment might rise a little because of the warm food, it is well worth it for safety's sake and for maximum nutrition retention. Cover all dishes tightly with wrap or transfer the food to smaller containers with lids.

Special care must be taken with egg- or cream-rich dishes. Cover and refrigerate any foods prepared with raw eggs, such as eggnog, and eat within the same day. Foods made with cooked eggs or cream, such as custards, quiches, casseroles, cream pies, or mousses, must be refrigerated as soon as they are slightly cool and served within a few days. Refrigerate or freeze leftover poultry and stuffing separately within two hours.

If possible, it is a good idea to heat leftovers thoroughly before serving. All foods will lose some of their nutrients with time. To prevent further vitamin loss, reheat vegetables in a double boiler with a bit of water to keep them moist. Or you can add cooked vegetables to soups. Boiled rice can be transformed into fried rice, and leftover cooked cereal can be added to meat loaf. Boil leftover soups and gravies for several minutes **before** serving.

Food	Recommended Storage Time	Handling Hints
Meat, Poultry, Fish, Eggs		
Meats		
beef, lamb, pork, and veal roasts, chops, steaks	3-5 days	All meat, poultry, and fish, when bought in plastic wrapping (from self-service counters), should be stored in original packages.
ground meat, stew meat	1-2 days	
variety meats (liver, heart, etc.)	1-2 days	At home, poke a small hole in the wrapper of prepackaged, uncured meats to allow air circulation.
Poultry		
chicken, duck, turkey	1-2 days	
Fish	1 day	
Cured and smoked meats		
hard sausage	2 weeks	
frankfurters, hot dogs	1 week	
hams, whole	1 week	
hams, canned, unopened	6-12 months	Check label: most require refrigeration.
luncheon meats	3 days	Keep tightly wrapped.
Eggs		
in shell	1-2 weeks	Time limit for best quality; safe longer. Store covered. Keep small ends down to center yolks.
Dairy Products		
Butter, margarine	2 weeks	Freeze for longer storage.
Cheese		
cottage	7-10 days	Keep all cheese tightly wrapped. If mold forms, discard entire package.
cream	10-14 days	
natural, hard	1-3 weeks	
processed	5 weeks	
Cream		
fresh	1 week	Check pull date for keeping time unopened.
sour	1 week	
Milk	1 week	Check for signs of spoilage: cream and milk will start to smell; yogurt begins to separate.
Yogurt	3 weeks	
Other		
Opened canned foods	3 days	After a few days, transfer to glass, ceramic, or plastic container to avoid metallic taste. Keep covered.
tomato-based	5 days	
Fresh or reconstituted juices	1 week	Keep covered.
Leftover gravy and broth	1-2 days	Keep covered.
Mayonnaise	3 months	Refrigerate after opening; keep covered.
Nuts, unshelled	6 months	Freeze for longer storage.

Keeping Foods Fresh
In the Freezer

When it comes to managing your personal food supply, foods that are stored properly frozen are second only to fresh foods in nutritional value. However, loss of taste and nutrition occurs rapidly if foods are partly thawed and then refrozen or if the freezer temperature is not 0 degrees or lower. If your freezer or refrigerator-freezer does not maintain 0 degrees throughout, keep frozen foods for less than the recommended time. Freezing does not kill bacteria in foods, it only stops them from multiplying.

Depending on their use and type, freezers should be defrosted periodically. A collection of ice reduces storage space and may cause the temperature of your freezer to rise several degrees. Even self-defrosting freezers should be defrosted—usually once a year; consult the manufacturer's directions.

Commercially Frozen Food

When you buy food that is already frozen, you should take some precautions. If you are concerned about eating preservatives, avoid complicated foods packed in sauces. Choose, instead, simple, plain food. Be sure that the merchant's freezer is clean. Note the temperature if there is a thermometer in the freezer. It should be 0 degrees or lower. If it is an open cabinet, there may be a line marked on the side above which packages must *not* be stored. Purchase only from below this freezer line. Avoid any packages that are dirty, soft, and misshapen. Such conditions may indicate that the packages have been improperly handled or thawed and refrozen between the processing plant and the market. Fruits and vegetables that were frozen in individual pieces in bags should still be separate and not in lumps. Neither bags nor boxes should be punctured, torn, or stained. Always buy frozen food last when you shop. Ask for insulated bags or double paper bags at the checkout counter to put your frozen items in, and come home to your freezer immediately.

Do not neglect to pay proper attention to your frozen food once you have stored it. Check the date on your packages and use the oldest first. When you put new packages into the freezer, store under or behind what is already there. It is wise to keep a

Purchased Frozen Foods

Food	Approximate Storage Time (in months)	Food	Approximate Storage Time (in months)	Food	Approximate Storage Time (in months)
Fruits and Vegetables		**Meat**		mullet; ocean perch; sea trout; striped bass	3
Fruits: cherries; peaches; raspberries; strawberries	12	Cooked meat: meat dinners; meat pie; Swiss steak	3	Pacific Ocean perch	2
Fruit juice concentrates: apple; grape; orange	12	**Poultry**		salmon steaks	2
Vegetables: asparagus; beans; cauliflower; corn; peas; spinach	8	Chicken		sea trout, dressed	3
		cut up	9	striped bass, dressed	3
Baked Goods		livers	3	**Shellfish**	
Bread and yeast rolls		whole	12	clams, shucked	3
white bread	3	Duck, whole	6	crabmeat	
cinnamon rolls	2	Goose, whole	6	Dungeness	3
plain rolls	3	Turkey		King	10
Cakes		cut up	6	oysters, shucked	4
angel; chiffon	2	whole	12	shrimp	12
chocolate layer	4	Cooked chicken and turkey		Cooked fish and shellfish	
fruit	12	dinners (sliced meat and gravy)	6	fish with lemon-butter sauce	3
pound; yellow	6	chicken or turkey pies	6	fried fish dinner	3
Danish pastry	3	fried chicken	4	fried fish sticks, scallops, or shrimp	3
Doughnuts: cake type; yeast raised	3	**Fish and Shellfish**		**Frozen Desserts**	
Pies (unbaked): apple; cherry; peach	8	Fish fillets: cod; flounder; haddock; halibut;	6	Ice cream	1
				Sherbet	1

record of your freezer's contents. Frozen foods will not keep in good condition indefinitely, even when properly stored at 0 degrees. The chart at bottom left gives maximum home-storage periods for the best quality of commercially frozen foods. Since these products are "flash" frozen or can contain preservatives, the storage times are usually longer than for home-frozen goods.

Home Freezing

Compared to all other ways of preserving foods, home freezing is a relatively simple and rewarding method of storage. The main thing to remember is to freeze only top quality foods. Freezing can preserve the quality, but it does not improve it.

When preparing foods for the freezer, your hands and any surface that comes into contact with the food to be frozen must be kept scrupulously clean in order to minimize bacterial growth. Work quickly, wrap foods tightly, label packages carefully, including the date, contents, and number of servings.

Meat, Poultry, Fish. At one time or another most people find it convenient to freeze meats—possibly because they are unable to cook the meat or fish when they had originally planned or because fresh meat happens to be a good buy.

All meat that is to be frozen must be properly wrapped. Packaged meat or poultry from the market is not usually adequately wrapped for long-term freezer storage. It is therefore wise to rewrap meat when you get it home. Improperly wrapped meat is subject to freezer burn, which means that portions of the meat become dried out and unusable.

Since packaging is very important for preserving quality, here are some tips:

- Wrap meat, poultry, or fish in plastic wrap and then in moisture-resistant wraps.
- Remove bones to save freezer space.
- Pad pointed tips of bones with several layers of wrap to prevent holes in the outer wrapping.
- When freezing slices of fish or poultry or meat patties, separate pieces or layers with waxed paper or freezer wrap.
- Seal all packages with tape.

Storage times for meats, fish, and poultry are given in the chart at right.

Dairy Products. Some dairy products such as butter freeze well, whereas others such as sour cream will become watery. The chart above tells how long these products will keep.

Eggs. Eggs cannot be frozen in their shells, which will crack. You can blend the whites and yolks, place the mixture in a small, covered container with ½-inch of headroom, and freeze. You can freeze the whites just as they are, but yolks require the addition of corn syrup, sugar, or salt, and the quality may still be poor. Eggs will keep from six months to a year in the freezer. Once thawed, do not refreeze.

Home Frozen Foods	
Food	Approximate Storage Time (in months)
Meat, Fresh	
Beef, steaks or roasts	9-12
Beef, ground	4-6
Lamb	9-12
Pork	6-9
Pork sausage	1-3
Beef or lamb liver	3-4
Pork liver	1-2
Veal	4-6
Meat, Smoked	
Bacon, sliced	not recommended
Bacon, slab	1-3
Ham, whole	1-3
Poultry and Game Birds	
Chicken, ready-to-cook	6-7
Giblets	2-3
Turkey, ready-to-cook	4-5
Ducks	6-7
Geese	3-4
Game birds	6-7
Fish	4-6
Shellfish	3-4
Dairy Products	
Butter	5-6
Cheese	
cottage cheese, creamed	not recommended
cottage cheese, uncreamed	1-2 weeks
cream cheese	not recommended
hard or semihard	6-12
soft	4
Cream	
heavy	3-6
light	not recommended
sour	not recommended
whipped	3-6
Milk	1

Keeping Foods Fresh
In the Freezer

What To Do When the Freezer Fails

Once you learn how to store food properly, your freezer can be like a faithful friend. But what happens when it breaks down or the power goes out? Try to find out how long it will be before your freezer is working again. Keep the freezer door closed. Don't keep opening and closing it to "check on the food." A fully loaded freezer will stay cold enough to keep food frozen for two days. A half-full freezer will only keep food cold for a day. Meats that still contain ice crystals or have been maintained at 45 degrees F or below for less than two days may be safely refrozen. Some quality may be lost, but the product is still wholesome. Throw out any food that has an unusual color or odor. Never refreeze ice cream.

If it looks as though the power will be off for a long time or your freezer won't be repaired for a while, use dry ice. If dry ice is placed in the freezer soon after the power goes off, 25 pounds should keep the temperature below freezing for 2 to 3 days in a 10-cubic-foot, half-full freezer and 3 to 4 days in a full freezer of the same size.

Handle dry ice carefully. Be sure the room is well ventilated, and never touch dry ice with your bare hands. Place the dry ice on cardboard or small boards on top of packages, and do not open the freezer again except to put in more dry ice or to remove it when your freezer is working again.

If using dry ice is not possible, move the food to a food locker. Carry it to the locker in insulated boxes or thick layers of paper to prevent thawing. Or possibly a neighbor may be willing to store some of your food until your freezer is working.

Can Thawed Foods Be Safely Refrozen When They Are:	Completely Thawed But Still Are Cold (45°F or lower)	Completely Thawed But Are Warm (above 45°F)
Uncooked Foods		
Fruits	Yes	Probably safe—but may have fermented.
Fruit juice concentrates	Yes, but flavor may be poor, and juice may separate.	No. May have fermented.
Vegetables	Yes	Questionable. Safer not to refreeze, especially corn, peas, and beans.
Meat	Yes, if odor is normal. If there is any off odor, discard.	Do not refreeze.
Milk and milk products	Yes, if odor is normal. If there is any off odor, discard.	No
Variety meats (liver, kidney)	Yes, if odor is normal. If there is any off odor, discard.	No
Poultry	Yes, if odor is normal. If there is any off odor, discard.	No
Fish and shellfish	Yes, if odor is normal. If there is any off odor, discard.	No
Pre-Cooked and Prepared Foods		
Cooked meat, poultry, fish	No	No
Combination dishes (meat, poultry, and pot pies, casseroles, whole meals)	No	No
Soups	No	No
Ice cream and sherbet	No	No
Fruit pies	Yes	Yes, but quality may be poor.
Baked goods		
bread	Yes	Yes, but texture may be poor.
plain cake and cookies	Yes	Yes, but texture may be poor.
cream-filled cake and cookies	No	No

Fruits and Vegetables. If you are lucky enough to have a garden, pick your vegetables and fruits just before you plan to freeze them, when they are at their nutritional peak. However, there is more work involved than simply packaging and putting the produce in the freezer. Some fruits are better packed with sugar; others should be dry packed. Most vegetables must be scalded, or blanched, before freezing. This process inactivates the enzymes that could affect the texture and flavor of vegetables. Scalding times vary depending on the vegetable. Many cookbooks have a section devoted to freezing fruits and vegetables.

Precooked Foods. One way to save time is to cook a double portion of soup or lasagna and freeze half. It is usually more economical to make your own frozen foods rather than to buy commercially prepared ones.

The U.S. Department of Agriculture gives the following advice regarding home freezing.

Prepare the food in the usual way and cook it until almost done. Frozen meats and vegetables easily become overcooked when reheated if they were completely cooked before freezing. Season lightly when you prepare the recipes because pepper, cloves, and synthetic vanilla tend to become strong and bitter when used in frozen foods. You can always add more seasoning just before serving.

Crumb and cheese toppings should be added to the frozen food just before reheating.

Here is some information to help you select combination main-dish recipes for freezing:

- Cooked chicken or turkey in casseroles freezes well.
- Almost any type of cooked meat, stew, ragout, or goulash—beef, lamb, pork, or veal can be frozen. Most vegetables used in these combination foods, such as peas, carrots, celery, or onions, also freeze well.
- Add a rich, flaky pastry topping to a good meat and vegetable stew, and you have a delicious meat pie. The unbaked pastry topping may be added before freezing, or it may be made fresh and placed on the pie when it is heated for serving.
- You can freeze meat loaf. Make enough for several meals and freeze the extra loaves. Meat loaf has better quality if frozen baked rather than unbaked.
- Cooked dry beans freeze especially well. Because freezing softens beans somewhat, cook them until barely tender for the best quality product.

Certain foods should not be frozen because their flavor or texture changes during the freezing process. For example:

- Cooked egg white toughens.
- Salad greens lose their crispness and become soggy.
- Raw tomatoes change in flavor and color and become limp and watery.
- Raw apples and grapes become soft and mushy.
- Fried foods tend to have a warmed-over taste when reheated.

Other foods may be successfully frozen if you follow some guidelines:

- New potatoes are better than mature potatoes in most frozen dishes. Mature potatoes tend to disintegrate or become watery when boiled and then frozen.
- Gelatin mixtures should be made stiffer than usual to lessen the chance of separating.
- Thoroughly combine the flour and fat in sauces and gravies. These foods may appear curdled while thawing but will usually recombine when stirred.

Packaging Materials. Be sure to wrap food carefully before freezing to prevent exposure to air and loss of moisture during freezing and storage. Exposure to air will cause changes in color and flavor and will permit delicate foods to absorb strong flavors and odors given off by other foods. Suitable packaging is particularly important in frost-free freezers that have a fan blowing air over the food, drawing moisture from the package.

Coated or laminated freezer papers, plastic wrap (or polyethylene films), and heavy-weight aluminum foil are good materials for freezing. Rigid plastic containers may be used for food that is cool when poured into the containers. Ceramic, metal, or glass containers may be used for hot or cold foods.

When freezing combination main dishes in baking pans, line the pans with a freezer wrap. Allow enough extra wrap to fold over the top. Use a nonmetallic wrap for acid foods such as tomatoes.

Cooling and Packaging Food. When hot food is ready to be frozen, it must be cooled quickly to stop the cooking, to retard growth of bacteria, and to help retain the natural flavor, color, and texture.

To cool food quickly, put it into 8- by 8-inch pans lined with heat-resistant freezer wrap. (If 8- by 8-

Keeping Foods Fresh
In the Freezer

inch pans are not available, use any ovenproof pan.) Use one pan for each six servings. Pack food tightly to avoid air pockets. Then let it stand at room temperature for 30 minutes.

Do not pour boiling hot foods into pans with plastic wrap because the wrap might melt.

To wrap, fold ends over the top and seal with freezer tape. Label with name of the food, date of freezing, and last date the food should be used for best eating quality. See storage chart below.

Freezing. Spread the pans or packages of food in freezer so food will freeze rapidly. Allow a 1-inch space around packages for air circulation. Follow freezer manufacturer's directions for placing food in the coldest section. You can freeze 2 to 3 pounds or one 8- by 8-inch pan of food per cubic foot of freezer space at one time. Leave the food for 10 to 12 hours until it is completely frozen. Then remove wrapped food from the pans. Check the wrappings to make sure they are airtight and secure before stacking.

Home-Prepared, Pre-Cooked Foods

Food	Approximate Storage Time (in months)	Food	Approximate Storage Time (in months)
Breads, Quick		**Fruits**	
Baked biscuits	1-2	Baked apples	4
Baked fruit and nut breads	1-2	Cranberry relish	8-12
Baked muffins	1-2	**Meals, Whole**	
Storage life on frozen, unbaked quick breads is shorter than those baked before freezing.		Foods chosen should retain quality for approximately the same length of time and should reheat in the same amount of time.	½-1
Breads, Yeast		**Meats and Poultry**	
Loaves and rolls, baked	2 weeks; edible for 12 months, but quality decreases the longer held	Broiled or fried	1-3
Brown-and-serve rolls, partially baked		Roasted, large pieces or sliced, covered with gravy	beef and poultry, 4-6; pork, 1-3
		Meat loaf, baked or unbaked	1-2
Cakes		**Pies**	
Layer and loaf cakes, baked and made with fat	4-6	Fruit, baked or unbaked (preferred)	3-4
Baked angel and sponge cakes	4-6	Unbaked pastry	1½-2
Baked fruit cake	12	Pecan, baked	3-4
Frostings and cakes are best frozen separately		*Pie meringue is not recommended for freezing.*	
Cookies		**Salads**	
Baked, all types except meringue	2 weeks; edible for 12 months, but quality decreases the longer held	Most salads do not freeze well. Combinations of fruit, cream, or mayonnaise (often with added gelatin) make acceptable frozen products.	4-6
Unbaked, refrigerator type			
Combination Dishes, Cooked		**Sandwiches**	
Baked beans, chili, chop suey, chow mein, curried lamb, meatballs with sauce, ravioli, stew	½-1	*Avoid fillings with hard-boiled egg whites, jellies, or raw vegetables.*	1-2
Casseroles		**Soups**	
Unbaked, but made from cooked ingredients; lasagna, Spanish rice, etc.	2-6	Chicken noodle, chowder, fish, meat stock, split pea, vegetable	1-3
Desserts		**Vegetables**	
Baked, cheesecake	4	Cooked, with sauces	½-1
Frozen desserts, ice cream, and fruit ice	1-6	Potatoes, baked, stuffed, or French-fried	½-1
Steamed pudding	1-6	Purees	½-1

Other Long-Term Storage

Three other methods of keeping foods over long periods of time are canning or preserving, dehydration, and where climate permits, winter storage in basement or root cellar.

Canning and Preserving. After decades of being out of fashion, home canning has become increasingly popular in recent years. Whether you wish to preserve garden produce or take advantage of a bumper crop at the farmer's markets, you will reap a rich sense of satisfaction when you view jars of homemade pickles or tomatoes.

Canning, however, is not a casual activity. The step-by-step directions for canning each food must be followed precisely to ensure food safety. Many cookbooks include a section on home canning. There are also books on the subject and booklets issued by the U.S. Department of Agriculture or by manufacturers of canning equipment.

To prevent botulism, home-canned, low-acid foods such as vegetables, meats, and poultry *must* be processed in a pressurized canner. Before serving, low-acid foods should be boiled for 15 to 20 minutes. If there is any foaming or off odor, discard in a safe manner. However, since so many nutrients are destroyed in canning these foods, it is usually wiser to freeze them. Plan instead on canning pickles, jams, preserves, acid fruits, and tomatoes (you can add 1 tablespoon of lemon juice to each quart of tomatoes to assure acidity). These foods can be processed safely in the simpler boiling-water bath canner and do not require pressure cooking.

Store jars in a dark, cool, dry place such as the basement and check them periodically. If the temperature of your storage area is below 65 degrees, the nutrient loss is minimal. Humid storage areas are unsuitable; the moisture may cause the canning lids to rust. Discard any jars with broken seals or in which the contents are leaking or discolored.

Drying. The process of removing moisture from fresh foods is one of the most ancient methods of preserving food. However, drying can be expensive and time consuming and may not be a practical choice for everyone. Although many foods can be dried, most people choose fruits and vegetables because the results here can be more satisfying.

There are three basic methods of drying—in the sun, in the oven, and in a dehydrator. Each requires some special equipment: from drying trays to the dehydrator itself. The drying times vary from as little as 3 to 4 hours for oven drying to several days if air drying in the sun.

Drying is a multistaged process in which each step is important to a successful product. Most vegetables must be steam blanched before they are processed for drying, and many fruits need to be treated with sulfur or they will lose their bright color.

In most parts of the United States, especially in the Northeast, artificial heat is needed to dry foods. Air drying by the heat of the sun will work only in areas where the climate is hot and dry. Since this method is directly tied to the weather, it is largely unpredictable.

Most herbs, however, can be air dried without much fuss. If possible, pull up the entire plant when it is mature. Always wash the herbs thoroughly and, if possible, hang outdoors in the sun for a few hours until the plants begin to wilt or dry. To continue the drying indoors, put each plant or a section of a plant in a paper bag that has been punched in a few places to permit air to circulate. Hang bags in a warm airy place such as the attic. When herbs are dry, put into jars and store away from light.

Home-drying methods can never remove as much moisture as commercial ones, which shortens the shelf life of home-dried foods. Sufficiently dehydrated foods will not mold. Dried foods must be stored in covered, moisture-proof containers in a dry, cool place—away from the light.

Root Cellars. If you have the space, you may want to plan a root cellar for wintering-over some of your autumn harvest. (An unheated cellar or the bulkhead to the basement have been used successfully for years for long-term storage.) Such storage is not possible unless you live where outdoor winter temperatures average 30 degrees or lower.

Root cellars provide ideal winter storage for root vegetables such as carrots, potatoes, beets, and turnips. Fruits such as apples, pears and, surprisingly, grapes, can also be kept in this way. Since fruits absorb odors from strong vegetables and can in turn affect them, keep fruits as far away from vegetables as possible or store separately.

There are numerous other ways to store produce outdoors, including storage pits, trenches, and mounds. If you want to find out more about this type of storage, you can get information about which method is suitable for your area from your local USDA County Extension Agent.

Preparation Techniques/Handle with Care

When preparing and cooking foods the major concerns are how to retain their nutritive value, the proper handling for food safety and, of course, taste.

Consider first how the food will be served—raw or cooked? If the food is to be cooked, which cooking method is the best (the various methods are discussed on the following pages)? Cooking is essential for certain foods. For instance, meat, poultry, and eggs can harbor harmful bacteria that are destroyed by the proper heat. The temperature guide below shows which temperatures inhibit or promote the growth of bacteria and toxins. A good rule to keep in mind is: keep hot foods hot (above 140 degrees) and cold foods cold (below 40 degrees). Do not hold foods at temperatures between 60 and 125 degrees for more than a few hours.

Before you begin. Keep all work surfaces and utensils scrupulously clean. Bacteria from the preparation of raw foods can infect cooked foods if the cutting boards and surfaces are not thoroughly cleaned with soap and water after each use.

Fruits and vegetables. A quick rinse under cold water is usually sufficient for cleaning most fruits and vegetables. The less contact there is with water, the fewer the losses of water-soluble vitamins and minerals. Leafy vegetables such as spinach may need several changes of water to rid the leaves of all sand. Some fruits and vegetables (apples, cucumbers) are treated with a protective coat of wax before shipping to help retain moisture. *To remove the wax*, hold the fruit or vegetable under warm running water and scrub lightly with a vegetable brush. This is a matter of personal preference, and there is no evidence to date to indicate that the wax coating is harmful.

Whenever possible, wash and cut vegetables and fruits immediately prior to serving or cooking. This will preserve the nutrients as well as the texture. If it is necessary to prepare them ahead of time, storage is important. Wrap greens in a damp towel and refrigerate. Sprinkle lemon juice over cut fruits that might darken, and refrigerate in a covered dish. Store cut vegetables in a slightly open plastic bag. Keeping peeled potatoes covered with water may prevent discoloration, but it will leach out nutrients. By just peeling the potatoes you will be throwing away valuable nutrients. If possible, do not peel vegetables because the skins usually contain vitamins and minerals.

Frozen foods. Generally, vegetables and prepared foods can be cooked while still frozen, but meats, poultry, and fish should be thawed first. Once foods are thawed, they lose nutrients rapidly, and bacterial growth can occur. It is best to thaw foods in the refrigerator (the cold slows down bacterial growth and moisture loss). However, this method can take a long time. Allow about 24 hours for steaks and chops; 2 days for roasts. Although it is possible to cook frozen meat, it will take about half again as long as roasting fresh meat.

Do not thaw seafood at room temperature or in warm or hot water as there is too much risk of surface spoilage. The best method for thawing seafood quickly is to place the entire package under running, cold tap water. If properly wrapped, the package should be watertight. As soon as the package contents can be pulled apart, the remainder of the thawing can be done in the refrigerator. Some prepared fish products must be cooked while frozen, so be sure to read the instructions.

What to do about mold. Never eat any food that has even a spot of mold. At one time it was thought that surface mold on food, especially cheese, should simply be cut away and that the rest of the food was still edible. However, food experts now know that the mold threads go deep into foods and advise that you return any moldy package to the store or discard it.

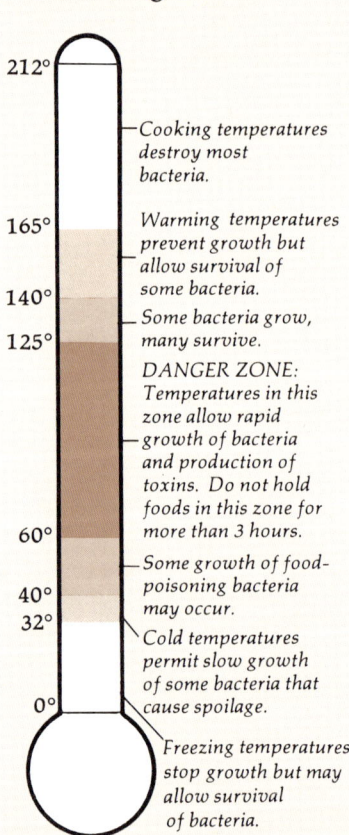

Controlling Bacteria

- 212° — Cooking temperatures destroy most bacteria.
- 165° — Warming temperatures prevent growth but allow survival of some bacteria.
- 140° — Some bacteria grow, many survive.
- 125° — DANGER ZONE: Temperatures in this zone allow rapid growth of bacteria and production of toxins. Do not hold foods in this zone for more than 3 hours.
- 60° — Some growth of food-poisoning bacteria may occur.
- 40°
- 32° — Cold temperatures permit slow growth of some bacteria that cause spoilage.
- 0° — Freezing temperatures stop growth but may allow survival of bacteria.

Choosing a Cooking Method

All cooking, like storage, destroys some nutrients. In general, the shorter the cooking time, the less the nutrient loss.

The way in which you cook a food depends on the food, the recipe, what cooking equipment you own, and your personal taste preference. Usually, cooking methods fall into the following categories: dry-heat methods, moist-heat methods, and special methods such as sautéing, stir-frying, and deep-fat frying. However, sometimes two methods are combined in one technique; for example, before a food is braised in liquid, it is usually first browned by sautéing.

Dry-heat cooking methods. As opposed to moist-heat types of cooking, dry-heat techniques do not require liquids to make foods palatable. Dry heat is best for cooking tender cuts of meat, whereas moist heat is more suited for tougher cuts.

Roasting originally meant turning food on a spit over an open fire. Today, baking and roasting are essentially the same, the primary difference being the foods that are associated with each technique. For example, hams, fish, foods with leavening agents such as breads, cakes, and soufflés are baked, whereas meats and whole poultry are roasted.

According to one school of thought, it best to first sear meat that is to be roasted over high heat and then to lower the temperature for the rest of the cooking time. This, however, results in excessive shrinkage and uneven cooking. A better method is to cook the food at one constant but lower temperature to retain moisture.

Roasting is best done on a rack in a shallow pan, a method that allows the heat to cook all sides of the food. Also, the rack will prevent foods from being cooked in the drippings.

During roasting the heat can slowly penetrate and cook whole poultry and thicker pieces of meat. *Broiling* or *grilling,* however, is suited to thinner cuts of beef and lamb, chicken, fish, and even some fruits and vegetables such as grapefruit, pineapple, and peppers.

Grilling is usually done on a barbecue and, as with broiling, heat is controlled by altering the distance of the broiler or grilling rack from the source of heat. In general, charcoal heat is hotter than broiler heat, which is provided by a conventional gas or electric oven unit. For foods about 1 to 2 inches thick, the usual distance from the heat is about 3 inches. Thicker cuts should be cooked about 5 inches from the heat so that the outside does not burn during the longer cooking time.

Before broiling or grilling meat, trim off the excess fat, which will splatter when heated. If necessary, grease the rack so that foods will not stick to it. With most foods the rack should not be preheated, but this is beneficial with fast-cooking foods or thin pieces of fish or meat that do not need turning because the heat from the rack will cook the part of the food that it comes in contact with faster than the remainder of the piece.

Sautéing, stir-frying, deep-fat frying. Of these quick-cooking methods *sautéing* is suitable for preparing eggs, hamburger, veal, and fish. Since this is done over direct heat with a small amount of cooking

---

Convection and Microwave Cooking

Two types of ovens that are becoming increasingly popular are the convection oven and the microwave oven. A convection oven is a conventional oven with the addition of an electric fan to circulate the heat. This circulation of heat cooks the food more evenly and in less time than does an oven without the fan.

A microwave oven, on the other hand, emits high-frequency electromagnetic waves that penetrate the food and cause the water molecules in the food to vibrate, producing heat that cooks the food. Getting the kinds of results you want with a microwave oven may take some practice. Usually the quantity and the composition of the food determine the cooking time. For example, although a single potato may take 4 minutes to bake, each additional potato will increase the total cooking time by another 4 minutes. For best results, follow the manufacturer's instructions and take advantage of the special microwave recipes. Cooking results are slightly different from those of a conventional oven, especially when it comes to browning foods. Also, because some uneven cooking is to be expected, it is best to avoid cooking pork in a microwave oven. Pork requires thorough, even cooking to kill the trichina parasite.

Preparation Techniques
Choosing a Cooking Method

oil, the shorter the cooking period the less fat the food will absorb. If sautéing for a longer time, keep draining off the fat so that the amount of fat a food might absorb will be kept to a minimum. The oil should be hot enough to cook the food but not so hot as to exceed the smoking point (see chart below).

Another quick-cooking method that is fast gaining in popularity is *stir-frying*. This technique uses a minimum of fats and liquids and retains the flavor and texture of meats or vegetables because the ingredients are quickly tossed or stirred as they fry. The major part of the work is the preparation of the foods to be cooked. In cooking vegetables, for example, all vegetables must be cut into even-sized pieces. Meat can be cut into ⅛-inch-thick pieces on the diagonal grain to the cut. It is easier to slice the meat while it is still slightly frozen. Although a specially designed pan with high, sloping sides called a wok is best to use for this type of cooking, good results can be achieved with a skillet.

Once the foods are all cut, add a small amount of oil to the pan (1 to 2 tablespoons of oil per pound of food) and turn on the heat. When the oil is hot, start by adding the ingredients that take the longest to cook, and stir to coat all pieces with oil. If stir-frying meats with vegetables, partially cook the meat and push it aside while starting the vegetables. Keep stirring and adding until all pieces are heated through but not wilted, usually in only a few minutes. Occasionally it may be necessary to cover for an additional few minutes. The addition of liquids and seasonings will depend on the recipe.

Although many shun *deep-fat frying*, when done properly (that is, quickly), deep-fat fried foods absorb very little fat. The oil you use for frying should have a high smoking point so it will be able to withstand the high temperatures (325 degrees to 400 degrees). Fill the pot just under half full with oil and use enough so that the food will have space to move around during cooking.

Heat the oil, using a deep-fat-frying thermometer clipped inside the pot to read the temperature of the oil. If you do not have a frying thermometer, drop a ⅝-inch bread cube into the oil when you think the oil is hot enough. If the cube turns golden brown in 30 seconds, the oil is ready for frying. If you deep-fat fry foods before the oil is sufficiently hot, the food will absorb too much oil and it will not cook properly. When done properly, the hot oil seals the outside of the food and the food is then cooked by the heat from the oil as well as by the moisture trapped in the food. If adding more food to the oil, let the oil reheat to the proper cooking temperature. Do not let the oil smoke, and keep removing bits of food that have collected in the oil. To reuse the oil, let it cool and then strain it through cheesecloth to remove all food particles. Refrigerate the oil until ready to use again. If properly strained each time and not overheated, the oil can be used six or seven times. Do not use the oil if it becomes dark or smells rancid.

Moist-heat cooking methods. All moist-heat cooking methods involve a cooking liquid such as water, stock or broth, or wine or beer. Moist-heat

Cooking Oils

When used properly, cooking with oils is not detrimental to good nutrition. To begin with, choose an oil that is low in saturated fats (see below). Saturated fats tend to increase the amount of cholesterol in the blood; unsaturated fats, especially polyunsaturated fats, tend to lower the blood serum cholesterol level. It is also very important to use an oil with a high smoking point so it can withstand the high temperatures of cooking before reaching the smoking point. When an oil smokes, it is beginning to decompose which, in turn, forms acrolein, a compound that gives fat an objectionable flavor and odor, and peroxides, substances that are destructive to vitamins. Butter is more saturated and has a lower smoking point than any of the oils listed. Margarine and salad oils vary too much by brand in their composition to be predictable.

Oil	Percentage of Saturated Fat	Smoking Point (°F)
Corn oil	17	475°
Olive oil	10	375°
Peanut oil	20	440°
Safflower oil	6	510°
Sesame oil	13	420°
Soybean oil	15	495°
Sunflower oil	8	485°

Percentage of Vitamin C Loss During Boiling*

Vegetable	Cooking Time (in minutes)	Percentage of loss	Vegetable	Cooking Time (in minutes)	Percentage of loss
Bean, snap	45	30-40	Collards	30	79
Bean, snap (frozen)	15	28	Lima beans	30	18
Bean, snap (canned)	10	63	Potatoes	60	50-60
Broccoli (frozen)	11	45	Potatoes	90	83
Broccoli (frozen)	2	36	Rutabagas	26-36	40-42
Cabbage	17-19	65-73	Spinach	7	42
Cabbage	60	20	Squash, summer	20-30	50
Cauliflower	12	85	Sweet potatoes	20	31
Chard, Swiss	14	71-75	Sweet potatoes, whole	35	24
Chard, Swiss	10	54-58	Turnip greens	slow	24-37
Collards	5	40	Turnip greens	rapid	16-23

*These results were obtained in the course of several experiments.

cooking tenderizes the tougher cuts of meat and fibrous vegetables. When *boiling*, *poaching*, or *stewing*, the food is often immersed in the cooking liquid. *Braising* requires a small amount of liquid, and in *steaming* and *double-boiler cooking* the food does not come into contact with the liquid. Keep checking the level of liquid as the liquid evaporates in boiling, and replenish when necessary.

Methods involving boiling or *simmering* (including poaching and stewing) are usually the most destructive of water-soluble nutrients because the nutrients are drawn into the cooking liquid. Therefore, it is a good idea to try to use the cooking liquid as part of the meal by using it in gravy or freezing it for later use in soups and stews. (One way is to freeze the liquid in ice cube trays and use the cubes as needed.) The chart above illustrates the amount of vitamin C loss that can occur with boiling certain vegetables. Methods in which little or no liquid touches the food are usually the most protective of the nutrients. Avoid adding salt, which tends to draw out the nutrients.

A partial cooking method associated with boiling is *blanching* or *parboiling*. With this method, food is dropped into boiling water and cooked for a short time—a few minutes or even less. Blanching is often a preliminary step to another preparation or cooking technique. Blanching vegetables before freezing them helps preserve quality. Also, tomatoes can be blanched to remove their skins before stewing.

Steaming is an excellent method for cooking most vegetables because nutrient loss is minimal and the flavor of the food is not diluted. To steam food, bring a small amount of water to a rolling boil, place the steamer basket with food into the pot, lower heat to a simmer, and cover the pot. Steam the food until it is just tender (not soggy). The steamer basket usually rests on small legs so that the water does not touch the food. Unless you like your vegetables very crunchy, steaming will usually take longer than boiling the same food. Fish, too, can be steamed by using a special fish steamer and oiling it lightly before using.

A fast and also very nutritious way of cooking foods is *pressure cooking*. Pressure cookers have the distinct advantage of cooking foods in half the time or less than it would take by conventional means. For example, a 2-pound pot roast that takes nearly three hours to cook in the oven will be ready to eat in about one hour if cooked under pressure. Pressure cooking is best suited for one-pot dishes but can also be used for steaming custards and casseroles. By using a timer you can keep the foods from overcooking. As its name implies, pressure cooking uses steam pressure to soften foods. Always follow manufacturer's instructions in using this equipment—*never remove the lid while the food is cooking.*

Preparation Techniques
Useful Facts and Figures

The charts and figures shown on these two pages are facts that you can refer to when cooking; for the most part, each unit is self-explanatory.

The list of equivalents and yields gives the approximate measure of a food when presented in a different form. For example, 1 pound of apples measures about 3 cups when sliced; 1 pound of spaghetti yields about 6 to 8 cups when cooked.

The list of substitutions, on the opposite page, gives foods that can take the place of others in a recipe if you don't have a particular ingredient on hand. Thus, if a recipe calls for dried breadcrumbs but you do not have any in the pantry, you can use bread or cracker crumbs instead.

If you live in a high altitude, some foods will take longer to cook. Below is a brief explanation of how the altitude affects cooking times.

The column on the far right shows how to convert cups and ounces to their metric equivalents and how to convert back and forth from Fahrenheit to Celsius temperatures.

High-Altitude Cooking

At sea level, water freezes at 32°F, simmers at about 195°F, and boils at 212°F. However, the higher you are above sea level, the lower is the boiling point of water. In fact, for each 500 to 550 feet above sea level, the boiling point of water drops by 1°F. For example, at 2,000 feet, water boils at 208°F.

High-altitude cooking has negligible effects on roasting but can require adjustments in time and ingredients in any liquid-based recipe, especially cake recipes. Although it takes less time for the liquid to reach the lower boiling point, the liquid is also less hot and therefore foods take longer to cook through. You will also probably need to add more liquid to compensate for the liquid that evaporates during cooking. In regard to home canning, high altitudes have an effect on the time and pressure needed to destroy harmful microorganisms so that the canned food will be safe to eat. For more specific advice on high-altitude cooking, you can consult your local home extension service.

Equivalents and Yields

Apples	1 lb	3 c pared, sliced
Bananas	3-4 med	1 lb or 1¾ c mashed
Beans, green, fresh	1 lb	3 c uncooked or 2½ c cooked
Beans, kidney, dried	1 lb	2½ c uncooked or 6 c cooked
Beans, navy, dried	½ lb	1 c uncooked or 3 c cooked
Broccoli	1 lb	2 c cooked
Butter	4 oz	8 tbsp or ½ c
Butter, whipped	1 lb	3 c
Cabbage	1 lb	4 c shredded
Carrots	1 lb	3 c shredded or 2½ c diced
Cheese	¼ lb	1 c shredded
Cheese, blue	4 oz	1 c crumbled
Cheese, cottage	½ lb	1 c
Cheese, cream	3 oz	6 tbsp
Chicken, broiler, fryer	3½ lbs	about 2 c cooked, diced
Chocolate	1 oz	1 square or 4 tbsp grated
Coffee	1 lb	40-50 6-oz c
Coffee, instant	2 oz	25 6-oz c
Flour, all purpose	1 lb	4 c sifted
Flour, cake	1 lb	4½ c
Honey	1 lb	1⅓ c
Lemon	1 med	2-3 tbsp juice; 2 tsp grated rind
Macaroni	1 lb	6-8 c cooked
Milk, instant, nonfat dry	1 lb	about 4 qts reconstituted
Milk, whole, dry	1 lb	14 c reconstituted
Mushrooms, canned	4 oz	⅔ c
Mushrooms, fresh	8 oz	about 1 c sliced, cooked
Noodles	1 lb	6-8 c cooked
Oatmeal	1 c	1¼ c cooked
Onion	1 med	½ c chopped
Oranges	1 med	6-8 tbsp juice; 2-3 tbsp grated rind
Peaches, pears	1 med	¼ lb or ½ c sliced
Peas, dried, split	1 lb	2¼ c uncooked or 5 c cooked
Peppers, green	1 lge	1 c diced
Potatoes	3 med	1 lb or 2¼ c cooked or 1¾ c mashed
Prunes, dried	1 lb	2½ c
Raisins, seedless	1 lb	2¾ c
Rice	1 c	½ lb or 3 c cooked
Spaghetti	1 lb	6-8 c cooked
Spinach	1 lb	1½ c cooked
Sugar, brown	1 lb	2¼ c
Sugar, confectioners	1 lb	3½ c
Sugar, granulated	1 lb	2 c
Tea	1 lb	125 c
Yeast, active, dry	1 pkg	1 tbsp

Substitutions

Baking powder	1 tsp	¼ tsp baking soda plus ⅝ tsp cream of tartar
Biscuit mix	1 c	1 c flour plus 1½ tsp baking powder plus ½ tsp salt plus 1 tbsp shortening
Butter *or* margarine	1 c	about 1 c vegetable shortening plus ½ tsp salt
Buttermilk	1 c	1 c yogurt
Breadcrumbs	1 c	4 slices bread *or* ¾ c cracker crumbs
Chocolate, unsweetened	1 oz	3 tbsp cocoa plus 1 tbsp butter *or* fat
Cream, half and half	1 c	3 tbsp butter plus about ¾ milk
Cream, heavy	1 c	⅓ c butter plus about ¾ c milk
Cream, sour	1 c	3 tbsp butter plus ⅞ c buttermilk *or* yogurt
Flour, all purpose	1 c sifted	1 c plus 2 tbsp sifted cake flour
Flour, cake	1 c sifted	⅞ c sifted all-purpose flour
Flour, self-rising	1 c	1 c flour plus 1¼ tsp baking powder plus ⅛ tsp salt
Garlic	1 clove	⅛ tsp garlic powder
Herbs, fresh	1 tbsp	⅓ tsp dried
Honey	1 c	1 c sugar plus ¼ c liquid
Lemon juice	1 tsp	½ tsp vinegar
Lemon rind, grated	1 tsp	½ tsp lemon extract
Milk, skim	1 c	⅓ c instant nonfat dry milk plus ice water to make 1 c
Milk, sour	1 c	1 tbsp vinegar *or* lemon juice plus about 1 c milk; let stand 5 minutes
Milk, whole	1 c	½ c evaporated milk plus ½ c water *or* ¼ c dry whole milk plus ⅞ c water
Mustard, prepared	1 tsp	⅓ tsp dry *or* powdered
Onion	1 small	¼ c frozen chopped *or* 1 tbsp instant
Sugar, brown	1 c	¾ c granulated plus ¼ c molasses
Sugar, confectioners	1¾ c	1 c granulated (not for baking)
Sugar, superfine	1 c	1 c granulated
Tomato paste	1 tbsp	1 tbsp tomato catsup
Tomato sauce	1 c	6 tbsp tomato paste plus ⅔ c water plus seasonings
Yogurt	1 c	1 c buttermilk

Equivalent Weights and Measures in Metric

U.S. Liquid Measures and Metric Equivalents

1 tsp = ⅓ tbsp = ⅙ fl oz = 5 mL
1 tbsp = 3 tsp = ½ fl oz = 15 mL
1 c = 8 fl oz = ½ fl pt = 237 mL (approx. ¼ L)
1 fl pt = 2 c = ½ fl qt = .473 L (approx. ½ L)
1 fl qt = 2 fl pt = ¼ gal = .946 L (approx. 1 L)

To convert ounces to milliliters (mL), multiply ounces by 29.57.

U.S. Weight Measures and Metric Equivalents

1 oz = 1/16 lb = 28.35 g = .028 kg
1 lb = 16 oz = 454 g = .454 kg
1 g = .035 oz = .002 lb = .001 kg
1 kg = 2.2 lb = 1000 g

To convert ounces to grams, multiply grams by 28.35.

Temperatures

Fahrenheit	Celsius
32° water freezes	0°
195° water simmers	90.6°
212° water boils	100°
300°	149°
350°	177°

To convert degrees from Celsius to Fahrenheit or vice versa, use the following formula:

$$C = \frac{(F - 32) \times 5}{9}$$

$$F = \left(\frac{C \times 9}{5}\right) + 32$$

The rule of thumb for converting oven temperatures to degrees Celsius is to halve the Fahrenheit temperature. For example, 400°F becomes 200°C.

Cooking the Nutritious Way

The following collection of recipes, selected and adapted from more than 45 cookbooks, was compiled with the Dietary Guidelines in mind (see pages 96-97). These guidelines, set forth by the U.S. Departments of Agriculture and Health and Human Services, recommend that Americans modify their diets by eating a greater variety of foods and by cutting back on sugar, salt, and fat. The guide to meal planning on pages 278-279 offers suggestions for including these nutritious recipes in your daily food choices.

To encourage you to eat more complex carbohydrates and less refined or processed foods, many of the recipes call for fresh fruits and vegetables, including the often-neglected but nutritious dried legumes and grains. By consuming larger portions of these carbohydrates and smaller portions of meat, you will be eating a healthier diet, and probably saving money as well.

Of course, meat, poultry, and seafood play an important role in the diet, too, and there are more than 40 dishes that include these foods as one of the main ingredients.

In the recipes that require rice or flour, brown rice and whole-wheat flour have been suggested because in some ways they are slightly superior in nutritive value to white rice and white flour.

Consistent with the Dietary Guidelines, the recipes suggest modest amounts of salt. For those especially concerned about their sodium intake, salt may be omitted altogether; instead, herbs and spices can be added to enhance the taste (see chart on pages 178-179). Also, in most recipes margarine can be substituted for butter, and vegetable oil can be used in place of olive oil.

Some of the recipes call for wine and other spirits. In most types of cooking, particularly if the dish is simmered for a long time, much of the alcohol evaporates in the process. Or if desired, you can eliminate the wine and substitute other liquids such as water or broth.

The note at the end of a recipe provides helpful hints on what to serve with the dish and ways to vary the recipe by changing one or more of the ingredients or by using an alternate cooking method.

The serving sizes in the recipes are designed to maintain ideal body weight in healthy persons. Very active people might require larger portions, whereas sedentary people may need smaller amounts.

Appetizers

CHILI BEAN DIP

2 cups cooked dried red kidney beans or 16-ounce can, drained
1 tablespoon red wine vinegar
¾ teaspoon chili powder
⅛ teaspoon ground cumin
2 teaspoons minced onion
2 teaspoons minced fresh parsley
2-3 cups raw vegetable sticks such as carrots, white turnips, or green beans

MAKES ONE AND ONE-THIRD CUPS

1. Place beans, vinegar, chili powder, and cumin in blender. Blend until smooth.
2. Remove mixture from blender. Stir in onion and parsley.
3. Serve with raw vegetables.

If you prefer a dip that is more moist, reserve a bit of the liquid from the beans and add to mixture.

BROILED TOMATO HALVES

4 ripe but firm tomatoes, 2½-3 inches in diameter
Freshly ground black pepper to taste
3 tablespoons grated Parmesan cheese
3 tablespoons fresh breadcrumbs
2 tablespoons butter, cut into 8 pats, ⅛ inch thick

MAKES FOUR SERVINGS

1. Remove the grid from your broiling pan and set the pan in the broiler about 5 inches from the source of heat. Then turn on the broiler at its highest setting to heat for 15 minutes.
2. Cut the tomatoes in half crosswise. Then arrange them on the cold grid, cut sides up, and sprinkle them with a few grindings of black pepper. Combine the cheese and breadcrumbs in a small bowl and pat the mixture evenly over the tomatoes. Place a pat of butter on each tomato half.
3. Set the grid in the preheated broiling pan. The tomatoes should be about 3 inches from the source of heat.
4. Broil the tomatoes for 6 to 8 minutes, watching

carefully for any sign of burning; lower the heat or move the broiling pan farther from the heat if needed.

5. When the topping is golden brown, test the tomatoes for doneness by pressing their sides gently. They should yield only slightly; if broiled beyond that point, they may fall apart. Quickly lift the tomatoes from the grid with a large spatula and serve them on a warm platter.

Tomatoes can be broiled ahead of time and served at room temperature.

CARROT, CELERY, AND EGG SALAD

½ pound carrots
¾ pound celery
2 hard-boiled eggs
¼ cup mayonnaise
3 tablespoons lemon juice
½ teaspoon salt
Freshly ground black pepper to taste
Boston lettuce leaves or spinach,
 washed (optional)

MAKES FOUR SERVINGS

1. Grate carrots on the large holes of a hand grater or in a food processor. Place in a bowl. Grate celery and, with your hands, squeeze out as much liquid as possible. Add celery to carrots.

2. Dice eggs into small pieces and add to carrots and celery. Blend lemon juice into mayonnaise and add to salad. Season with salt and pepper and mix ingredients together. Refrigerate until ready to use.

3. Serve this on Boston lettuce or spinach, if desired.

Be sure to squeeze out all the liquid from the celery or you will dilute the dressing. Serve this as a first course, or as a side dish.

PEANUTS-GO-LIGHTLY DIP

Mix together 2 cups unsalted, roasted peanuts, finely chopped, ½ cup plain yogurt, and ¼ teaspoon finely grated lemon rind. Season lightly with salt. Serve with raw vegetables.
             MAKES TWO AND ONE-HALF CUPS

EGGPLANT SALAD

2 young, firm eggplants, about 2 pounds
1 tablespoon peanut or vegetable oil
2 tablespoons cider vinegar
 or white wine vinegar
2 teaspoons brown sugar (optional)
2 small cloves garlic, minced
2 tablespoons minced onion
2 teaspoons grated fresh ginger or
 ½ teaspoon powdered ginger
2 teaspoons fresh lemon juice
¼ teaspoon salt

MAKES FOUR SERVINGS

1. Preheat oven to 400 degrees. Prick the eggplants in several places with a fork and roast them, on a baking sheet, for 1 hour or until they are quite soft.

2. When the eggplants are cool enough to handle, cut them in half and scrape the pulp carefully from the skin. If the seeds are dark brown and starting to separate from the eggplant, they will be bitter and must be removed. If the seeds are pale and small, leave them.

3. Drain the eggplant pulp thoroughly in a large sieve and mince the eggplant. Combine the minced eggplant in a bowl with all the remaining ingredients. Mix well, cover, and chill for several hours.

4. Serve small portions of the chilled eggplant on lettuce leaves as a first course, or with unsalted crackers as a dip.

This salad is a good accompaniment to cold roasts such as pork or chicken.

MARINATED LEEKS

8-10 slender leeks, about ¾ pound
⅓ cup olive oil
½ cup white wine vinegar
½ cup white wine
2 small inner stalks celery
2 bay leaves
10-12 black peppercorns
10-12 whole coriander seeds
½ teaspoon salt
3 sprigs fresh parsley

MAKES FOUR TO SIX SERVINGS

1. Cut off the roots and remove any withered leaves from the leeks. Trim off all the dark-green parts of

Cooking the Nutritious Way
Appetizers

leeks. If the white parts are very long, cut them in 3-inch lengths. Carefully spread the sections apart and wash them very well to remove all grit.

2. Arrange the leeks in a shallow enameled fireproof casserole. Pour the olive oil, wine vinegar, and wine over them. Add enough water to cover the leeks.

3. Cut the celery stalks in 3-inch lengths, then slice them lengthwise into strips the size of green beans. Add them to the leeks, along with all the remaining ingredients. Simmer, covered, over medium heat for about 20 minutes; then cool, cover, and chill overnight.

If your market has only large, plump leeks, cut the leeks into quarters lengthwise. If you cannot find leeks at all, substitute whole scallions, but simmer only for 10 to 15 minutes. This dish could also be served as a summer salad, garnished with fresh, quartered tomatoes. Reminder: You may want to substitute vegetable oil for olive oil.

Marinated Chick-Peas

3 cups cooked dried chick-peas
　or 20-ounce can, drained
½ cup vegetable oil
3 tablespoons vinegar or
　juice of 1 lemon
½ cup chopped fresh parsley
¼ cup chopped scallions
2 cloves garlic, minced
¼ teaspooon freshly ground black pepper

MAKES FOUR TO SIX SERVINGS

1. Combine all ingredients and allow to marinate in the refrigerator for at least 2 hours. Drain.

2. Serve with toast rounds, or as part of an antipasto

Melon and Ginger

Cut a cantaloupe or honeydew melon into 4 wedges and loosen flesh with a grapefruit knife. Combine 2 teaspoons of sugar with ½ teaspoon powdered ginger and sprinkle on melon. Garnish with fresh mint leaves if available.

MAKES FOUR SERVINGS

French Cauliflower Pie

1 medium cauliflower, about 1½ pounds
2 cups milk
½ cup grated Swiss cheese
⅛ teaspoon nutmeg
½ teaspoon dried tarragon
½ teaspoon salt
¼ teaspoon freshly ground black pepper
4 large eggs, lightly beaten
1 teaspoon butter

MAKES EIGHT SERVINGS

1. Steam the cauliflower for about 5 minutes, or until it is still rather firm. Let cool for 10 minutes. Remove the core and chop the rest coarsely.

2. Preheat oven to 375 degrees. Stir the cauliflower and all other ingredients, except the butter, into the eggs. Grease a 2-quart mold or deep pan, such as a soufflé dish, with the butter, and pour the cauliflower mixture into it.

3. Bake for about 45 minutes to 1 hour, or until the center seems firm when shaken and the top is beginning to turn golden.

Using the same method, you can substitute other vegetables such as broccoli, cabbage, or potatoes in place of the cauliflower. Reminder: You may want to substitute margarine for butter.

Ricotta Cheese Souffles

1 tablespoon butter
⅓ cup ricotta cheese
1 teaspoon prepared mustard
1 teaspoon oregano
Pinch of cayenne pepper
¾ cup Parmesan cheese, grated
3 tablespoons milk
3 eggs, separated
Pinch of salt

MAKES SIX SERVINGS

1. Preheat oven to 400 degrees.

2. Butter six custard-cup molds or ramekins, each one about ½ cup capacity. Set aside.

3. In a bowl mix until well blended the ricotta cheese, mustard, oregano, cayenne pepper, Parmesan cheese, milk, and the three egg yolks.

4. In a clean bowl, and with clean beaters, whip the egg whites with the salt until stiff. Do not overbeat or your soufflés will be dry. Fold the egg whites into the cheese batter. Work quickly so that you do not deflate the egg whites. Divide the batter among the molds. Place them in a baking pan filled with enough hot water to come three-quarters of the way up the sides of the molds. Bake for 15 minutes. The centers should be soft.

5. Serve from the molds.

These soufflés will rise only slightly, not like the average soufflé. Reminder: You may want to substitute margarine for butter.

POLENTA CHEESE SQUARES

3 teaspoons vegetable oil
5 cups cold water
½ teaspoon salt
1½ cups white or yellow cornmeal, preferably stone-ground
1 cup sharp Cheddar cheese, grated
⅓ cup Parmesan cheese, grated

MAKES EIGHT SERVINGS

1. With 2 teaspoons oil, lightly grease a 9 by 9 by 2-inch baking pan and set aside. In a large, heavy saucepan, bring cold water and salt to a boil. Add cornmeal very slowly, stirring constantly with a wire whisk or long wooden spoon until mixture is thick and free from lumps. This should take about 7 minutes.

2. Transfer cornmeal mixture to top of double boiler. Place over boiling water and cook, covered, for 30 minutes, stirring occasionally. Cornmeal is finished when it leaves sides of pan.

3. Remove from heat and turn cornmeal into the prepared baking pan. Cool, refrigerate until stiff enough to cut (3 to 4 hours or overnight).

4. Preheat oven to 400 degrees. With 1 teaspoon of the remaining oil, grease a baking dish. Cut polenta into 16 squares. Arrange in the baking dish. Sprinkle with Cheddar and Parmesan cheese.

5. Place in preheated oven, and bake for 15 minutes or until cheese is melted and nicely browned. Serve immediately.

This dish is delicious with a homemade marinara sauce (see recipe on page 261—Pasta Marinara). For a light meal, serve with a fresh vegetable salad.

Soups

PARSLEY SOUP

1 cup coarsely chopped parsley (including tender stems), tightly packed
1½ cups water or chicken broth, preferably homemade (recipe on page 226)
1 tablespoon butter
1 tablespoon unbleached white or whole-wheat flour
1 cup milk
½ teaspoon salt
White pepper to taste

MAKES TWO TO FOUR SERVINGS

1. Bring parsley and chicken broth or water to boil in a 2-quart pot. Lower the heat and simmer, covered, for 7 minutes.

2. Pour the mixture into an electric blender and whirl briefly. Add remaining ingredients and blend again. Return to pan. Simmer for 5 minutes.

Parsley, most often used as a garnish, can also be eaten as a vegetable. It is rich in vitamins A and C.

TOMATO BOUILLON

½ bay leaf
2 whole cloves
¼ teaspoon dill seed
¼ teaspoon dried basil or 1 tablespoon chopped fresh basil
¼ teaspoon dried marjoram
¼ teaspoon dried oregano
Freshly ground black pepper to taste
4 cups tomato juice
4 tablespoons chopped fresh parsley

MAKES FOUR TO SIX SERVINGS

1. Place all herbs except parsley in the tomato juice and let stand for 1 hour to allow flavors to blend.

2. Heat tomato and herb mixture to boiling point. Remove from heat and strain. Pour into serving bowls. Garnish with parsley.

To serve cold, add 1½ cups finely diced vegetables such as green peppers, cucumbers, carrots, and scallions with tops. You could use the bouillon as broth for soups and stews.

Cooking the Nutritious Way
Soups

CREAM OF VEGETABLE SOUP

6-8 cups shredded Romaine lettuce, about 1 large head
3 bunches watercress, with stems
2 bunches scallions, green and white parts, sliced
2 cups diced potatoes, scrubbed and unpeeled
6 cups hot chicken broth, preferably homemade (recipe on page 226)
½ teaspoon salt
Freshly ground black pepper to taste
1-2 tablespoons butter or margarine
½ cup thinly sliced cucumbers or zucchini (optional)

MAKES FOUR TO SIX SERVINGS

1. Combine Romaine, watercress, scallions, potatoes, and broth in a large 3-quart saucepan. Bring to the boiling point, reduce heat and simmer, covered, for 10 to 15 minutes or until potatoes are tender.
2. Puree soup in a blender or strain through a food mill. Season with salt and pepper. Stir in the butter. Sprinkle cucumber or zucchini slices on top.

If watercress is unavailable, use equal amount of parsley. Instead of Romaine, try spinach or some other dark, leafy green such as turnip greens or kale, and simmer the soup for 5 minutes longer.

BUTTERMILK GAZPACHO

2 hard-cooked eggs, peeled and halved
1 12-ounce can vegetable or tomato juice
1-1½ cups buttermilk
½ cup chopped Spanish or Bermuda onion
½ cup diced celery
½ cup diced sweet green pepper
1 tablespoon minced fresh dill or ¼ teaspoon dill weed
Freshly ground black pepper to taste
1 lime or lemon, sliced thin

MAKES FOUR SERVINGS

1. Sieve the egg yolks and place in a mixing bowl. Add the vegetable juice, buttermilk, onion, celery, green pepper, and seasonings and stir to mix.
2. Mince the egg whites, then wrap and refrigerate until ready to use. Also refrigerate the gazpacho for several hours to blend the flavors.
3. To serve, spoon a little minced egg white into the bottom of four soup cups, pour in the gazpacho, and garnish with lime or lemon slices.

FIVE-MINUTE SOUP

4 cups chicken broth, preferably homemade (recipe on page 226)
Half a raw cucumber, peeled and sliced very thin
4 raw mushrooms, sliced
2 cups shredded raw green-leaf vegetable such as spinach, lettuce, or cabbage
1 tomato cut into ½-inch dice
½ cup leftover lean meat or poultry, shredded (optional)
Freshly ground black pepper to taste

MAKES SIX SERVINGS

1. Heat the chicken broth. Add the vegetables and meat. Bring to a boil and simmer for 5 minutes. Season with pepper.

VEGETABLE CHOWDER

2 tablespoons chopped onion
¼ cup chopped celery
2 tablespoons chopped green pepper
1 tablespoon butter or margarine
½ cup diced potatoes, scrubbed, unpeeled
1 cup water or stock (beef or chicken)
⅛ teaspoon dried marjoram
¼ teaspoon salt
¼ teaspoon freshly ground black pepper
1 cup corn kernels, fresh or frozen
½ cup green beans cut into 1-inch pieces
2 tablespoons flour, preferably whole wheat
1½ cups milk

MAKES FOUR SERVINGS

1. Cook onion, celery, and green pepper in butter or margarine for 5 minutes or until almost tender.
2. Add potatoes, water or stock, and seasonings.

Cover and simmer until potatoes are tender, about 20 minutes.

3. Add corn and beans. Cover and simmer for 10 minutes longer or until beans are tender.

4. Mix flour with a small amount of milk; add to remaining milk. Stir milk mixture into cooked vegetable mixture. Cook, stirring constantly until slightly thickened.

MINESTRONE

4-5 cloves garlic, minced
1 cup chopped onion
3 tablespoons olive or vegetable oil
1 teaspoon salt
1 cup chopped carrots
1 cup chopped celery
1 cup chopped eggplant or zucchini
1 teaspoon oregano
¼ teaspoon freshly ground black pepper
1 teaspoon dried basil or
    1 tablespoon fresh basil
1 cup chopped green pepper
3½ cups water or beef stock
2 cups tomato puree
1½ cups cooked dried split peas or
    cooked chick-peas
3 tablespoons dry red wine
1 cup fresh chopped tomatoes
½ cup dry pasta
½ cup fresh chopped parsley
½ cup grated Parmesan cheese

MAKES SIX TO EIGHT SERVINGS

1. In a 4-quart soup kettle, sauté garlic and onion in olive or vegetable oil until soft and translucent.

2. Add ½ teaspoon salt, carrots, celery, and eggplant. (If you use zucchini, add it with the green pepper.) Add oregano, pepper, and basil. Cover and cook over low heat for 5 to 8 minutes.

3. Add green pepper, water or stock, tomato puree, cooked peas, and wine. Cover and simmer for 15 minutes.

4. Add tomatoes and remaining salt. Keep at lowest heat until 10 minutes before you plan to serve.

5. Then heat the soup to a boil, add pasta and boil gently until pasta is tender, for about 10 minutes. Serve immediately, topped with parsley and freshly grated Parmesan cheese.

S'CHEE
(Russian Cabbage Soup)

3 pounds boneless chuck
3 pounds beef marrow bones, cracked
1 large onion, peeled
2 carrots, scrubbed
1 parsnip, scrubbed
1 white or yellow turnip, scrubbed
8 cups boiling water
1 20-ounce can tomatoes, drained
1½ tablespoons tomato paste
Bouquet garni: 5 sprigs parsley; 2 leeks,
    washed; 2 celery tops; 2 bay leaves;
    5 sprigs fresh dill; all tied together
    in cotton cheesecloth
1 tablespoon salt
4 tablespoons vegetable oil
1 cup finely chopped onion
½ cup finely chopped celery
½ cup finely chopped carrots
1 teaspoon minced garlic
1 pound sauerkraut, fresh or canned,
    well washed to remove brine
7 cups shredded cabbage, about 2 pounds
4 tablespoons sugar (optional)
3 tablespoons lemon juice
2 cups yogurt
¼ cup finely chopped fresh dill

MAKES EIGHT TO TEN SERVINGS

1. Preheat oven to 500 degrees. In a large, shallow roasting pan arrange, in one layer if possible, the meat, bones, onion, carrots, parsnip, and turnip. Roast for 20 minutes, turning meat and vegetables from time to time so that their surfaces brown evenly. Then transfer meat, bones, and vegetables to a large soup kettle. Discard the fat left in the roasting pan.

2. Into the roasting pan pour the 8 cups of boiling water. With a large spoon scrape up and mix into the water all the brown particles clinging to the bottom and sides of the pan. Empty the mixture into the soup kettle. If the meat and vegetables are not quite covered, add a little more water.

3. Start the soup cooking over moderate heat, and remove the foam and scum that will persistently rise to the surface for quite a while. When the stock reaches the boil, turn the heat down to the barest simmer. Skim once more, then add the tomatoes, tomato paste, bouquet garni, and salt. Partially cover the pot and simmer slowly for about 2 hours, skimming whenever necessary.

4. In the meantime, in a large, heavy frying pan,

Cooking the Nutritious Way
Soups

heat vegetable oil. Add the chopped onion, celery, carrots, and garlic and sauté them for about 15 minutes. Squeeze the washed sauerkraut dry, chop it coarsely, and add it to the pan. Cook for 2 minutes, lower the heat and mix in the shredded cabbage. Cook, over moderate heat, until cabbage begins to wilt. Half cover the pan, add a spoonful of stock from the soup kettle every 8 minutes or so to moisten the vegetables, and let them slowly braise for 30 minutes. Remove the pan from the heat and put it aside, half covered.

5. When the soup in the kettle has cooked for about 2 hours, discard all the vegetables and bouquet garni. In their place add the braised cabbage and vegetables. Stir in the sugar, if used, and lemon juice; bring the soup to a boil, then reduce and simmer gently for another 1½ hours.

6. Turn heat off, remove bones and dislodge their marrow, which you add to the soup. Let the soup rest and skim off all fat from top. Serve with a dollop of yogurt and garnish with dill.

You can make this soup a few days in advance.

BLACK-EYED PEA SOUP

2 cups dried black-eyed peas
1 small ham hock (optional)
4 cups boiling water
1 bay leaf
2 ribs celery, coarsely chopped
1 onion, studded with 2 whole cloves
½ teaspoon salt
4 whole black peppercorns
4-6 thin slices lemon
Paprika
1 tablespoon minced parsley

MAKES FOUR TO SIX SERVINGS

1. Place the black-eyed peas in a 2-quart kettle.
2. Add the ham hock, if used, boiling water, bay leaf, celery, onion, salt, and peppercorns and bring to a boil. Cook until peas are tender, 2 to 2½ hours. As the soup cooks, skim the surface as necessary.
3. Remove the ham hock, if used, and bay leaf and puree the soup either through a sieve or in an electric blender. Spoon into hot soup plates and top each with a slice of lemon. Dot the center of each lemon slice with a little paprika and parsley.

Omit salt if using ham hock. Instead of celery, try 2 thinly sliced carrots.

SPRING PEA SOUP

1 tablespoon butter
1 cup diced potatoes
3 cups chicken broth, preferably homemade (recipe on page 226), or water
1 cup freshly shelled green peas or frozen and thawed peas
1 tablespoon chopped chives or scallions
Freshly ground black pepper to taste

MAKES SIX SERVINGS

1. Melt the butter in a 2-quart soup pot and swirl the potatoes around in it. Add the chicken broth or water and simmer until the potatoes are soft, about 20 minutes.
2. Purée in a blender and return soup to the pot. Bring to a boil and put in the fresh green peas. Cook them until just tender—test by eating one—and stir in the chives or scallions before serving. Season with pepper.

YANKEE BEAN CHOWDER

1 cup dried pea beans or navy beans
1 medium onion, finely chopped
1 cup diced carrots
1 green pepper, diced
1½ cups canned tomatoes
½ teaspoon salt
½ teaspoon freshly ground black pepper
1 cup diced potatoes, unpeeled
2 cups milk

MAKES SIX SERVINGS

1. Pick over and wash the beans. Cover with cold water and bring to a boil. Simmer for 2 minutes. Remove from heat, cover, and let beans soak for 1 hour.
2. Drain the beans and place in a kettle with 1½ quarts fresh cold water.
3. Add the onion and bring to a boil. Cover and simmer until beans are barely tender, about 30 minutes. Add the carrots, green pepper, tomatoes, salt, and black pepper and cook for 10 minutes. If desired, soup can be put through an electric blender or food mill at this point.
4. Add the potatoes and milk and cook for 15 minutes longer, or until the potatoes are tender. Check seasoning.

Black Bean Soup

2 cups dried black beans
6 cups vegetable broth (recipe on
   page 227) or water
2 tablespoons safflower or other oil
1 onion, chopped
4 cloves garlic, minced
1 stalk celery, with leaves, chopped
½ teaspoon salt
Freshly ground black pepper to taste
Juice of 1½ lemons
1 teaspoon celery seed
3 to 4 tablespoons dry sherry (optional)
Paper-thin lemon slices
1 hard-boiled egg, chopped, optional

MAKES SIX TO EIGHT SERVINGS

1. Wash the beans and soak in the broth or water overnight or for several hours.
2. In a large, heavy-bottomed stock pot or Dutch oven, heat the oil and sauté the onion, garlic, and celery until tender. Add the beans and their liquid and bring to a boil. Add the salt, reduce the heat, cover, and simmer for two hours, or until the beans are tender.
3. Remove half the beans from the pot and puree in a blender, with soup liquid to cover, adding the pepper and celery seeds.
4. Return the puree to the pot and reheat, stirring, until it thickens slightly. Stir in the lemon juice and sherry, if desired.
5. Serve garnished with lemon slices and, if desired, chopped, hard-boiled egg.

Haddock Chowder, Passamaquoddy Bay

2-pound piece of haddock
2 cups, about ¾ pound, raw potatoes,
   cut into 1-inch cubes
¼ cup minced salt pork or 3 tablespoons
   vegetable oil
1 medium onion, sliced
2 cups milk
1 tablespoon butter
1 teaspoon salt
Freshly ground black pepper to taste

MAKES SIX TO EIGHT SERVINGS

1. Bring to the boil in a 4-quart heavy saucepan about 4 cups or enough water to cover the fish. Then put the fish in and simmer for 15 minutes or until cooked through. Remove the fish from the pot. Remove the skin and bones, and flake the flesh. Strain and reserve 3 cups of broth.
2. To this broth add the potatoes and cook them until they are tender but not soft. Meanwhile, crisp the salt pork, if used, in a skillet and then brown the onion in the hot fat or vegetable oil for about 10 minutes.
3. Now add to the fish broth and potatoes, the contents of the skillet, the flaked fish, and the remaining ingredients. Heat almost to the boiling point before serving. Season with pepper.

To make the salt pork less salty, simmer in boiling water for a few minutes. You can substitute 3 strips of lean bacon for the salt pork.

French Fish Soup

1 fish head from a snapper, bass, or flounder
1 flounder carcass, chopped
1 teaspoon salt
Freshly ground black pepper to taste
1 tablespoon flour
2 medium boiling potatoes
2 medium onions
7 teaspoons olive oil
2 fresh tomatoes, quartered, or
   ⅔ cup drained canned tomatoes
1 teaspoon thyme
3 2-inch pieces orange rind
1 bay leaf
1½ quarts water or 5 cups water mixed
   with 1 cup dry white wine
3 slices white or whole-wheat bread
½ teaspoon saffron or 1 teaspoon
   sweet paprika
1 garlic clove, crushed
½ cup grated Parmesan or Swiss cheese
½ cup very thin vermicelli (optional)

MAKES EIGHT SERVINGS

1. Rinse and dry the fish head and bones. Sprinkle them with salt, pepper, and flour and set aside. Dice the potatoes into 1-inch pieces. Peel and grate the onions or mince them finely.
2. In a heavy 4-quart pan, heat 6 teaspoons olive oil and add the onions. Sauté gently for 3 minutes, add the fish head and bones and sauté for another 3 minutes. Add the potatoes, tomatoes, thyme, orange rind,

Cooking the Nutritious Way
Soups

bay leaf, and cook for 5 minutes. Add the water or water and wine and bring to a boil. Simmer for 30 minutes. While soup is simmering, cut the bread into triangles and dry them out for 30 minutes in a 350-degree oven.

3. Crush the saffron between your fingers over the soup or add the paprika. Cook the soup for another 2 minutes. Remove bay leaf.

4. Place a food mill over a pan and pour 2 ladlefuls at a time of the soup mixture into it. Add broth whenever necessary to help grind fish. Discard the residue left in the food mill.

5. Reheat the soup over medium heat. Add the garlic, the remaining teaspoon of olive oil, salt, and pepper to taste.

6. If you want a more substantial soup, add the vermicelli 10 minutes before serving. Serve the soup over the bread triangles; sprinkle with cheese.

Fish heads and carcasses can be obtained, usually free of charge, from a fish market.

CHICKEN BROTH

3-4 pounds chicken parts, such as wings, backs, and gizzards
2 cups chopped celery, stalks and leaves
1 medium onion, chopped
1 large carrot, chopped
½ cup fresh parsley leaves
1 or 2 teaspoons salt
6 whole black peppercorns
7 cups boiling water

MAKES SIX TO EIGHT SERVINGS

1. Remove all visible fat from the chicken parts, but leave the skins. Place chicken in a large kettle. Add all the remaining ingredients. Bring to the boiling point. Lower heat to very low and skim. Cover the kettle and simmer over low heat for 2 hours, skim the soup as needed.

2. Strain the soup through a sieve into a bowl. Let soup come to room temperature, then place in refrigerator to settle the fat by chilling. When the fat is solid, remove it and throw it away. (Or remove the fat from the hot broth by first spooning off as much as possible.) Scrape all the vegetables off the chicken pieces and remove and discard all skin, bones, and remaining fat. Use the meat for other dishes.

It is tastier and cheaper to use fresh vegetables for your chicken broth than packaged soup greens.

CHICKEN IN A POT

4-5 pound stewing fowl, trussed
2-3 quarts water or chicken broth, preferably homemade (recipe on page 226)
2 pounds leeks, washed: green parts in the bouquet garni (see below); white parts tied in a bundle
1 pound carrots, cut into 2 to 3-inch lengths
½ pound white turnips, washed and halved
Bouquet garni: 1 stalk celery; leek greens; 1 teaspoon thyme; 1 bay leaf; 8 parsley sprigs; wrap in cotton cheesecloth and tie with string
1 head garlic, superficial husk removed, left whole
1 teaspoon salt
1 small green cabbage, about 1½ pounds
1 pound small new potatoes, unpeeled, washed
Accompaniment: dried slices of French or Italian bread, freshly grated Parmesan cheese, Dijon mustard, fresh horseradish

MAKES SIX TO EIGHT SERVINGS

1. Remove as much fat from chicken as possible. Place chicken in a 6 to 8-quart heavy pot. Pour over stock and water to cover; bring slowly to a boil and skim as necessary. Add the leeks, carrots, turnips, the bouquet garni, the head of garlic, salt, and maintain the liquid at the barest simmer, lid slightly off, until the chicken is cooked and tender, 1½ to 3 hours. Skim off the fat.

2. While the chicken is cooking, remove the outer leaves from the cabbage, quarter it, and arrange the quarters in a large saucepan. Pour over boiling water to cover and parboil for 10 minutes. Drain, keeping the quarters intact and pressing them gently to rid them of the maximum amount of liquid. Return them to the saucepan and ladle over enough bouillon from the surface of the chicken pot to barely cover them. Simmer, covered, for about 45 minutes.

3. Half an hour before serving the dish, cook the potatoes in their skins.

4. Serve first a tureen of the bouillon, with slices of bread on the bottom of each soup plate. Sprinkle bread with cheese if you wish. Discard garlic and the bouquet garni; clip and remove strings from chicken and leeks. Serve the chicken and the vegetables on separate plates. Keep the bouillon at the table, pouring a ladleful over each serving of meat and vegetables. You may serve mustard and fresh horseradish on the side.

This chicken recipe is two dishes in one—the soup course and the main course with vegetables.

GOULASH SOUP

2 pounds beef chuck, trimmed of all fat,
  and cut into ½-inch cubes
½ teaspoon caraway seeds
2 tablespoons sweet paprika
1 teaspoon minced garlic
1½ cups chopped onion
2 quarts cold water or chicken broth,
  preferably homemade (recipe on page 226)
2 teaspoons salt (only if water is used)
½ pound potatoes, cut into 1-inch cubes
1 large green bell pepper, diced
4 carrots, thinly sliced
1 1-pound can tomatoes, drained
Freshly ground black pepper to taste

MAKES SIX TO EIGHT SERVINGS

1. Preheat oven to 400 degrees. Place the meat cubes in a 3 to 4-quart casserole that has a tight-fitting cover.
2. Sprinkle the caraway seeds over the meat; add the paprika, garlic, and onions. Pour the water or broth over the ingredients. If you use water, add the salt.
3. Place the casserole, uncovered, over high heat and bring to a boil. Remove the foam with a slotted spoon. Cover the casserole and transfer it to the lower middle shelf of the oven. Bake the soup for 1 hour.
4. Add the potato cubes and continue to bake the soup for 30 minutes. Add the diced pepper, the carrots and tomatoes, and bake the soup 30 minutes longer. Add freshly ground pepper to taste. Serve very hot.

VEGETABLE BROTHS

An easy way to make vegetable broths is to save the water from steamed vegetables. Use the cooking liquids instead of chicken or beef broth. You can also save the liquids from cooked beans and other dried legumes. These add body to your soups and stews. Freeze broths as soon as the liquid cools; they will keep 6 to 8 months in the freezer.

Fish and Shellfish

TROUT COOKED ON A PLATE

4 brook trout, about 2 pounds, cleaned,
  gutted, heads off, boned (fillets)
Juice of ½ lemon
¼ cup dry white wine
2 teaspoons olive oil
½ teaspoon salt
Freshly ground black pepper to taste
4 sprigs parsley, coarsely chopped

MAKES FOUR SERVINGS

1. In a small bowl, combine lemon juice, wine, olive oil, and salt and pepper.
2. Oil a large fireproof plate and on it place the trout, with their skins on. Pour the lemon juice mixture over the trout and sprinkle the parsley on top. Wrap the plate completely in aluminum foil.
3. Put a large quantity of water in a large pot and set it on the heat. When the water reaches the boiling point, lower the flame to a simmer and place the plate on top of the pot. Let the fish steam for 16 to 18 minutes.
4. Remove the plate from the pot, carefully unwrap the foil, and serve immediately.

Plate should fit over the pot like a lid. Reminder: You may want to use vegetable oil instead of olive oil. Try this method of steaming with other fish fillets.

SCANDINAVIAN DRY-BAKED FLOUNDER

4-pound whole flounder or sole, cleaned
  and gutted
½ cup grated fresh horseradish (optional)
½ cup chopped fresh parsley or dill
Coarse salt
Melted butter
Lemon wedges
Freshly ground black pepper to taste

MAKES FOUR TO SIX SERVINGS

1. Preheat oven to 200 degrees. Wash and dry the fish and place it in a baking dish without adding any butter, salt, or water. Bake, uncovered, for 1 hour.
2. Carefully transfer the fish to a heated serving

Cooking the Nutritious Way
Fish and Shellfish

platter. Discard the liquid that will have accumulated in the baking pan.

3. Remove the skin. Serve the fish with small dishes filled with the horseradish, if available, parsley or dill, coarse salt, melted butter, lemon wedges, and freshly ground black pepper.

Reminder: You may want to substitute margarine for butter.

WHOLE FISH BAKED ON A BED OF AROMATIC VEGETABLES

1 small celery root, peeled and diced, or 2 stalks celery, diced
6 small carrots, sliced
2 small onions, thinly sliced
2 to 2½-pound whole fish such as flounder, grey sole, red snapper, cod, sea bass, or whiting, cleaned, with head and tail left on
½ teaspoon salt
Freshly ground black pepper to taste
½ cup dry white wine
2 tablespoons chopped fresh basil or parsley
2-3 tablespoons butter (optional)

MAKES FOUR SERVINGS

1. Preheat oven to 350 degrees. Choose an oval casserole, with a tight-fitting lid, large enough to hold the fish without bending it.

2. Separately, steam celery, carrots, and onions for 5 minutes each. Cover the bottom of the casserole with these steamed vegetables.

3. Wash the fish under cold running water, then dry it and lightly sprinkle its inside with salt and pepper. Lay the fish on the bed of vegetables and pour over it ⅓ cup of the wine. Cover the casserole and set in the oven for 40 minutes.

4. Check the fish for doneness. When perfectly cooked, the flesh at the center should be firm, flaky, and opaque. If it is done, baste the fish with the juices from the bottom of the casserole. If not quite done, bake a few more minutes.

5. Transfer the fish to a hot serving platter and keep warm while you prepare the sauce. Puree the vegetables in a hand food-mill, a blender, or a food processor. Transfer puree to a saucepan. Taste and adjust seasonings. Add part or all of the remaining wine if the sauce is too thick. Bring to a simmer. Stir in chopped basil or parsley. You may stir in the butter to enrich the sauce. Pour the sauce into a sauceboat and serve.

BOMBAY-STYLE SOLE

1½ pounds fillet of sole, flounder, or any other flatfish, skinned
1 cup yogurt
1 teaspoon paprika
1 teaspoon ground cumin
1 teaspoon ground coriander
½ teaspoon salt
Freshly ground black pepper to taste

MAKES FOUR SERVINGS

1. Put the fish in a rectangular oven-proof glass or earthenware dish.

2. In a blender, combine the yogurt, paprika, cumin, and coriander; blend until well mixed. Pour over the fish, cover with plastic wrap, and let marinate for a couple of hours in the refrigerator, turning fish occasionally.

3. Preheat the broiler and broil the fish for 4 minutes; turn and broil on the second side for 4 minutes more. Season with salt and pepper. Serve immediately with more yogurt if desired.

You can also bake the fish instead of broiling it. Preheat oven to 350 degrees and bake the fish in a lightly greased pan for 10 to 15 minutes.

WRAPPED FISH

4 boneless 6-ounce cod, bass, or halibut fillets
1 tablespoon melted butter
4 parboiled rings of green pepper
4 paper-thin slices of onion
4 slices of tomato
¼ cup lemon juice
1 teaspoon dried oregano
½ teaspoon salt
Freshly ground pepper to taste
4 small bay leaves
Water

MAKES FOUR SERVINGS

1. Preheat oven to 400 degrees. Put each fish fillet on a piece of oiled aluminum foil large enough to enclose it. Brush with butter and top with green pepper, onion, and tomato. Sprinkle with lemon juice and oregano. Season with salt and pepper. Place a bay leaf on top of each fillet. The bay leaf is mainly for effect. Fold the foil over the top of the filling and crimp the edges together securely.

2. Put the fillets in a baking dish just large enough to hold them. Pour in ¼ inch of water and bake for 15 to 20 minutes. Check the fish after 15 minutes and bake a few minutes more if necessary.

3. Serve the fish in its wrappings.

Tomato Crown Haddock

1½ cups water
2 tablespoons lemon juice
1½ pounds haddock, halibut, or cod fillets
½ teaspoon salt
⅛ teaspoon pepper
2 large fresh tomatoes, sliced ¼ inch thick
½ medium green pepper, finely chopped
2 tablespoons finely chopped onion
¼ cup dry breadcrumbs
½ teaspoon dried basil
1 tablespoon vegetable oil

MAKES SIX SERVINGS

1. Combine water and lemon juice. Pour over fish fillets and let stand for 30 minutes. Drain fillets. Place fish in an oiled baking dish. Season with salt and pepper. Preheat oven to 350 degrees.

2. Place tomato slices on fish and sprinkle with green pepper and onion.

3. Combine breadcrumbs, basil, and oil, blending well. Spread seasoned crumb mixture evenly over tomatoes. Bake, uncovered, for 15 to 20 minutes, or until fish is firm and flakes easily

---

Bluefish with Citrus Juices

3-3½ pounds bluefish, cleaned, with
  head and tail left on
1 cup orange juice
2 tablespoons lemon juice
2 limes
1 teaspoon salt
½ teaspoon freshly ground black pepper
1 cup finely chopped onions
2 tablespoons chopped parsley

MAKES FOUR TO SIX SERVINGS

1. Wash fish inside and out under cold running water. Pat dry.

2. Combine orange and lemon juices in a cup. Cut each lime into 4 wedges for garnish and set aside in refrigerator.

3. Make 4 slashes on each side of fish. Rub fish inside and out with salt and pepper.

4 Scatter ½ cup onions on bottom of large, shallow baking dish. Place fish on top of onions and pour orange and lemon juices over fish. Scatter remaining onions on top of fish. Let fish sit for 30 minutes.

5. Preheat oven to 400 degrees. Bake fish for 30 minutes, or until the flesh flakes easily when tested with a fork. Sprinkle with parsley. Serve with lime wedges and juices remaining in baking dish.

Florida Keys Red Snapper

3-4-pound red snapper or sea bass,
  cleaned and scaled
Peanut or vegetable oil
½ teaspoon salt
Freshly ground black pepper to taste
¼ cup butter
½ cup finely chopped onion
¼ cup finely chopped celery
¼ cup finely chopped green pepper
2 scallions, including green part, chopped
2 cups toasted fresh breadcrumbs
¼ cup finely chopped parsley
¼ cup coarsely chopped toasted almonds
6 thin tomato slices
6 thin onion slices
6 thin orange slices
6 thin lime slices
Juice of ½ lime

MAKES SIX TO EIGHT SERVINGS

1. Preheat oven to 350 degrees. Rub the fish lightly with oil and sprinkle inside and outside with salt and pepper.

2. Melt the butter and cook the onion, celery, green pepper, and scallions in it until onion is wilted. Stir in the breadcrumbs, parsley, and almonds. Season to taste with salt and pepper. Stuff the fish with the mixture and tie with string.

3. Place the fish on a length of aluminum foil and cover with alternating, slightly overlapping, slices of tomato, onion, orange, and lime. Sprinkle with salt, pepper, and lime juice. Bring up the edges of the foil and secure it envelope style. Bake for 30 minutes, or until fish flakes easily when tested with a fork.

Cooking the Nutritious Way
Fish and Shellfish

BROILED FISH

4 fish fillets, such as bluefish, weakfish, or flounder, each about ½ pound
2 tablespoons peanut, vegetable, or corn oil
¼ teaspoon paprika
2 tablespoons melted, unsalted butter or margarine (optional)
Lemon halves
2 tablespoons finely chopped parsley

MAKES FOUR SERVINGS

1. Preheat the broiler to high.
2. Place the fish on a flat, shallow baking dish and pour the oil over. Turn the fillets in the oil. Arrange them skin side down and sprinkle with paprika. Brush with a pastry brush to spread the oil and paprika evenly over them.
3. Place the broiler rack so that the fish will be 4 or 5 inches from the source of heat. Place the fish under the broiler. Keep the broiler door open while the fish is cooking. Broil for 6 or 7 minutes, or until fish has lost its raw texture. Do not overcook. The fish does not have to be turned.
4. Serve, if desired, with melted butter or margarine, lemon halves, and finely chopped parsley.

For added flavor, sprinkle fish with ¼ teaspoon cumin.

BAKED OYSTERS OR CLAMS

12 oysters or 24 Little Neck clams on the half shell
2-4 tablespoons butter
1 cup fresh breadcrumbs
½ teaspoon finely chopped garlic
2 tablespoons finely chopped scallions
2 tablespoons chopped fresh parsley
Pinch of salt
Freshly ground black pepper to taste
Lemon wedges

MAKES FOUR SERVINGS

1. Preheat oven to 425 degrees. Set each oyster or clam in its half shell on a dish, and set aside.
2. Melt the butter in a 10-inch skillet over medium heat. When the butter is very hot, add the breadcrumbs. With a wooden spoon, stir them constantly as they toast, darkening evenly to pale gold, for 4 to 6 minutes. Stir in the garlic. Alternate stirring the mixture and shaking the pan for about 1 minute. Stir in the scallions, then the parsley—just to heat them through—and remove from heat. Immediately scrape the contents of the skillet into a bowl.
3. Cover the top of each oyster or clam with some of the mixture, distributing all of it equally. Sprinkle each topping lightly with salt and pepper. Transfer the oysters or clams to a baking sheet large enough to hold them without crowding. Place the baking sheet on the middle shelf of the oven and cook for 10 minutes.
4. Remove the baking sheet from the oven. With a metal spatula, transfer the shellfish to serving dishes. Serve hot, with lemon wedges.

To make fresh breadcrumbs, remove crusts from 3 slices of fresh (not dry) white or whole-wheat bread; reduce bread to crumbs in a blender or in a food processor.

MUSSELS

4 pounds large mussels, in their shells
4 tablespoons butter
½ cup finely chopped onion
½ teaspoon dried thyme
½ teaspoon freshly ground black pepper
1 cup dry white wine
½ cup water
½ teaspoon salt (optional)
¼ cup chopped parsley

MAKES FOUR TO SIX SERVINGS

1. First remove hairlike beard from the mussels. Scrub mussels under cold running water with wire brush. Remove all sea growth with sharp knife.
2. Melt butter in an 8- to 10-quart pot over medium high heat. When butter is very hot and stops bubbling, add onions and cook, stirring all the while for 3 to 4 minutes. Add thyme, pepper, white wine, and water. Bring liquid to a boil. Add mussels.
3. Bring liquid back to a boil, cover pot, and reduce heat. Steam mussels for about 10 minutes, or until shells open.
4. Remove opened mussels to soup plates. Discard mussels that have not opened. Taste broth for salt; add chopped parsley and spoon over mussels.

Reminder: You may want to substitute margarine for butter.

Poultry

Chicken Cacciatore

½ cup chopped onion
¼ cup boiling water
8-ounce can tomatoes
½ cup tomato puree
1 garlic clove
1 teaspoon oregano
½ teaspoon celery seed
¼ teaspoon freshly ground pepper
4 skinless chicken-breast halves

MAKES FOUR SERVINGS

1. Cook onion in boiling water until tender. Do not drain. Add tomatoes, tomato puree, garlic, oregano, celery seed, and pepper to onions. Simmer for 10 minutes to blend flavors.
2. Place breast halves in heavy frying pan. Pour tomato mixture over chicken. Cook, covered, over low heat until chicken is tender, about 1 hour. Remove garlic before serving.

Stuffed Chicken Breasts

3 whole chicken breasts, boned, skinned, and halved
6 thin slices country ham
¼ cup freshly grated Parmesan cheese
¾ cup chopped parsley
½ cup blanched, slivered almonds
3 tablespoons butter
½ cup dry white vermouth
2 tablespoons brandy
¼ cup chicken broth
Pinch of salt
Freshly ground black pepper to taste

MAKES FOUR TO SIX SERVINGS

1. On the thickest side of the chicken breast, cut a pocket. It does not need to be very big, but try not to have any tears or holes in it.
2. Line each pocket with a slice of ham. Combine cheese, parsley, and almonds and stuff each pocket with some of the mixture.
3. Heat butter in a large skillet. Sauté chicken breasts, about 5 minutes per side, starting with pocket side down. Cook slowly so little stuffing comes out. Turn carefully. Add vermouth and brandy. At this point dish may be refrigerated until serving time.
4. To serve, cover skillet and bring liquid to a boil, simmer gently for 10 minutes. Remove breasts to a warm platter. Add broth to skillet; stir and heat through. Season with salt and pepper. Pour liquid from skillet over chicken breasts.

If country ham is unavailable, use prosciutto instead. Secure the pockets with toothpicks if necessary.

Chicken with Wine Vinegar

3-pound roasting chicken, cut into 8 pieces
½ teaspoon salt
Freshly ground black pepper to taste
3 tablespoons butter
15 garlic cloves, unpeeled
1¾ cups red wine vinegar
2 ripe tomatoes, peeled, cored, and chopped or ½ cup drained canned tomatoes
1 tablespoon tomato paste
1 cup chicken broth, preferably homemade (recipe on page 226)
Parsley sprigs for decoration

MAKES FOUR TO SIX SERVINGS

1. Season the pieces of chicken with salt and pepper. In a 12-inch skillet, heat 1 tablespoon of the butter and add the pieces of chicken, skin side down, starting with the legs and thighs because they need the longest cooking. After 3 or 4 minutes, when they begin to brown, add the wing pieces and finally the breast pieces. When all are brown, turn them over and brown the other sides for 1 to 2 minutes.
2. Add garlic cloves, cover, and cook over low heat for 20 minutes. Pour off the excess fat, add the vinegar and simmer, over low heat, for about 10 minutes, uncovered, until well reduced. Turn chicken over, add the tomatoes, tomato paste, and simmer, covered, for 10 minutes more.
3. Transfer the chicken to a platter and keep warm. Add the stock to the pan and boil until very well reduced and concentrated in flavor. Taste for seasoning and strain through a sieve, pressing hard on the garlic.
4. Reheat sauce, skim off the fat, remove from heat, and stir in the remaining butter. Taste for seasoning and adjust. Pour the sauce over the chicken and decorate with sprigs of parsley.

Cooking the Nutritious Way
Poultry

ROMANIAN CHICKEN STEW

3½-pound chicken, cut into 8 pieces
1 onion, thinly sliced
3 carrots, thinly sliced
2 stalks celery, thinly sliced
1 cup chicken broth, preferably homemade (recipe on page 226)
½ teaspoon salt
Freshly ground black pepper to taste
1 cup cooked peas
1 20-ounce can white kidney beans, drained, or 2 cups cooked dried beans
1 tablespoon softened butter
2 tablespoons flour

MAKES FOUR SERVINGS

1. Soak a clay pot or casserole (see note below) in cold water for 10 minutes.
2. Place the chicken, onion, carrots, celery, and broth in the pot. Season with salt and pepper.
3. Cover and place in a cold oven; adjust heat to 450 degrees and cook for 1 hour.
4. Add the peas and beans. Combine the butter and flour and stir into the pot juices. Cover and continue cooking for 15 minutes.

A clay pot is an excellent utensil for cooking food that is practically fat free. It preserves and enhances the natural flavors of the fresh ingredients. If you do not own a clay pot, preheat the oven to 350 degrees, place the chicken, onion, carrots, celery, broth, and salt and pepper in a fireproof casserole. Bring liquid to a simmer on top of the stove, cover, then transfer pot to oven and proceed as above.

BROILED CHICKEN BREASTS WITH LIME JUICE

Wash and dry 2 chicken breasts, each one about 1¼ pounds. Split them down the middle so that you have 4 halves. Heat charcoal fire for about 30 minutes or broiler for 15 minutes. Rub juice of 1 lime on chicken breasts. Season with salt and pepper to taste. Broil, skin side up, on lightly oiled grill for 5 minutes on one side and 10 minutes, skin side down, on the other. Sprinkle with fresh-chopped or dried tarragon.

MAKES FOUR SERVINGS

CHICKEN WITH CITRUS FRUITS

3½-pound chicken
½ teaspoon salt
2 lemons, thinly sliced and each slice cut in half
2 limes, thinly sliced and each slice cut in half
1 thick-skinned orange, thinly sliced and each slice cut into quarters
1 tablespoon vegetable oil
1 teaspoon paprika

MAKES FOUR TO SIX SERVINGS

1. Preheat oven to 350 degrees. Put the salt inside the chicken cavity along with a few of the lemon, lime, and orange slices. Arrange half the remaining slices in a baking dish. Truss the chicken, brush it with oil, sprinkle with paprika, and put it in a baking dish.
2. Bake the chicken for about 1½ hours or until done. Cut the chicken into serving pieces and garnish with the remaining fresh fruit.

COUNTRY CAPTAIN

3 tablespoons butter
1 small onion, finely chopped
1 small carrot, finely chopped
½ small green pepper, finely chopped
2 garlic cloves, finely chopped
2 tablespoons vegetable oil
½ cup flour
½ teaspoon salt
1 teaspoon freshly ground black pepper
2½-3-pound chicken, cut into 8 pieces
12-ounce can peeled Italian plum tomatoes, drained
2 cups chicken broth, preferably homemade (recipe on page 226)
2 tablespoons curry powder
¼ cup raisins
½ teaspoon salt (optional)
Freshly ground black pepper to taste
¼ cup slivered, toasted almonds

MAKES FOUR TO SIX SERVINGS

1. Melt the butter over medium-low heat in a straight-sided skillet large enough to hold all the chicken in one layer. When hot, add the onion, carrot, green pepper, and garlic and sauté for about 6 minutes, until

tender. Transfer vegetables to a saucepan. Add the oil to the skillet.

2. Combine the flour, salt, and pepper in a bowl. Roll the chicken pieces in this, shaking off any excess flour. Arrange the chicken in the skillet, skin side down and sauté for 6 to 8 minutes, turning occasionally, until the chicken is nicely browned on all sides.

3. While the chicken is sautéing, add the tomatoes, broth, and curry powder to the saucepan with the sautéed vegetables. Bring to a simmer.

4. When the chicken has finished sautéing, skim off excess fat and pour the simmering sauce over it. Cover, reduce the heat to low, and simmer for 15 minutes. Stir in the raisins and simmer for 5 minutes more. Taste the sauce, and season with salt, if desired, and pepper.

5. Arrange the chicken in a serving bowl and garnish with toasted almond slivers. Serve with rice.

Tandoori Chicken
(Indian Barbecued Chicken)

3 chickens, about 2¼ pounds each, quartered
⅓ cup lemon juice
2 large garlic cloves
1 tablespoon chopped fresh ginger or 1 teaspoon powdered ginger
1 teaspoon ground cumin
½ teaspoon ground cardamom
¼–½ teaspoon red pepper
1 tablespoon paprika
⅓ cup plain yogurt
Vegetable oil for basting

MAKES SIX SERVINGS

1. Pull away the skin of the chicken. Prick the chicken all over with a fork. Make diagonal slashes, ½-inch deep, 1 inch apart on one side of the meat. Put the meat in a large bowl. Add lemon juice and rub it into the chicken. Cover and marinate for ½ hour.

2. Put all the remaining ingredients, except the oil, into the container of a blender or food processor and blend until reduced to a smooth sauce. Pour this marinade over the chicken pieces and mix, turning and tossing to coat all the pieces well. This can be done up to 2 days in advance, and kept refrigerated, or marinated for 4 hours at room temperature.

3. Take the chicken from the refrigerator at least 1 hour before cooking. Preheat oven to highest setting (500 or 550 degrees). Take the chicken out of the marinade. Brush it with oil and place it in an extra-large, shallow roasting pan, preferably with a wire rack. Set the pan in the middle level of the oven, and roast for 25 to 30 minutes, or until meat is cooked through. There is no need to baste while the chicken is roasting.

To broil the chicken outdoors, place the chicken pieces, slashed sides up, on the grill, and cook 2 to 3 inches from the heat for 30 minutes, turning once.

Chicken and Vegetables in Aspic

3 cups chicken broth, preferably homemade (recipe on page 226)
2 packages (2 tablespoons) unflavored gelatin
1¼ cups cooked chicken, cut into small pieces
1¼ cups green beans, cut into small pieces and steamed
1 cup cooked peas
1 cup diced tomatoes, with seeds removed
2 tablespoons finely chopped parsley

MAKES FOUR SERVINGS

1. Pour 1 cup of cold chicken broth into a small saucepan and sprinkle the gelatin over the surface. Let stand for 5 minutes. Place over low heat until the gelatin has dissolved and a clear liquid has formed. Stir in the remaining chicken broth.

2. Stir in all the remaining ingredients and divide between 4 ramekins or glass custard dishes, each one of about 1¼ cup capacity. Chill for 4 hours and serve from ramekins or unmold onto a bed of lettuce leaves. Top each serving with mayonnaise, if you wish.

Roast Chicken

Preheat oven to 400 degrees. Sprinkle 3-pound chicken inside with salt and pepper and rub with a peeled garlic clove. Dust the outside with salt and pepper and rub garlic clove thoroughly into skin. Squeeze the juice of 1 lemon and rub the juice on the inside and the outside of the chicken. Truss, and roast on a rack with some water poured in roasting pan. Cook for 1 hour, without opening the oven door. Allow chicken to rest for 5 to 10 minutes. Before carving, pour pan juices over bird.   MAKES FOUR SERVINGS

Cooking the Nutritious Way
Poultry

ROAST CHICKEN WITH CANADIAN BACON AND COTTAGE CHEESE

3-pound roasting chicken
8 slices Canadian bacon
1 cup cottage cheese
½ teaspoon salt
Freshly ground black pepper to taste

MAKES FOUR TO SIX SERVINGS

1. Preheat oven to 350 degrees. Beginning at the neck of the chicken, run your finger beneath the skin to lift it from the chicken meat. Slide a piece of Canadian bacon beneath the skin. Use four slices for the breast, making sure each slice is flat and smooth. Arrange the remaining slices beneath the thigh skin.

2. Fill the cavity of the chicken with cottage cheese. Truss the cavity. Place on a rack in a roasting pan, breast side up. Season with salt and pepper.

3. Bake for about 1¼ hours or until a meat thermometer registers 180 degrees, or until the juices run clear without any traces of pink when the thigh is pricked with the point of a knife.

If you want to omit bacon, add 1 tablespoon tarragon and half a clove of minced garlic to the cottage cheese.

ROAST TURKEY WITH SAUSAGE DRESSING

12-14-pound turkey
1 pound sausage meat
8 cups stale bread-cubes, preferably whole-wheat bread
2 cups diced celery
1 onion, finely chopped
2 teaspoons grated orange rind
½ teaspoon grated lemon rind
1 teaspoon salt
Freshly ground black pepper to taste
1 teaspoon thyme
½ teaspoon marjoram
½ teaspoon sage
¼ cup chopped parsley
¼ cup orange juice
½ cup melted butter

MAKES FOURTEEN SERVINGS

1. Wash and dry the turkey and season the cavity with salt. Preheat oven to 325 degrees.

2. In a skillet, cook the sausage, breaking up the lumps as it cooks, until lightly browned. With a slotted spoon, transfer the meat to a large bowl and mix with the bread cubes and celery. Drain off and discard all but 2 tablespoons of the fat from skillet. Add the onion to the skillet and sauté until tender.

3. Add the onion, orange and lemon rinds, salt and pepper, thyme, marjoram, sage, parsley, and orange juice to the bread mixture. Stuff neck and body cavities of turkey. Close with skewers and string. Truss turkey, brush with some of the butter, and place, breast side down, on a rack in a shallow roasting pan. Roast for 2½ hours, basting often with remaining butter.

4. Turn breast side up and roast, basting frequently with butter and pan drippings, for 1½ to 2 hours more or until the internal temperature of a thigh joint is 180 degrees. Cover with aluminum foil if turkey browns too much. Let turkey set in a warm place for 20 to 30 minutes before carving.

Reminder: You can substitute margarine for butter.

CRISP-FRIED TURKEY BREAST

½ cup flour, preferably whole wheat
1 teaspoon thyme
1 tablespoon paprika
½ teaspoon salt
Freshly ground black pepper to taste
8 thin slices turkey breast, leftover or uncooked
2 eggs, lightly beaten
2 tablespoons milk
1 tablespoon mustard, preferably Dijon
1 cup fine breadcrumbs
2 tablespoons butter
1 tablespoon oil

MAKES FOUR TO SIX SERVINGS

1. Combine flour, thyme, paprika, salt, and pepper to taste. Dredge the turkey breast in the seasoned flour. Shake off excess flour.

2. Dip floured turkey breasts in eggs combined with milk and mustard. Dredge in breadcrumbs.

3. Heat the butter and oil together in a large frying pan. Fry leftover, cooked turkey over moderately high heat for 4 minutes on each side until the crust is crisp and golden. Allow an additional 2 minutes on each side for raw turkey slices.

This dish can also be made with raw veal scallopine or leftover slices of rare roast beef.

Meats

Basic Pot Roast of Beef

4 pounds chuck, rump, or round roast
2 tablespoons flour
3 tablespoons vegetable oil or butter
1 onion stuck with 2 whole cloves
1 bay leaf
1 teaspoon freshly ground black pepper
½ tablespoon salt
1½ teaspoons thyme
1 cup beef broth or water
6 carrots, cut into 2-inch lengths
12 small white onions, peeled
2 small white turnips, quartered

MAKES EIGHT SERVINGS

1. Rub the roast with flour. Heat the oil or butter in a pan large enough to hold the roast. When hot, sear all sides of the roast.
2. When well colored, add the onion, bay leaf, pepper, salt, thyme, and broth or water. Bring to a boil and simmer, covered, atop the stove or in a 300-degree oven for 2 hours.
3. Test the meat, and if it is on the way to being tender, add the remaining vegetables. Cook for about 1 hour more, until the vegetables are tender. Remove meat to a carving board and keep it warm.
4. Skim off the fat from the sauce and taste for seasoning. Carve meat into thin slices and serve.

Peppered Roast Beef

2½ pounds round roast, well trimmed
2 tablespoons oil
1 teaspoon freshly ground black pepper
1 medium onion, sliced
1 medium carrot, sliced
1 large stalk celery, sliced
½ cup dry red wine

MAKES EIGHT TO TEN SERVINGS

1. Preheat oven to 350 degrees. Rub meat with oil and pepper and place in an open roasting pan. Insert a meat thermometer so bulb reaches the center of thickest part.
2. Arrange onion, carrot, and celery slices around meat. Pour red wine over all. Roast, uncovered, for about 1½ hours or until thermometer registers desired degree of doneness.
3. If more liquid is needed, baste with additional wine during roasting. Do not use drippings. Skim fat from pan juices and discard. Let roast rest for 15 minutes before carving, and spoon pan juices over thinly sliced meat.

Paris Broil

2 pounds flank steak
1 cup dry red or white wine
Lots of coarsely cracked black pepper
1 large clove garlic, minced
½ teaspoon thyme
1 tablespoon butter or vegetable oil
½ teaspoon salt

MAKES FOUR TO SIX SERVINGS

1. Pick out a nonmetallic casserole just big enough to hold the meat when folded in thirds. In it mix together the wine, pepper, garlic, and thyme. Do not add salt because it draws out the juices of the meat.
2. Roll the steak in the marinade to coat all sides; then fold it in thirds and press it down into the casserole. Cover and leave at room temperature for 3 or 4 hours, turning the meat occasionally. Refrigerate 1 hour before broiling.
3. Preheat the broiler to red hot. Dry off steak, rub it with salt and butter or oil, and lay it on the hot broiler rack. Broil as close to the flame as possible but taking care it does not flame up. Broil for about 5 minutes per side, maximum. Remove to a carving board and carve into thin diagonal slices, serving some of the natural juices on each helping.

Broiled Hamburgers

Mix 1 pound lean, chopped round beef with 1 tablespoon minced onion, 3 tablespoons toasted wheat germ, and salt and pepper to taste. Form into 1-inch-thick patties and broil for about 4 minutes per side. Garnish with parsley.

MAKES FOUR SERVINGS

Cooking the Nutritious Way

Meats

BEEF TACOS

Brown 1 pound lean ground beef and ¼ cup chopped onion in a frying pan. Drain off excess fat. Stir in an 8-ounce can tomato sauce and 2 teaspoons chili powder. Simmer for about 15 minutes, uncovered, stirring occasionally, until mixture is dry and crumbly. Fill 12 taco shells with the meat mixture. Combine 1 cup chopped tomato, 1 cup shredded lettuce, and ½ cup shredded sharp Cheddar cheese. Top each taco with about 2 tablespoons of this mixture.

MAKES SIX SERVINGS

BEEF WITH ONIONS AND TOMATOES

2 tablespoons olive oil
2 onions, minced
2 tomatoes, chopped, or 1 cup canned, drained
2 tablespoons beef broth or water
1 teaspoon red wine vinegar
1 garlic clove, peeled and minced
1 bay leaf
½ teaspoon grated nutmeg
⅓ cup chopped parsley
Salt to taste
Freshly ground black pepper to taste
6-8 slices or 3 cups chopped cooked beef or lamb
2 teaspoons capers
⅓ cup fresh breadcrumbs, preferably homemade (recipe on page 268)

MAKES SIX SERVINGS

1. Preheat oven to 375 degrees. Oil a shallow baking dish.
2. Gently heat 1 tablespoon of the olive oil in a 9-inch skillet. Cook the onions over a low flame, covered, for about 10 minutes. Add the tomatoes and cook, covered, for 10 minutes more.
3. With a wooden spoon, stir in the broth and vinegar. Add the garlic, bay leaf, nutmeg, parsley, and salt and pepper. Simmer, uncovered, for 10 minutes.
4. Remove the bay leaf and pour half the sauce into the oiled baking dish. Put the slices of beef or lamb and the capers on the sauce and pour the rest of the sauce over them. Sprinkle with breadcrumbs and the remaining olive oil. Bake for 30 minutes.

Reminder: You may want to substitute vegetable oil for olive oil.

ORIENTAL BEEF

2-4 tablespoons soy sauce
2 teaspoons cornstarch
1 teaspoon sugar
½ teaspoon ginger
1 pound flank steak, trimmed, cut in 2-inch by ⅛-inch strips
3 tablespoons vegetable oil
1 cup (about 1 medium) green pepper, cut into thin strips
20-ounce can pineapple chunks, in own juice, drained

MAKES SIX SERVINGS

1. Mix soy sauce, cornstarch, sugar, and ginger.
2. Coat meat with soy-sauce mixture.
3. Heat 1 tablespoon oil in large frypan.
4. Add green pepper strips. Cook for 2 minutes, stirring constantly. Remove green pepper from pan.
5. Heat remaining 2 tablespoons oil.
6. Add meat. Cook for 1 to 2 minutes, stirring constantly, until beef is lightly browned.
7. Add green pepper and pineapple. Heat through.

BEEF GOULASH

2 pounds lean, boneless, sirloin steak
Freshly ground black pepper to taste
1 tablespoon paprika
2 tablespoons vegetable oil
1 tablespoon unsalted butter or margarine
½ cup chopped onion
2 tablespoons all-purpose flour
½ cup red wine
¼ cup crushed, canned tomatoes
1 cup plain yogurt
½ teaspoon dried thyme

MAKES FOUR TO SIX SERVINGS

1. Cut meat into thin strips about 2 inches long and

¼ inch wide. Sprinkle the strips with a generous grinding of black pepper and the paprika.

2. Heat the oil in a large, heavy skillet and add half the meat, cooking and stirring over high heat until meat is browned, about 3 minutes. Using a slotted spoon, transfer the meat to another skillet. In the first skillet, add the remaining beef and cook rapidly over high heat until browned. Transfer this meat to the other skillet.

3. Pour off any fat remaining in the first skillet. Add the butter or margarine and onion to the skillet and cook until the onion wilts. Sprinkle onion with flour and stir. Add the wine and tomatoes, stirring. Cook for about 4 minutes, uncovered. Add the yogurt, stirring rapidly. Add any juices that have accumulated around the meat. Add the thyme and cook for about 5 minutes, stirring constantly.

4. Place a strainer over the meat and strain the sauce into the skillet, stirring with a wooden spoon or spatula to push through as much of the solids in the sauce as possible. Heat and serve with noodles or rice.

Veal Stew

2½ pounds stewing veal
1 onion, finely chopped
2 cloves garlic, finely chopped
3 carrots, cut into 2-inch lengths
2 tomatoes, cut into wedges and seeds removed
1 green pepper, cut into ¼-inch strips
1 cup chicken broth, preferably homemade (recipe on page 226)
2 teaspoons tomato paste
½ teaspoon salt
Freshly ground black pepper to taste
2 tablespoons softened butter
3 tablespoons flour
2 tablespoons minced parsley

MAKES SIX SERVINGS

1. Place all the ingredients except the butter, flour, and parsley in a casserole. Preheat oven to 300 degrees. Bring the mixture to a simmer on top of the stove. Transfer to the oven and bake for 1½ to 2 hours or until meat is very tender.

2. Ten minutes before the total cooking time has elapsed, combine the butter with the flour and stir the mixture into the juices in the casserole. Continue cooking for the remaining 10 minutes, until the sauce has thickened. Garnish with parsley.

Lemon Lamb Roast

2-4 cloves garlic, peeled
Whole leg of lamb
2-4 tablespoons lemon juice
1-2 teaspoons oregano or rosemary
1 teaspoon salt
Freshly ground black pepper to taste

MAKES SIX TO TEN SERVINGS

1. Slice the garlic lengthwise into slivers. With a sharp-pointed knife, insert the garlic slivers into the meat and push them in with the tip of the knife. Arrange the roast on a rack in a shallow roasting pan. Sprinkle the meat liberally with lemon juice, oregano or rosemary, and salt and pepper.

2. Place the roast in a cold oven and set the temperature at 300 degrees. Roast for 2 hours for rosy, rare lamb or 3 hours for well done. Baste occasionally. Allow roast to stand for 10 to 20 minutes before carving to allow juices to retreat into flesh.

Cook half leg of lamb for 1½ hours for rosy lamb or 2½ hours for well-done. Try leftover lamb, sliced thinly, in sandwiches made with rye bread, mayonnaise, lettuce, and tomato.

Roast Lamb and Beans

1 boned lamb shoulder, in one piece
2 teaspoons ground cumin
4 garlic cloves, cut into slivers
1 pound potatoes, scrubbed
3 large carrots, scrubbed
1 parsnip, scrubbed
1 medium white turnip, peeled
½ teaspoon salt
Freshly ground black pepper to taste
6 medium onions, quartered
2 cups white beans, such as Great Northern, soaked and drained
2 tablespoons yogurt
Watercress or parsley for garnish

MAKES SIX TO EIGHT SERVINGS

1. Preheat oven to 375 degrees. Trim away as much of the outside fat from lamb as possible. Rub cumin into flesh of the lamb.

2. Make little nicks in the surface of the lamb and tuck in the garlic slivers. Place lamb in a large roasting

Cooking the Nutritious Way
Meats

pan, big enough to accommodate lamb and surrounding vegetables.

3. Cut potatoes, carrots, parsnip, and turnip into 1-inch pieces; add to roast with 2 cups of water. Season lightly with salt and pepper. Roast for 1 hour, basting frequently. After an hour, add onions, and continue to cook for 1 hour more, basting occasionally.

4. Meanwhile, cover the beans with 1 inch of water and season with salt and pepper. Cook, partially covered, for 1 hour, or until tender. Drain.

5. To serve, spread the beans in a thick layer on a large platter. Arrange the vegetables on top; slice the meat and arrange on top of vegetables.

6. Put the roasting pan on top of stove and skim off fat from surface of pan juices. Bring pan juices to a simmer and reduce them, for about 1 minute, over medium-high heat. Remove from heat and whisk in yogurt; adjust seasoning. Pour this over meat and vegetables to moisten them. Garnish platter with sprigs of watercress or parsley.

Most butchers will bone the lamb shoulder for you, or you may be able to find it in your market already boned, rolled, and tied. A boned shoulder roast usually weighs 3 to 4 pounds.

SHOULDER LAMB CHOPS BRAISED WITH ONIONS AND PEPPERS

6 shoulder chops, arm or blade, about 1-inch thick
4 medium onions, thinly sliced
3 medium green peppers, seeded and thinly sliced
½ teaspoon salt
Freshly ground black pepper to taste
1 cup tomato sauce
1 teaspoon dried basil or 1 tablespoon fresh basil

MAKES SIX SERVINGS

1. Trim as much fat from chops as possible.
2. Rub a 12-inch skillet with some lamb fat. Sear the chops for about 2 to 3 minutes per side. Add the onions, green peppers, salt, pepper, and tomato sauce. Cover and simmer 25 to 30 minutes.
3. Add the basil and cook, covered, for another 5 to 10 minutes. Remove chops, spoon sauce into a bowl, and remove as much fat as possible. Correct the seasoning. Quickly reheat chops in sauce.

LAMB SHISH KEBAB

1 pound lean, fat-trimmed, boneless lamb, preferably leg, cut into 1½-inch cubes
¼ cup lemon juice
1 clove garlic, minced
1 teaspoon oregano
⅛ teaspoon ground cinnamon
⅛ teaspoon ground nutmeg
2 teaspoons olive oil

MAKES FOUR TO SIX SERVINGS

1. Combine all ingredients, except oil, in a glass or stainless bowl. Cover and marinate for 1 hour at room temperature or for several hours in the refrigerator.
2. Thread meat on skewers, reserving marinade. Add oil to remaining marinade and brush meat.
3. Barbecue or broil meat for about 10 minutes, turning occasionally. Brush meat with marinade each time you turn it.

PORK SAUSAGE PATTIES

¾ pound lean ground pork
¼ teaspoon pepper
¼ teaspoon basil
¼ teaspoon sage
¼ teaspoon oregano
⅛ teaspoon allspice
⅛ teaspoon nutmeg
⅛ teaspoon dill weed
⅛ teaspoon chili powder (optional)
⅛ teaspoon Tabasco sauce (optional)
½ teaspoon minced garlic
1 egg white
2 tablespoons water

MAKES FOUR PATTIES

1. Combine all ingredients and mix thoroughly. Shape into 4 patties and place on a rack in a shallow pan. Broil 2 to 4 inches from the heat for 10 to 15 minutes. Turn patties and broil for 5 to 10 minutes or until well done.

Whenever a recipe calls for fresh pork sausages, you can use this mixture. You might wish to vary the seasonings according to taste. The recipe can easily be doubled. Shape meat into patties, place them between squares of aluminum foil, wrap tightly, and freeze.

Pork Chops Baked with Orange

6 center-cut loin pork chops, about 2 pounds
½ teaspoon salt
Freshly ground black pepper to taste
Flour for dredging pork chops
3-4 tablespoons butter
1 large orange or 2 small ones
½ cup fresh orange juice
1 bunch watercress

MAKES SIX SERVINGS

1. Preheat oven to 350 degrees. Rub the chops on both sides with salt and pepper. Dredge lightly in flour, shaking off excess. Heat the butter in a large frying pan. Over moderately high heat, quickly brown chops on both sides. Transfer browned chops in one layer to a large, shallow baking dish.
2. Peel the orange, making sure all the white pith is removed, and cut the orange into thin slices. Top each chop with 1 or 2 slices. Add orange juice to pan. Put cover on baking dish or wrap in aluminum foil. Bake for about 1 hour or until tender. Serve in a heated serving dish lined with washed watercress.

Pork Chops with Spinach

¼ cup flour
½ teaspoon salt
4 large pork chops, trimmed
2 tablespoons olive oil
1 clove garlic, minced
2 tablespoons minced parsley
1 tablespoon chopped onion
¼ cup dry white wine
½ teaspoon prepared mustard, preferably Dijon
1 pound fresh spinach, well washed and chopped, or a 10-ounce package frozen chopped spinach, partially defrosted

MAKES FOUR SERVINGS

1. Combine the flour and ¼ teaspoon salt. Dredge the pork chops into this mixture and shake off excess. Heat oil in a 10-inch skillet and brown chops, about 2 minutes per side. Cover and cook for 10 minutes over low heat. Transfer chops to a shallow casserole.
2. Preheat oven to 375 degrees. Add garlic, parsley, and onion to skillet and cook until onion is wilted. Add the wine, mustard, spinach, and remaining salt.

3. Cook, covered, for 4 minutes. Drain off excess liquid. Puree the spinach mixture in an electric blender or force through a sieve. Pile spinach over chops. Cover casserole and bake for 20 to 25 minutes or until chops are cooked through.

Ham Steak Baked in Milk

1½-inch-thick center-cut ham steak, about 2½ pounds
2 teaspoons brown sugar
½ teaspoon dry mustard
½ teaspoon ground ginger
About 1 quart of whole milk

MAKES SIX SERVINGS

1. The ham steak should have a round center bone and about a ½-inch layer of fat surrounding it. Trim off fat and use a small piece of it to grease a baking dish not much larger than the meat.
2. Preheat oven to 350 degrees. Rub half the brown sugar, mustard, and ginger into one side of the ham steak. Place it in the greased baking dish and rub the other side with the remaining flavorings.
3. Pour in enough milk just to cover the ham steak. Place in oven and bake for about 2 hours. When done, all the milk will have evaporated and there will be a dark-brown crust over the meat and sticking to the pan. Include a piece of this crust with each serving.

The crust will not form if you use skim milk.

Sauteed Liver with Wheat Germ

⅔ cup toasted plain wheat germ
½ teaspoon salt
1 teaspoon dried oregano or thyme
Freshly ground black pepper to taste
4 teaspoons fresh lemon juice
4 teaspoons sesame oil or vegetable oil
1½ pounds calves' liver, cut into ½-inch-thick slices
¼ cup sesame oil or unsalted butter
4 wedges of lemon

MAKES FOUR SERVINGS

1. Combine the wheat germ, salt, oregano or thyme,

Cooking the Nutritious Way
Meats

and pepper on a large plate and toss gently to mix.

2. Blend together the lemon juice and sesame or vegetable oil, and brush or rub it into the liver. Lay the oiled liver onto the seasoned wheat germ and turn to coat both sides. Pat the wheat germ into the liver. Set dredged liver onto a fine-meshed rack and allow to set for 10 minutes.

3. Heat the oil or butter over a low-medium heat, in a large skillet. Add the slices of liver and sauté for about 4 minutes, turning once, until the liver is medium-rare. Transfer to a plate and serve immediately, with lemon wedges.

Wheat germ and sesame oil are available in specialty-food stores, if your supermarket does not carry them.

LIVER WITH LENTILS AND YOGURT

1 onion, thinly sliced
1 carrot, thinly sliced
⅔ cup lentils
⅔ cup brown rice
1 bay leaf
1 teaspoon salt
½ teaspoon freshly ground black pepper
½ pound calves' liver, cut into
    2- by ½-inch pieces
1 tablespoon oil
1 teaspoon dry mustard
¼ cup plain yogurt
1 bunch watercress

MAKES FOUR SERVINGS

1. Put the onion and carrot into a saucepan with the lentils, rice, bay leaf, salt, and pepper. Pour in 2 cups of water and bring to a boil. Cover the pan and simmer for 45 minutes. Check occasionally, and add more water if mixture becomes too dry; there should be just a hint of moisture by the time the rice and lentils are tender, without the need to drain.

2. When the lentils and rice are done, remove bay leaf and quickly sauté the liver in the oil for about 2 minutes per side. Take the pan off the heat. Stir the mustard into the yogurt; then turn this mixture into the slightly cooled liver. Make a nest of the lentils and rice and put the liver mixture in the middle. Decorate with watercress.

This is an example of how to stretch an expensive cut of meat by complementing it with an inexpensive source of protein such as legumes and grains.

One Dish Meals

PIZZA RUSTICA

Pastry
2 cups flour, preferably half whole wheat
½ teaspoon salt
½ teaspoon sugar
¾ cup butter or margarine
Lemon juice
1-3 tablespoons iced water
Filling
5 eggs
1 pound ricotta cheese
2 tablespoons chopped onion
1 tablespoon chopped parsley
1 cup grated Parmesan cheese
Salt to taste
Freshly ground black pepper to taste
2 tablespoons olive oil
2 cloves garlic, minced
¼ teaspoon marjoram
½ teaspoon oregano
10 ounces canned tomato puree
4 ounces canned tomato paste
⅔ cup sliced black olives
½ pound thinly sliced mozzarella cheese
1 very large bell pepper, seeded and cut into
    matchstick pieces

MAKES EIGHT TO TEN SERVINGS

1. Make the pastry first. Mix the flour, salt, and sugar in a bowl. Cut in the butter or margarine, using 2 knives or a pastry cutter, until the mixture resembles coarse cornmeal. Sprinkle over it a few drops of lemon juice and a very small amount of ice water—no more than 3 tablespoons—and toss lightly until it begins to come together. Form it quickly into a ball and chill for 2 hours.

2. Lightly grease a deep-dish 10-inch pie plate. Divide dough in half. Roll out one half and place in pie plate. Cover and refrigerate the other half.

3. Beat the eggs; stir in the ricotta cheese, onion, parsley, and Parmesan cheese and season with salt and pepper. Set aside. Preheat oven to 425 degrees.

4. Heat the olive oil in a small saucepan. Add the garlic and herbs. When the garlic is clear and begins to turn gold, stir in the tomato puree, tomato paste, olives, and season with salt and pepper. Slice the mozzarella thinly.

5. Spread half of the ricotta mixture in the prepared

pie shell. Arrange over it half the mozzarella slices. Cover with half the tomato sauce and spread half the green pepper over it. Repeat all the layers. Roll out the other half of the dough and place on top. Pinch the edges of the bottom and top crusts together, and flute. With a sharp knife, make 3 long, parallel slashes through the top crust. Bake for 35 to 40 minutes or until it is well browned. Let stand for ½ hour before serving.

This is so tasty and filling that it is perfect as a main course served with a mixed green salad. If you prefer to make a single-crust pie, with no top crust, make only half the pastry recipe. If you wish you can use a ready-made frozen pie shell.

Lasagna

¾ pound lasagna noodles, preferably whole wheat
½ teaspoon salt
½ cup chopped walnuts, almonds, or sunflower seeds
½ pound fresh spinach
3 cups tomato sauce (recipe on page 261—Pasta Marinara)
Freshly ground black pepper to taste
1 cup cottage cheese, or ¾ cup ricotta cheese mixed with ½ cup skim milk
¼ cup grated Parmesan cheese
12 thin slices mozzarella or Swiss cheese

MAKES SIX TO EIGHT SERVINGS

1. Cook noodles in boiling salted water until tender but still somewhat firm. Drain. Preheat oven to 350 degrees.
2. Toast nuts or seeds in oven, stirring a few times for about 10 minutes or until roasted.
3. Wash and dry spinach and chop into bite-size pieces.
4. Spread ¾ cup of the tomato sauce in bottom of an 8 by 8-inch baking dish. Place ⅓ of the noodles on top and season lightly with salt and pepper. Cover with ⅓ of the spinach, ¼ of the nuts, ¼ cup cottage cheese or ricotta cheese-milk mixture, 1 tablespoon Parmesan cheese, and a layer of mozzarella slices. Repeat layers twice. Spread the last cup of sauce and the remaining nuts and cheeses on top.
5. Bake for 40 minutes, and let stand for 10 minutes before cutting.

Kasha Pie

Pie crust pastry (recipe on page 240—Pizza Rustica)
2 eggs, beaten separately
1 cup unroasted buckwheat groats
2½ cups vegetable broth (recipe on page 227) or water
½ teaspoon salt
1 carrot, sliced
1 onion, chopped
1 rib celery, chopped
Freshly ground black pepper
½ cup chopped almonds or pecans
⅔ cup cooked beans, such as soy or kidney
2½ cups tomato sauce (recipe on page 261—Pasta Marinara)

MAKES SIX TO EIGHT SERVINGS

1. Make the pie crust, then line a deep pie pan with half the crust and save the other half for a top crust. Refrigerate for 2 hours.
2. Place one of the beaten eggs in a bowl. Combine with the buckwheat groats and stir together until all the grains are coated with egg.
3. Heat a heavy pan over moderate heat and pour in the groats-egg mixture. Keep stirring the mixture with a wooden spoon until the egg is absorbed and the grains begin to toast; it is important that the egg be absorbed completely or you will have unattractive strings of cooked egg in the kasha.
4. Bring the broth to a boil and pour it into the kasha. Add the salt, carrot, onion, and celery and bring to a second boil. Lower the heat, cover, and cook slowly for 35 minutes. Remove lid and continue cooking until liquid is absorbed. Season to taste with more salt, if desired, and freshly ground black pepper.
5. Ten minutes before refrigeration time is up, preheat oven to 350 degrees. Brush the crust with some of the other beaten egg and prebake the pie crust for 5 minutes.
6. Combine the cooked groats with the almonds or pecans and the cooked beans.
7. Fill the prebaked pie crust with the kasha mixture and pour the tomato sauce over. Roll out the top crust and cover the pie; pinch the top and bottom crusts together. Slash or pierce the top to allow steam to escape. Brush with the remaining beaten egg.
8. Bake for 30 to 40 minutes or until top crust is golden.

If raw buckwheat groats are unavailable, you can substitute roasted buckwheat called kasha.

Cooking the Nutritious Way
One Dish Meals

SWISS CHARD AND CHEESE PIE

3 pounds fresh Swiss chard
2 cups low-fat cottage cheese
2 eggs, lightly beaten
Juice of 1 lemon
½ teaspoon salt
2 tablespoons chopped chives (optional)
½ cup whole-grain breadcrumbs
Paprika

MAKES SIX TO EIGHT SERVINGS

1. Lightly grease an 8 by 8-inch baking pan. Wash chard and remove the stems, then chop into bite-size pieces. Cook quickly in a heavy pan with no added water, stirring constantly until wilted. Drain very well, saving the juice for other soups or casseroles.
2. Preheat oven to 350 degrees. Beat together the cottage cheese, eggs, lemon, salt, and the chives, if used. Stir a cup of this mixture into the chard. Put into the greased baking pan and press down firmly with a fork. Spread remaining cottage cheese mixture evenly over the top and sprinkle with breadcrumbs and paprika. Bake for 30 minutes, or until set. Allow to stand several minutes before cutting into squares and serving.

If Swiss chard is unavailable, substitute other greens such as spinach, kale, or mustard greens. For a summertime supper, chill the pie and serve garnished with crumbled blue cheese, sliced tomatoes, and minced parsley. To use chard stems, steam and use as you would celery.

GRATIN OF SPINACH AND HARD-BOILED EGGS

1 large onion, finely chopped
3 tablespoons butter
2 pounds fresh spinach, stemmed, steamed, squeezed, and chopped, about 2 cups
1 tablespoon flour
2 cups milk
½ teaspoon salt
Freshly ground black pepper to taste
⅛ teaspoon nutmeg
3 hard-boiled eggs
½ cup breadcrumbs, preferably whole wheat

MAKES FOUR TO SIX SERVINGS

1. Stew the onion in 2 tablespoons of butter in a heavy saucepan over low heat for about 15 minutes, stirring frequently, until soft and yellowed. Add the spinach, continuing to cook over low heat for 15 minutes longer, stirring and respreading the mass out on the bottom of the saucepan by tapping into it with the side of a wooden spoon.
2. Sprinkle with the flour, stir well, and begin adding the milk in small quantities at a time, stirring and waiting until it has been thoroughly absorbed by the spinach before adding more. Wait another 15 minutes or so for the spinach to absorb all the milk. Season to taste with salt, pepper, and nutmeg. Preheat oven to 400 degrees.
3. Add the hard-boiled eggs, coarsely cut up. Stir well and turn out into a large, buttered gratin dish, spreading the mixture smoothly to no more than 1-inch thickness. Sprinkle evenly with breadcrumbs and dot the top with remaining tablespoon of butter. Bake for about 15 minutes or until heated through.

Serve this with whole-grain bread, cheese, and a steamed vegetable, for a complete meal. Reminder: You may want to substitute margarine for butter.

CASSEROLE OF SPRING GARDEN VEGETABLES

2 tablespoons butter
6 medium carrots, cut into thin matchsticks, about 2 inches long
1 turnip, cut into thin matchsticks, about 2 inches long
2 small onions, thinly sliced
4 tender celery stalks, thinly sliced
⅓ cup white vermouth or dry white wine
½ teaspoon salt
Freshly ground black pepper to taste
Parsley for garnish

MAKES SIX SERVINGS

1. Preheat oven to 325 degrees.
2. Melt butter in a small casserole. Combine the vegetables and place them in the casserole. Add the wine and season with salt and pepper.
3. Butter a circle of wax paper and place on top and touching the vegetables. Cover casserole and cook for 1 hour or until vegetables are tender. Top with parsley.

The wax paper will keep the vegetables from drying out. You can change the vegetables and use parsnips, rutabaga, chard stems, or anything that is in season.

Eggplant Parmesan

6 tablespoons olive or vegetable oil
1 onion, chopped
3 cloves garlic, minced
1 green pepper, chopped (optional)
4 cups peeled chopped tomatoes
1 12-ounce can tomato paste
½ teaspoon salt
Freshly ground pepper to taste
1 tablespoon fresh basil or 1 teaspoon dried basil
1 teaspoon oregano or less to taste
Pinch of ground cinnamon
1 large or 2 small eggplants
½ cup whole-wheat flour
1 pound mozzarella cheese, sliced
½–1 cup breadcrumbs, preferably whole wheat
1 cup freshly grated Parmesan cheese

MAKES SIX TO EIGHT SERVINGS

1. In a large saucepan heat about 2 tablespoons of the olive oil and sauté the onion with half the garlic and the optional green pepper until tender.
2. Add the tomatoes, remaining garlic, tomato paste, ¼ teaspoon salt, and pepper and let simmer for 1 hour while you prepare the eggplant. Add the basil and oregano after the first half hour. Toward the end of the cooking time, add the cinnamon to the sauce and correct the seasoning; you may wish to add more oregano or basil.
3. Preheat oven to 500 degrees. Cut eggplant in half lengthwise. With a sharp knife, make 2 lengthwise slits in each half, cutting through *to* the skin but not through it. Oil a baking pan generously. Place the eggplant flat side down in the pan and bake for 15 minutes; remove from the oven. The skin will have shriveled and the eggplant will be soft and fragrant.
4. When the eggplant is cool enough to handle, slice it in lengthwise pieces about ¼-inch thick. Meanwhile, in a bowl, combine the flour and ¼ teaspoon salt. Dip the eggplant slices in this mixture, a few at a time, and sauté on both sides in the remaining olive oil until crisp. Drain well. When the slices are cool enough, cut them in half crosswise. Turn oven down to 350 degrees.
5. Oil a 2½ or 3-quart casserole. Place ¼ inch of tomato sauce on the bottom, then add a layer of eggplant slices. Cover with some of the mozzarella, a thicker layer of sauce, a sprinkling of breadcrumbs, and then of Parmesan cheese. Continue in this order, finishing with a lavish helping of sauce, breadcrumbs, and Parmesan cheese. Bake for 30 to 40 minutes and serve immediately.

Vegetable Paella

2 cups raw brown rice
6 cups vegetable broth (recipe on page 227), chicken broth (recipe on page 226), or water
2 onions, thinly sliced
4 cloves garlic, minced
3 green peppers, seeded and sliced thin
2 tomatoes, sliced
¼ cup olive oil
½ teaspoon salt
1 teaspoon saffron threads (optional)
1 bay leaf
2 cups cooked chick-peas
2 cups peas, lightly steamed
1 cup sliced black olives
8 pimientos, sliced
½ cup almonds, whole or cut in half

MAKES SIX TO EIGHT SERVINGS

1. Cook the rice, covered, in 3 cups of broth or water until the liquid is absorbed.
2. In a large heavy-bottomed skillet, or flameproof casserole, sauté the onion, garlic, peppers, and tomatoes in the olive oil until the onion is tender.
3. Stir in the rice, remaining stock or water, salt, saffron, bay leaf, and chick-peas. Cover and cook over low heat until the water is nearly absorbed, about 30 minutes. Add the peas, olives, and pimientos; do not stir. Continue cooking, uncovered, until all the water is absorbed.
4. Garnish with the almonds.

Mushroom, Egg, and Barley Casserole

¼ cup uncooked barley
2 cups boiling water
3 tablespoons chopped green pepper
2 cups sliced mushrooms
3 tablespoons butter
2 tablespoons flour
2 cups milk
¼ cup grated Parmesan cheese
4 eggs, hard-boiled
½ teaspoon salt
Freshly ground black pepper to taste

MAKES FOUR SERVINGS

1. Preheat oven to 350 degrees. Pour barley slowly

Cooking the Nutritious Way
One Dish Meals

into boiling water and cook for about 30 minutes, until tender; drain and set aside.

2. Sauté green pepper and mushrooms in 1 tablespoon butter for 5 to 6 minutes.

3. Meanwhile, in a 1½ to 2-quart flameproof casserole melt 2 tablespoons butter, stir in the flour and cook, over gentle heat, stirring constantly, for about 2 minutes. Remove from heat, blend in milk, then return to heat and whisk until smooth and thickened.

4. Stir cheese into the sauce, then mix in the hard-boiled eggs, drained barley, sautéed vegetables. Season to taste with salt and pepper. Bake for 30 to 40 minutes until crusty surface forms.

Reminder: You may wish to substitute vegetable oil for olive oil.

ITALIAN SOYBEAN-GRAINS CASSEROLE

1 onion, chopped
2 garlic cloves, minced
¼ cup olive oil
8 tomatoes, chopped
6-ounce can tomato paste
1 teaspoon oregano
1 tablespoon chopped fresh basil or
    1 teaspoon dried basil
½ teaspoon salt
2 medium zucchini, sliced
2 cups cooked soybeans
2 cups cooked bulgur or brown rice
4 ounces Cheddar cheese, sliced or grated
½ cup toasted wheat germ

MAKES SIX TO EIGHT SERVINGS

1. Sauté the onion and garlic in 2 tablespoons of the olive oil until the onion is tender. Add the tomatoes, tomato paste, and seasonings; then cover and simmer for 30 minutes.

2. Sauté the zucchini in the remaining oil until just beginning to be translucent. Sprinkle with salt.

3. Preheat oven to 350 degrees; oil a 2-quart casserole. Combine the soybeans and grains with 1 cup of the sauce and spread them over the bottom of the prepared casserole. Layer the zucchini over the grains and beans. Pour on the remaining sauce, sprinkle on the cheese, and top with wheat germ. Bake for 30 minutes.

This is a model meatless protein dish. The combination of grains and soybeans makes a complete protein.

SPANISH CASSEROLE

2 chicken breasts, boned, split, and skinned
⅓ cup vegetable oil
1 onion, finely chopped
1 cup raw long-grain brown rice
¼ cup pimiento, diced
½ cup green or red pepper, diced
1 cup chicken broth, preferably
    homemade (recipe on page 226)
1 cup canned tomatoes, drained
1 teaspoon thyme
Freshly ground black pepper to taste
½ cup cooked green peas

MAKES FOUR SERVINGS

1. Preheat oven to 350 degrees. Sauté chicken in oil for about 5 minutes on each side or until browned. Remove to a 1½- to 2-quart casserole. Add onion and rice to oil and sauté for a couple of minutes; remove to casserole.

2. Add pimiento, pepper, broth, tomatoes, and seasonings to chicken and rice mixture. Bake, covered, for 40 minutes or until rice is cooked.

3. Garnish with peas and serve.

CALDO GALLEGO
(Portuguese Stew)

1½ cups dried navy or other white beans
¼ pound lean salt pork, diced
1 cup diced cooked ham
1 cup chopped onion
½ cup chopped celery
½ cup chopped green pepper
½ cup chopped scallions, with tops
2 cups peeled, chopped fresh tomatoes
2 cloves garlic, minced
1 meaty ham bone
2 quarts water
¼ teaspoon oregano
3 cups diced raw potatoes
½ pound Swiss chard or spinach

MAKES EIGHT SERVINGS

1. Pick over the beans and place them in a large heavy pot. Add water to cover and bring to a boil. Boil 1 minute. Remove from heat and soak, covered, for 1 hour. Drain beans and discard soaking water.

2. In this same pot, brown the salt pork, then add

ham and brown. Add the onion, celery, green pepper, and scallions, and continue to cook, over medium heat, stirring frequently, until vegetables are limp.

3. Add tomatoes and garlic, mix well, and cook for 5 minutes more. Return the beans to the pot, and add the ham bone, water, and oregano. Cover and bring water to the boil, then reduce heat and cook, covered, until the beans are tender, about 1½ hours. Add more water, if necessary, but not too much—the stew should be rather thick.

4. During the last half hour, add the diced potatoes. During the last 5 minutes, add the Swiss chard or spinach, torn into smallish pieces. Serve very hot.

GARBURE
(French Vegetable Soup with Meat)

1 cup dried small white beans
1 pound smoked turkey, chicken, or ham
1 small head cabbage, coarsely shredded
½ pound string beans, cut into ½-inch pieces
1 white turnip, cut into ½-inch cubes
1 onion, stuck with 4 whole cloves
2 pounds potatoes, washed and cut into ½-inch thick slices
¼ teaspoon marjoram or oregano
½ teaspoon thyme
4 sprigs parsley
½ head garlic, still attached to core and unpeeled (about 12 cloves)

MAKES FOUR TO SIX SERVINGS

1. A day ahead, or the morning you plan to serve the garbure, bring 2 quarts of water to a rolling boil in a 3-quart saucepan. Add the beans and boil for 2 minutes. Remove from heat, cover, and let stand 1 hour. Return to heat and simmer 30 minutes or until beans are just tender, but not fully done. Drain and reserve beans.

2. In a 6-quart pot, bring 3 quarts of water to a rolling boil. Add the turkey, chicken, or ham and simmer for 10 minutes.

3. Slowly add the remaining ingredients in the order listed so that the water never stops boiling completely. Lower heat and simmer slowly for 1½ hours.

4. Remove the whole onion and the half head of garlic. Discard the onion. Squeeze the pulp out of the garlic and add to the soup.

5. Remove the meat and cut into cubes and return to soup. Serve immediately.

Sauces and Relishes

SIMPLE VINAIGRETTE

¼ cup herb or white wine vinegar
1 tablespoon lemon juice
1 teaspoon prepared Dijon mustard or ¼ teaspoon dry mustard
¼ teaspoon salt
Freshly ground black pepper to taste
½ cup olive or vegetable oil

MAKES THREE-QUARTERS CUP

1. Mix together the vinegar, lemon juice, mustard, salt, and pepper. Add oil, a little at a time, beating with a whisk until the mixture emulsifies.

2. This sauce may also be made in the blender or food processor. Simply put all ingredients into the container and blend at high speed for a minute. Serve on salads and on raw or cooked vegetables.

This keeps for months in the refrigerator. If the oil separates from the other ingredients, shake the container to mix before serving. To alter the recipe, add 2 tablespoons of minced fresh herbs or a finely chopped clove of garlic to the vinaigrette. Increase the oil if you prefer a milder dressing.

TARRAGON-BUTTERMILK DRESSING

¾–1 cup buttermilk
½ cup tarragon vinegar
1 tablespoon olive oil
2 tablespoons minced fresh chives or scallions
½ teaspoon crumbled dry tarragon
½ teaspoon salt
¼ teaspoon freshly ground black pepper
1-3 tablespoons grated Parmesan cheese (optional)

MAKES ONE AND THREE-QUARTERS CUPS

1. Place all the ingredients in a 1-pint shaker jar and shake vigorously to blend. Refrigerate for several hours before using. Shake well again before using.

This is a good way to use leftover buttermilk and Parmesan cheese. Serve this dressing with crisp green salads, cold chicken, or cold poached sole.

Cooking the Nutritious Way
Sauces and Relishes

High-Protein, Low-Calorie Dressing

Puree in a blender or food processor ¼ teaspoon chopped garlic, 1 cup yogurt or buttermilk, 1 cup low-fat cottage cheese, 1½ teaspoons vinegar, ½ teaspoon salt, ¼ teaspoon dill weed, and ¼ teaspoon freshly ground black pepper. Use this dressing for green vegetable salads or serve with cold chicken.   MAKES TWO CUPS

Tomato Ketchup

12-ounce can tomato paste
½ cup cider vinegar
½ cup water
½ teaspoon salt
1 teaspoon oregano
⅛ teaspoon ground cumin
⅛ teaspoon nutmeg
¼ teaspoon freshly ground black pepper
½ teaspoon mustard powder
½ teaspoon minced garlic

MAKES ONE AND THREE-QUARTERS CUPS

1. Mix all the ingredients together very well.

This does not taste like the commercial varieties, but it is a wholesome version without sugar or preservatives. It will keep for two weeks in a covered jar in the refrigerator. Freeze for longer storage.

Broccoli Dressing

Puree in a blender or food processor, 1 cup cooked broccoli, mainly flowerets, ¼ cup vegetable oil, ¼ cup white wine vinegar, a dash each of basil, dill weed, ground cumin, and freshly ground black pepper, 1 tablespoon tomato sauce, and ¼ teaspoon salt. Refrigerate until needed. If you find this too thick for a dressing, use it as a dip for fresh raw vegetables, cold steamed vegetables, or cold meats.   MAKES ABOUT ONE CUP

Mustard Sauce

1½ cups milk
2 tablespoons unsalted butter
2 tablespoons chopped onion
1 teaspoon dry mustard
2 tablespoons flour
½ teaspoon salt
2 teaspoons prepared mustard

MAKES ABOUT ONE AND ONE-HALF CUPS

1. Heat milk in a small saucepan until bubbles form around the edge.
2. Melt butter in a medium-sized saucepan over low heat. When butter is hot, add onion and cook for 3 minutes.
3. Stir in dry mustard and flour. Cook over low heat for 2 minutes. Remove pan from heat.
4. With a wire whisk, slowly beat hot milk into the flour mixture. Add salt and prepared mustard. Return mixture to high heat and continue to beat with a wire whisk until sauce comes to a boil.
5. Reduce heat and let sauce simmer for 2 minutes. Strain through a sieve.

Serve this sauce with poultry and fish.

Onion Sauce

2 tablespoons butter or margarine
2 tablespoons onion, finely chopped
2 tablespoons flour
1½ cups vegetable broth
   (see recipe page 227) or water
2 teaspoons soy sauce
½ teaspoon salt
Freshly ground pepper to taste

MAKES ONE AND ONE-HALF CUPS

1. Melt butter or margarine over moderate heat. Cook onion until lightly browned.
2. Stir in flour.
3. Remove from heat.
4. Stir in rest of ingredients. Cook and stir until thickened. Thin with a little water if needed.

Serve this sauce with meat loaf made from your favorite recipe. To add flavor to steamed Brussels sprouts or cooked pearl onions, cover with onion sauce, sprinkle with grated Parmesan cheese, and place under broiler until lightly browned.

Cold Vegetable Sauce

5 tablespoons cucumber, cut into ¼-inch dice
2 tablespoons green pepper, cut into ¼-inch dice
⅓ cup onion, cut into ¼-inch dice
2 tablespoons seeded tomatoes, cut into ¼-inch dice
1 teaspoon olive oil
3 tablespoons red wine vinegar
½ teaspoon Worcestershire sauce
½ teaspoon Dijon-type mustard
1 tablespoon minced sour pickles
1 scant tablespoon pickled capers
1 whole clove garlic, peeled and split
½ teaspoon thyme
½ bay leaf
¼ teaspoon salt
Freshly ground black pepper to taste

MAKES ONE CUP

1. Combine all the vegetables in a bowl.
2. Combine the remaining ingredients and pour over vegetables. Store, covered, in the refrigerator for at least 3 days before using.

This is a wonderful accompaniment to hot or cold broiled or grilled meats and fish.

Barbecue Sauce

1 cup dry white wine
¼ cup olive oil
2 tablespoons butter
1 medium onion, minced
1 crushed clove of garlic
¼ teaspoon salt
¼ teaspoon paprika
3 teaspoons fresh rosemary or 1 teaspoon dried rosemary
2 teaspoons minced parsley

MAKES ONE CUP

1. Combine all ingredients in a 1-quart nonaluminum saucepan. Bring to a boil. Lower to a simmer and cook for 30 minutes. Use as a barbecue sauce for chicken or turkey or for basting roasts.

This sauce will keep well in the refrigerator for a week, or it can be frozen.

Mayonnaise

Place 1 whole egg in the bowl of a blender or food processor. Add ½ teaspoon dry mustard and 1–2 tablespoons vinegar or lemon juice. Cover and blend on low speed for about 30 seconds. Then, slowly, in a thin steady stream, pour in 1 cup of polyunsaturated oil. When all the oil has been added, replace the cover and blend for another minute or until the mayonnaise is thick. Add salt, pepper, and herbs to taste. This will keep in the refrigerator for one week.

MAKES ONE AND ONE-QUARTER CUPS

Curry Marinade

1 cup chicken broth (recipe on page 226)
1 cup water
1 cup dry white wine
1 medium onion, sliced
2 tablespoons fresh ginger, coarsely chopped, or 1 tablespoon dry ginger
3 tablespoons curry powder
Grated peel of ½ lemon

MAKES THREE CUPS

1. Combine all ingredients, mix well, and store in a covered jar in the refrigerator.

Use for marinating chicken, beef, or pork.

Pickled Peppers

4 large bell peppers
4 cups water
1 cup cider vinegar
½ cup sugar
2 teaspoons pickling spice
1½ tablespoons salt
1 clove garlic, peeled

MAKES ABOUT ONE QUART

1. Cut the bell peppers into thick strips or 1-inch squares.
2. Heat the water in an enameled saucepan with the vinegar, sugar, pickling spice, salt, and garlic. Add the peppers and let simmer gently for about 15 minutes, or

Cooking the Nutritious Way

Sauces and Relishes

until just tender. Turn off the heat and let stand for 15 minutes.

3. Transfer the peppers to a jar, strain the liquid, and pour in as much as is needed to cover the peppers completely. Cover the jar and let stand for 24 hours.

ONION AND ROASTED TOMATO RELISH

2 medium-sized onions
1 medium-sized ripe tomato
¼ teaspoon salt

MAKES SIX TO EIGHT SERVINGS

1. Preheat oven to 500 degrees. Peel the onions, and cut them in half from top to bottom. Slice each half into ⅛-inch slices. Separate the shreds, and wash them in several changes of water, squeezing them slightly. Do not squeeze too hard, or you may crush the shreds. Put them in a bowl and set aside.

2. Wash the tomato, wipe dry, and smear a little oil over it. Place the tomato in a small oven-proof dish. Bake, uncovered, in the middle level of the oven, for 15 minutes or until the tomato is fully cooked and very soft and the skin is cracked and charred. Take the dish from the oven and let the tomato cool briefly. Then carefully peel off the skin. Mash the pulp with a fork or spoon. Be careful not to overmash; the pulp must remain a little lumpy. Mix onion and tomato pulp in a small serving bowl. Add salt and serve.

GRATED CUCUMBER RELISH

Peel 3 medium-sized cucumbers and cut in half lengthwise. Scrape out the seeds with a spoon and discard. Grate the cucumbers into a bowl. Cover and refrigerate up to 4 hours in advance of serving. When ready to serve, add 1 tablespoon lemon juice, ¼ teaspoon salt, and freshly ground black pepper to taste.

Serve as a low-calorie snack or as a salad with cold fish or meat. Add 1 tablespoon of chopped fresh dill, if desired.

MAKES SIX TO EIGHT SERVINGS

Vegetables

BEETS AND GREENS

6 medium beets and their greens
Juice of 1 lemon
Salt to taste
Freshly ground black pepper to taste
1 tablespoon fresh thyme or
   1 teaspoon dried thyme
2 tablespoons butter, cut in small pieces

MAKES FOUR TO SIX SERVINGS

1. Rinse the beets and cut off and reserve the leaves. Steam beets, covered, in about 1 inch of water for about 25 minutes or until just tender.

2. Preheat oven to 350 degrees. Meanwhile, wash the beet greens and remove the ribs. When the beets are cooked, drain them. Immediately add beet greens to water in which the beets were steamed. Cook for about 2 minutes. Drain and cool.

3. Place the beets in cold water. Peel off the outer skin and cut beets into matchstick pieces, about 2 inches by ½ inch.

4. Squeeze water from the greens and chop fine. Scatter beets and greens in a small baking dish. Add lemon juice, salt, pepper, and thyme. Disperse butter over the top and bake for 15 minutes.

Reserve the water from steaming beets and greens, and use for stocks or soups. Freeze as soon as the liquid cools; use within 6 to 8 months.

BROCCOLI HARLEQUIN

1 small head cauliflower
2 small bunches broccoli
4 tablespoons butter
2–3 tablespoons plain yogurt (optional)
2 tablespoons grated Parmesan cheese
¼ teaspoon salt
Freshly ground black pepper to taste
¾ cup breadcrumbs, preferably made
   from whole-grain bread

MAKES SIX TO EIGHT SERVINGS

1. Break the cauliflower into flowerets and remove most of the white stalks. Steam the cauliflower for 3 to 4 minutes or until still firm.

2. Steam the broccoli for about 6 minutes or until soft enough to puree. Preheat oven to 350 degrees. Puree broccoli with butter and optional yogurt.

3. Lightly grease a 6-cup oven-proof dish, mound the cauliflower in it, and sprinkle with the cheese, salt, and pepper. Season the broccoli puree with salt and pepper; then spoon it over the cauliflower and sprinkle the top with the breadcrumbs. Bake for 20 minutes.

Reminder: You may want to substitute margarine for butter.

BRUSSELS SPROUTS WITH WATER CHESTNUTS

1½ quarts Brussels sprouts
1 quart chicken broth
  (recipe on page 226) or water
8½-ounce can water chestnuts, drained
4 tablespoons melted butter

MAKES TWELVE SERVINGS

1. Preheat oven to 350 degrees. Cut off the ends of the sprouts and trim as necessary. With the tip of a sharp knife, cut a cross about ¼-inch deep in the base of each sprout. Bring the stock to a boil in a large saucepan and cook the sprouts, uncovered, for 5 to 7 minutes, until just tender. Drain sprouts.

2. Butter a 2-quart casserole. Put the sprouts and water chestnuts in the casserole and pour the butter over them. Bake, uncovered, until thoroughly heated, about 20 minutes.

Save the broth or water and use for stock or soup. This is a dish appropriate for a buffet because it can be prepared ahead of time to the baking stage.

BROCCOLI WITH EGGS

Steam 4 stalks of broccoli until tender, and cut into thin strips. Soft-boil 4 eggs for 4 minutes. Lay the broccoli strips on a plate. Shell the eggs and chop them in a bowl. Blend in 4 to 6 tablespoons lemon juice with salt and pepper to taste. Spread this over the broccoli; garnish with paprika. Serve immediately.

MAKES FOUR SERVINGS

OVEN-ROASTED SWEET CORN IN THE HUSK

6 medium-sized ears fresh sweet corn,
  in the husk
Butter (optional)
Salt to taste
Freshly ground black pepper to taste

MAKES SIX SERVINGS

1. If corn husks seem dry, sprinkle lightly with water. Preheat oven to 400 degrees.

2. Lay ears one layer deep in a large, shallow roasting pan and roast, uncovered, in a hot oven for 30 minutes or until kernels are tender; to test, peel husks back on one ear and pierce a kernel with a toothpick—if no milky juices run out, corn is done. The kernels should be firm, tender, and taste faintly nutlike.

3. Remove ears from oven; husk and remove silks, and serve hot with butter, salt, and pepper.

PUEBLO CAULIFLOWER

1 head of cauliflower
½ cup toasted pumpkin seeds (optional)
¼ cup almonds
½ teaspoon cumin seeds, or ¼ teaspoon
  ground cumin
3 small, green, canned Tabasco peppers
1 large garlic clove, minced
4 tablespoons minced parsley
1 cup chicken broth, preferably
  homemade (recipe on page 226)
⅓ cup Monterey Jack cheese, grated

MAKES FOUR SERVINGS

1. Preheat oven to 350 degrees. Steam cauliflower for about 15 minutes, until just tender. Cool and break into flowerets.

2. Put pumpkin seeds, if used, almonds, and cumin seeds in a blender; spin until gritty. Remove seeds from canned peppers, add peppers to contents of blender, with garlic and parsley, and spin long enough to make a smooth paste.

3. Put this in a saucepan and add stock, a little at a time, while bringing mixture to a boil. Simmer for about 5 minutes and add drained cauliflower.

4. Mix well and turn into a baking dish; top with grated cheese. Bake for 10 minutes, until the cheese bubbles.

Cooking the Nutritious Way
Vegetables

PUREED CELERIAC

4 celeriac, about 2 pounds
2 potatoes, about 1 pound
½ teaspoon salt
Freshly ground white pepper to taste
½ cup milk

MAKES SIX TO EIGHT SERVINGS

1. With a stainless-steel knife or vegetable peeler, peel the celeriac and potatoes and cut into 2-inch cubes.
2. Steam them, covered, for about 25 minutes.
3. Pass the vegetables through a food mill or a food ricer. Season with salt and pepper to taste and stir in the milk to give the mixture a light consistency. Serve at once or keep warm in a double boiler over simmering water.

If you cannot find celeriac, make a puree from carrots and potatoes, or broccoli and potatoes. Do not use the food processor, which makes the potatoes gummy.

RED CABBAGE

3-pound head of red cabbage
2 tablespoons butter or vegetable oil
½ cup chopped onion
2 tart apples, such as Granny Smiths, peeled and cut into ½-inch dice
3 tablespoons red wine vinegar
2 teaspoons sugar
½ teaspoon salt

MAKES SIX SERVINGS

1. Preheat oven to 325 degrees. Remove any bruised leaves from the cabbage and discard them. Wash the head of cabbage under cold running water. Quarter it, then cut out and discard core. One at a time, lay each quarter on one flat side and shred it thinly.
2. Over medium heat, melt the butter or oil in a 4 to 6-quart casserole that has a tight-fitting cover. When the fat is very hot, stir in the onion and let it cook until lightly browned. Add the cabbage, apples, vinegar, sugar, salt, and 1 cup of water. Mix all the ingredients together, then remove the casserole from the heat.
3. Cut a circle of wax paper or brown paper large enough to fit into the casserole. Press it down onto the cabbage mixture. Cover the casserole and place it in oven. Braise for 1½ hours or until the cabbage is very soft. As the cabbage braises, check it from time to time; if it seems dry, add ½ cup water.

Leftover red cabbage will lose its color while stored in the refrigerator. To bring it back to its original color, stir in 1 or 2 tablespoons of red wine vinegar while reheating it. This technique works as well with green cabbage, but use white wine vinegar.

GREEN BEAN CASSEROLE

1½ pounds green beans, cut into 1½-inch lengths
1 tablespoon oil
2 tablespoons butter
1 clove garlic, finely minced
¾ cup chopped onion
¾ cup chopped green pepper
¼ cup chopped pimientos
2 cups tomato sauce, preferably homemade (recipe on page 261—Pasta Marinara)
Tabasco sauce to taste (optional)
1 cup grated sharp Cheddar cheese

MAKES SIX SERVINGS

1. Preheat oven to 350 degrees.
2. Rinse and drain the beans and put them in a 4-cup saucepan with cover. Add the oil. Do not add water or salt. Cover the beans and cook them over medium heat, shaking the pan occasionally so the beans do not stick. Cook for 5 to 10 minutes, depending on the age of the beans, until they are crisp-tender. Pour beans into a baking dish.
3. Meanwhile, melt the butter and cook the garlic, onion, and green pepper until the onion is translucent. Stir occasionally.
4. Add the pimientos, tomato sauce, and Tabasco sauce, if desired, to the onion mixture. Simmer briefly and pour the sauce over the beans. Sprinkle with the cheese and bake for 25 minutes.

GREEN CABBAGE AND GARLIC

Remove core and heavy stems from a small green cabbage and shred it. Place in a heavy saucepan with 2 peeled cloves of garlic, crushed, ¼ cup cider vinegar, and 1 cup of water. Cover and steam over low heat for 18 minutes. It should be a little crispy.   MAKES FOUR SERVINGS

Carrots with Dill

Preheat oven to 350 degrees. Cut 18 medium carrots in half lengthwise and slice them. Overlap the slices on a sheet of aluminum foil. Add 3 tablespoons butter, 1 tablespoon chopped fresh dill or 1 teaspoon dried dill, ½ teaspoon salt, and pepper to taste. Seal the carrots in the foil tightly. Cook on a baking sheet for 45 minutes or until tender. MAKES EIGHT SERVINGS

Stir-Fried Watercress with Carrots

8-ounce bunch watercress
2 tablespoons vegetable oil
½ pound carrots, grated
½ teaspoon salt
Freshly ground black pepper to taste

MAKES FOUR SERVINGS

1. Rinse the watercress in cold water; you do not have to dry it. Remove and discard 2 inches from stems, and chop what is left into 2-inch pieces.
2. In a 10-inch skillet, heat the oil. Stir in the carrots and sauté, over high heat, for about 30 seconds. Add watercress and stir it around until just wilted. Season with salt and pepper and serve immediately.

Other greens such as spinach or escarole can also be used instead of the watercress.

Baked Carrots and Apples

4-5 medium-sized carrots, unpeeled, cut into quarters lengthwise
1-3 apples, such as McIntosh or Delicious, unpeeled, quartered, cored, and sliced thinly
2 tablespoons butter
½ teaspoon salt
1 teaspoon grated lemon rind

MAKES FOUR SERVINGS

1. Combine carrots and apples in a heavy skillet.
2. Top with bits of butter, salt, lemon rind, and cover with 3 tablespoons of hot water.
3. Bring to a simmer, cover, and cook gently for about 20 minutes or until tender.

Instead of lemon rind, add a few tablespoons of toasted wheat germ for flavor.

Assorted Greens

4 pounds collard, mustard, turnip, or mixed greens
¼ pound salt pork, finely chopped
1 onion, minced
Pinch of crushed red pepper
Salt to taste

MAKES EIGHT SERVINGS

1. Remove large stems from greens and wash the greens thoroughly.
2. Put all ingredients and 2 cups of water in a large pot. Bring to a boil and simmer for 30 minutes to 1 hour, depending on the greens; the collards take the longest. They should be very tender.
3. Drain the greens and chop them fine. You can reserve the liquid from the greens for soups.

If fresh greens are not available, substitute 4 10-ounce packages of frozen greens and simmer them, without adding water, for about 20 minutes.

Baked Kale

2½ pounds fresh kale, spinach, or turnip greens
2½ tablespoons butter
2½ tablespoons all-purpose or whole-wheat flour
1 cup milk, scalded
½ cup grated Swiss or Jarlsberg cheese
½ teaspoon salt
½ teaspoon freshly ground black pepper
½ teaspoon ground nutmeg
Dash of hot pepper sauce
½ cup breadcrumbs, preferably whole grain

MAKES FOUR TO SIX SERVINGS

1. Preheat oven to 425 degrees. Wash kale several

Cooking the Nutritious Way
Vegetables

times under cold water. Discard faded or yellowing leaves; remove tough center ribs. Steam, covered, for about 15 minutes or until tender. Cool and press out liquid from the kale. Chop kale finely.

2. Melt butter in a heavy saucepan, over low heat; whisk in flour. Cook and stir for 2 minutes. Whisk in the milk. Add ¼ cup of cheese and the salt, pepper, nutmeg, and hot pepper sauce. Cook, stirring constantly, until thick. Add the chopped kale.

3. Transfer mixture to a buttered baking dish; sprinkle with breadcrumbs and remaining cheese. Bake until golden brown and bubbly, 15 to 20 minutes.

MUSTARD GREENS AND ONIONS

1 tablespoon vegetable oil
1 large red onion, finely chopped
2-3 broccoli stalks
1 bunch mustard, turnip, or collard greens, about ½ pound
2 teaspoons soy sauce

MAKES FOUR SERVINGS

1. Heat the oil in a large skillet over medium heat. Sauté onion for 2 to 3 minutes or until transparent.

2. Trim coarse ends from broccoli stalks, slice stalks thinly, on the diagonal, and add to onions. Sauté for 2 minutes.

3. Trim ends from greens, chop coarsely, and stir into mixture. Combine ¼ cup water with soy sauce and pour over vegetables.

4. Reduce heat, cover and steam for about 10 minutes or until cooked to taste. Toss gently and serve immediately.

PEAS AND LETTUCE

Place 1½ cups freshly shelled, or frozen, peas, along with 1 small head of Boston lettuce, cut in fourths, ¼ cup dry white wine, ¼ cup water, and ¼ teaspoon salt and pepper to taste in a heavy saucepan. Bring to a simmer and cook gently for 10 minutes, covered.   MAKES FOUR SERVINGS

LETTUCE AND ASPARAGUS STEW

1½ pounds asparagus
1 firm Boston lettuce
2 tablespoons butter
3 small bunches scallions, trimmed and thinly sliced, green and white parts
½ teaspoon salt
Freshly ground pepper to taste
1 tablespoon minced fresh herbs such as parsley, chives, or tarragon
4 slices whole-grain toast

MAKES FOUR SERVINGS

1. Break the asparagus at its tender point and cut stalks into 2 or 3 pieces.

2. Give the lettuce core a hard knock on the edge of a counter and twist it out. Rinse lettuce, discarding any blighted outer leaves. Dry and cut into thin strips.

3. Melt butter and gently stew the scallions until they start to become tender. Add the asparagus and scatter the lettuce over all. Season with salt and pepper, cover the pan, and turn up the heat to medium high. Shake the pan from time to time. In 4 or 5 minutes the asparagus should be just cooked, and the lettuce will have melted down into the onions, forming a delicious stew. Stir in the herbs and serve on toast.

BRAISED JERUSALEM ARTICHOKES

2 pounds Jerusalem artichokes
Vinegar or lemon juice
2 cups dry red wine
4 tablespoons butter
½ teaspoon salt
Freshly ground black pepper to taste
2 tablespoons finely chopped parsley

MAKES SIX TO EIGHT SERVINGS

1. Preheat oven to 350 degrees. Peel the Jerusalem artichokes—a good, sharp paring knife is essential—and put them in a bowl of water with a little vinegar or lemon juice until they are all ready for cooking. Then drain them.

2. Put the Jerusalem artichokes, wine, butter, and salt and pepper in a heavy pan with a tight-fitting lid. Bring to a boil on top of the stove, then cover and cook in the oven for 30 minutes. Test for doneness with a fork or toothpick. They should be firm like properly done potatoes.

3. Take Jerusalem artichokes out of the liquid with a slotted spoon. Over high heat, reduce the liquid in the pan to ¾ cup and pour it over the artichokes. Serve them at room temperature, sprinkled liberally with chopped parsley.

Peppers and Eggplant

3 tablespoons olive oil
1 medium red onion, cut into 1-inch pieces
4 green or yellow sweet peppers, seeded and cut into ½-inch rings
2 medium eggplants, cut into 1-inch pieces
1 cup canned tomatoes, with juice
Salt to taste
Freshly ground black pepper to taste

MAKES SIX SERVINGS

1. Put olive oil in a flameproof casserole. Add onion to the casserole. Make a layer of peppers on top of onion in the casserole. Place eggplant pieces on top of the peppers. Add the tomatoes and sprinkle with salt and pepper. Do not mix.
2. Cover the casserole with a lid and place it on a medium flame. Simmer for 20 minutes without mixing; then mix thoroughly and taste for salt and pepper.
3. Simmer for 15 minutes more, uncovered, mixing every so often with a wooden spoon. Transfer to a serving dish.

Reminder: You may want to substitute vegetable oil for olive oil.

Steamed New Potatoes in Broth

1 pound unpeeled new potatoes, scrubbed and sliced
2 tablespoons lemon juice
¼ cup chicken broth, preferably homemade (recipe on page 226)
¼ cup minced parsley or scallions
½ teaspoon salt
Freshly ground black pepper to taste

MAKES FOUR SERVINGS

1. Steam the potatoes, covered, over 1 inch of simmering water for about 15 minutes, or until they are tender.
2. Heat together the lemon juice, broth, parsley or scallions, salt, and pepper. Put steamed potatoes into a bowl, toss with broth mixture, and serve.

Potato-Tomato Bake

2 large potatoes, scrubbed
2 large onions, sliced thin
3 large tomatoes, cut into fairly thick slices
2 tablespoons butter
¾ cup grated Romano or Parmesan cheese
1 teaspoon cayenne pepper or, if you do not like it hot, 2 teaspoons paprika
½ teaspoon salt

MAKES FOUR SERVINGS

1. Preheat oven to 375 degrees. Boil or steam the potatoes in their jackets, until firm, and slice them.
2. In a well-greased baking dish, place layers of onions, potatoes, and tomatoes, dotting each layer with butter and a sprinkling of cheese. End with potatoes, again dotting with butter and sprinkling with the rest of the cheese, cayenne pepper or paprika, and salt.
3. Bake for 1 hour, until the onions are well cooked and the tomatoes have released their juice and the potatoes have absorbed it.

Reminder: You may want to substitute margarine for butter.

Roasted Onions

As an accompaniment to meat or poultry, try these instead of deep-fried onion rings. Heat 1 tablespoon of oil in a heavy 10-inch skillet. When smoking hot, add 1 pound Spanish onions, cut into ¾-inch slices. Do not stir but let the onions sizzle and roast undisturbed for 30 seconds. Now stir, and keep roasting, tossing and turning for 2 minutes, just until onions are translucent. Fold in 2 tablespoons coarsely chopped parsley. The onions should be crisp and sweet, not limp.   MAKES SIX SERVINGS

Cooking the Nutritious Way
Vegetables

RUTABAGA PANCAKES

1 egg
2 tablespoons milk or yogurt
½ teaspoon salt
Freshly ground black pepper to taste
2 cups, about ½ pound, coarsely grated peeled rutabagas, white turnips, or daikon radish
½ cup finely chopped scallions or onion
2-4 tablespoons vegetable oil

MAKES EIGHT PANCAKES

1. In a small bowl, whisk together the egg, milk or yogurt, salt, and pepper. Stir in grated rutabaga or other root vegetable and scallions or onion.
2. Heat oil in a heavy iron skillet. Make 4 pancakes, each with a quarter cupful of the mixture. Put mixture into skillet and press down with a spatula. When brown on bottom, turn over and brown on second side, again pressing down with the spatula. When brown, remove to a baking dish large enough to hold the pancakes.
3. Preheat oven to 350 degrees. Repeat the procedure for the other 4 pancakes. Put baking dish in oven and let pancakes finish cooking for 8-10 minutes.

These pancakes are delicious served with pork, turkey, or roast chicken.

TURNIP-POTATO PUREE

4 cups diced yellow or white turnips
4 cups diced potatoes
2 cups boiling chicken broth, preferably homemade (recipe on page 226)
1 tablespoon light-brown sugar
¼ teaspoon freshly ground black pepper
2 tablespoons finely grated onion
½ cup finely grated sharp Cheddar cheese
3 tablespoons butter

MAKES SIX SERVINGS

1. Place the turnips and potatoes in a saucepan. Add the broth and sugar. Cover and simmer until vegetables are tender, about 15 minutes. Drain well and mash.
2. Add the remaining ingredients and beat well.

To vary this dish, use sweet potatoes instead of white potatoes, and omit the sugar.

CRISP SHREDDED TURNIPS

Shred 4 to 6 medium, unpeeled turnips, and simmer them, covered, in a skillet with two tablespoons hot milk for five minutes. Season with ½ teaspoon salt, freshly ground black pepper, and cayenne pepper.

MAKES FOUR SERVINGS

SPINACH CREAMED WITH PEACHES

2 pounds fresh spinach, stalks removed
¼ teaspoon salt
2 medium peaches, preferably very ripe
2 teaspoons lemon juice
Freshly ground black pepper to taste

MAKES FOUR SMALL SERVINGS

1. Thoroughly wash the spinach in cold water, without shaking the water off the leaves. Put at once into a big pot, over high heat. As it sizzles and steams, salt and mash down with a wooden spoon. This should take about 2 to 3 minutes.
2. Turn off heat and let cool enough to handle, then take handfuls of the spinach and squeeze out as much water as possible. You may reserve this "water" for soups or stews. Chop drained spinach finely and reserve.
3. Plunge peaches into boiling water for 2 minutes. When cool enough to handle, remove skins. Remove stones and chop peaches coarsely.
4. Put the spinach and peach pieces into the bowl of a food processor, blender, or a hand food-mill. Puree until mixture is smooth, but do not let it become liquefied.
5. Transfer this mixture to a skillet and set it over medium heat until it begins to bubble merrily. Stir almost continuously to avoid the danger of burning. Let it continue to bubble until you have evaporated enough water to bring the puree to the stiffness you want—about 5 minutes. Finally, work in the lemon juice and season to taste with pepper.

For another low calorie and nutritious idea, instead of peaches, try creaming spinach with pears. It is just as delicious.

Acorn Squash and Cranberries

2 firm medium-sized acorn squash
2 tablespoons butter
2 tablespoons sherry
1 cup cooked cranberries, fresh or canned

MAKES FOUR SERVINGS

1. Preheat oven to 375 degrees. Wash squash and cut them into halves, but do not remove seeds and pulp.
2. Bake squash, in a little hot water, in a shallow baking pan until they are tender, usually about 30 to 40 minutes.
3. Scoop out seeds and pulp, and fill cavity of each squash with butter and sherry. Return to oven for a few minutes. At serving time, fill cavity with cooked cranberries.

Squash and Onions

1 butternut squash, about 2 pounds
1 tablespoon corn or vegetable oil
3 medium, yellow onions, thinly sliced
½ teaspoon oregano
½ cup vegetable broth or water
½ teaspoon salt

MAKES SIX SERVINGS

1. Scrub the squash and cut into 2-inch pieces.
2. Heat the oil in a 2-quart saucepan, add the onions and sauté until transparent.
3. Add the squash and oregano and sauté for another 2 to 3 minutes. Add the broth or water and salt. Reduce heat, cover, and cook for 25 minutes.

Zucchini and Fresh Dill

1½ pounds unpeeled, washed zucchini
1 tablespoon white wine vinegar
2 tablespoons minced fresh dill
¼ teaspoon salt
Freshly ground black pepper to taste

MAKES FOUR SERVINGS

1. Cut the zucchini into 2 by ¼-inch strips.
2. Steam zucchini for about 3 minutes or until it is just cooked and still bright green. Drain and pat dry.
3. Arrange zucchini in a serving bowl and toss quickly with vinegar, dill, salt, and pepper. Serve immediately as this cools quickly.

Grated Zucchini

2 pounds zucchini or yellow summer squash
½ teaspoon salt
2 tablespoons butter
½ small onion, finely chopped
Freshly ground black pepper to taste
½ lemon
2-3 tablespoons chopped parsley

MAKES FOUR SERVINGS

1. Scrub the zucchini or yellow summer squash and cut off the ends. Grate and put into a colander. Toss lightly with salt and leave to drain for 30 minutes.
2. When ready to cook, squeeze the zucchini in a potato ricer to extract all liquid, which you can reserve for another use.
3. Melt the butter in a large heavy skillet and sauté the onion over low heat until soft. Add zucchini and cook over medium-high heat, stirring and tossing constantly, for 3 to 4 minutes, until cooked but still crisp. Season with salt, if necessary, pepper, juice of the lemon, and the parsley. Serve immediately.

If you don't have a potato ricer, lay zucchini on a piece of cheesecloth, make a ball, and squeeze out the liquid.

Baked Cherry Tomatoes

3 pint-size baskets cherry tomatoes
⅓ cup or more olive oil
½ teaspoon salt
Freshly ground black pepper to taste
Chopped fresh parsley
Chopped fresh basil or other fresh green herbs

MAKES TWELVE SERVINGS

1. Preheat oven to 350 degrees.

Cooking the Nutritious Way
Vegetables

2. Put the tomatoes in one layer in a rectangular cake pan or a small roasting pan. Brush with olive oil, shake pan, and brush the uncoated sides until the tomatoes are lightly but completely coated with oil. Sprinkle with salt and pepper and bake for about 10 minutes. Begin checking at 8 minutes. Tomatoes should cook long enough to warm through and soften a bit, but do not bake until the skins begin to split.

3. Put in a warm serving dish and sprinkle with parsley and basil.

Reminder: You may want to substitute vegetable oil for olive oil.

Vegetable Stew

2 medium-sized onions, sliced thinly
3 cloves garlic, peeled and crushed
2 medium unpeeled potatoes, cut into 1-inch dice
1 small eggplant, cut into 1-inch dice
4 tablespoons butter
½ teaspoon salt
Freshly ground black pepper to taste
2 stalks celery, thinly sliced
1 stalk fresh broccoli, sliced
3 medium-sized carrots, thinly sliced
½ cup dry red wine
2 small zucchini, cut into 1½-inch chunks
3 tablespoons tomato paste
3 fresh tomatoes, peeled and diced
½ pound fresh mushrooms, thinly sliced
3 tablespoons molasses
1 tablespoon fresh dill weed

MAKES SIX TO EIGHT SERVINGS

1. In a heavy stew pot, sauté onions, garlic, potatoes, and eggplant in the butter. Season lightly with salt and pepper.

2. After 10 minutes, or when the potatoes begin to get tender, add celery, broccoli, carrots, and wine. Cover and steam over low heat for about 5 minutes.

3. Then add the zucchini, tomato paste, tomatoes, mushrooms, molasses, and dill. Cover and simmer over low heat for 20 minutes. Remove cover and correct seasoning.

Freeze leftover tomato paste in a small, tightly covered container. If fresh dill is unavailable substitute 1 teaspoon of dried dill.

Colache
(Mexican Vegetable Medley)

2 tablespoons vegetable oil
1 pound unpeeled, washed zucchini, thinly sliced
1 small onion, thinly sliced
½ cup diced green or red pepper
⅔ cup diced fresh tomato
1½ cups corn kernels, fresh or frozen
Freshly ground black pepper

MAKES EIGHT SERVINGS

1. Heat oil in a heavy, large skillet. Sauté zucchini, onion, and pepper until limp, about 10 minutes. Stir occasionally to prevent burning.

2. Add ½ cup water, tomato, and corn. Cover and cook for 5 minutes or until squash is tender, adding more water if necessary. Season heavily with pepper.

Mediterranean Ratatouille

2 medium-sized onions, peeled and sliced
1 garlic clove, minced
5 tablespoons olive oil
2 small zucchini, about 1-pound size, washed and thinly sliced
2 small eggplants, about 1-pound each, peeled and cubed
2 medium-sized green peppers, washed, stems and seeds removed, cut into 1-inch strips
5 medium-sized tomatoes, peeled and quartered, or 2 cups canned tomatoes, coarsely chopped
2 tablespoons freshly snipped basil or 1 teaspoon dried basil leaves
2 tablespoons freshly snipped parsley
½ teaspoon salt
¼ teaspoon freshly ground black pepper

MAKES EIGHT TO TEN SERVINGS

1. Using a large, heavy skillet, sauté onions and garlic in 2 tablespoons oil for 5 minutes.

2. Add zucchini, eggplant, and green pepper to skillet, adding more oil as needed. Stir gently but thoroughly. Sauté mixture for 10 minutes.

3. Stir in the tomatoes, basil, parsley, salt, and pepper. Reduce heat, cover skillet tightly, and continue to simmer for 15 minutes longer. Serve immediately.

This is also good cold or as a first course.

Salads

Asparagus Salad

2 tablespoons vegetable oil
2 tablespoons sesame seeds
2 teaspoons honey (optional)
3 tablespoons cider vinegar or
   white wine vinegar
1 teaspoon soy sauce
1-1½ pounds fresh asparagus

MAKES FOUR SERVINGS

1. Sauté sesame seeds in oil for about 1 minute, or until lightly browned; remove from heat. Stir in honey, if used, and allow to cool. Blend in vinegar and soy sauce. Set aside.
2. Meanwhile, break asparagus at lower end of stalks, where the green top merges with the white bottom, and discard ends. Steam for 5 minutes or until tender but not limp. Pour sauce over hot asparagus, turning stalks to cover evenly. Refrigerate.
3. Serve on a bed of cold, cooked brown rice.

Bean Sprout Salad

1 cup carrots, shredded
½ cup sweet red pepper, shredded
2 scallions, white and green parts,
   thinly sliced
2 cups mung bean sprouts
¼ cup pine nuts or almonds
5 tablespoons red wine or rice vinegar
2 tablespoons soy sauce
½ tablespoon sesame-seed oil
3 tablespoons peanut oil
¼ teaspoon freshly ground black pepper

MAKES FOUR TO SIX SERVINGS

1. Refrigerate the vegetables until ready to use.
2. Preheat oven to 350 degrees and roast the nuts for 15 minutes.
3. For the salad dressing, mix the remaining ingredients in a bowl. Just before serving, toss the dressing with the vegetables and nuts until well mixed. Serve immediately.

Try other raw vegetables such as snow peas, green pepper, and broccoli.

Israeli Carrot Salad

In a bowl combine 1 pound carrots, washed and grated, ½ cup orange juice, 2 tablespoons sesame seeds (optional), ½ cup raisins, 2 oranges, peeled and sectioned. Chill. Serve on lettuce leaves.

MAKES FOUR SERVINGS

Bean Salad

1 cup cooked dried, or canned, drained
   kidney beans
1 cup cooked dried, or canned, drained
   chick-peas
½ cup sliced carrots
¼ cup chopped onion
3 tablespoons chopped sweet pickle
¼ teaspoon salt
⅛ teaspoon freshly ground black pepper
½ teaspoon dry mustard
3 tablespoons red or white wine vinegar
1 tablespoon honey (optional)
¼ cup vegetable oil

MAKES FOUR SERVINGS

1. Mix vegetables and pickle in a bowl.
2. Thoroughly mix remaining ingredients and pour over vegetable mixture. Mix gently.
3. Chill at least 1 hour before serving.

This improves with marinating time. You could also serve this as a first course.

White Rabbit Salad

In a bowl combine 3 cups cottage cheese with 2 small apples, chopped, ¼ cup raisins, ½ cup chopped toasted nuts, ¼ cup toasted sunflower seeds, 2 teaspoons poppyseeds, 1 to 2 tablespoons honey, and juice of ½ lemon. Serve very cold on greens. Among optional additions are fresh, firm pears or peaches, green seedless grapes, orange sections, or melon.

MAKES SIX SERVINGS

Cooking the Nutritious Way
Salads

LOUISIANA SWEET POTATO SALAD

To 1 cup grated, peeled, raw sweet potato, add 2 cups diced apples, ½ cup broken pecans, ¾ cup seedless raisins, ¼ cup diced celery, and ½ cup mayonnaise. Serve chilled, on lettuce.

MAKES FOUR TO SIX SERVINGS

CRISP RUTABAGA SALAD

½ cup grated raw rutabaga
   or white turnip
½ cup thinly sliced celery
2 scallions, including green part, chopped
2 radishes, sliced paper thin
3 cups shredded Romaine lettuce
3 tablespoons olive or vegetable oil
1 tablespoon white wine vinegar
½ teaspoon salt
½ teaspoon freshly ground black pepper
⅛ teaspoon dry mustard
¼ teaspoon sugar (optional)
¼ teaspoon dried basil or
   1 tablespoon fresh basil

MAKES FOUR SERVINGS

1. Combine the rutabaga, celery, scallions, radishes, and Romaine in a bowl. Chill well.
2. Combine the remaining ingredients in a jar and shake. Chill. Toss the salad with the dressing just before serving.

FENNEL SALAD

Remove the green stalks and tough outer leaves from fennel heads. Slice the tender white hearts into wafer-thin slices. Sprinkle with a little salt and pepper, olive oil, and lemon juice to taste. Let stand for 1 to 2 hours before serving.

ONE HEAD OF FENNEL MAKES TWO SERVINGS

BEETS WITH TUNA

2 cups sliced steamed beets
1 small red onion, sliced
1 7-ounce can tuna, packed in olive oil
   or water
Juice of ½ lemon
1 tablespoon minced parsley
Salt to taste
Freshly ground black pepper to taste
2 tablespoons olive oil (optional)

MAKES FOUR SERVINGS

1. Mix all ingredients together. If you use tuna packed in water, add the optional olive oil.
2. Serve at room temperature.

POTATO SALAD TZAPANOS

3 pounds boiling potatoes, preferably
   new potatoes
1½ pounds carrots
¼ cup olive oil
⅓ cup white wine vinegar
2 teaspoons salt
4 teaspoons dried dill weed, or
   3 tablespoons minced fresh dill
2 cloves garlic, minced

MAKES EIGHT TO TEN SERVINGS

1. Steam the potatoes in their jackets until they are just tender. Drain them immediately and allow them to cool.
2. Scrape the carrots, cut them into large pieces and steam or boil them until they are tender; drain them and let them cool.
3. Cut the potatoes into ½-inch dice and coarsely chop the carrots. Combine them in a large bowl with all the remaining ingredients and toss the mixture until thoroughly blended. Chill the salad for several hours and toss it once more before serving.

To vary the recipe, add either 1 cup fresh green beans, washed, cut, and steamed, or ½ head cauliflower, separated into flowerets, and steamed, or 1 large cucumber, peeled, seeded, and diced. Or add all three of these and make extra dressing. Instead of dill you could substitute ¼ cup chopped fresh parsley or a combination of fresh herbs such as basil and tarragon.

Rice Salad Vinaigrette

⅓ cup finely diced carrots
¾ cup string beans, cut into ¼-inch bits
¼ cup diced celery
¼ cup diced green bell pepper
½ cup chopped red onion
3 tablespoons minced fresh parsley
2½ cups cooked rice, preferably brown, warm or cold
4 tablespoons grated Parmesan cheese
4 tablespoons olive oil
3 tablespoons white wine vinegar
Pinch of salt and pepper
Pinch dried thyme, basil, and oregano

MAKES FOUR TO SIX SERVINGS

1. Steam the carrots and green beans until they are barely tender, and drain immediately.
2. Combine the first 7 ingredients in a large bowl and toss together.
3. Combine the cheese, olive oil, vinegar, and seasonings and whisk until smooth. Pour the dressing over the salad, toss, and chill for several hours.

Gado Gado
(Indonesian Salad)

2 large potatoes, cut into 2-inch dice
½ cup water
3 medium carrots, sliced thin
½ pound string beans, cut into 1-inch-long pieces
1 cup shredded cabbage
1 cup mung bean sprouts
1 medium cucumber, diced
1 small green pepper, seeded and diced
4 hard-cooked eggs, each cut in half lengthwise
6 tablespoons unhomogenized peanut butter
2 teaspoons molasses
1 large garlic clove, minced
¼ teaspoon cayenne pepper
1–1½ cups beef broth
½ teaspoon salt
1 or more teaspoons lemon juice to taste

MAKES SIX TO EIGHT SERVINGS

1. In a 3-quart saucepan, combine the potatoes and water. Cover and simmer for about 3 minutes.
2. Add the carrots and string beans. Cover and simmer for 2 minutes.
3. Add cabbage and simmer for another 5 minutes. Drain well.
4. On a large platter, arrange a bed of the steamed vegetables. In a decorative pattern, arrange the remaining vegetables—the sprouts, cucumber, and pepper—on top of the steamed ones. Arrange the egg halves in the center or on the outer edge. Serve with peanut-butter sauce.
5. To make sauce, in a small saucepan combine all the remaining ingredients and, stirring constantly, bring to a simmer. (If you do use peanut butter with added oil, use less liquid.) The sauce should be thick but pourable. Remove from heat and serve warm.

Tabouli
(Middle Eastern Salad)

1 cup dry bulgur or cracked wheat
1½ cups boiling water
1 teaspoon salt
¼ cup fresh lemon or lime juice
1 generous teaspoon minced fresh garlic
¼ cup olive or vegetable oil
½ teaspoon dried mint
½ cup chopped scallions, including greens
2 medium tomatoes, diced
1 packed cup chopped fresh parsley
½ cup cooked chick-peas
1 chopped green pepper (optional)
½ cup coarsely grated carrot (optional)
1 chopped cucumber or summer squash (optional)
Freshly ground black pepper to taste

MAKES SIX TO EIGHT SERVINGS

1. Combine bulgur or cracked wheat, boiling water, and salt in a bowl. Cover and let stand for 15 to 20 minutes, or until the bulgur or cracked wheat is chewable.
2. Add lemon or lime juice, garlic, oil, and mint and mix thoroughly. Cover and refrigerate for 2 to 3 hours.
3. Just before serving add the vegetables and mix gently. Correct seasonings.

Bulgur or cracked wheat is available in specialty food stores. If you cannot find it, substitute 1 cup brown rice, boiled or steamed until tender. Serve as filling in Middle Eastern pita, or pocket, bread.

Cooking the Nutritious Way
Salads

HALIBUT SALAD WITH DILL

1 quart water
1 large stalk celery with a few leaves
1 thick slice lemon
6 peppercorns
2 tablespoons salt
3 pounds halibut, preferably cut in a thick steak or chunk, with center bone in
3 teaspoons lemon juice
½ teaspoon ground white pepper
2 tablespoons minced fresh dill
¾ cup mayonnaise, as needed
Boston or Romaine lettuce

MAKES SIX SERVINGS

1. Bring water to a boil with celery, lemon slice, peppercorns, and salt. Gently lower the fish into the boiling water, then cover and reduce the heat until the water is at a barely perceptible simmer. Poach the halibut for 10 to 12 minutes, depending on thickness, until firm and white through to the bone.
2. Remove the fish from the liquid and drain. Let cool. Trim off the skin and break the fish away from the bone. Remove all small bones from the edges if there are any. Working with 2 forks, break the cooled fish into small clumps or pieces. Try not to shred or mash it. Sprinkle with lemon juice and a pinch of salt and pepper. Add the dill and toss lightly. Add the mayonnaise and fold it in gently with a wooden spoon, being careful not to break the fish any more than you have to. There should be just enough mayonnaise to bind the mixture. Check the seasoning. Chill thoroughly for 5 to 7 hours. Serve on cold, crisp, lettuce leaves.

To vary the recipe, substitute cooked shrimp, crab meat, or lobster meat for the halibut.

CHICKEN SALAD

To 2 cups leftover cold chicken, cut into bite-size pieces, add 1 carrot, thinly sliced, 3 tablespoons white wine vinegar, ½ teaspoon salt, 2 cloves, pinch of mace or nutmeg, and pinch of pepper. Marinate overnight in white wine to cover. Next day, drain, remove cloves, and toss with 2 tablespoons olive oil. Arrange on spinach leaves.
MAKES TWO SERVINGS

Pasta, Grains, Legumes

SPAGHETTI ALLA MATRICIANA

4 cups fresh ripe tomatoes
¼ cup diced bacon
1 medium onion, chopped
Hot pepper to taste
1 pound spaghetti
½ cup grated Parmesan or Romano cheese

MAKES SIX SERVINGS

1. Drop tomatoes into boiling water. Quickly remove them and slip off their skins. Cut tomatoes into pieces and run through food mill, food processor, or blender.
2. Cook bacon until fat is rendered. Add onion and continue to simmer, uncovered, until onion is translucent. Add tomatoes and pepper. Simmer, uncovered, for 5 to 10 minutes.
3. Cook spaghetti until firm but cooked through. Drain, and serve with sauce and grated cheese.

PASTA E FAGIOLI
(Noodles and Beans)

4 slices bacon or 4 tablespoons vegetable oil
2 medium onions, roughly chopped
2 cloves garlic, minced
1 carrot, chopped
1 green pepper, seeded and chopped
1 15-ounce can tomatoes, drained and roughly chopped
4 cups water, more if necessary
2 cups dried red or brown lentils
2 bay leaves
2 teaspoons dried thyme
1 tablespoon dried oregano
3 tablespoons chopped fresh basil or 1 tablespoon dried basil
1 pound thin spaghetti, plain or whole wheat
Freshly grated Parmesan cheese, about ½ cup

MAKES EIGHT SERVINGS

1. In a large heavy kettle, sauté the bacon or heat the oil. When crisp, or when oil is hot, add the onion,

garlic, carrot, and green pepper. When the onion is golden, add the tomatoes and water and bring to a boil.

2. Reduce to a simmer, then add the lentils gradually, stirring constantly.

3. Add the herbs and simmer for 1 hour or more, until the lentils are tender.

4. Add the thin spaghetti and more water, if necessary. Cook for 8 minutes more, or until the spaghetti is cooked al dente (firm to the bite). Remove bay leaves. Serve in bowls, with a side dish of freshly grated Parmesan cheese.

Pasta Marinara

4 cups canned Italian plum tomatoes, drained
 and roughly chopped, or 4 cups peeled,
 seeded, and chopped fresh tomatoes
3 tablespoons olive oil
4 medium onions, finely chopped
2 cloves garlic, minced
½ teaspoon salt
Freshly ground black pepper to taste
1 tablespoon chopped fresh oregano or
 1 teaspoon dried oregano
1 tablespoon chopped fresh basil or
 1 teaspoon dried basil
1 bay leaf
1 pound spaghetti
½ cup grated Parmesan cheese (optional)

MAKES ONE QUART OF SAUCE
OR FOUR TO SIX SERVINGS

1. Put the tomatoes through a food mill and set aside.

2. Heat oil in a heavy saucepan and sauté the onion until golden, stirring occasionally. Add the garlic and sauté for 2 minutes more, then add the tomatoes, salt, pepper, and herbs and simmer for 30 minutes, partially covered.

3. Boil the pasta in water until firm. Drain well, put into a serving bowl, and serve with the sauce and freshly grated Parmesan cheese on the side.

This is a wonderful sauce to serve with roast chicken or turkey, with broiled fish such as bluefish, and with many other dishes that call for tomato sauce. Make double the amount and freeze the other half in 1-cup portions. The sauce will keep for a week in the refrigerator and for months in the freezer. Reminder: You may want to substitute vegetable oil for olive oil.

Linguine with Broccoli

1 bunch broccoli, about 1¼ pounds
6 tablespoons olive or vegetable oil
2 teaspoons minced garlic
½ teaspoon crushed red pepper
½ cup chicken broth, preferably
 homemade (recipe on page 226)
Freshly ground black pepper to taste
1 pound linguine, preferably whole grain

MAKES EIGHT SERVINGS

1. Cut broccoli flowerets off stems. Cut stems into bite-size pieces. There should be about 6 cups of stem pieces and flowerets.

2. Steam broccoli for about 3 minutes and drain. Do not overcook; broccoli must remain crisp. Run cold water over broccoli to chill quickly.

3. Heat oil in a large skillet and add garlic. Cook briefly without browning. Add broccoli and toss to heat through. Add crushed red pepper, broth, and black pepper and bring to a boil.

4. In a separate large pot, bring 4 quarts of water to a boil. Cook linguine until cooked through but still firm, or follow package directions.

5. Drain pasta and toss with hot broccoli mixture. Serve immediately on warm plates.

Whole-grain pastas can be found in specialty food stores and in some supermarkets.

"Dirty" Rice

2 cups long-grain white rice
6 cups chicken broth, preferably
 homemade (recipe on page 226) or water
1 bay leaf
1 cup finely chopped onion
2 tablespoons vegetable oil
¼ pound chicken livers
¼ pound chicken gizzards
1 clove garlic, finely minced
¾ cup finely chopped scallions, including
 green part
½ cup finely chopped parsley
½ teaspoon salt
Freshly ground black pepper to taste

MAKES SIX TO EIGHT SERVINGS

1. Preheat oven to 350 degrees. Place the rice in a

Cooking the Nutritious Way
Pasta, Grains, Legumes

1½-quart saucepan and add 4 cups of broth or water and the bay leaf. Cover, bring to a boil, and simmer for exactly 15 minutes.

2. Cook the onion in the vegetable oil until almost brown. Chop the livers and gizzards fine and add them. Cook, stirring, until brown, about 10 minutes. Add the garlic, scallions, and parsley. Season with salt and pepper and add the remaining broth. Combine the partially cooked rice and the chicken-giblet mixture and pour all into a baking pan. Bake for 15 minutes.

Brown rice can be used. Cook the rice for about 40 minutes before baking it.

BLACK BEANS AND RICE

2 cups dried black beans, about 1 pound
1½ teaspoons salt
2 tablespoons vegetable or olive oil
2 large onions, chopped
2 large garlic cloves, minced
1 pound ground chuck beef
1 teaspoon dried thyme
1½ tablespoons ground cumin
3 tablespoons chili powder
2 cups beef broth or water
6 cups fluffy cooked rice,
    preferably brown

MAKES SIX TO EIGHT SERVINGS

1. Cover beans with 6 cups of water. Bring to a boil, simmer for 1 minute, turn off heat, cover, and soak beans for 1 hour. Drain beans and discard soaking water.

2. Cover drained, soaked beans with 2 quarts water, bring to a boil and simmer for ½ hour; add 1½ teaspoons salt and simmer for ½ hour more.

3. Meanwhile, heat the oil in a heavy skillet and sauté the onion, garlic, and ground beef for about 5 minutes. Stir in thyme, cumin, and chili powder and stir fry for a couple of minutes. Pour in broth or water, stir, simmer briefly, and set aside.

4. Preheat oven to 325 degrees. After 1 hour of simmering, put beans and their liquid in a deep ovenproof casserole with a cover. Stir the meat and onion mixture into the beans. There should be ½ inch of liquid above the beans; if there is not, add some boiling water.

5. Set the casserole, covered, in the middle of the oven and bake for about 1½ hours or until the beans are tender. Serve with rice and salad.

INDIAN KEDGEREE
(Rice and Lentils)

1 large onion, sliced
1½ tablespoons olive oil
2 teaspoons curry powder
1 cup long-grain rice, preferably brown
1 cup lentils
2½ cups chicken broth (recipe on page 226)
    or water
1 bay leaf
½ teaspoon salt
Freshly ground black pepper to taste
2 large hard-boiled eggs, sliced
Chopped parsley
Lemon quarters

MAKES FOUR TO SIX SERVINGS

1. Preheat oven to 350 degrees. In a 3-quart flameproof casserole, sauté the onion in the olive oil for about 5 minutes. Add the curry powder, stir in the rice, and cook for 2 to 3 minutes.

2. Add the lentils, broth, bay leaf, and salt and pepper, and bring to a simmer. Cover and transfer casserole to oven and cook for about 40 to 45 minutes or until all the broth is absorbed and lentils are tender.

3. Serve steaming hot, garnished with eggs, chopped parsley, and surrounded with quarters of lemon to squeeze on top.

This also makes a delicious one dish meal.

GREEN RICE

Place 2 cups of long-grain brown rice with 1 quart of water and ½ teaspoon salt in a heavy saucepan. Bring to a boil, cover, and simmer for 45 minutes, until firm but not hard on the inside. Preheat oven to 325 degrees. Transfer rice to a baking pan, cover with a clean towel, and bake for 30 minutes. Correct the seasoning and stir in ½ cup packed, finely chopped fresh parsley. MAKES SIX TO EIGHT SERVINGS

Haitian Black Beans

2 cups dried black beans, soaked
2 cups chopped onion
1 cup chopped green pepper
2 large garlic cloves, mashed
2 medium bay leaves
½ teaspoon salt
Freshly ground black pepper to taste
¼ teaspoon oregano
¼ teaspoon thyme
3 tablespoons vinegar, preferably cider
4-ounce jar pimientos, chopped

MAKES SIX TO EIGHT SERVINGS

1. Simmer the soaked and drained black beans in 4 cups of water for 30 minutes.
2. Add onion, green pepper, garlic, bay leaves, salt, pepper, oregano, and thyme and continue to simmer for 1½ hours.
3. Add the vinegar, mixing thoroughly, and simmer for another minute.
4. Fifteen minutes before serving, mix in the pimientos and stir often during this final period to avoid scorching. Serve with brown rice.

Hoppin' John
(Black-Eyed Peas and Rice)

2 ham hocks (optional)
1 bay leaf
2 onions, chopped
1 celery stalk, diced
½ teaspoon crushed red pepper
2 cups dried black-eyed peas
4 cups cooked rice, preferably brown

MAKES TEN SERVINGS

1. Place ham hocks in a large saucepan. Add water to cover and simmer for about 30 minutes. (If you do not use ham hocks, omit this step and add vegetables and flavorings to simmering peas.)
2. Add bay leaf, onions, celery, and red pepper.
3. Sort out and discard any discolored or damaged peas. Rinse remainder well and add to the pot. If necessary, adjust water level so that the peas are well covered. Simmer slowly until tender and liquid level is low, about 2 hours.
4. Fluff rice into peas. Adjust seasoning and cook over low heat until all the liquid is absorbed.

Boston Baked Beans

¼ pound salt pork
1 small onion, sliced
1½ cups dried navy or pinto beans, soaked
¼ cup molasses
½ teaspoon dry mustard
½ teaspoon salt
Freshly ground black pepper to taste

MAKES SIX SERVINGS

1. Preheat oven to 325 degrees. Simmer the salt pork in boiling water for 15 minutes, drain, cut off the rind, and cut the salt pork into small pieces.
2. Put the onion and pork into an oven-proof baking pot, preferably earthenware.
3. Add the drained beans, molasses, and mustard. Pour in water to 1 inch above the beans and bake, covered, for about 6 hours, taking care to keep enough liquid in the pot.
4. Fifteen minutes before serving, season with salt and pepper. Serve with whole-grain bread such as whole wheat or cornmeal.

If you wish to omit the salt pork, add 1 more chopped onion and 2 cloves of garlic, minced, for flavor.

White Beans in Olive Oil

2 cups dried white beans, soaked
4 garlic cloves, crushed
2 medium onions, chopped
2 medium carrots, finely diced
½ cup olive oil
½ teaspoon salt
2 tablespoons white wine vinegar or fresh lemon juice
2 teaspoons sugar
3 tablespoons chopped fresh parsley

MAKES EIGHT TO TEN SERVINGS

1. Place soaked and drained beans in a large saucepan with 4 cups of water, or enough to cover by 1 inch, and simmer, covered, for 45 minutes.
2. Add garlic, onions, carrots, olive oil, and salt. Continue to simmer slowly, covered, until beans are tender, about 45 minutes more.
3. Stir in vinegar or lemon juice and sugar and cook for another 5 minutes. Serve at room temperature or cold, in a large bowl, garnished with parsley.

Cooking the Nutritious Way
Pasta, Grains, Legumes

KIDNEY BEANS WITH RED CABBAGE AND APPLES

1 small red cabbage, about 5 inches in diameter, shredded
3 onions, sliced
1 pound cooking apples, cored, quartered, and sliced
2 cups cooked red kidney beans
¼ teaspoon allspice
¼ teaspoon ground cinnamon
¼ teaspoon thyme
2 cloves garlic, minced
1 teaspoon finely grated orange rind
½ teaspoon salt
Freshly ground black pepper to taste
2 tablespoons brown sugar
1¼ cups red wine
2 tablespoons red wine vinegar

MAKES SIX SERVINGS

1. Preheat oven to 325 degrees. Steam the cabbage, covered, for 5 minutes.
2. In a deep casserole, layer the cabbage, onion, apples, and beans, seasoning each layer with the spices and the thyme, garlic, orange rind, and salt and pepper. Sprinkle brown sugar over the top, then add the wine and wine vinegar, diluted in a little hot water.
3. Cover and simmer slowly, in the oven, for 30 to 45 minutes, or until tender but not too mushy, adding a little more wine if necessary.

ROASTED CHICK-PEAS

1 clove garlic, peeled
3 tablespoons olive oil
1 pound dried chick-peas
½ teaspoon salt

MAKES FOUR CUPS

1. Place the flat side of a knife blade over the garlic and press down hard. Put crushed clove in oil and leave to steep.
2. Cover chick-peas generously with water and bring to a boil. Boil for 2 minutes, turn off heat, cover and let soak for 1 hour. Drain and pat dry. Preheat oven to 350 degrees.
3. Place chick-peas in an uncrowded baking pan. Remove garlic and pour oil over the beans, making sure each is lightly moistened. Sprinkle with salt and bake for about 40 minutes.
4. Blot any excess oil. Serve as a snack and as a light hors d'oeuvre with radishes.

Reminder: You may want to substitute vegetable oil for olive oil.

GRATIN OF CHICK-PEAS WITH SPINACH

2 pounds spinach, picked over, stems removed, and washed
2 medium tomatoes, peeled, seeded, and coarsely chopped
3 tablespoons olive oil
3 cloves garlic, peeled and sliced paper thin
½ cup chopped parsley
Pinch of dry, crumbled savory
¼ teaspoon salt
12 almonds
2 hard-boiled eggs
Pinch of cayenne
2 cups cooked chick-peas
½ cup stale bread, preferably whole wheat, crusts removed, crumbled

MAKES FOUR TO SIX SERVINGS

1. Steam spinach for a couple of minutes in water that clings to the leaves. Drain and press out liquid, which you can save for later. Chop and reserve, covered, in a bowl, until later.
2. Stew the tomatoes gently in olive oil with the garlic, parsley, and savory for about 15 minutes. Season lightly with salt.
3. In a blender or food processor, pound the almonds to a paste with egg yolks and cayenne; slice the egg whites thinly.
4. Preheat oven to 400 degrees. Combine the chick-peas, tomato mixture, almond and egg-yolk mixture, and the sliced egg whites with some of the reserved spinach liquid. Bring to a simmer and stir, crushing some of the chick-peas to lend greater body to the sauce. Mix in the spinach and add salt, if desired.
5. Pour the mixture into a lightly oiled baking dish. Sprinkle crumbled bread on top and bake for 20 minutes or until the mass is bubbling hot.

If fresh spinach is unavailable, you can substitute two 10-ounce packages of frozen spinach. Let thaw before adding to the mixture.

Vegetarian Nut Patties

1 cup soft breadcrumbs, preferably whole grain
1 tablespoon butter, melted
1 cup cooked long-grain rice, preferably brown
1 teaspoon sage
½ teaspoon paprika
¾ cup chopped cashews or pecans
¾ cup chopped walnuts
2 eggs, beaten
½ teaspoon salt
¼ teaspoon celery seed or salt
1 teaspoon minced onion
2 tablespoons vegetable oil

MAKES FOUR TO EIGHT SERVINGS

1. Combine thoroughly all the ingredients except the oil. Adjust seasoning.
2. Form into small patties and sauté in the oil for about 2 or 3 minutes on each side. They should be golden brown. Serve hot.

This makes 8 servings as an appetizer but 4 as a main course.

Kasha and Red Peppers

3-4 medium-sized red sweet peppers or a combination of red and green
1 medium-large onion, cut into ½-inch dice
2 tablespoons olive oil
1 egg
1½ cups whole-grain kasha (roasted buckwheat groats)
½ teaspoon salt
1 teaspoon dried, summer savory leaves, crumbled
2¼ cups boiling water
Freshly ground black pepper to taste

MAKES SIX SERVINGS

1. Steam peppers for about 5 minutes. Run under cold water to cool. Gently remove stems, ribs, and seeds. Cut into ½-inch dice.
2. In a heavy saucepan, cook the onion in the oil until slightly softened. Add the peppers and cook for a minute over medium heat. Scrape into a dish and set aside. Keep the saucepan handy.
3. In a small bowl, beat the egg. Add the kasha and stir until all the grains are coated. Scrape the mixture into the pan in which the vegetables were cooked. Stir over moderate heat for a few minutes or until all the grains are dried and separated. Add salt, savory, boiling water, pepper, and the vegetables. Return to a boil.
4. Turn the heat to its lowest point, cover the pan, and cook for 15 minutes. Remove from the heat and let stand for 15 minutes or so. Turn into a fairly wide, oven-proof serving dish, fluffing the grains. Let rest at room temperature, or refrigerate, covered, overnight.

To serve hot or to reheat the next day, preheat oven to 375 degrees, cover the kasha with foil, and leave until heated through, about 30 minutes if chilled, slightly less if room temperature.

Kasha Stuffing

2 cups kasha (roasted buckwheat groats), preferably fine, but medium will do
4 large eggs, lightly beaten
4 cups boiling water
½ teaspoon salt
3 tablespoons vegetable oil
1 medium onion, chopped
¼ pound fresh mushrooms, coarsely chopped
Freshly ground white pepper to taste

MAKES ABOUT FOUR CUPS OF STUFFING

1. Put the kasha in a bowl and add ½ the beaten eggs, stirring until eggs are absorbed. Turn into a cold skillet and slowly heat, stirring frequently, until the kasha grains are dry and separate and just beginning to brown. Pour in the boiling water and salt. Stir once, then simmer, covered, over moderately low heat until all the water is absorbed and the kasha is half cooked, about 10 minutes.
2. Heat the oil in a skillet and in it slowly sauté the onion until it begins to soften; do not brown. Add the mushrooms, raise the heat, and sauté for a minute or two, or until the liquid evaporates.
3. Combine the sautéed onion and mushrooms with the kasha and stir. Taste and adjust the seasoning with salt and pepper. Stir in the remaining beaten eggs.

This stuffing may be used for chicken, turkey, or other poultry, and breast of veal. It can be prepared ahead and refrigerated, but do not stuff the bird until just before roasting. This recipe makes enough stuffing for a 10 to 15-pound turkey.

Cooking the Nutritious Way
Pasta, Grains, Legumes

BULGUR WHEAT WITH YOGURT

2 tablespoons vegetable oil
1 onion, finely chopped
2 celery stalks, finely chopped
1 cup bulgur wheat
1½ cups chicken broth, preferably homemade (recipe on page 226) or water
¼ teaspoon salt
Freshly ground black pepper to taste
2 tablespoons plain yogurt
2 tablespoons minced fresh parsley

MAKES FOUR SERVINGS

1. Heat oil in a 9-inch skillet. When hot, add onions and celery and sauté over medium heat for about 5 minutes or until onions are translucent.
2. Add bulgur wheat and continue to sauté for 1 minute more. Add broth or water, salt, and pepper. Cover and simmer, over low heat, for 15 minutes or until the wheat is tender. If it is not tender enough, just simmer it a bit longer. Taste for seasoning and adjust.
3. Turn off heat and stir in yogurt and parsley.

Bulgur wheat is available in specialty food stores and in some supermarkets.

FRUITED BULGUR

¼ cup butter
1 large onion, minced
¾ cup slivered blanched almonds
1 pound bulgur wheat
4½ cups beef, chicken (recipe on page 226), or vegetable (recipe on page 227) broth
¾ cup dried apricots, cut up
¼ cup raisins or currants

MAKES TEN SERVINGS

1. Preheat oven to 350 degrees. Melt the butter in a large heavy skillet. Sauté the onion and almonds in the butter until golden. Add the bulgur and cook until the bulgur begins to turn golden.
2. Add the stock, apricots, and raisins or currants and place in a deep baking dish. Bake for 40 to 45 minutes, until all the liquid is absorbed.

Serve this as an accompaniment to meat or poultry instead of rice. Bulgur wheat is available in specialty food stores and some supermarkets.

FARINA DUMPLINGS

2 eggs, beaten
2 tablespoons melted butter or margarine
¼ teaspoon salt
1 cup farina or cream of wheat
¼-⅓ cup milk

MAKES EIGHT DUMPLINGS

1. Bring a pot of salted water to a boil.
2. Meanwhile, combine eggs, butter or margarine, salt, and farina or cream of wheat in a bowl; mix well. Add milk, enough to make a stiff dough.
3. Turn heat off under boiling water, and drop the mixture by spoonfuls into water.
4. Turn heat on, bring to a simmer and cook, covered, for 10 to 15 minutes or until tender. Test by tearing one dumpling apart with 2 forks. The inside should be moist and fluffy; if not, simmer for a couple more minutes. Serve hot with melted butter or yogurt.

This makes a fine accompaniment to main courses that have a lot of sauce or gravy, such as pot roast.

BARLEY CASSEROLE

2 tablespoons butter
2 tablespoons minced shallots or onion
¼ pound fresh mushrooms, finely chopped
1 cup medium pearled barley
2-2½ cups chicken broth, preferably homemade (recipe on page 226)
Pinch of salt
Freshly ground black pepper to taste
¼ cup thinly sliced scallions
2 tablespoons chopped fresh parsley

MAKES SIX SERVINGS

1. Preheat oven to 350 degrees. Over medium heat, melt the butter in a 2-quart casserole that has a tight-fitting cover. When the butter is hot, stir in the shallots or onion and cook until they are transparent. Add the mushrooms and cook until they are soft. Stir in the barley and pour in 2 cups of the chicken broth. Add salt and pepper to taste. Bring the mixture to a boil over high heat and immediately remove from heat.
2. Cover the casserole, place it on the middle shelf of the oven, and bake for 45 minutes or until all the broth has been absorbed and the barley is tender. If the barley looks too dry, add the other ½ cup broth, cover

the casserole, and bake for 15 minutes longer.

3. Remove the casserole from oven. With a fork, lightly stir the scallions and parsley through the barley; serve from the casserole.

SCALLION-CHEESE CEREAL

1 cup thinly sliced scallions
¼ teaspoon salt
Freshly ground pepper to taste
1 cup whole-grain cereal
1 cup creamed cottage cheese

MAKES FOUR CUPS

1. Bring 3 cups of water, scallions, salt, and a grating of black pepper to a boil in a heavy 1½-quart pot.

2. Stir in cereal, bring to a boil, then lower heat and simmer, uncovered, for 5 minutes. Turn off heat, cover pan, and let stand for 5 minutes. Stir in cottage cheese.

This makes a good and nourishing breakfast on a cold morning or a side dish to meat and fish.

GRANOLA

3 cups rolled oats
1 cup sesame seeds
1 cup sunflower seeds
1 cup chopped almonds (optional)
1 cup chopped walnuts
½ cup wheat germ
½ cup unsalted peanuts
⅓ cup oil
½ cup honey
2 cups raisins
1 cup chopped dried apricots

MAKES ELEVEN CUPS

1. Preheat oven to 250 degrees. Combine oats, sesame seeds, sunflower seeds, almonds, walnuts, wheat germ, and peanuts with oil and honey and just enough water to moisten, about ¼ cup.

2. Spread mixture in 2 baking pans or on cookie sheets and roast slowly for about 1 hour. Turn heat up to 350 degrees and roast for another 15 minutes or until dark brown. Cool.

3. Add raisins and apricots and store, covered, in the refrigerator.

Breads

PANCAKE MIX

1 cup rye flour
1 cup whole-wheat flour
2 cups all-purpose flour
½ cup yellow cornmeal, preferably stone-ground
2 tablespoons baking powder
1½ teaspoons salt
½ teaspoon baking soda

MAKES THREE BATCHES, EACH SUFFICIENT FOR 12 TO 14 FOUR-INCH PANCAKES

1. Sift the flours, cornmeal, baking powder, salt, and soda into a bowl, using a wide-meshed sieve. With a large whisk, mix them very thoroughly for at least 30 seconds.

2. Measure the mix into three plastic bags or other containers, putting 1¾ cups into each. If any mix is left over, divide it among the bags. Close the containers and store them at room temperature.

You can vary this mix by using 2 cups of whole-wheat flour and omitting rye, or by increasing the cornmeal by ½ cup and decreasing one of the flours by ½ cup.

OATMEAL PANCAKES

1⅓ cups milk
1 cup rolled oats
2 tablespoons vegetable oil
2 eggs, beaten
½ cup whole-wheat flour
1 tablespoon brown sugar
1 teaspoon baking powder
¼ teaspoon salt

MAKES TEN TO TWELVE FOUR-INCH PANCAKES

1. Combine the milk and rolled oats in a bowl and let them stand at least 5 minutes.

2. Add the oil and beaten eggs, mixing well. Then stir in the flour, sugar, baking powder, and salt. Stir just until the dry ingredients are moistened.

3. Cook on a hot, lightly oiled griddle, using ¼ cup of batter for each pancake. Turn them when the tops are bubbly and the edges slightly dry.

Cooking the Nutritious Way
Breads

BUTTERMILK PANCAKES

1 batch pancake mix (recipe on page 267)
¼ teaspoon baking soda
2 eggs
1⅔ cups buttermilk, or more if needed
2 tablespoons melted butter or vegetable oil

MAKES 12 TO 14 FOUR-INCH PANCAKES
1. Sift the mix and the soda together.
2. In a mixing bowl, beat the eggs with a whisk until well mixed, then whisk in the 1⅔ cups of buttermilk and the melted butter or oil.
3. Add the sifted dry ingredients and mix with a fork just until the dry ingredients are moistened. Leave the batter lumpy (add more buttermilk if too thick).
4. Bake the pancakes on a hot griddle, greased or not, depending on the manufacturer's instructions, ladling out a scant ¼ cup of batter for each cake. Turn the pancakes when 1 or 2 of the bubbles on top have burst and the edges begin to lose their gloss. Then bake the second side until no more steam rises, or until the light touch of a finger leaves no imprint. Serve the pancakes on warmed plates with warm honey.

To make pancakes with milk, use only 1¼ cups of milk, and omit the soda.

CORNBREAD

2 cups cornmeal, yellow or white, preferably stone-ground
1 tablespoon baking powder
¼ teaspoon salt
1 egg, lightly beaten
1 cup milk
2 tablespoons honey
¼ cup vegetable oil

MAKES EIGHT PIECES
1. Preheat the oven to 400 degrees. Grease an 8 by 8 by 2-inch baking pan.
2. Mix cornmeal, baking powder, and salt thoroughly. Mix egg, milk, honey, and oil. Add to cornmeal mixture.
3. Stir only until dry ingredients are moistened. Batter will be lumpy. Pour into pan and bake for 20 minutes or until lightly browned. When cool, cut into 8 pieces, 2 by 4 inches each.

Stone-ground cornmeal is available in specialty food stores and in some supermarkets.

SEASONED BREADCRUMBS
To 3 cups of fresh breadcrumbs, preferably made from whole-wheat bread, add 3 tablespoons wheat germ, ¼ teaspoon marjoram, thyme, or sage, 2 teaspoons black pepper, 1 teaspoon salt, and 1 teaspoon grated lemon or lime rind. Keep in a tightly sealed container for 1 week in refrigerator, or frozen for longer periods of time.
MAKES THREE AND ONE-HALF CUPS

CORN PONE

2 cups white cornmeal, preferably stone-ground
1 teaspoon baking powder
½ teaspoon salt
⅔ cup cold water
½ cup milk
1 tablespoon melted butter

MAKES FOUR PONES
1. Preheat oven to 375 degrees. Sift the cornmeal, baking powder, and salt into a mixing bowl.
2. Add the water and milk. Stir well. Add melted butter and let the mixture rest for 10 minutes.
3. Shape the batter into round forms by cupping both hands together and patting it into form.
4. Place each pone upon a baking sheet, 1 inch apart from the others, and bake for 15 to 20 minutes, no longer, or the bread will dry out.

WHOLE-WHEAT BAKING POWDER BISCUITS

2 cups whole-wheat flour
2 teaspoons baking powder
½ teaspoon salt
¼ cup butter or margarine
¾ cup milk, buttermilk, or yogurt

MAKES TWENTY BISCUITS
1. Preheat oven to 450 degrees. Stir together flour, baking powder, and salt.
2. Cut in butter or margarine, blending in with a

fork until dough has the consistency of cornmeal. Add milk, buttermilk, or yogurt and stir well.

3. Turn dough onto a lightly floured board and pat lightly with floured hands until dough is ½-inch thick. Cut into 2-inch rounds with a floured glass or a biscuit cutter. Place on a slightly greased baking sheet, close together for soft sides, or about 1 inch apart for crusty sides, and bake for about 12 minutes.

For a lighter biscuit use 1 cup whole-wheat flour and 1 cup all-purpose white.

BREAD STUFFING

⅓ cup chopped celery
1 small onion, chopped
1 garlic clove, peeled
¼ cup vegetable oil
2 medium tart apples, washed, cored, and coarsely grated
2 cups stale bread, preferably whole wheat, cut into cubes
¼ teaspoon nutmeg
¼ teaspoon freshly ground black pepper
1 tablespoon brown sugar

MAKES FOUR SERVINGS

1. Slowly sauté celery, onion, and garlic in 1 tablespoon of oil for about 10 minutes. Remove the garlic.
2. Preheat oven to 350 degrees. Add remaining oil, apples, bread, nutmeg, pepper, and brown sugar to celery mixture and mix together lightly.

This makes enough stuffing for an 8- to 10-pound turkey—or bake as a side dish for 25 minutes.

CROUTONS

Preheat oven to 350 degrees. Remove crusts from 4 medium slices of bread, preferably whole grain. Spread bread very thinly with butter or margarine. Then sprinkle on about 1 teaspoon of herbs and spices of your choice, if you wish. Cut bread into ½-inch cubes and bake on a cookie sheet for about 20 to 25 minutes or until golden. Remove and cool. Use immediately or store, covered tightly, in the refrigerator.

MAKES ABOUT TWO CUPS

OATMEAL-BANANA MUFFINS

1½ cups rolled oats
¾ cup milk
1 egg, beaten lightly
½ cup vegetable oil
⅓ cup firmly packed light or dark-brown sugar
1 large ripe banana, peeled and mashed
1¼ cups sifted all-purpose flour or unsifted whole-wheat flour
4 teaspoons baking powder
¼ teaspoon salt

MAKES EIGHTEEN MUFFINS

1. Preheat oven to 425 degrees. Soak the oats in the milk in a mixing bowl for 30 minutes, or until all the milk has been absorbed.
2. Combine the egg, oil, sugar, and mashed banana, beating until smooth, and stir into the oat mixture.
3. Combine the dry ingredients in a second mixing bowl and make a well in the center. Pour in the banana-oat mixture and stir lightly—just until the dry ingredients are moistened. Do not overbeat, or your muffins will be tough and shot through with tunnels.
4. Grease muffin pans or line with crinkly paper cupcake liners and spoon in the batter, half filling each cup. Bake for 15 minutes or until the muffins are lightly browned and springy to the touch.

BANANA-NUT BREAD

1¾ cups whole-wheat flour
½ cup sugar
1 tablespoon baking powder
¼ teaspoon salt
½ cup chopped walnuts
⅓ cup vegetable oil
2 eggs
2 medium bananas, mashed, about 1 cup

MAKES ONE LOAF: EIGHTEEN SLICES

1. Preheat oven to 350 degrees. Grease a 9 by 5 by 3-inch loaf pan.
2. Mix flour, sugar, baking powder, salt, and nuts.
3. Mix oil and eggs together. Mix in bananas.
4. Add dry ingredients to banana mixture; stir until just smooth and pour into loaf pan. Bake for 45 minutes or until firmly set when lightly touched on top.
5. Cool on rack; remove from pan after 10 minutes.

Cooking the Nutritious Way
Breads

Baking Yeast Breads at Home

Because of the renewed interest in whole grains and the concern in adding fiber to our diet, more people are once again baking their own bread.

Bread is a simple food. Few ingredients and little equipment are needed to make it. The basic ingredients are yeast, flour, and water or other liquids: yeast to make the dough rise, flour to provide substance and structure, and liquid to give the bread moisture. Sweeteners add flavor, help in browning, and activate the yeast. Many recipes call for white cane sugar, but molasses, brown sugar, and honey can also be used. Shortening makes bread more tender, provides additional flavor, improves keeping quality, and helps form a brown crust. Butter, margarine, or any bland cooking oil such as vegetable oil can be used. If the bread recipe is especially rich in heavier flours such as rye, or eggs, candied fruit, or nuts, it will take longer to rise. Salt adds flavor and slows down the action of the yeast, thereby preventing it from rising too quickly.

The incomparable smell, taste, and texture of a loaf of homemade, preservative-free bread is well worth the effort, especially since breadmaking is not nearly as time-consuming as many believe. Measuring, mixing, kneading, and shaping can be accomplished in 30 minutes or less. Rising takes longer; but this is a process that occurs by itself.

You may have to make a few loaves before you bake the perfect one. Every step is important, but the instructions in *italic* throughout this section are keys to the success of the finished product.

Mixing the Ingredients. Be sure that all ingredients are at room temperature when you begin. If the flour and yeast have been refrigerated, allow time to bring them to room temperature.

To begin, sprinkle the yeast over the lukewarm liquid in a large mixing bowl that has been rinsed in hot water and then dried (a warm bowl will help the action of the yeast). *The temperature of the water in the bowl should be between 105 and 115 degrees. A temperature higher than 115 degrees will kill the yeast and the bread will not rise.* To test the temperature, put a few drops of water on your wrist; it should feel only slightly warm, not hot. Use a candy thermometer that registers below 115 degrees if you are not confident with the water-on-your-wrist method.

Let the yeast and water mixture stand for 5 to 10 minutes "to proof," or "prove," the yeast—that is, to test if it is active. Active yeast produces small bubbles or foam on the surface of the water. If no bubbles or foam appear, the yeast is dead. Start over again with another package or cake of yeast. It is more economical to throw out the yeast-water mixture than to discard a batch of dough that did not rise.

Once the yeast has proofed, stir in the lukewarm liquid (not over 115 degrees), shortening, sweetener (if used), and salt.

Now you are ready to add the flour. With a wooden spoon or an electric mixer, gradually beat in one cupful of flour at a time. *Thorough mixing distributes the yeast and develops the gluten in the flour.* When the dough is too stiff to beat, work in the remaining flour with your hands. If you are using a heavy-duty mixer with a dough hook, continue to add the flour and let the dough hook do the final mixing.

One of the most important secrets of making bread is to use as little flour as possible and still be able to handle the dough. You may not need all the flour called for in the recipe. The dough should feel slightly damp, but not sticky. Any flour added beyond this point will make the bread heavy. Remember that the amount of flour given in a bread recipe can only be approximate, since flours vary greatly in their capacity to absorb moisture, and differ from one locale to another. Experience will help you judge the correct amount.

There are tasty and nutritious flours and meals such as rye, barley, soy, buckwheat, oat, and corn that are heavier than regular all-purpose wheat flour and have little or no significant gluten content. If you vary the basic recipe on page 272 by using a larger amount of such flours or meals, add approximately ¼ cup of gluten flour to your recipe to help the dough rise. Gluten is the protein portion of the wheat grain and can be bought in most specialty food stores. It is expensive, but a little goes a long way and it can be stored in your refrigerator.

Kneading the Dough. Kneading helps to distribute the yeast throughout the dough and develops the texture. The gluten in the flour makes a kind of network that traps the yeast bubbles. Turn out the dough onto a lightly floured board, marble slab, or counter-top. Sprinkle the dough lightly with flour. One method of kneading is to vigorously push the dough away from you, with the heels of your hands. Fold the dough in half, give it a quarter turn, and repeat the pushing, folding, and turning for about 10 minutes or until the dough is smooth and elastic. Another method of kneading is to hold the edge of the dough with only one hand and push with the other, then repeat the pushing, folding, and turning as above. Whichever method you use, try to develop a rhythmic motion. About every fifth turn or so, break your rhythm. Lift the dough about 2 feet above the work surface and crash it down on the board. This helps to develop the gluten even more. Generally, about 10 minutes of kneading is sufficient. If you use a heavy-duty machine with a dough hook, 5 minutes of kneading is usually sufficient. Form the dough into a ball.

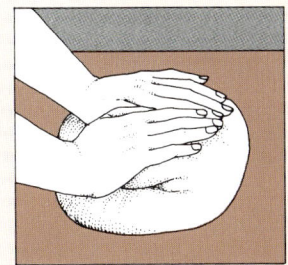
Kneading, method one.

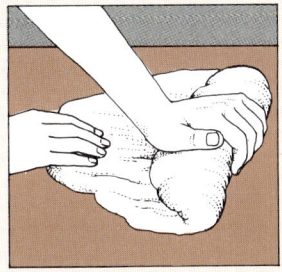
Kneading, method two.

First Rising. Grease a large, clean mixing bowl with about 1 tablespoon of oil or softened butter. Place the ball of dough into the bowl, turn the dough over, and roll it in the bowl so that its whole surface is greased. This will keep the dough from drying out and cracking as it rises. Cover with a clean, slightly damp kitchen towel or plastic wrap and let rise in a warm, draft-free place (80 to 85 degrees) for about 1½ to 2 hours or until doubled in bulk—that is, until it is twice the original size. If the room is cold, place the bowl in a pilot-lighted oven, or on a rack over (not in) a pan of hot water in a cold oven, or place the bowl inside a larger bowl containing warm water (not above 130 degrees), cover, and replace warm water as it is needed.

Because dough that has doubled in bulk is difficult to judge accurately by the eye, it is best to use the following test. *Make an indentation by pressing a finger into the dough about ½ inch deep. If the dough does not spring back, it has risen enough.*

If the dough has failed to rise at all after an hour and a half, do not despair. Dissolve a fresh packet of yeast in a small amount of lukewarm water and work it well into the ball of dough. Grease the surface of the dough with oil or softened butter and set it in the bowl to rise again.

When risen sufficiently, punch the dough down with your fist to deflate it. Pull the edges toward the center and turn it out on a lightly floured board. Knead well for a few moments or pound the dough with your fist to force out the gas bubbles.

If the dough has risen at an inconvenient time for you to shape and bake it, let it rise again and then proceed with the shaping, as described above.

Cut the dough in half with a sharp knife and shape each half into a smooth ball. Cover with a towel or plastic wrap and let rest about 5 minutes to make it easier to shape.

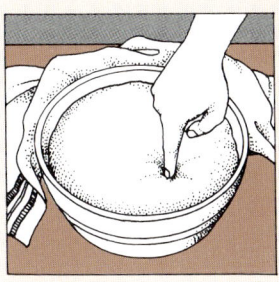
Testing the dough.

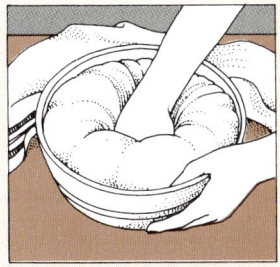
Punching down risen dough.

Shaping the Dough. Use a rolling pin or your fists to flatten each ball of dough into a rectangle about 2 inches wider than the length of the pan you are using and about 12 inches long. (A popular size loaf pan measures 8½ inches by 4½ inches by 2 inches.) Roll the dough up tightly from the short side like a jelly roll. Next, press the ends together to seal them, and fold about 1 inch of each end underneath the roll. *Lift the loaves carefully and place them in greased pans with their seam sides down.*

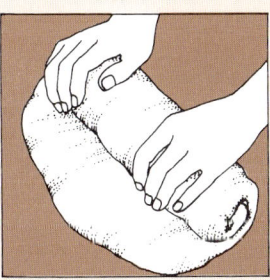
Rolling the dough.

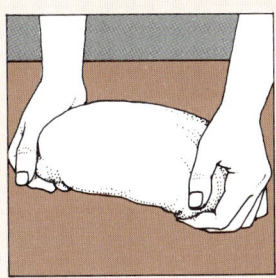
Shaping the loaf.

Cooking the Nutritious Way
Breads

Second Rising. Cover the pans with a clean towel or waxed paper. Do not use plastic wrap at this stage because it may stick to the dough and cause it to collapse when the plastic is removed. *As before, let the dough rise in a warm, draft-free place until it has doubled in bulk.* If it has not risen enough, the bread will be heavy. If it has risen a little too much, the bread will not be seriously affected; however, excessive rising can change texture and flavor and result in a bread that is full of large holes. *To test, press your finger about ½ inch deep into the edge of the dough. If the dent remains, the dough is ready for baking.* The purpose of this second rising is to give the dough a finer grain. This rising will take less time than the first rising—¾ to 1¼ hours is typical.

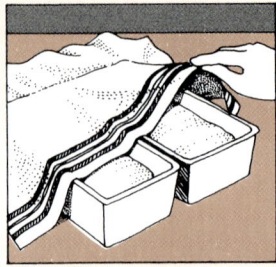
Start of the second rising.

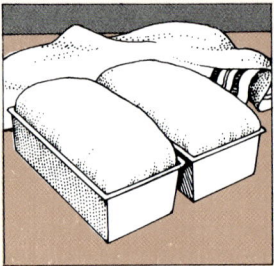
Loaves ready for baking.

For an old-fashioned look, dust the bread lightly but evenly with white flour just before baking.

Baking the Bread. Preheat oven to 375 degrees. Place the bread pans so that their tops are as close to the center of the oven as possible. You may have to place the loaves on the lower rack of the oven so that the tops will be in the center. To permit adequate circulation of hot air, the pans should not touch each other or the sides of the oven. Bake the length of time suggested in the recipe you are following. If the bread begins to brown too much, lower the oven temperature.

To test for doneness, take a potholder in each hand, turn the loaf out of the pan, and tap the bottom of the bread with your finger; it should sound hollow. If it is soft on the bottom, return the loaf to the pan, and bake an additional 5 to 10 minutes, and test again. Some home bakers return the bread to the oven without the pan. This method will make the bread crisper.

Remove the pans from the oven and immediately turn out the loaves on their sides on a wire rack to cool in a draft-free location. Let cool completely—about 2 to 3 hours—before slicing.

Storing. Freshly baked breads can be stored at room temperature for a few days either in the bread box or covered with a towel; or they can be wrapped in plastic or waxed paper and refrigerated for about a week. For longer storage, wrap breads in aluminum foil and freeze; they will keep for months in the freezer. To improve the texture of refrigerated bread, sprinkle lightly with water, wrap in foil, and reheat in a moderate oven for about 10 to 15 minutes. Frozen loaves can be taken directly from the freezer and reheated in the foil in a moderate oven for about 35 minutes.

WHOLE-WHEAT BREAD

1 package active dry yeast
½ cup lukewarm water (105 to 115 degrees)
1 cup milk
1 cup boiling water
2 tablespoons shortening
2 tablespoons molasses, preferably blackstrap, honey, or sugar (optional)
2 teaspoons salt
Approximately 3 cups all-purpose flour, preferably unbleached
Approximately 3 cups whole-wheat flour, preferably stone-ground
1 tablespoon shortening (for greasing the bowl)
⅛ cup gluten flour (optional)

1. Sprinkle the yeast over the lukewarm water. Stir. Let stand for 5 to 10 minutes to proof.
2. In a separate bowl, mix the milk, boiling water, shortening, molasses, honey, or sugar, if used, and salt. Let cool to lukewarm (105 to 115 degrees) and add to the yeast mixture. Wash, dry, grease the second bowl and set aside.
3. With a wooden spoon or electric mixer, gradually beat in the all-purpose flour—about 1 cup at a time. Then gradually beat in the whole-wheat flour. When the dough becomes too stiff to beat, work in the remaining flour by hand. You may not need to use the entire amount.
4. Knead, let rise.
5. When double in bulk, punch down the dough. Grease 2 baking pans (8½ by 4½ by 2 inches).
6. Shape dough into 2 loaves and place loaves in baking pans. Let rise again.
7. Preheat oven to 375 degrees.
8. Bake for about 50 minutes.

Desserts

POACHED FRESH PEACHES WITH RASPBERRY SAUCE

¾ cup sugar
2 cups water
1 tablespoon vanilla extract
6-8 whole peaches, peeled
1 cup fresh raspberries or a 10-ounce
  package frozen raspberries

MAKES SIX TO EIGHT SERVINGS

1. Combine sugar, 2 cups water, and vanilla in a saucepan. Bring to a boil and simmer for 5 minutes. Add peaches, and simmer until tender when pierced with the point of a sharp knife. Baste occasionally. Chill peaches in syrup.
2. Combine in the container of an electric blender all except a few raspberries for garnish with ¼ cup of poaching syrup. Blend and strain to eliminate seeds. If you are using the frozen raspberries, thaw them first, then puree in electric blender or food processor, without additional syrup, and strain.
3. Arrange chilled peaches in serving dish. Just before serving, cover with raspberry sauce and garnish with raspberries.

Freeze the remainder of the poaching liquid if you wish, and use to poach other fruit.

GINGER PEARS

4 cups dry white wine
2 tablespoons sugar
Strip of orange rind, about 2 inches
  in length
10 paper-thin slices fresh ginger,
  (about a 1-inch piece)
1 tablespoon vanilla extract
2 teaspoons orange liqueur
½ lemon
8 medium-sized pears

MAKES EIGHT SERVINGS

1. Place wine, sugar, orange rind, ginger, vanilla, and liqueur in a straight-sided skillet that will hold the pears snugly. Bring the wine to a boil, reduce heat, cover, and simmer this syrup for 15 minutes.
2. Meanwhile, fill a large mixing bowl with water, and squeeze in the juice of the lemon half. Peel the pears, leaving the stems intact. Remove a slice from the bottom of each pear, to insure that it will stand upright, and drop them into lemon water to keep them from turning brown.
3. Place the pears in the simmering syrup, cover, and poach for 15 to 20 minutes. Do not overcook. Remove the pears to a bowl and discard the orange rind and ginger slices. Serve the pears warm, cool, or chilled, with the syrup.

MIXED FRUIT

4 large eating oranges
1 fresh ripe pineapple
2 tablespoons finely chopped fresh mint
1 tablespoon fresh lemon juice
1 tablespoon unsweetened pineapple juice
¼ cup dry sherry (optional)
Mint sprigs

MAKES EIGHT SERVINGS

1. Cut away all rind and bitter white pith from oranges. Separate oranges into segments.
2. Peel, remove the core of the pineapple, and cut it into 1-inch cubes.
3. Combine orange sections and pineapple cubes and toss them with mint, lemon juice, pineapple juice, and optional sherry. Serve in fruit cocktail cups garnished with sprigs of mint.

If you do not want to use as much sherry, either use half the amount or omit it entirely; the flavor of the dessert will still be good.

PEARS WITH GORGONZOLA

Wash 3 ripe, but not mushy, pears. Halve and remove centers with teaspoon. Also remove woody part, but leave stems intact. Into each pear cavity, spoon about 2 tablespoons of softened Gorgonzola or blue cheese. Cover and refrigerate but bring back to room temperature about 15 minutes before serving.

MAKES SIX SERVINGS

Cooking the Nutritious Way
Desserts

FRUIT WITH HONEY-LIME DRESSING

Cut 2 medium peaches or nectarines into wedges; cut 1 small honeydew or cantaloupe into bite-size cubes. In a bowl, combine the fruit mixture with 1 cup blueberries, ⅓ cup honey, and 3 tablespoons fresh lime juice. Cover and refrigerate for 1 hour. Garnish with fresh mint if available.   MAKES SIX SERVINGS

ORANGE-PINEAPPLE CUP

1 cup fresh orange sections, cut from 2 fresh navel oranges
8-ounce can unsweetened pineapple chunks, in own juice
½ cup seedless grapes
½ cup unsweetened coconut (optional)
Fresh mint leaves

MAKES FOUR SERVINGS

1. Mix fruit and coconut together gently. Chill until serving time and garnish with mint leaves.

Unsweetened coconut can be found in specialty food stores. If you omit the coconut, substitute ½ cup of chopped walnuts.

FRUIT SNOWBALL

1 cup strawberries or other seasonal fruit
1 medium banana
¼ cup orange juice or other fruit juice

MAKES FOUR SERVINGS

1. Rinse and hull the berries or rinse and cut the fruit into 1-inch pieces. Place them in a plastic bag or box and put them in the freezer to freeze solid.
2. Peel the banana, cut it into 1-inch chunks and immediately roll tightly in plastic wrap; place in freezer to freeze solid.
3. At serving time, place the frozen fruit in the container of a food processor, pour on the juice and process with the metal blade. At first the fruit will be chopped into small bits and will then amalgamate into a creamy pink mass. Serve at once.

If you do not have a food processor, puree the fruit in a blender, using a little more liquid and blending the fruit mixture in very small batches to keep blender from clogging.

RHUBARB COMPOTE

1 pound rhubarb
3 medium apples
1 by 1-inch strip orange rind, chopped fine
½ cup sugar
¼ cup unsweetened apple juice
Pinch nutmeg

MAKES SIX SERVINGS

1. Trim the rhubarb, pulling off any thick fibers, and cut into 1-inch pieces. Peel the apples, cut into quarters, and core. Reserve several strips of the peel. Place the fruit in a mixing bowl, sprinkle on the orange rind and sugar, and mix with your hands to distribute the flavors. Cover and set aside for 15 minutes.
2. Transfer the fruit to a heavy nonaluminum pot. Pour the apple juice into the bowl and swirl it around to dissolve any residual sugar, then add the juice to the pot with the nutmeg. Tuck in the reserved apple peelings, which will help intensify the rosy color.
3. Place on medium heat and bring juice to a boil. Reduce the heat, cover, and simmer for 7 to 10 minutes, or until fruit is soft. Do not overcook. Discard apple peels and cool the compote. Serve warm or chilled.

ROAST PINEAPPLE

Preheat oven to 400 degrees. Slice 1 medium pineapple in half lengthwise and score the flesh with a sharp knife. Spoon 1 tablespoon honey over each half, and roast for 20 minutes. Cut each half in 3 pieces and serve.

MAKES SIX SERVINGS

Red Plum Compote

⅔ cup sugar
1 cup dry white wine
4 whole cloves
3-inch stick cinnamon
Grated rind of ½ lemon
18 firm, ripe, red plums, stemmed
    and rinsed

MAKES SIX SERVINGS

1. Combine sugar, wine, 1 cup water, cloves, cinnamon, and lemon in a saucepan large enough to hold plums. Bring ingredients to a boil and cook, uncovered, for 5 minutes.
2. Add plums and bring mixture to boil; lower heat and simmer the plums for 10 to 20 minutes, depending on their ripeness, until they are tender but still hold their shape.
3. Some plums will be cooked before others. Remove cooked fruit. Then, when all are cooked, return all the plums to the syrup.
4. Chill plums in syrup and serve.

For a festive dessert, serve chilled compote over vanilla ice cream.

Figs in Wine

1 pound dried figs
2 cups sweet red wine such as port
    or Madeira
2 small branches fresh thyme or
    ½ teaspoon crumbled dried thyme
2 tablespoons honey
Almonds or other nuts, coarsely
    chopped (optional)

MAKES FOUR SERVINGS

1. Cut off the dry stems from the figs, then simmer with the wine, thyme, and honey, in a covered pot, for about 30 minutes. Turn the figs once, halfway through the cooking process.
2. With a slotted spoon, remove the figs. Turn up the heat and continue to cook the syrup, uncovered, for a few minutes, stirring until it thickens a bit.
3. Pour the syrup on the figs, and serve. Add coarsely chopped almonds or other nuts to the syrup at the last moment, if desired.

Baked Apples

Preheat oven to 400 degrees. Wash apples, remove cores, without cutting through to bottoms. Slit skin horizontally around the middle of each apple to prevent bursting. Place in a shallow 9-inch baking dish. Stuff each apple with 4 raisins and 2 almonds; sprinkle with cinnamon and fill the cavities with water. Pour about ¾ cup of water into baking dish. Bake for 30 minutes or until apples are soft.

MAKES FOUR SERVINGS

Fresh Fruit Cake

1 tablespoon butter or margarine
1 cup vegetable oil
1 cup chopped walnuts
1 cup chopped almonds
1 cup raisins
2 cups rolled oats
3 cups crushed, fresh-fruit pulp
    and juice of your choice
1 teaspoon vanilla
1 cup all-purpose flour
1-1½ cups whole-wheat flour
½ pound pitted dates

MAKES TWELVE TO SIXTEEN SERVINGS

1. Lightly grease 2 round, 9-inch cake pans with butter or margarine. Preheat over to 350 degrees.
2. Mix all ingredients, except the dates, to form a soft and slightly crumbly dough. Press into greased pans. Bake for 40 to 50 minutes until sides and bottom are golden brown.
3. Let cool in pans for 10 minutes. Turn out onto plate or board for further cooling.
4. Place dates in saucepan with water to cover. Simmer for 10 to 15 minutes or until soft. Mash into a paste with a hand masher, or in a food processor or blender. Spread the filling on one layer and put the other layer on top. Let the cake stand at room temperature for a couple of hours before serving. This cake improves with age and will keep, tightly wrapped and refrigerated, for 10 days.

The best fruits to use are strawberries, pineapple, or ripe peaches.

Cooking the Nutritious Way
Desserts

GINGER COOKIES

¼ cup brown sugar
¼ cup unsalted butter or margarine
1 egg, lightly beaten
¼ teaspoon vanilla extract
1 teaspoon ground ginger
¼ teaspoon allspice
¼ teaspoon cinnamon
¼ teaspoon ground cloves
⅓ cup plus 1 tablespoon flour

MAKES THREE DOZEN COOKIES

1. Preheat oven to 375 degrees. Combine the sugar and butter or margarine in the bowl of an electric mixer. Beat well until the butter is creamed.
2. Beat in the egg and vanilla. Stir in the spices and ⅓ cup flour.
3. Lightly grease a baking sheet and sprinkle with 1 tablespoon flour. Shake off any excess. Spoon small amounts of the batter onto the sheet, leaving about 2 inches between each drop. Bake for 6 to 7 minutes. Cool the cookies on a cake rack.

OATMEAL SNACKS

1 egg
½ cup melted butter
½ cup honey
1 cup flour, preferably whole wheat
½ teaspoon baking soda
¼ teaspoon salt
½ teaspoon cinnamon
1½ cups rolled oats, not the quick-cooking variety
½ cup chopped walnuts or almonds

MAKES TWO DOZEN COOKIES

1. Preheat oven to 325 degrees. Lightly grease 2 baking sheets.
2. Beat egg. Add butter and honey and blend thoroughly. Stir flour with baking soda, salt, and cinnamon, making sure there are no lumps. Add to liquid mixture and mix well. Stir in oats and nuts.
3. Drop by tablespoonfuls onto baking sheets. Bake for 12 to 15 minutes. Remove the cookies to a cake rack after 5 minutes.

These oatmeal cookies are chewy and not too sweet. They are not the usual crisp kind you might be used to making.

INDIAN PUDDING

4 cups milk
⅓ cup yellow cornmeal, preferably stone-ground
2 tablespoons butter
¼ cup molasses
¼ cup brown sugar, firmly packed
½ teaspoon salt
½ teaspoon ground ginger
½ teaspoon cinnamon
1 egg, beaten

MAKES EIGHT SERVINGS

1. Preheat oven to 325 degrees. Lightly grease a 1-quart baking pan and set aside.
2. Pour the milk into the top of a double boiler and heat over boiling water.
3. When hot, stir in the cornmeal. Cook over simmering water, stirring frequently with a wooden spatula, for 10 minutes. Stir in all the remaining ingredients, except the egg, and continue cooking, with an occasional stir, for 10 minutes longer.
4. Transfer the mixture to a bowl and whisk in the egg. Pour into the baking dish and bake for 2 hours.

You could add ½ cup raisins or 1½ cups sliced apples when the egg is added.

ITALIAN CARROT TORTE

1 tablespoon butter
9 tablespoons sugar
4 eggs, separated
3 cups finely grated, peeled carrots
2 cups finely grated almonds
¼ teaspoon ground allspice
2 teaspoons Marsala wine or brandy
Whipped cream (optional)

MAKES EIGHT SERVINGS

1. Preheat oven to 275 degrees. Butter a 9-inch, round cake pan.
2. Beat the sugar with the egg yolks until thick. Stir in the grated carrots, almonds, allspice, and Marsala.
3. Beat egg whites until stiff, and fold into the carrot mixture. Turn into cake pan and bake for 1 hour. Serve warm, with whipped cream, if desired.

Reminder: You may want to substitute margarine for the butter.

Gingerbread

1 tablespoon butter
⅓ cup vegetable oil
⅓ cup light molasses
⅓ cup sugar
2 egg whites, slightly beaten
1 cup unsifted whole-wheat flour
¼ teaspoon baking soda
¼ teaspoon salt
1 teaspoon baking powder
1 teaspoon ground ginger
½ teaspoon cinnamon
¼ teaspoon nutmeg

MAKES EIGHT SERVINGS

1. Preheat oven to 350 degrees. Butter an 8 by 8 by 2-inch baking pan. Flour the pan and shake out excess.
2. Mix vegetable oil with ⅓ cup water. Add molasses, sugar, and egg whites. Stir until sugar is dissolved. Mix flour, baking soda, salt, baking powder, and spices. Add to liquid mixture and beat until smooth.
3. Pour into pan and bake for 30 minutes or until surface springs back when touched lightly.

Store unused egg yolks in the freezer for 2 months.

Austrian Curd Cake

4 tablespoons butter, at room temperature
⅓ cup honey
2 large eggs, separated
1½ cups creamed, large-curd cottage cheese
⅓ cup farina or granulated tapioca
3 tablespoons lemon juice
½ cup raisins

MAKES SIX TO EIGHT SERVINGS

1. Lightly grease an 8 by 8-inch baking pan. Preheat oven to 350 degrees.
2. Blend butter and honey in a bowl. Add yolks, then whisk in cottage cheese, ½ cup at a time. Whisk in farina or tapioca; then mix in lemon juice and raisins.
3. With an egg beater, whip egg whites until very stiff and white. Stir a large spoonful of beaten whites into the cottage-cheese mixture; then use a rubber scraper to cut and fold in the remainder.
4. Pour batter into baking pan and bake for 50 minutes. Cake will rise hardly at all. When baked, set pan on rack to cool. Serve warm or cold from the pan.

Drinks

Melon Cooler

1 small cantaloupe
1 20-ounce can crushed pineapple, packed in its own juice
1 cup crushed ice
Unsweetened pineapple juice
Mint sprigs (optional)

MAKES SIX SERVINGS

1. Peel and seed cantaloupe; cut into chunks.
2. In an electric blender, or food processor, combine about ⅓ of the cantaloupe cubes, all of the crushed pineapple, and the ice. Blend at high speed, adding the remaining cantaloupe cubes gradually. Stop blender and push large pieces of fruit away from sides of blender. Blend until smooth.
3. Thin the mixture with unsweetened pineapple juice to consistency desired. Pour into glasses and serve, garnished with mint sprigs.

As a variation, use honeydew melon or watermelon in place of the cantaloupe. This makes a delicious start to breakfast. Also this cooler may be served as a cold summertime soup.

Orange Smoothee

6-ounce can frozen orange juice concentrate
1 cup milk
1 cup water
¼ cup sugar (optional)
½ teaspoon vanilla
10 ice cubes

MAKES SIX SERVINGS

1. Place all ingredients in a blender.
2. Cover and blend until smooth.
3. Serve immediately.

You may want to use low-fat milk instead of whole milk or, for thicker consistency, an 8-ounce container of plain yogurt. If you prefer vanilla-flavored yogurt, omit the vanilla that is called for in the recipe. Try this for breakfast or as a mid-afternoon snack.

Cooking the Nutritious Way
Adding Variety to Meals

The menus given below will help guide you in planning interesting and nutritious meals that take advantage of the recipes, marked with an asterisk*, in the preceding section. (The index to the recipes begins on page 411.) When creating your own menus, be sure to refer to the recommended number of servings per day from each of the Basic Four Food Groups, as explained on pages 96-105.

For many people, reducing the amount of fat, sugar, and salt in their diets, as recommended in the Dietary Guidelines, and increasing the amount of complex carbohydrates mean a change in eating habits. Of course, it is impossible and perhaps even undesirable to make all these changes overnight. Rather, you may want to introduce new dishes one at a time or experiment with a whole day's meals before trying a completely new weekly menu. If you want to plan a meatless day, see the suggestions in

MENU 1	MENU 2	MENU 3
Breakfast Orange or tangerine sections Bran muffin with peanut butter Milk	**Breakfast** Fresh fruit and plain yogurt topped with wheat germ Whole-wheat baking powder biscuits* or whole-wheat toast and jam	**Breakfast** Tomato or other vegetable juice Scrambled egg with chives or herbs Banana-nut bread* Milk
Lunch Yankee bean chowder* Mixed green salad with tarragon-buttermilk dressing* Cornbread* Baked apples*	**Lunch** Chicken salad* on black bread Fresh or baked cherry tomatoes* Potato Salad Tzapanos*	**Lunch** Spaghetti alla Matriciana* Fresh spinach and mushroom salad with vinaigrette dressing* Orange-pineapple cup*
Dinner Roast chicken with kasha stuffing* Acorn squash and cranberries* or baked carrots and apples* Austrian curd cake*	**Dinner** Scandinavian dry-baked flounder* Steamed new potatoes in broth* Grated cucumber relish* or sliced tomatoes Fresh fruit cake*	**Dinner** Five-Minute Soup* with leftover meat Whole-wheat baking powder biscuits* or whole-wheat crackers Italian carrot torte*
Snacks Gingerbread* and milk or Orange Smoothee*	**Snacks** Chili bean dip with raw vegetables* Tomato juice	**Snacks** Home-popped plain popcorn

Menu 5. Use the menus below as a guide and vary them according to the occasion, the availability of fresh foods at the market, and the amount of time you have to prepare a meal.

Beverages have been omitted from these menus except for milk at breakfast, because milk is an important part both of this meal and of a balanced diet. Low-fat milk will help reduce your consumption of fat. You can, of course, also drink milk at other meals or choose from among fruit or vegetable juices, water, coffee, or tea.

If you are eating away from home, you will usually be able to find meals similar to the ones given here at restaurants. For further guidance on eating out, see page 305. In addition, some of the breakfasts and lunches can be packed in bags or containers to take along with you. For more brownbag lunch ideas, see pages 312-313.

MENU 4	MENU 5	MENU 6	MENU 7
Breakfast Chilled grapefruit half Unsweetened cold cereal with raisins and milk	**Breakfast** Applesauce with cinnamon Hot oatmeal with honey Milk	**Breakfast** Cantaloupe wedge topped with blueberries Granola* and milk	**Breakfast** Chilled orange juice Buttermilk pancakes* with maple syrup
Lunch White Rabbit Salad* Whole-wheat bread or muffins Tomato juice	**Lunch** Tabouli* Pita, or pocket, bread Plain yogurt mixed with strawberries or bananas	**Lunch** Broiled hamburger* on a toasted bun Coleslaw or bean salad* Fresh fruit with honey-lime dressing*	**Lunch** Beets with tuna* served on lettuce Breadsticks Melon cooler
Dinner Oriental beef* Stir-fried watercress with carrots* Bean sprout salad* or brown rice Roast pineapple	**Dinner** Vegetable chowder* Swiss chard and cheese pie* Ginger cookies*	**Dinner** Minestrone* Lasagna* Mixed green salad with vinaigrette dressing* Fruit snowball*	**Dinner** Basic pot roast of beef* Farina dumplings* Red plum compote*
Snacks Fresh fruit in season	**Snacks** Dry-roasted peanuts Milk	**Snacks** Roasted chick-peas* Milk or fruit juice	**Snacks** Oatmeal snacks* Milk or fruit juice

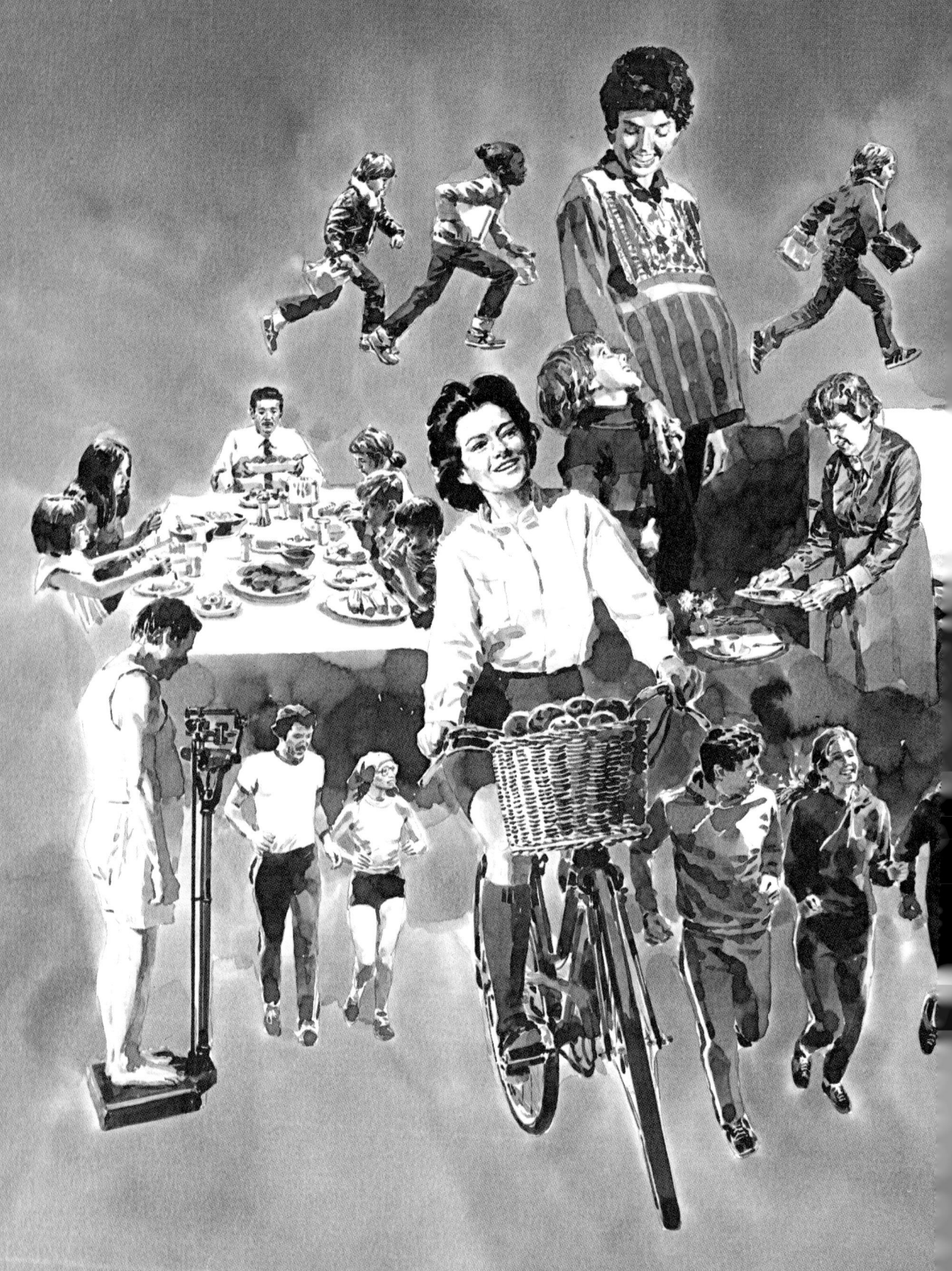

3. EATING FOR GOOD HEALTH

The American concern with weight: a review of reducing diets, spas, and support groups. How to change your habits and learn to eat sensibly. Diet suggestions for all the members of your family. Plus a special section: Fitness Through Exercise.

Dealing with Overweight
    Reducing Diets 282
        How Appetite Works 283
        Appraising the Diets 284
        Extreme Measures 287
        Drugstore Diets 288
    Spas and Support Groups .. 293
Eating Sensibly 296
    Finding Your Ideal Weight
      and Caloric Needs 298
    Changing Your Eating Habits 300
    If You Want To Gain
      Weight 301
    Balanced Meal Planning 302
    Cooking for One 304
    Eating Out 305
    A Diet for Pregnant Women 306
    Feeding Your Baby 308
        Introducing Solid Food ... 309
    What Children Need To Eat . 310
        Brownbag Lunches 312
    The Critical Adolescent Years 314
    The Advancing Years 318

Fitness Through Exercise
    Getting into Shape 320
        Exercise Myths 321
    Testing Your Dynamic
      Fitness 322
        Rating Physical Activities . 323
    What's Best for You 324
    The Exercise Routine 326
    Calisthenics for Conditioning 328
    Calisthenics Therapy 330
        The Joy of Movement 331
    Resistance Training 332
    Aerobic Conditioning 334
    Running for Health 336
    The Fitness Trail 338
    Touring Sports 340
    Swimming 342
        Exercise Afloat 343
    Aquaexercises 344
    Court and Field 346
    Adding Variety to Exercise .. 348
    Exercise in Your Daily
      Routine 350

Dealing with Overweight/Reducing Diets

To speak of Americans as being obsessed by food is neither exaggeration nor accusation but the simple truth. It is an obsession that gets us coming and going: we worry whether we are getting enough of the "right" foods, those that will ensure that we look and feel our best; and we worry whether we eat too much food, too much for health or beauty. It's an obsession, furthermore, that is reinforced at every turn. We are bombarded with insidious, seductive messages everywhere we look. Television commercials and billboards, newspaper and magazine ads, fill our minds with images of beautiful, healthy, *thin* people—all happily, guiltlessly EATING!

Who are all those thin people on television anyway, the ones cavorting on a sunny island, sipping rum drinks, consuming high-fat French cheeses with never a thought to cholesterol counts? How come none of them wind up with beer bellies, jelly thighs, or arteriosclerosis? What's in that container of yogurt that makes the blonde model carrying it across a waving meadow look so sexy? And what does she eat when she isn't eating yogurt? If food is so good for us, why does it also make us so miserable? And how are we to know when it is the one thing, and when it will lead to the other?

In fact, the issue of food is so muddled in most of our minds that the actual relationship between it and its effects is frequently forgotten. Perhaps in no respect is this truer than in the American custom of dieting. As most of us have known since adolescence or earlier, weight loss (barring serious illness) results from one process only: the accumulation, over time, of a calorie deficit. In other words, from eating less and/or doing more. There simply is no other way, as anyone who has ever gasped at his swelling image in a mirror and sworn "I've got to stop eating" intuitively knows. It is one of the simplest equations to comprehend but one of the most difficult to practice in daily life.

An adult of normal weight carries from 10 to 25 percent of his body weight as fat, with the average somewhat lower for men than women. If 30 to 40 percent of your body weight is fat, you are overweight; if your body weight is more than 40 percent fat, you are obese. Although a weight-height chart is given on page 298, your physician can more accurately judge your weight condition.

The physiological costs of overweight are many, and by now, familiar. Too much extra weight strains the body in a variety of ways: it aggravates diabetes, high blood pressure, and heart disease, and contributes to digestive and kidney diseases; it increases one's vulnerability during surgery; moreover, statistics show, seriously overweight people are more susceptible to certain cancers and fatal accidents.

The economic penalties of overweight are also considerable: excessive food costs, higher insurance premiums, reduced job opportunities, eventually fewer chances for promotion.

For the estimated 80 million Americans who are overweight, including the 20 million who are by one definition obese, the painful social and emotional penalties that are part of the package hardly need listing. These, more than any other factors, are what drive most people to attempt losing weight. And attempt it they do. Repeatedly. They do it on doctors' orders, on the advice of a friend or member of the family, out of a feeling of guilt. They do it the "right" way and the wrong way and in ways that leave one breathless.

There is a "diet" in circulation to suit every taste, every budget, and every misconception. There are fat farms and diet pills, "miracle" waist trimmers, and sugarless fudge. There are "natural" approaches and unabashedly unnatural ones. There are mental attitudes and behaviorial methods, reducing groups that combine the rituals of the confessional and the pep rally. Acupuncture is touted by some, hypnosis by others. And for the desperate, there are truly desperate measures: sleep cures, jaw wiring, even gastric stapling.

It would be incorrect to say that all this activity benefits no one. One study shows that only 12 out of 100 dieters succeeded initially—though 10 regained weight. But without a doubt, the single largest group to benefit from America's addiction to dieting is made up of the purveyors of diet books and weight-control products or services.

One obesity expert speaks knowingly of an "epidemic of slimming": it has been estimated that the typical overweight American "goes on a diet" 15 separate times between the ages of 20 and 50. *The Washington Post* reported the case of a 48-year-old woman who had been dieting on and off for 37 years. She had embarked on 20 separate diets, including a protein-sparing modified fast, and had become dependent on diet pills. As her weight bounced up and down from a high of 183 pounds to a twice-reached low of 124 pounds, the woman lost a total of 375 pounds but never succeeded in maintaining her desired weight. To add insult to exhaustion, her lifetime purchases in the endless, stalemated war against fat had cost her $14,288 or $38 per lost (even if regained) pound.

That such persistence, multiplied by the experience of millions, would go so consistently unrewarded suggests that something is terribly askew in our attitudes toward dieting and even more fundamentally awry with our attitudes toward food.

Dieting, it seems clear, is for most people a frustrating and recurring preoccupation, a demoralizing cycle of denial followed by indulgence, of pounds and inches lost and regained. Most significantly, dieting appears to have a life of its own, to take place outside the context of the dieter's "normal" life. A person diets, and when he has succeeded (or failed) in shedding the unwanted pounds, he returns to eating the kinds and amount of food that led to overweight in the first place. In a relatively short time, any lost weight is back, and the cycle begins again. It is what the noted nutrition authority Jean Mayer calls "the rhythm method of girth control."

Between those two points—beginning a diet and returning, victorious or defeated, to old habits of eating—is a vast field of self-denial, self-delusion and, in some cases, a serious abuse of health. In the following pages, we take a look at how America attempts to lose weight. What are the most popular diets? How do they work, what do they entail, how effective are they in taking weight off and keeping it off, and what do they mean in terms of health? What other methods—diet pills, support groups—are popular? Are they safe? Are they effective?

How Appetite Works

Most of us eat when we are hungry—though few of us experience actual hunger since our eating schedule is dictated more by habit and custom.

Hunger is a complex of unpleasant sensations that build slowly in the stomach, throat and mouth, and head and increase in intensity the longer you go without eating.

Appetite is the not unpleasant desire for a specific food and may have nothing to do with hunger. One may feel full but still have room for dessert.

Satiety, the active mechanism in weight control, is the subconscious, often abrupt signal to stop eating. Both hunger and satiety are regulated by the interaction of a number of areas in the brain responding to various stimuli. In most adults this mechanism maintains an ideal weight within a pound or two for 40 years or more. However, overweight people have disconnected this mechanism; their urge to eat is generally governed not by physical need but by external factors—such mental states as boredom or fatigue and such incidental stimuli as remembering that leftover cake in the kitchen.

Diets by the Dozens

Walk into any bookstore and you are certain to find, as likely as not cheek-by-jowl with an ever-expanding collection of cookbooks, a competing display of diet manuals with catchy titles and promises of success. Dozens are on the market at any moment; one or two are always near the top of the best-seller list. These are richly supplemented by an apparently endless stream of diets published in women's magazines, in the form of the diet of the month, the "spring shape-up," the "just in time for the holidays" diet, the "seven-day, two-week, or weekend" diet, the "let's face the music last chance" diet—all of which add up to literally thousands of diets over the years, a great many of them undertaken, in sequence, by the same frustrated dieters apparently unaware that there are no breakthrough diets—and never will be—and that there are no scientific secrets to losing weight.

How can there be so many routes to a single goal? And how is one to choose among them? A few definitions are in order.

The six most important words in a dieter's vocabulary are *carbohydrates*, *fats*, *proteins*, *vitamins*, *minerals*, and *calories* (although a good argument could be made for *restraint* and *patience*). All food is composed of the first three, singly or in a variety of combinations; the body needs vitamins and minerals; and all food can be assigned a caloric value, a calorie being nothing more complicated than the amount of heat needed to raise the temperature of one gram of water one degree centigrade at sea level (but see also page 12). Translated into the energy required to run the human body, calorie counting is a simple way of keeping track of what otherwise seems a mysterious process—the conversion of food

Dealing with Overweight
Reducing Diets

Appraising the Diets

Type of Diet	Examples	Appeal
Unbalanced Diets. Stress or limit one of the basic food groups, altering recommended ratio of protein/carbohydrate/fat; permitted foods may be unlimited, others restricted in calories or amounts; may extol a "miracle enzyme" or chemical breakthrough; should be limited to 1 to 2 weeks; dramatic results promised.		A radical change in eating habits defines "dieting," provides control; weight is lost quickly and easily; no hunger cravings in ketogenic diets.
Fasting: no food for hours, days, or longer; no-calorie liquids allowed.		Cheap, quickest, and easiest; no choices; appetite soon lost.
Protein-sparing modified fasts (PSMFs): medically supervised fasts plus a balanced formula to "spare" protein depletion.	Optifast	If obesity is a health hazard, may be the quickest way.
Protein supplements: over-the-counter liquid or powdered protein products measured and flavored to provide some 500 calories.	Last Chance	Little temptation from unappealing and monotonous substance.
Low carbohydrate: restricts carbohydrates to cut calories; some say all you can eat of permitted foods; may have 600 to 1,200 calorie limit or require "carbo-counting"; vitamin and mineral supplements may be advised.	Drinking Man's	Quick, easy, weight loss (mostly water); meat is popular whereas starch is considered fattening; all-you-can-eat limited by normal satiation levels, thus reducing calorie intake automatically; no appetite.
High protein: eliminates most carbohydrates, unlimited protein; 2 quarts of water daily.	Doctor's Quick Weight Loss Scarsdale I Love New York	Loss of appetite from ketosis. Food choices limited.
High fat: high protein with fat intake encouraged.	Diet Revolution	Fat takes longer to digest, postponing hunger pangs.
Fad: only one or a few foods permitted, often represented as having magical properties.	Grapefruit, Rice, Banana, Ice Cream, Hamburger diets	Easy to remember; no calorie counting; boredom limits intake; grapefruit, bananas are healthy.
High carbohydrate: increased complex carbohydrates; reduced sugar, saturated fats, protein. **High fiber:** stress roughage, bran, fruit, vegetables; may permit low-fat meat and poultry; no sugar.	Rockefeller Watermelon Quick Inches-Off Beverly Hills Pritikin Save Your Life	No calorie counting; weight loss can be rapid; fruit, vegetables, grains are healthy, natural, nonfilling but nonfattening; low in cholesterol and fat; none of the hazards of ketogenic diets.
Balanced Diets. Nutritional balance of protein/carbohydrate/fat; protein ratio may be boosted; sugar and fat reduced; may have 1,000 to 1,200 calorie limit; exercise often recommended for weight losses of 1 to 2 pounds a week.		Weight loss is safe, steady; can be lifetime diet; normal and varied foods allowed.
Vegetarian/lacto-ovo: allows dairy products, eggs, but no meat.	Seventh Day Adventist Weight Watchers Vegetarian	For "natural" food advocates; low fat protects heart, prolongs life.
Hypocaloric, anticoronary: low saturated fat and sugar; whole dairy products, egg yolks, calories may be limited.	Prudent Redbook Wise Woman's	Heart protection and health often prime objective; 75 percent keep weight off.

Drawbacks

Weight loss mostly water unless diet sustained; unsafe unless limited to brief periods; eating problems unresolved; willpower required in limiting portion size; nutritional deficiencies trigger disorders, fatigue, dizziness.

See "carbohydrate deficiency" below; 70% regain weight.
Medical supervision only, still possibly unsafe. Protein-only diets may not "spare" vital tissue; no long-term weight loss; low blood pressure and dizziness.
Supplements often of poor quality, lacking essential amino acids; have caused heart failure and death.

Carbohydrate deficiency causes body to raid vital tissues for energy; conversion causes ketosis, nitrogen loss, acidosis; elevated blood uric-acid level exacerbates gout; liver and kidneys overworked; fatigue, loss of coordination and concentration; nausea, bad breath, chills.

Constipation, frequent urination, bad breath, fatigue, dizziness.

Fat is fattening, elevates serum cholesterol; vitamin supplements inadequate.

Not even grapefruit can make pounds "melt away"; malnutrition soon results from vitamin and mineral deficiencies.

Protein deficiency leads to soft bones, dizziness, muscle degeneration, hunger cravings because feel full but not satisfied; often deficient in iron, calcium, niacin, Vitamin A. Fiber brings gas, frequent bowel movements, may result in malabsorption of nutrients; nondairy lacks calcium.

No miracles are promised or realized; weight loss is slow; where calories or amounts not specified willpower is required to limit portion size; too much like everyday diet.

Possible undernourishment; vegetarians often diet conscious, strict.

No sweets.

---

into energy, necessary body proteins, or excess fat. It takes 3,500 calories to add a pound of fat to your body and a deficit of 3,500 calories to shed a pound.

Although most commonly thought of in terms of meat, fish, milk, and eggs—all animal products—protein actually derives from many food sources, and in most parts of the world people get their required protein from combinations of such staples as legumes, grains, and vegetables. Because animal protein contains in ready-made form the best balance of the amino acids the body needs, it is often called complete protein. Most nonanimal sources of protein, on the other hand, are usually low in one or more of the essential amino acids and thus are called incomplete. All this means is that the latter must be eaten in combination, which is precisely the solution that most of the world follows.

Countering the convenience of animal protein is the hidden fat it contains. As Ronald M. Deutsch points out in *The Fat Counter Guide*, the caloric value of the protein in many foods is dwarfed by the caloric value of its fat content. Deutsch gives as an example a 6-ounce slice of prime rib roast with a total calorie count of 748. Protein accounts for only 135 calories; the remainder is all fat. Trimming all visible fat from the meat helps—Deutsch rids the slice of 340 calories that way. But the slice still contains "invisible" fat, the marbling that gives beef its flavor, and accounts for more than half the remaining calories. In contrast, tofu, or pressed soybean cake, a staple in both Chinese and Japanese diets, is low in calories but has 40 percent the protein of an equivalent slice of rib roast.

In the lore of dieting, probably no food group has been more unjustly, or counterproductively, maligned than carbohydrates. For years, scrupulous dieters have been passing up bread, potatoes, rice, beans, cereals, and spaghetti while consuming protein-rich foods in quantity and confidence. In so doing, they have robbed themselves of a useful source of energy available for the body to do its work. Carbohydrates are divided into two groups, complex and simple (see pages 13–17), but many of the foods we think of as primarily carbohydrates—such as beans and rice—also contain high-quality protein if used in combination. In addition, the fiber needed for proper digestion and elimination is to be found in no other class of foods.

On the other hand, it is no accident that we label

Dealing with Overweight
Reducing Diets

fattening those foods we believe make us fat. Whereas 1 gram of either protein or carbohydrate represents 4 calories, every gram of fat equals 9 calories. So, whereas too much of any kind of food, including protein and carbohydrates, can add pounds, gram for gram, fats do it faster.

Fats are not total villains. The body needs a small amount of fat in the diet to obtain linoleic acid, which should account for 1 to 2 percent of total calories in order to ensure proper growth and healthy skin. Fat in human tissue also cushions vital organs and helps prevent rapid body-heat loss. But fats *are* treacherous for the dieter, "hiding out" in foods and adding unwanted calories to otherwise good sources of protein.

All diets, whether designed for weight loss or medical reasons, fall into one of two categories: those that are balanced and those that are unbalanced. In a balanced diet, daily food intake provides all the protein, carbohydrates, fats, vitamins, and minerals needed for health, needs that vary somewhat with age and sex but which, by and large, can be accommodated by choosing from among a wide variety of foods.

An unbalanced diet, by comparison, is one that radically departs from this standard by overloading one food group at the expense of others. With a finite number of calories permitted on a low-calorie diet, the dieter can easily shortchange himself on important nutrients by favoring proteins at the expense of carbohydrates or vice versa. Extremely unbalanced diets are dangerous and can have short-term ill effects or even impair health over the long range. This is why advocates of unbalanced diets usually caution their followers to discontinue the diet after a period of two weeks. Furthermore, an unbalanced diet reinforces the self-defeating notion that "dieting" entails a peculiar, or aberrant, form of eating, one that has nothing to do with the way you eat normally; as such it is a poor preparation for a lifetime of eating ahead.

The argument for a balanced diet is unassailable, except on one count: for many dieters, it does not work. It does not work because it requires a major change in attitude toward weight loss and eating habits; because for most it does not bring results quickly enough; and because, again for most dieters, the slow, balanced approach is not different enough from "real" life to keep the dieter's mind off eating.

Instead, dieters cling to short-term, unbalanced diets that promise a quick fix, and that, in wrenching a dieter out of last week's eating habits, provide, at least temporarily, sufficient attraction for the dieter to be able to stick with them. Hence the popularity of such regimes as the Scarsdale diet (a promised weight loss of a pound per day or up to 20 or more pounds in two weeks), the Doctor's Quick Weight Loss, or Stillman, diet (7 to 15 pounds the first week, an average of 5 a week thereafter), or the 9-Day Wonder diet, which promises a loss of up to 15 pounds from one weekend to the next.

Most of the popular, unbalanced diets on the market today fall into one of three categories: low-carbohydrate (often called high-protein, and just as appropriately called high-fat); liquid, no food, or fasting diets, undertaken with or without supplements; and high-carbohydrate. Fad diets that promote particular foods as "fat-burning" or promise to "melt" cellulose are simply variations on one or another of the basic unbalanced models, a sampling of which are listed in the chart on pages 284-285.

Low-Carbohydrate Diets

The progenitor of the modern quick-weight-loss diet was promulgated in the late 19th century by a British surgeon named William Harvey, whose prescription for weight loss was to restrict severely his patients' intake of carbohydrates while permitting 5 ounces of meat and fish at every meal. His most famous patient was the corpulent coffin maker William Banting, who had come to Harvey with an ear complaint, and whose trouble Harvey divined to be too much fat pressing on a channel to the inner ear. Banting lost 46 pounds in one year and went on to publish a pamphlet in which he extolled the success of Harvey's diet.

The Scarsdale diet is perhaps the most popular and representative low-carbohydrate, or ketogenic, diet of recent years. Such diets vary only in their particulars and all should result in short-term weight loss accompanying a process called ketosis. Ketosis occurs when the amount of carbohydrate fuel—the fuel that is needed to run the body—drops below a critical level, forcing the body to turn first to protein and then to fat reserves to do the work carbohydrates normally do. When protein is deflected in this manner, it releases nitrogen into the blood stream, placing a burden on the kidneys as they try to excrete excessive urinary water due to sodium loss. When fat is likewise deflected, the breakup releases fatty acids, or ketones, into the bloodstream, further burdening the kidneys. If ketosis continues for long periods of time, serious damage to the liver and kidneys can occur, which is why most sponsors of these diets recommend only short-term use, and why many nutritionists caution their patients—especially women in the early stages of pregnancy—against following them at all.

The great appeal of the basic ketogenic diet is that it generally produces results: follow it scrupulously and you will lose weight. What's more, for many dieters the ketogenic diet provides a badly needed framework, clear rules, and a prescription for accomplishing something that seems beyond their individual powers. Some dieters feel incapable of making the correct choices of foods and portion sizes, of controlling themselves when handling or serving food. Exact definitions, lists of forbidden or recommended foods, and other particulars that characterize many of the popular ketogenic diets fulfill the dieter's need for discipline and direction.

But possibly most important to the majority of dieters is the relative speed with which one can lose weight on a ketogenic diet. Because of the rapid water loss that attends the ketogenic process, the illusion of weight loss exceeds the actual loss, and that psychological boost, particularly at the outset, is of real value to dieters. The sensation of bloating that often accompanies overweight and is in fact due to water retention (an especially common problem with women) is alleviated early in a ketogenic diet, so that the dieter striving to "think thin" will in fact "feel" thinner too, if only by virtue of having shed a few uncomfortable pounds of water.

Although there is much that is attractive to dieters in the ketogenic approach, anyone concerned with health should be clear about its disadvantages and dangers as well. Of the latter, the most significant is clearly the risk associated with ketosis itself. It cannot be emphasized too strongly that pregnant women, alcoholics, or persons suffering from kidney or liver disease should never undertake a ketogenic diet.

Other potentially serious and certainly discomforting side effects associated with ketogenic diets include temporary dizziness, headache, lethargy, weakness and, in extremis, diarrhea and nausea. In

Extreme Measures

The enormity of the dieting problem for some overweight people is sharply demonstrated by the number of what must be called "last-ditch" methods of weight control—all of which are based on the conviction that the dieter who is incapable of helping himself requires outside help to lose weight.

Hypnosis has lately been tested for a variety of medical and psychiatric purposes. Smokers and overeaters, to name two compulsive types, are using hypnosis in an attempt to gain mastery over their despised habits.

Acupuncture, the ancient Oriental art of needle stimulus, is one of the latest developments in the diet business. A sharp needle is painlessly inserted into that part of the ear containing vagus nerve fibers. The vagus nerve runs from the ear down through the neck and chest to the stomach. This nerve stimulus supposedly inhibits stomach pangs, thereby depressing appetite.

Jaw wiring is the equivalent of placing a padlock on the refrigerator door, except that one's own mouth is the aperture that is rendered unopenable. The procedure entails serious potential damage to the teeth, in addition to the more obvious risks associated with a prolonged fast.

Intestinal bypass surgery enables a patient to fast while continuing to eat as before. In this radical approach to weight control, a section of the small intestine is surgically bypassed and with it the body's capacity to absorb nutrients from food consumed. Weight loss can be substantial, even though the patient may continue to eat as before. Side effects, however, are many and often severe: continuous diarrhea, liver and kidney complications, arthritis.

Gastric stapling is a somewhat less dangerous but nevertheless radical surgical procedure. Stainless-steel staples are implanted across the top of the stomach leaving only a small opening through which food can pass into the reduced stomach pouch and intestinal tract. After surgery, patients can eat about 56 grams of food comfortably, but more than 84 grams causes pain, and an intake of 112 grams will induce vomiting.

Dealing with Overweight
Reducing Diets

addition, a person on a diet extremely low in carbohydrates, fiber, and many vitamins and minerals is liable to feel cranky, sluggish, and deprived.

The widely publicized links between cholesterol and heart disease have not been proved to the satisfaction of many nutritionists and cardiologists, but there is little doubt about the deleterious effects of excessive levels of fat in the diet. Any low-carbohydrate (high-protein) diet is a high-fat diet as well, a little recognized, and never advertised, catch that comes as a surprise to most dieters. Since most animal protein comes literally nature-packed in fat, and since on diets very low in calories one must in fact increase the proportion of protein in the diet, in order to ensure sufficiency, special care must be taken in the selection of protein in order to avoid accompanying fat.

The final disadvantage of ketogenic dieting is that it bears little or no resemblance to real life. By diverging so radically from normal patterns of eating, the ketogenic approach does little or nothing to alter the dieter's overall dietary habits. At the end of

Drugstore Diets

In their search for a quick and easy way to lose weight, Americans spend more than $200 million a year on dietary aids. What are these products, do they work, and are they safe?

For one thing, all these dietary aids are but temporary measures. In addition, none of them will produce a true weight loss unless accompanied by a diet and exercise plan. Indeed, many over-the-counter diet aids contain familiar instructions in fine print for reducing calorie intake and increasing exercise.

Anorectic drugs suppress the appetite. One type, *amphetamines*, are available only with a prescription; their use as a dietary aid has been banned in some states. Amphetamines increase wakefulness and physical activity and dull the senses of taste and smell. They are habit forming, and a tolerance for the drug develops with its use. If the dose is increased, such undesirable side effects as nervousness, insomnia, and depression also increase, with the possibility of "amphetamine psychosis," which is indistinguishable from acute paranoid schizophrenia. Withdrawal reactions include depression, anxiety, lassitude, prolonged sleep, nightmares, cramps, disorientation, and ravenous appetite.

Most over-the-counter diet pills today contain an amphetaminelike drug known as *PPA* (phenylpropanolamine). Some of the PPA diet pills also contain caffeine. The PPA supposedly suppresses the appetite and the caffeine acts as a mild stimulant and diuretic. The user of PPA diet pills is cautioned to discontinue use if dizziness, nervousness, rapid pulse, sleeplessness, or palpitations occur.

There is also a warning that PPA should not be taken by those who suffer from heart disease, high blood pressure, diabetes, thyroid or kidney disorders, or are pregnant, being treated for depression, or are under 18 or over 60 years old. Most PPA diet pills deliver the maximum daily dose of the drug (75 milligrams). However, PPA is also a common ingredient of cold remedy preparations and, if you are taking one of these remedies as well as a PPA diet pill, you could overdose. Users of PPA have been hospitalized for severe hypertension, convulsive seizures, and acute psychosis.

Some drugs not intended for use as dietary aids have been used to promote weight loss. The cardiac stimulant *digitalis*, prescribed for heart patients, induces side effects of anorexia, nausea, and vomiting—which could contribute to loss of appetite and weight. *Thyroid hormones*, beneficial to those with a hypothyroid condition, can—if used indiscriminately—disrupt the normal activity of a healthy thyroid and reduce lean tissues to dangerous levels. Such weight loss is undesirable.

Laxatives and *diuretics*, as beneficial as they may on occasion be, should not be used to promote weight loss.

Diet candy and *gum* usually contain a mild local anesthetic such as Benzocaine, which temporarily deadens your taste buds so that if you cannot taste what you are eating, perhaps you will eat less.

The bulking agent *methylcellulose* is a nondigestible material that, when ingested, swells slowly in the stomach. This eventually makes you feel full but does not diminish appetite significantly. Use can lead to intestinal disorders and bloody diarrhea.

two weeks (the usual period prescribed by popular diet plans) he is once again on his own, equipped with no new insights and in command of no new habits.

Up to this point, the ketogenic diet has been treated principally as a generic item in these pages. But most dieters are likely to come upon a ketogenic diet in the form of a widely advertised, flashily presented "new" diet for sale in a drugstore or bookstore. Though all rely on ketosis, there are differences among them. Some are more restrictive of fats than others; some strictly prohibit, or limit the inclusion of, certain foods; some list allowances of permitted foods by grams or estimated portions; others prescribe meal by meal; some count calories and others do not. The chart on pages 284-285 draws some distinctions between several popular versions of the old meat-and-no-bread diet first peddled more than 100 years ago in London.

Liquid Protein and Protein Supplements

In recent years a variety of diets containing the words "liquid" or "protein," separately or together, have become confused in the public mind. *Liquid diets* contain varying amounts of carbohydrates, protein, and fats in a liquid form. *Liquid protein* is, obviously, protein in a liquid form. *Protein supplement* is protein in a liquid or solid form. The misnamed liquid protein diets are actually hydrolysates of amino acids made from such protein-intense but aesthetically unappealing ingredients as pulverized animal hides and bones. The best known of these was Prolinn, available through physicians and advocated by its inventor, Dr. Robert Linn, author of *The Last Chance Diet.* Such concoctions have been the objects of strong criticism from nutritionists and other health experts.

Much of the alarm generated by the use of protein hydrolysates came in 1977 in the wake of some 50 deaths among users. The victims were mainly women, young and middle aged, severely obese, who had been on the liquid protein diet for periods of up to eight months. In 16 cases, death was caused by cardiac arrhythmia, or irregular heartbeat. The Food and Drug Administration proposed that manufacturers of liquid protein affix warning labels on their products stating that serious illness or death could result from use of the product.

Despite the unfavorable publicity, protein products continue to sell as dieters seek a quick solution to their problems of weight control. The attractions are unmistakable: protein hydrolysate diets offer quick weight loss and freedom from having to choose, plan, and manage one's daily food intake; and they depress appetite after prolonged use, thereby alleviating a major concern of the dieter.

Yet, after sustained use of hydrolysates and in the absence of all food, there can be a serious danger to the heart. Moreover, such low-residue diets are dangerous unless supplemented by such high-residue but low-calorie foods as celery and lettuce to maintain bulk in the lower intestines. In broader terms, protein hydrolysates are counterproductive to the dieter in need of losing weight and keeping it off since they do nothing to alter lifetime eating habits—which should be the dieter's goal.

Fasting

All the major religions of the world observe periods of penitential fasting, and fasting for political reasons has been common in both Eastern and Western cultures. With its philosophical and religious underpinnings, fasting is seen by many as a possibly purifying and edifying experience and it is free. As a quick weight-loss program, it is unquestionably highly effective, resulting in losses of up to a pound a day. By any standard, however, fasting is an extreme dietary measure, not to be undertaken lightly or without consulting your doctor.

The line between fasting and starvation is thin. Doctors who prescribe it for their most-resistant-to-diet patients frequently hospitalize them in order to monitor for such common side effects as lowered blood pressure, anemia, and postural hypotension—a dramatic drop in blood pressure brought on by a sudden change of body position, such as standing up quickly from a seated or lying position.

As in high-protein dieting, the mechanism of weight loss in fasting is ketosis. Dehydration is a danger, and must be averted through conscientious consumption of water. Fasting also depletes the body's store of potassium, sodium, calcium, magnesium, and phosphate.

Only after several days is appetite effectively suppressed, so that fasts of shorter duration must be recognized as food respites, useful for reducing total calorie intake (assuming one does not "make up" for fast days with increased consumption before and

Dealing with Overweight
Reducing Diets

after) but not equivalent to an extended fast. And though dramatic results are possible with a strict, long-term fast, the consequences to health and the prognosis for keeping weight off suggest that this is a dangerous and unwise method for losing weight. Follow-up studies on fasting show that most dieters return to their previous weight within two years of completing a fast.

High-Fat Diets

Quite understandably, no diet guru is going to make his fortune off a scheme billed as a "high-fat diet." Even the most disconsolate, lifelong battler against excess weight would pass such a title by. Yet a number of ketogenic diets that advertise themselves as "high-protein" or "low-carbohydrate" are in fact extremely *high-fat* diets with dangerous implications for the dieter.

The two diets that have generated the most attention—and presumably the greatest number of followers—are the Calories Don't Count diet, first promulgated in 1961 by Dr. Herman Taller, and Dr. Atkins' Diet Revolution, which appeared in 1972. Both books have been the subject of repeated trouncings by nutritionists and the American Medical Association. Dr. Fredrick Stare, former chairman of Harvard's department of nutrition, has been quoted as saying the Atkins' program "borders on malpractice" and amounts to "planned malnutrition," and the respected *Medical Letter* has pronounced it "unbalanced, unsound, and unsafe." Despite such negative reactions to Atkins' diet and despite the fact that every nutritionist knows calories *do* count, both these high-fat diets achieved sizable pieces of the market, demonstrating that health is a minor consideration when dieting becomes an obsession.

High-Carbohydrate Diets

Though less numerous than their high-protein cousins, diets based on high levels of carbohydrates have also been in circulation for years, with a special appeal to dieters who believe they cannot face life without pasta or fresh fruits and vegetables. Such diets buck the prevailing pro-protein sentiment and, because carbohydrates have been so consistently denigrated by diet "experts," have even acquired something of an illicit aura. Recent nutritional findings have rescued the high-carbohydrate approach as a whole from the gimmick category, but the development of popular, balanced high-carbohydrate diets lags far behind.

Although there are many advantages to a balanced vegetarian plan (see pages 392-396), an unbalanced high-carbohydrate diet can be quite dangerous, the chief difficulty being the risk of protein deficiency. In order to obtain sufficient protein to maintain health, one must choose carefully from among the vegetable group and supplement the diet with grains, legumes, eggs, or dairy products. No vegetable by itself provides the complete proteins the body needs. Informed selection is the key.

Two high-carbohydrate diets, each of which has enjoyed some popularity but which unfortunately do not take advantage of the available intelligence, are the Doctor's Quick Inches-Off diet and the Zen Macrobiotic diet. The former is the flip side of Dr. Stillman's Quick Weight Loss diet. Whereas the Quick Weight Loss diet is an all-you-want high-protein plan, Stillman's Inches-Off diet emphasizes vegetables, fruits, grains, pasta, and water. The diet bans all animal protein, but does not make up for it with vegetable protein: although it is a vegetarian regimen, those plant sources that provide needed protein in highest proportions—beans, rice, nuts—are also banned or severely restricted. In short, this is an unhealthy vegetarian diet.

The Zen Macrobiotic diet peaked in popularity during the 1960s, particularly among the young, who adopted it in search less of slimness than of serenity. As defined by its Japanese founder, George Ohsawa, the Zen macrobiotic approach actually includes 10 diet levels, or ways of eating, through which a novice is expected to progress. The lowest level diet, −3, is composed of 10 percent cereal, 30 percent vegetables, 10 percent soups, 30 percent animal products, 15 percent salads and fruits, and 5 percent desserts, and presents no nutritional problem to the dieter. Similarly, diets up to level 0 are nutritionally sound and could be considered an improvement in many respects over the average American diet. The higher levels of the Zen macrobiotic scheme, however, tend to the extreme, with the highest, −7, a diet of unpolished rice and nothing else, disturbingly unsafe.

Balanced Diets

For many dieters, the path to a balanced weight-reducing plan is long, circuitous, and thick with pounds lost several times over in a series of short-term diets with disappointing long-term results. Giving good sense a try seems to come only after bitter experience. But when a dieter *is* ready to face the truth about dieting, it is time for a balanced diet that will yield slow, steady progress, on the order of a pound or two a week, and which will also introduce the dieter to a new way of eating.

One can be a vegetarian or a meat eater, enjoy ethnic foods, eat out (with foresight), eat with others, and eat inexpensively. Eating for good health does not mean being miserable. Neither does being on a diet.

Of the many balanced diets that have been put together over the years by nutritionists and doctors, none has earned such unanimous praise—nor been as universally imitated—as the Prudent diet, published in a 1952 book *Reduce and Stay Reduced*. Devised in the early 1950s by Dr. Norman Jolliffe, director of the New York City Bureau of Nutrition, Department of Health, for a group of middle-aged men believed to be at high risk of heart disease, the diet is actually a carefully thought-out system of low-cholesterol eating that is applicable to persons of all ages, male and female. (*Redbook* magazine has been publishing its adaptation of Jolliffe, under the heading "The Wise Woman's Diet," for the past 15 years.)

The Jolliffe approach insists on informed eating. Any reader of this book, updated several times since its original publication (but not to be confused with the *I Love New York Diet*), will come away with an improved understanding of nutrition as well as a new view of his own personal eating habits. Jolliffe instructs the beginning dieter to measure food portions carefully until he is able to estimate accurately by sight, and to study caloric and nutritional values. In the first half of the book, Jolliffe presents the basic elements of nutrition and diet, disposing of a number of myths along the way, and provides detailed instructions for calculating one's daily caloric expenditure at current weight and the approximate caloric deficit necessary to achieve steady weight loss.

In the book's second half, Jolliffe presents his system of food values, or exchanges, by food group, calorie count and portion size, and the "patterns" which are the daily prescriptions for eating. There are 8 diet patterns for adults, based on daily calorie totals of 600 (to be undertaken only under a doctor's care), 800, 1,000, 1,200, 1,500, 1,800, 2,000, and 2,500. There are also patterns for teenagers (applicable for pregnant women or anyone requiring 4 cups of milk daily), with caloric values ranging from 1,600 to 3,000. Each pattern lists the daily calorie allotment broken into food groups, with portion size and calorie counts specified.

Three suggested daily menus are given for each diet pattern, as are the approximate fat, carbohydrate, and protein values for each. This is an eminently healthy diet, one that guarantees variety, accommodates personal preference, and requires no intolerable deprivation while promising slow, steady, and safe weight loss. By encouraging the reduction of fats and the substitution of polyunsaturated for saturated fats, it falls within the Dietary Guidelines of 1980. Finally, it permits one to diet within a family and among friends.

Some nutritionists would argue for a protein ratio lower than Jolliffe recommends, on the basis of recent studies showing that a shift in favor of more complex carbohydrates increases both overall health and long-term weight loss.

How To Rate a Diet

Consumer Guide suggests the following guidelines.

1. Has the author tried it on hundreds of overweight people, objectively compared the results against a similar number of people on regular or other weight-reducing diets, and published the findings in a reputable medical journal?
2. Is the diet based on some "secret" just discovered? These "secrets" do not exist.
3. Is the diet well-balanced nutritionally? Only well-balanced diets are safe.
4. Is the person promoting the diet known to be knowledgeable in nutrition? Simply being a physician does not qualify one in nutrition.
5. Is the proponent of the new diet challenging the recommendations of the best authorities? A valid challenge has to be backed up by new findings available for scrutiny.
6. Does the diet allow for individual preference, practice, and taste? Rigid diets that tell you what and when to eat and give you no nutritional information are doomed to fail.
7. Could you live on this for the rest of your life? Weight control is a lifelong effort.

Dealing with Overweight
Reducing Diets

Dieters in search of a more radical, but still balanced, approach to weight loss and health might look to the Pritikin Program for Diet and Exercise, a regimen based on what Nathan Pritikin calls "an essentially Third World" diet, and a total departure from the average American diet.

On the Pritikin reducing plan, one eats as often as 8 times a day, but consumes no more than 600 calories per day, largely in the form of complex carbohydrates—vegetables and grains—and fruits, with the foods that make up the bulk of the ordinary American menu reduced to virtual condiment status. Fats, oils, sugar, and honey are strictly forbidden, as are coffee, tea, tobacco, and alcohol, while meats, eggs, poultry, dairy products, and even fish, traditional dieters' friends, are doled out by ounces: no more than 3½ ounces of meat, 2 ounces of cheese, and 8 ounces of milk per day.

Pritikin bills his diet as a life saver, and has drawn most of his followers—many of whom have been willing to pay $5,000 and up in order to spend 26 days learning new habits of diet and exercise at Pritikin centers in Santa Monica and Santa Barbara, California—from the ranks of cardiovascular patients or those who believe themselves headed in that direction. A principal goal of the Pritikin plan is to reduce cholesterol in the diet and prevent its collection in the arteries. Even after one has reached a desired weight (Pritikin claims average losses of 13 pounds in 26 days), there is no return to old ways of eating, only a modest increase in the total calories permitted per day.

Critics of Pritikin have focused less on the principles of eating he proposes—which, though bordering on protein deficient, are generally quite sound nutritionally—and more on the extravagance of his claim to be able to reverse active heart disease through diet and exercise. Within the medical establishment, few are willing to grant the measure of success that Pritikin, a layman, claims. And many who evince interest in his methods are reluctant to try to persuade patients to adopt them, conscious of how spartan a program it is. (The weight-loss diet of 600 calories a day should not be started except under a doctor's care.) The Pritikin diet requires that one forswear lifelong tastes and habits—for many a nearly impossible undertaking. Nonetheless, as we shall see beginning on page 296, losing weight means reassessing one's eating habits.

Before You Pick a Diet

"All diets should be made to suit the patient," Dr. Norman Jolliffe wrote in *Reduce and Stay Reduced*, "and not the patient made to fit the diet." Following are Dr. Jolliffe's suggestions for determining whether or not a diet is satisfactory for you.

1. The reducing diet should contain sufficient high-value protein to prevent vital body tissues (organ and muscle) from being utilized for protein. Without an adequate amount of such high-value protein as meat, fish, poultry, shellfish, eggs, or milk included in each meal, the reducer may develop weakness, nervousness, fatigue, and other symptoms of protein depletion. With adequate protein intake, these symptoms occur less frequently, and when they do are probably psychological.

2. The reducing diet should contain less than 30 percent of its calories as fat. This means a diet not high in fat; it does not necessarily mean a low-fat diet. It is recognized that a small amount of fat in the diet is necessary.

3. The reducing diet should contain 50 grams of carbohydrate, or 1 gram for each 3 pounds of ideal body weight, whichever is the larger. This minimum amount of carbohydrate will prevent such rapid burning of fat as to cause acidosis. It also will prevent too rapid withdrawal of fat from the body's fatty tissues, which may cause unusual lipemia (too much fat in the blood).

4. The reducing diet should contain sufficient minerals and vitamins to ensure optimum health [a full discussion of this subject is given on pages 30-49].

5. A reducing diet should form the basis for your dietary re-education so that proper eating habits will continue after the desired loss of weight has been attained. For this reason, high-fat diets, low-protein diets, skipping meals, and uncommon or trick diets that do not furnish a sound basis for permanent dietary habits are not recommended.

To be completely satisfactory, a reducing diet should meet the above standards. A diet that fails to do so should be followed for only the most compelling medical reasons as decided by your physician.

Spas and Support Groups

No matter what diet they try, and no matter how many times they try, some people can't seem to lick the problem of overweight alone. The well-to-do with that sort of problem take themselves off to "fat farms," spas where every morsel and every movement are accounted for and lack of willpower doesn't count against them. The combination of expense (over $200 a day at some spas), prearranged meals, programmed exercise, the company of other dieters, and the absence of reminders of real life back home seems to do for some dieters what the prospect of a solitary diet stretching without end into the future somehow never does. For veterans of the diet wars, a spa may provide a much deserved vacation from solitary misery.

The range of styles in spas is quite broad, from the unabashedly plush like The Greenhouse, between Dallas and Fort Worth, Texas, to the diet camps run by one of the mutual support groups at several locations around the country. The majority of spas offer low-calorie meals and a program of exercise including facilities for swimming, tennis, and other sports. Some have resident physicians, but not all do, an important fact to determine in advance. Certain spas bill themselves as "natural" or "health" resorts where, for example, one is offered "a controlled diet program, fasting in the conditions of peace and quiet, a personalized exercise program, and most important, a continued health education in the principles of right living. . . ."

Because each spa takes a slightly different approach, anyone contemplating a stay in one should get the facts straight before mailing off a check. But more fundamentally, one should take a realistic look at what is being offered and what one is likely to accomplish in a week or two of dieting anywhere. Those nubile bodies on the brochure covers didn't get that way because of a two-week visit to a spa; two weeks isn't likely to transform you, either. As a luxurious send-off to a new you, or possibly as a grand finale to diet well-observed over time, a spa may be just the thing. Reality, however, resides at home.

Not many dieters can afford the spa approach except in fantasy, but several of the elements that make it appealing turn up in a relatively recent and growing approach to dieting: support groups.

To hear their members tell it, support groups for weight loss may be the greatest diet discovery since water, and have been steadily growing in membership since 1948, when Esther Manz first organized a group of women neighbors in Wisconsin to form the nucleus of what was legally incorporated in 1952 as TOPS (Take Off Pounds Sensibly.)

TOPS was followed in 1960 by Overeaters Anonymous, in 1963 by Weight Watchers International, Inc., and in 1965 by Diet Workshop, Inc. These four groups are the biggest diet organizations, but new groups, smaller and often regionally based, appear each year. All operate on similar principles: weekly meetings for group support and discussion, careful diet and menu planning, exchange of diet tips, weigh-ins, goal setting, a recommended exercise program, and behavior modification techniques. The dieter is urged to examine closely his or her eating habits, in order to discover why and when overeating most typically occurs, how to handle social situations, how to win needed support from friends and relatives. Still, there are differences in attitude and approach among the clubs, and each is likely to have differences among its local chapters.

TOPS is modeled on Alcoholics Anonymous, with each "chapter" retaining a high degree of autonomy, electing its own leaders and running its own meetings. Members, who receive a monthly magazine and access to TOPS dietary research (paid for by members' fees and contributions), are encouraged to compete for most pounds lost.

Overeaters Anonymous, also based on AA principles, duplicates the language of AA when it declares that "compulsive overeating is an illness, a progressive illness, which cannot be cured but which like other illnesses, can be arrested. . ." The focus, therefore, is on overeating as an obsessive disorder and on treating the underlying problem rather than its physical manifestation, overweight. There is no membership fee in OA (as there is in TOPS), but members are invited at meetings to make donations to cover expenses. Members attend meetings as often as they need, depending on availability. OA is not in the "diet" business but is in the business of habit-fighting. It does not offer diet programming or weigh-ins, but recommends that members consult their own doctors. The basis for recovery is abstinence: abstaining from overeating one day at a time. As part of their recovery programs, overeaters are expected to be candid in sharing their experiences with other overeaters.

Dealing with Overweight
Spas and Support Groups

Weight Watchers International, Inc. (since 1978 a subsidiary of the H.J. Heinz Company) is a big business as well as a weight-loss system. Members pay for weekly meetings (including those that are missed) and are encouraged, along with the general public, to purchase Weight Watchers frozen meals, soft drinks, and other diet products. The organization recommends specific diet plans for reducing (at a rate of 1–2 pounds per week), leveling off, and maintenance. The diets offer full choice, limited choice, and no choice, and there is a vegetarian plan as well. Weight Watchers diets are based not on calories but on portion size and follow a protein, carbohydrate, fat ratio of 25:45:30. The protein ratio is slightly higher than those of the dietary goals to ensure adequate protein on a low-calorie diet. The program is quite strict, with certain foods declared "illegal"; wine and beer are permitted. Weight Watchers does not advocate diet pills, food substitutes, or dietetic products such as appetite suppressants and protein mixes.

As with TOPS, there is a weigh-in at the start of every meeting, followed by a lecture and a discussion period; emphasis is on behavior modification and group support. Weight Watchers offers an exercise program and publishes a monthly magazine.

Diet Workshop, Inc., like TOPS and Weight Watchers, was founded by overweight housewives. Co-founder Edith Berman weighed 221 pounds when she joined her fat friend Lois Lynns Lindauer to start the franchise operation. After 16 years of experience, Diet Workshop knows that weight control is a long-term commitment and is geared to weight maintenance as well as to initial weight reduction. Members pay a registration fee, plus weekly dues. Meetings provide group discussions and close, individual attention and support—"We Are with You All the Weigh" is one DW motto. DW offers two diets: the Beacon Hill Diet, a regimented, rapid weight-loss plan, and the Flexi-Diet for those who have gained some control over eating problems. It also offers a person-to-person counseling service, extending its philosophy of personal attention and support. Dieters who doubt their own resolve should know that DW does not give up easily, keeping up with members and vigorously pursuing dropouts. According to *Consumer Guide*'s 1981 diet review, DW offers more personal attention than its competitors.

Confessions of an F.F.H.

In her 1970 book *The Story of Weight Watchers*, Jean Nidetch described her personal route to permanent weight loss—and the beginning of the famous reducing organization she helped found.

F.F.H. That's me. A Formerly Fat Housewife once married to a Formerly Fat Bus Driver. I'm also a Formerly Fat Baby, a Formerly Fat Child, and a Formerly Fat Girl. I was fat until I was 38 years old, only I didn't call myself fat. I never said the word "fat." I weighed 214 pounds and I was "chubby." But "chubby" isn't for 38-year-olds, it belongs to 18. That's when I discovered I was "big-boned." I carried my "big bones" on a "large frame," and I "carried my weight" rather well. I was a perfect size 44. I surrounded myself with big-boned, large-framed people. I was married to a fat man. I had a fat dog and fat friends. My whole world was fat.

I found out that all big-boned people developed a disease. The disease we had was "glandular." I'm not even sure what "glandular" is, except my doctor said, "You don't have it." But I liked having "glandular" because it was a great sickness for me. I found that "glandular" develops into something more serious called "heredity." My fat was inherited. One of my aunts was very stout—even if she wasn't actually a blood relative.

Every night in the bathtub, I would make a promise. I used to promise that I would choke on the next cookie. When you are sitting in a bathtub, there is no place to look. When you look in a mirror, you learn never to look below the shoulders. You concentrate on the face. You tell yourself you have pretty eyes and a nice nose. When you buy clothes, you are very concerned with what's happening at the neckline. When you have your picture taken, there's always a child, a chair, a sweater, *something* to hide behind. But in a bathtub? It's all you and it's floating. You can't escape it. I never took a bath but that I wasn't sure I had been cursed.

After my bath, I'd make the terrible mistake of walking into my living room, where I was forced to look at my couch. Obviously, when you don't like your couch, you have to eat something. Some people think that's ridiculous. For them, it's the carpeting that makes them eat. Or the drapes that don't hang right. After looking at my couch, I would go into the kitchen and eat some chocolate-covered marshmallow cookies.

I weighed 214 pounds in 1961, only I never told

anybody. On my driver's license, I always wrote 145. I had never, in my adult life, weighed 145. That was me, Jean Nidetch, in 1961—214 pounds of big bones on a large frame, suffering from glandular heredity, making promises in the bathtub and breaking them in the kitchen.

I had dieted all my life. I dieted in preparation for birthday parties. I dieted for graduation. I dieted for my engagement party. I dieted for my wedding. I'm talking about crash diets, any fast method like black coffee with nothing. Or black coffee and cigarettes, or eggs and grapefruit. Oil capsules. Wafers that looked and tasted like dog biscuits. I took little red pills, little yellow pills, little green pills. I lost weight hundreds of times. You can lose weight if you eat watermelon for two weeks. Or bananas and milk, or cottage cheese and peaches. Sometimes you don't feel well, often you don't look well, but you always lose weight. After I'd lose 20 or 30 pounds, I'd always go off the diet. That's what a diet is, something to go on and then go off.

But this time, starting in late 1961, it was different. I discovered a new way of eating and a new way to live. And that was the beginning of the Weight Watchers story. I lost 72 pounds—but that's not my claim to fame because I probably could have done that on oil and evaporated milk. The important thing is that I've maintained that loss. I fluctuate a few pounds this side or that, but I never get panicky because I know I'll never be fat again.

I discovered a diet written by Dr. Norman Jolliffe many years ago [the Prudent diet, see page 291]. Desperation drove me to the New York City Department of Health Obesity Clinic in October 1961, and there I was handed a piece of paper with a diet on it. The first thought in my mind was that I would rewrite it, change it to suit myself. I would find a way to substitute cake for something else. I looked for a way to work in my favorite cookies.

But I wasn't allowed to substitute anything. I wasn't allowed to cut out anything. I had to go along with the entire program or I wouldn't be permitted to stay with the clinic. And I *had* to stay with the clinic because I was desperate. I was making one last effort to dig myself out of all that fat. I had been fat all my life and I wanted to get down to a size 20.

I did get down to a size 20, then a size 18, 16, 14, and finally 12. From a perfect 44 I went to an imperfect 12, and I've stayed that way. I now weigh 142, even less than what it used to say on my driver's license.

I lost all that weight on the obesity clinic's diet, but I added something. I added talk. I found that I couldn't do it on a diet alone. I had to be able to *talk* about my eating problems, to tell other people what I was going through. So I called up a few fat friends and asked them to come to my house to talk. They came. And then they came every week after that, bringing other fat people with them. It was our little group where we met to tell each other about being fat. Soon the group grew—40, 50, 60, 100 people—until now half a million people gather each week in classes run by formerly fat people like myself to talk about losing weight. There have been 11 million enrollments in Weight Watchers. My little private club has become an industry. I never intended it to. It was really just a group, a group for me and my fat friends.

I've heard people describe Weight Watchers as "group therapy." I have heard people say, "It must be brainwashing." It's been called "self-hypnosis," a "revival meeting," and "the fat man's Alcoholics Anonymous." One of our lecturers once said, "It's a place where you walk in fat and hope nobody notices you, and four or five months later, you walk out thin and hope that everyone notices you."

I prefer to call it a program, because it is not something you just forget about when you have lost your weight. It's a plan for managing your eating that will stay with you the rest of your life, if you want to remain thin. You learn to eat, in an intelligent, disciplined way, three meals a day with "legal" snacks in between.

So, you see, Weight Watchers is more than simply a diet. It's people gathering together to learn new eating habits. When they eat. Why they eat. How they eat. And to learn new attitudes about eating, so that food no longer will make them fat.

It works. Overeating can be an emotional problem, and because we recognized that, we developed a program that helps people handle their problems in better ways than stuffing food into their mouths.

The biggest reason Weight Watchers is such a success is that fat people can finally talk freely, openly, and honestly. We can reveal our real feelings to other people, and those other people will understand. I can say to a Weight Watchers class, "I remember sitting in a bathtub watching my fat floating," and there isn't a person there who can't relate to me at that moment. A thin person would never understand that.

Eating Sensibly

Eating is one of the great, necessary pleasures in life, one of those select activities that both feels good and is good for you. If food were not so important, then potatoes and carrots might taste like the dirt they are grown in, and our salivary glands would not begin working at the smell of a roasting chicken nearing doneness in the oven. In serving up life's sustenance in such glorious, tempting variety, Nature ensured that we would survive and flourish.

That food is both tasty and essential is impossible to argue, yet it is equally clear that, to a great extent for some people, to a lesser extent for many more, it has become something else—a source of inordinate unhappiness manifest in food anxieties, phobias, and obsessions, and too often the cause of serious medical problems as well.

Eating need not result in any of these unwanted consequences. It is possible to eat and enjoy eating; whether you eat well and with pleasure, or poorly, with guilt and anxiety, is up to you. Placing food in its proper perspective is the first step. Understanding its role in your life is the second. Creating a framework for eating sensibly is the third.

What we're talking about is the development of an informed philosophy of food that will see you healthily through a long life. There is no need to banish ceremonial or celebratory food from your table. But it is essential to introduce moderation and balance to your diet and critical to distinguish between eating to satisfy your energy and health needs and eating to satisfy emotional or other needs.

Healthy eating requires a basic understanding of nutrition and in particular of your own body's nutritional needs at different stages of life. It requires forethought, careful meal planning, and coordination. Initially, it means giving a lot of thought to how and when you eat and being determined to stick to your resolution. Before long, good eating will become second nature, by which we mean letting one's good—that is, informed—sense take over.

The problem for many people lies in distinguishing among competing, frequently confusing sources of information about what is best, and incorporating that information into daily life. For many adults, the occasion of parenthood makes nutrition a matter of interest for the first time. Few parents knowingly overlook the obligation to provide their children with proper nutrition, and often consult with a pediatrician about diet. It is a rare mother who does as much for herself. The strong conviction that nutrition matters seems to weaken when the subject in question is no longer a child but a parent or grandparent. All those good habits we try to instill in children are contradicted by our poor eating habits as adults. But proper nutrition is a lifelong necessity. It *is* important to start a child off right; it is just as important, for lifelong health and well-being, for adults to attend to their diets. Many of the conditions that most limit the freedom and reduce the quality of life for adults and the elderly are avoidable: proper diet is in many instances the means of avoiding such conditions.

Our purpose here is to help you reevaluate your family's eating habits and then develop a personal system of food management that not only ensures health but is appropriate to the food tastes, energy needs, daily habits, current or desired weights, and special short-term needs of everyone in the family, from an infant to its grandparent. The emphasis is on the practical, a plan for eating you can live with and enjoy and that accommodates the changing nutritional requirements of the body as it grows to maturity and begins to age.

For many readers, the first priority—and possibly the original impetus for rethinking one's eating habits—is reducing. In the next four pages, we show you first how to determine your ideal weight and calculate your daily calorie needs; and then, how to reduce safely and with real hope of success through a combination of conscientious, balanced dieting and the practice of behavior modification techniques that have helped many dieters change the self-defeating habits of a lifetime.

But before you read any further, take a moment to try to get a fix on how you and your family are doing right now by answering these questons:

• What is your primary reason for eating? Survival? Maintenance? Hunger? Something to do? Frustration? Anger? Depression? Boredom?

• Have you ever really surveyed the eating habits and nutritional needs of members of your family?

• Do you know that different age groups have different nutritional needs?

• Are you as aware of what your child eats as what you eat? What about grandmother or grandfather—do you know what and how much they eat?

• Do you know what members of your family are eating when they eat away from home? Do you try

Name: John R. Doe			Food Intake Record					Date: 9.14.82
Time Start-End	Place	Physical Position	With Whom	Eating Cues	Associated Activity	Mood	Degree of Hunger	Food Eaten and Amount
7:30 8:00	kitchen	sitting	family	breakfast time	making notes for work	rushed	0	3 cups coffee
10:00 10:30	office	standing	co-workers	coffee break	discussing report	tense	3	1 cup coffee, 1 apricot danish
12:30 1:45	restaurant	sitting	important business contact	lunch	discussing contract	nervous	2	1 martini, salad, roll, lasagna, 1/2 piece cheesecake
6:00	living room	sitting	wife	cocktail hour	discussing children's school	angry	4	2 beers, 1/2 cup peanuts
6:30 7:15	dining room	sitting	wife and kids	dinner	planning vacation	relaxed	3	steak, baked potato with sour cream, salad
10:30	bedroom	sitting	wife	T.V. commercial	watching T.V.	drowsy	1	slice of cake, glass of milk

to compensate for any possible imbalances in their diet with foods served at home?
• Does your family eat good breakfasts?
• What types of foods are most often thrown away? Why are they thrown away?
• Do you adjust the portion sizes for child, teenager, adult, senior citizen?
• Is dinner the main meal? Lunch?
• How soon after eating do you go to bed?
• Who snacks and when and on what?
• What are you doing about the poor eater in your family? The overeater?
• If your child's school has a school lunch program, do you see the weekly menus? Are the school lunches adequate? If not, do you pack lunches?
• Are meals eaten at the table or in front of the television?
• Do you sit down together to eat as a family? Do you avoid arguments at mealtime?
• If single, do you prepare full meals or just snacks? Do you skip meals?
• If you know you are going to eat out, do you plan your other meals as a nutritional complement?
• Are you able to say no to someone who tries to put too much food on your plate?
• Are there foods that you won't eat because they look strange? Do your children follow your example? Would you want your children to eat as you do when they grow up?

• Do you use food to bribe, reward, punish?
• How often do you shop and what do you buy?
• When do you do your shopping? After meals? When you are hungry, tired, with the children?
• Do you have a vegetable garden? Did the children help in the planning and maintenance of the garden?
• Do you allow junk food in the house? Always? Often? Rarely? Never?

Discovering that most of your weekday meals are eaten on the run, that your teenager eats six meals a day while your 2-year-old eats barely one, and your aging parent consistently skips protein in favor of sweets may give you some perspective on your family's assorted dietary gaps.

Another valuable method of evaluating food patterns is the food diary above. Simply keep a faithful record of everything you eat (get the others to keep their own diaries) for a week or two, noting the type and amount of food and drink, the time and place it's eaten, the physical position you're in, whether alone or with others, what else is going on, your emotional state, and the degree of hunger you were experiencing at the time, on a scale of 1 to 5. A week or two of scrupulously honest entries should give you all the information you need about what, when, and how you eat. Thus armed, you're well on your way to developing a new system of personal and family food management.

Eating Sensibly
Finding Your Ideal Weight and Calorie Needs

What kind of shape are you in? A good long look in a full-length mirror, muscles slackened, front, rear, and side views included, should give you a general idea. If you are overweight, those excess pounds will glow like neon: bulging thighs and an inflated derriere on a woman, a protruding belly and flabby chest on a man. Too thin? Can you circle your forearm close to the elbow with the fingers of one hand? Can you count your ribs by sight instead of by feel? Are you slightly uncomfortable sitting on a hard chair?

Chances are you already know, or think you do, whether you are overweight or under. The first question is by how much? The second, what can you do about it.

The modern concept of an "ideal" weight for each person is just that—a concept, not a fact. It derives chiefly from two sources of equally dubious authority. One is the standard of fashion, the other the height-weight charts issued by the insurance industry and based on data that correlate weight and longevity and nothing else. Both imply certain untruths—that a standard is possible or desirable, that thin is better than not thin, that weight-to-height is the primary measure of fitness.

The truth is that the range of what is normal, or health promoting, or even average is quite broad, as the charts on this page, which reflect current nutritional thinking, demonstrate. Weight alone tells us too little about fitness. A well-conditioned football player may be overweight by the charts, but in reality fit because his excess weight is muscle and bone, not fat. As for longevity and weight, studies have shown that life span is the result of many interwoven factors, of which weight is but one. Unless your weight is significantly under the minimum or over the maximum shown below, or unless you fail one of the sight or touch tests mentioned earlier, drastic action is not in order.

If, on the other hand, your weight is markedly low, or high, and you don't feel well to boot, you may want to consider changing your caloric intake.

Whatever your ideal weight, you probably attained it around the age of 20, at the end of your adolescent growth spurt. But, to maintain that weight, and health, through maturity and into old age requires a steady reduction of calories after reaching adulthood. How many men and women look up in surprise to discover themselves "fat" in their 30s, though they swear in good conscience that they haven't been eating any more than they did when in college? What happened? Age and less physical activity, not gluttony, did it.

Calories are energy: they come in the form of food and are spent in activity, the most fundamental measure of which is called the basal metabolism rate

Average and Range of Weight

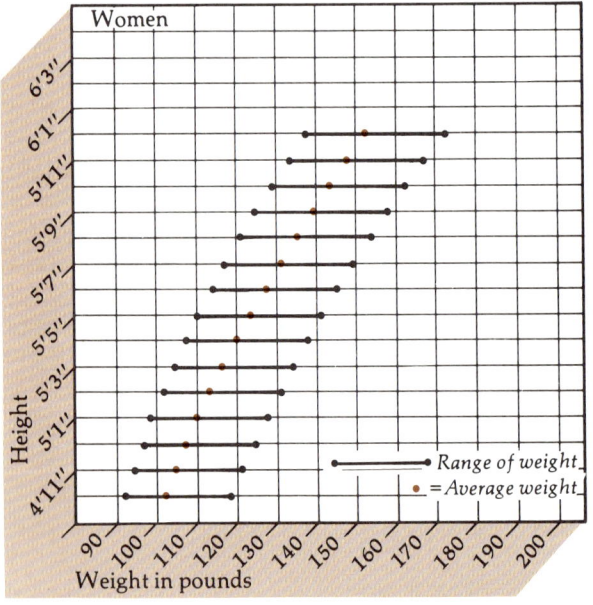
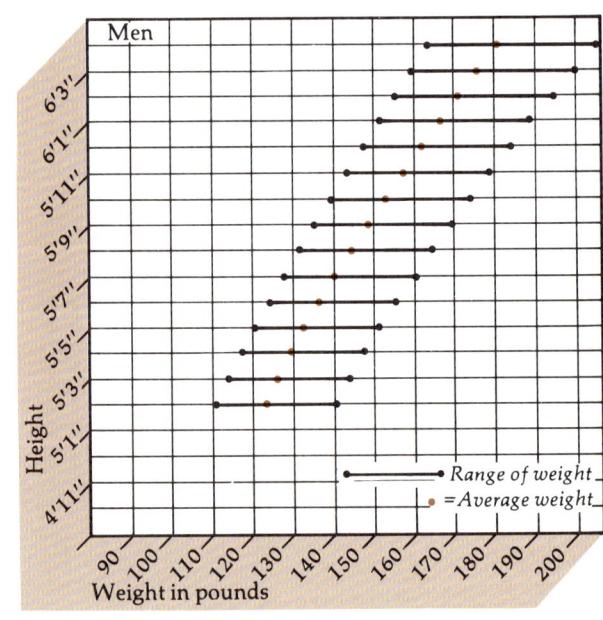

(BMR), or resting metabolism—a highly individual, and variable, measure of how many calories are required to fuel the body at rest. Although one can roughly calculate one's BMR by adding a zero to one's body weight, then adding that figure to one's weight (thus, 120 pounds becomes 1,200 + 120 = 1,320), the variance by age, sex, and condition is considerable. Big people, whether fat or large framed, simply spend more calories than small people. Because muscle needs more fuel than fat, athletes have a BMR higher than other people.

The BMR responds to many influences: it speeds up dramatically during pregnancy, when a woman's BMR rises by as much as 28 percent; it slows to conserve the body's resources in times of stress, deprivation, or illness. And, as the charts below (derived from the Recommended Dietary Allowances) show, it slows with age. At 25, a 154-pound man in good health consumes as many as 2,900 calories daily. His 65-year-old same-weight counterpart requires barely 2,200.

All these influences make calculating your individual BMR an inexact process, but you can get a fair idea of what your *total* daily expenditure of calories should be by multiplying your current weight by a factor of 13.6 if you are largely sedentary, by 16 to 18 if you are moderately active, and by 20 if you are very active.

With that estimate in mind, you can perform the basic math necessary to guide you in a weight-loss or weight-gain program. One pound of body weight is equivalent to 3,500 calories. To add a pound you must consume 3,500 more calories than you spend. To shed a pound you must spend 3,500 more than you take in. If you want to lose 5 pounds, you must create a deficit of 17,500 calories. Assume your daily intake is 2,100 calories. With a daily deficit of 500 calories, you will lose a pound a week and 5 pounds in 35 days. If you follow a 1,200 calorie per day program (the lowest safe diet recommended by nutrition experts), you will create a deficit of 900 calories a day and, theoretically, shed the 5 pounds in 20 days. If you add exercise you can hasten the weight loss without further calorie deficit.

The key word is "theoretically." Our bodies do not respond only to exterior signals. They have their own directives, and these are powerful. Some nutritionists talk of a "set point," a natural weight that one's body strives to maintain. The set point may explain why some of us seem to lose the same 5 or 10 pounds over and over again: we say 130, but our bodies answer 135. Before you break your spirit on a diet, close your eyes to fashion and listen to your body. Unless your doctor finds medical reasons for you to lose weight, you may decide—if you are only moderately overweight—to leave well enough alone.

Energy Needs by Age

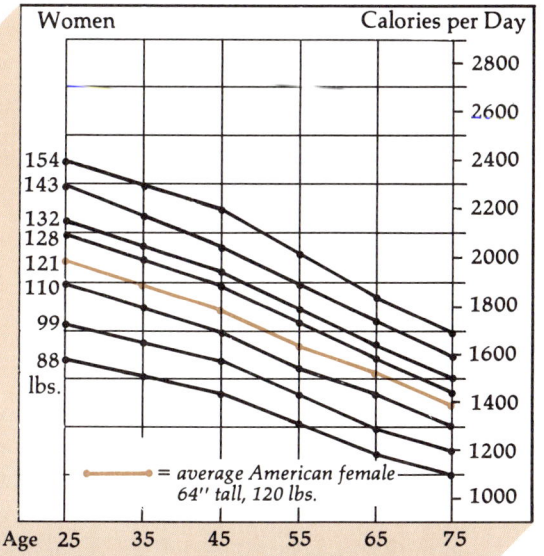

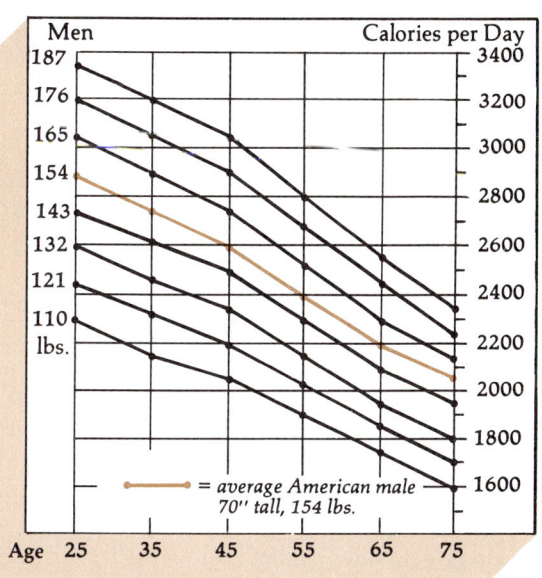

Eating Sensibly
Changing Your Eating Habits

"Diet" is a word that gives a lot of people trouble—whether they are trying to lose weight, are worried that they are not eating the right things, or attribute their poor health to bad eating habits. To most of us, "diet" means just one thing—miserable, punishing, and seemingly interminable deprivation, even when undertaken for a short time. A distinctly unhappy prospect, it is also an unnecessary one. The key is a change in attitude.

One who learned that lesson well is Jane Brody, personal health columnist for *The New York Times*. "I've spent much of my life watching my weight," she writes in *Jane Brody's Nutrition Book*. "From my early teens to my mid-twenties, it was mostly watching it go up. And nearly all that time, I was on a diet. . . . I tried them all—all the commercial versions of the day plus a few I devised on my own. . . . Then, fourteen years ago, desperate, disgusted, and fat, I made a decision: I stopped dieting and started to eat like a 'normal' person. I ate every meal, and I ate all the foods I loved. But instead of becoming even more like the Goodyear blimp, I started to lose. Slowly, to be sure . . . but painlessly. . . . After two years of not dieting, I weighed 35 pounds less than when I had lived from one best-selling weight-loss scheme to the next. And I never regained the lost pounds."

The key to Brody's success was neither a special food (added or forbidden) nor a special diet, but her decision to restore food to its proper place in her life. You can make a similar decision for yourself. Moreover, if you have children, your example will contribute heavily to the shaping of *their* lifelong attitudes toward food.

Begin by redefining the word "diet" so that it functions for you in a personal and positive way. Instead of focusing on restrictions, focus on choices. In place of abstinence and self-denial, try being good to yourself. Don't *diet*; eat well. Stop thinking of diet in terms of what some authority says you can't eat; that attitude will only make you resentful and rebellious. Think instead in terms of what *you* choose to eat in order to feel and look the way *you* want to. The goal is to design a personal food program that frees you from anxiety about eating. A diet needn't be something you go on for a while and then turn your back on; it can be a liberation, if you let it be.

Although most people undertake an overhaul of their diet with weight loss in mind, the task is equally appropriate to those who are underweight or *undernourished* at any weight. Many people who are thin or even "just-the-right" weight stay that way at real cost to their health. They too need to achieve balance by rethinking their dietary patterns.

Making It Work. In recent years the psychological approach called behavior modification has proved highly successful in treating eating disorders from the mild to the very serious. Because many experts believe that external stimuli, or cues in the environment, trigger eating, they have focused on altering habits that are, in fact, conditioned responses to false stimuli. What many people read as signals to eat are in fact symptoms—or sensations—of fatigue, anger, depression, anxiety, boredom, or tension. The aim of behavior modification is to teach you to recognize when you are most vulnerable to false stimuli and how to change your behavior to thwart inappropriate responses. By attending to *your* patterns, *your* habits, and *your* responses, you can avoid the feeling of helplessness that overtakes troubled eaters. These tips should help get you started.

• The first step is to decide you really do want to change. List the benefits you believe will result if you succeed in gaining control of your eating.

• Set realistic goals and realistic means of achieving them. (Weight gained over 10 years can't be lost in a week or two.)

• Focus on patterns, not pounds. You are teaching yourself new responses, not counting every bite.

• Avoid situations that cause anxiety—it leads to eating, which leads to more anxiety which leads. . . .

• Never use food as a reward or a tranquilizer, nor as a punishment.

• Don't collapse in guilt if you break down and have a brownie. Just put away the rest of the brownies and pat yourself on the back.

• Keep a food diary. Be honest and precise.

• When you've become aware of your personal danger zones, take action to avoid them: plan ahead; change your routine; avoid temptation.

• Eat three meals a day. Don't skimp. Have a good breakfast and make every meal an occasion.

• If you must snack, make it low calorie and make the most of it. Eat it slowly. Don't gobble.

• Eat only sitting down; and when at home, in a place designated specially for eating.

- Present food attractively. Divide meals into two or more courses, even if the second course is only coffee or tea.
- Avoid distractions at the table: no reading, no television. If with company, have a pleasant conversation. Avoid arguments and anger.
- Serve yourself small portions on a small plate. It will look less skimpy.
- Eat slowly. Taste your food. Put down your knife and fork after every two or three bites. Make each meal last 20 to 30 minutes.
- Postpone that second helping 20 minutes, time enough to realize you don't need it.
- Eat your favorite foods first so you don't stuff yourself at the end of the meal. Sip water between bites; this will not only fill you up but will also slow you down.
- Don't think you have to clean your plate. If you've piled it on too high, throw what you don't want into the soup pot.
- Never shop when hungry. Make a list and stick to it. Buy only what you need right now. Buy small packages, even if they aren't the best bargain. Buy foods that require preparation—and time to think about whether you really need to eat.
- Don't lay in snacks for uninvited visitors.
- Store food out of sight in cupboards.
- Stay out of the kitchen when not preparing or eating scheduled meals.
- Build support for success. Educate those close to you to reinforce your efforts. But weight control and eating habits are your responsibility. Don't ask someone else to control your actions.
- Act thin. Stand erect. Walk confidently at any weight and you'll look better, feel better.
- Look at yourself in the mirror once a day, but weigh yourself only every week or two. Weight fluctuates from day to day, and you could unfairly become discouraged by failure to lose or by suddenly gaining a pound or two. Get some form of exercise periodically, at least twice a week.

Once you reach your desired weight or state of health, don't revert to old eating habits. Remind yourself that you've just accomplished something terrific. And, if you do find your weight creeping back up, start keeping a diary again to find out where you're having trouble. You'll have had a lot of practice running your own life by then. It shouldn't take long to get yourself back on track.

If You Want To Gain Weight

Often, the reverse of advice for losing weight will help you put on desired pounds if you are underweight. Here are some tips from *Jane Brody's Nutrition Book*.

1. Try to increase your caloric intake by about 500 calories a day—that will put on a pound a week—by adding high-calorie foods to your meals or consuming them as between-meal snacks.
2. Fat is the most concentrated source of calories, so you might use more vegetable oils and polyunsaturated margarines.
3. Avoid bulky, low-calorie foods with your meals lest they fill you up before you've consumed an adequate number of calories. Eat your salad as a side dish after your main course and use lots of rich dressing.
4. Concentrate on high-calorie vegetables, such as winter squash, dried beans, and potatoes, and don't skimp on rice, pasta, and bread.
5. Don't drink water, tea, coffee, or other low-calorie drinks before eating or with your meal. However, a cocktail before dinner or wine with dinner can help you relax and may stimulate your appetite.
6. Snack two or three hours before meals so it won't ruin your appetite. An excellent time for a high-calorie snack is just before bed.
7. If you find you can eat only small amounts of food at a time, plan substantial meals and divide them into five or six "doses" over the course of your day rather than trying to eat a large, complete meal at one sitting.
8. Get some exercise on a regular basis. This will tone up your body, help you to relax, and improve your overall sense of well-being. Exercise will also help you to put on extra pounds as muscle rather than flabby fat. But don't go overboard on exercise or you'll end up burning more calories than you can consume, and losing weight instead of gaining it.
9. Be sure to get lots of rest. Taking daily exercise, avoiding caffeine-containing beverages, and perhaps drinking a glass of warm milk at bedtime will help to improve your ability to relax and sleep well.
10. If you're a smoker, quit, and try food when you want to put something to your lips.

Eating Sensibly
Balanced Meal Planning

Whatever the reasons for changing your eating habits—to lose weight, to improve health, to cut back on salt, fat, or sweets, or simply to start eating a balanced diet—the true test comes not as you contemplate the figures on a scale or scan the items on a grocer's shelf, but daily, and day after day, in the food you put on the table for yourself and your family.

To meet any caloric maximum or nutritional minimum requires forethought, as the previous pages have stressed. Few of us, however, have the time to spend toiling over menu plans, totaling grams of protein, vitamin units, and calories according to source. Still less likely is it that such minutiae will be worked out for all the different members of the family, each of whom is likely to have different nutritional needs. How, then, does one go about feeding a family practically and without bringing a calculator and food scale to the table?

As the sample menus opposite demonstrate, the answer lies in providing a nutritional base for all, with additions, exchanges or omissions designed to accommodate the specific needs of individual family members. A breakfast offering of orange juice, cereal or whole-grain bread with butter and jelly, and a glass of milk, for example, will provide that base for the whole family. The adolescent who requires 3,000 or more calories and four to six 8-ounce glasses of milk a day just to stay even nutritionally, however, can easily drink another glass of milk and eat an extra slice or two of toast at breakfast. His slightly overweight mother, on the other hand, might want to skip the butter and jelly on her toast and substitute skim milk for whole, whereas his little sister will probably eat only the basic, 2,000-calorie menu.

The first step in sketching a balanced family menu is to assess your family's individual and group needs. Working from the Dietary Guidelines (see pages 96-97) and the nutritive value charts beginning on page 51, you can establish a nutritional and caloric base for every member of the family, from infant through toddler and adolescent to adult and grandparent or other elderly relative if appropriate. If this is the first time you've ever attempted to survey your family nutritionally, you might begin by reading the special sections on the different age groups or special conditions that follow. The basic daily requirements, you'll find, will be similar for all members of the family, although volume, choice, and thus total caloric intake will vary considerably.

Using a chart like the one at right, above, block out the family's weekly allowance in each category. Once you have a clear picture of how much food from each category each member of the family is likely to consume in a given week, you can begin to plan menus.

Thinking in terms of weeks rather than days is not only efficient and economical—it makes practical nutritional sense as well. No food is required everyday, but certain nutrient-rich foods should be eaten occasionally—liver once a week for adolescent girls or pregnant women, milk-based desserts for reluctant milk drinkers of any age. A roast chicken served first on Sunday can return in Tuesday's soup or as the protein in a stir-fried Chinese-style meal or a chef's salad. Vegetarian suppers can alternate with meat-based ones, soup-and-sandwich dinners can be planned for evenings when some family members return home late. If you have a hard time getting some members of the family to eat leafy green vegetables, slip a broccoli soufflé into the middle of the week, chopped spinach into the cheese mixture of Thursday night's lasagna.

Alternate spicy items with bland, and keep in mind the lunchtime habits of your school-age children, yourself and your spouse if you both eat away from home. A lot of dining out will probably leave the diners short on fresh fruits and vegetables. Compensate. If you know your adolescents head straight from the dinner table to a movie or a party on Friday nights, assume they will be eating plenty of (a) fat, (b) sugar, and (c) calories, and prebalance the load with a light supper high in vegetables and complex carbohydrates: for instance, a plate of enriched pasta with tomato sauce and a green salad, or a bowl of lentil soup followed by carrot and raisin salad—and no dessert. (See also Adding Variety to Your Meals, pages 278-279.)

Even special diets can be worked into the family food plan: cutting down on salt is likely to be good for everyone, so if one member needs to cut down, cook without it and let the others add their own. Everyone can benefit from cutting back on sugar: halve the amount called for in recipes, and replace most desserts with fresh fruit.

Above all, remember that nutritional safety is best assured by variety: offer it at your table and encourage your family to develop adventurous appetites.

Weekly Food Budget

Foods	Amount	Total	Adult over 55	Adult	Child 6-8	Adolescent
Milk, Cheese, Ice Cream	qts	20 qts	3.4	3.4	5.8	6.6
Meat, Poultry, Fish	lbs	14½ lbs	3.2	4.1	2.6	4.6
Eggs	number	16	4	4	3.3	4
Vegetables, Fruits	lbs	23 lbs	6.2	5.5	4.8	6
Citrus, Tomatoes	lbs	11 lbs	3	3	2	2.7
Cereals, Grains, Legumes	lbs	15 lbs	2.5	3.8	2.7	6
Potatoes	lbs	5½ lbs	1.1	1.3	1.1	2
Fats, Oils	lbs	2.67 lbs	.45	.65	.5	1.07

A Menu for the Entire Family

	Overweight Adult	Child 4-6 or Adult	Child 6-8	Adolescent
Breakfast				
Orange juice	½ cup	¾ cup	1 cup	1 cup
Oatmeal, cinnamon, raisins	½ cup	½ cup	¾ cup	1 cup, sugar
Whole-wheat toast	1 slice	1 slice	1-2 slices	2 slices
Butter, jelly		2 tsp jelly	2 tsp jelly	2 tsp butter
Milk, whole or skim	½ cup skim	½ cup whole	1 cup whole	1 cup whole
Lunch				
Ham and cheese or				3 oz meat
Tuna fish sandwich, 2 slices whole wheat	2 oz tuna	2 oz tuna	2 oz tuna	
Mixed green salad, ½ tomato	salad	salad	salad	salad
French dressing		2 tsp (adult)	2 tsp	2½ tsp
Apple, grapes	apple	grapes	apple	apple
Tea, coffee, milk	coffee/tea	1 cup milk tea (adult)	1 cup milk	1 cup milk
Dinner				
Fruit cup, orange, pineapple, grapes	3 oz	½ cup	½ cup	1 cup
Pot roast, lean only	3 oz	4 oz	3 oz	4 oz
Broccoli, fresh or frozen	½ cup	½ cup	¼ cup, buttered	½ cup
Mashed potato	1 serving	1 serving	¼ cup	⅔ cup
Bread and butter		1 slice	1 slice	2 slices, 1 tsp butter
Spinach salad	1 cup		½ cup	1 cup
Angelfood cake or pudding		cake	pudding	cake
Milk, whole or skim	1 cup skim	1 cup skim	1 cup whole	1 cup whole
Snacks				
Crackers, peanut butter		4 crackers		4 crackers
Raw vegetable sticks, cucumbers, carrots		½ cup	½ cup	
Chili bean dip (page 218)		1 tbsp		1 tbsp
Juice, fruit, milk		1 peach	peach, banana	1 cup milk banana
Total Calories	1,200-1,300	1,800-2,000	2,400	3,000

Eating Sensibly
Cooking for One

According to the 1980 census, 17.2 million Americans—1 out of 13—live alone. Living alone, temporarily, or for long periods of time, is some people's idea of bliss; the resulting quiet, privacy, and absence of obligation are enviable conditions all—with the freedom to eat what one wants, when one wants, and wherever one wants. Others find that living alone depresses both spirit and appetite. In either case, healthy eating often suffers.

If you live alone, think about what is appropriate for you—rather than compare your situation to that of a family or a couple. Look on eating alone not as a chore but as a gift to yourself, the way you might a hot bath or a cool drink at the end of a long day. Establish a routine to ensure that your solitary meals are occasions of both pleasure and health.

The size and content of the meals you most often eat alone—breakfast and dinner—should take into account the quality of the meal you usually eat in company—for most working people that means lunch. Regardless of your other plans, start the day with a substantial, nutritious breakfast. If you are a light midday eater, plan something heartier for dinner. If you like a big meal in the middle of the day, your dinner need not be as substantial.

If you are one of those people who come home from work dying for a big meal, plan your week something like this: on the weekend, prepare a substantial soup or stew, stock up on staples (see Shelf List at right), perhaps cook up a sauce for pasta that will last the week. Three nights of the week, feast on your preprepared meals, supplemented by fresh vegetables, rice, noodles, or potatoes cooked that night. The other two nights, broil a quarter-split chicken (the rest can go in a soup, a stew, or the freezer), a piece of fresh or frozen fish, a steak or a hamburger patty from the freezer, and add a simple vegetable. A good meal doesn't take long to prepare. Deciding to treat yourself as someone worth pleasing is the trick.

If you are the type who really doesn't have much of an appetite at night but would like a little something for the comfort of it, as well as to promote health and sleep, take a different tack and fix yourself a nightly repast that more resembles a minimeal. Only instead of a plate of cookies, try a peanut butter and jelly sandwich (light on the jelly) on whole-wheat bread and a glass of milk. Or a couple of slices of black bread spread with ricotta or other low-fat cheese. A green salad or a plate of raw vegetables would be excellent choices on vegetable-short days.

Whether you go for a big meal or a mini, keep a few things in mind: the later in the evening you eat, the lighter your meal should be, for good digestion and a good night's sleep. Make your meals esthetically pleasant: set the table for one, but set it. You needn't be formal, but do be civilized. Take your time. Sit down, chew your food. Enjoy it. Or, if you would like nothing better than to climb into bed with your peanut butter sandwich, climb in. Exercise all the options of solitary living, remembering that treating yourself well means many things, including the pleasure of eating regularly and rewardingly.

Shelf List of Staples

Soups: broths, rather than cream soups, avoid salty brands; homemade chicken soup and beef stock; dried soup mixes for soup or for flavoring other dishes.

Vegetables: variety of frozen vegetables; canned whole tomatoes (for salad or cooking), tomato paste, corn, peas, potatoes, yams, mushrooms; sweet and hot peppers in jars; squashes, potatoes, onions (keep well fresh).

Pasta, Cereals: rice, noodles (green ones for company dishes), spaghetti, macaroni, rice cakes; oatmeal, wheat cereal, a variety of dry cereal (beware of those with added sugar).

Fish: canned tuna, sardines, mackerel, crabmeat, lobster, salmon.

Milk, Butter, Cheese: 1 pound butter or margarine; grated Parmesan cheese, yogurt, cottage cheese (in refrigerator—watch dates); evaporated milk or dry-milk powder.

Fruit: unsweetened concentrated juices, whole fruit in cans (as pineapple chunks or slices for salads or desserts), applesauce; oranges and lemons in refrigerator at all times; raisins, dried prunes, or apricots.

Nuts: canned water chestnuts, almonds, walnuts, etc., to add texture and variety to usual fare; unsalted peanut butter.

Spices: try new herbs and spices to perk up familiar fare—cumin, allspice, star anise, ginger root—as well as parsley, oregano, basil, onion flakes, garlic, paprika, dill.

Eating Out

Eating out, whether in a restaurant or at a friend's table, is a break from routine that everyone should be able to enjoy from time to time. For those whose professional or social life makes eating out an everyday event, and for those who have trouble controlling their diets, however, the treat can easily turn to threat. When one dines out, one is in the hands of others, forced to eat someone else's idea of lunch or dinner. One has lost control. Right? Only if you want it that way.

You needn't remain a prisoner in your own house in order to safeguard your health or your figure. Neither need you be a victim of a restaurant menu nor of your host and hostess. Plan ahead, use judgment and self-control, and you can eat out with self-confidence and enjoyment. If you're struggling to lose 50 pounds, or even 20, don't sabotage or torment yourself by frequenting restaurants that serve rich food. Pass up invitations from friends who force rich desserts on their guests—and won't take no for an answer. Self-control doesn't begin the moment your hand reaches for the second roll with soup or as your eyes light on the pastry tray. It begins now, in thinking through the pitfalls, and pleasures, of dining out.

Restaurants. Whenever possible, be the one to choose the restaurant. If you're concerned about calories, and especially high fat, pass up French and American restaurants, with their respective emphasis on cream sauces and butter, red meat, and fried foods. Consider Italian (a plate of pasta with a low-fat tomato sauce is filling, soothing, and far lower in calories than a steak—also much easier to sleep on), Chinese (high in vegetables and other carbohydrates, a trace of low-fat protein), Japanese (high in low-fat protein), or other low-calorie ethnic cuisines.

If the choice of restaurant is not yours, read the menu carefully for sensible selections. Don't be pressured by waiters or companions into choosing something you don't want. Just because the menu lists appetizers doesn't mean you have to order one. If you do, choose consommé over creamed soup, melon over pâté. Ask for fish or chicken, broiled plain, and served without sauce. Decline creamed vegetables in favor of steamed or sautéed, pass by French-fried potatoes and select baked or boiled. Most restaurants offer fruit desserts; if not, you can order the fruit cup or melon from the appetizer. But, if you are watching your weight, skip those tempting but rich desserts and be content to sip a cup of tea or coffee to finish the meal.

Travel Fare. For travelers whose diet is restricted by ethnic preferences, religious beliefs, weight control, or chronic illness, major airlines, railroads, hotels, and tour operators will provide special meals on 12- to 24-hour notice (kosher, low calorie, low carbohydrate, diabetic, low fat, vegetarian, nonmilk, gluten free, etc.)

The Good Guest. Being invited to dine at someone else's table can be a mixed blessing. If you have a dinner invitation (or brunch or lunch), make your other meals especially lighter that day, and the next. Don't plan a lunch with one friend if you're going to another's house for dinner that same night. If your hostess is filling everyone's plate without inquiring about portion sizes, let her. Just don't eat it all. If challenged, say that everything was delicious but you can't eat another bite. If you are serving yourself, keep portions small and eat slowly. When dessert comes, speak up and ask for a small portion. Even hostesses who bake their own pies will feel sufficiently rewarded if you taste their triumph—you don't need to wear it home. If you are on a strict diet, announce the fact and politely but firmly decline dessert.

Cocktail parties and buffets, while they can be most dangerous for the nervous or compulsive eater, also allow for plenty of self-protective shamming. In the mob you actually can get away with total abstinence, which may be the easiest way out for some. Remember: a few dips into the peanut bowl and you're 300 calories in the red; carrot sticks are fine, but beware the sour-cream dip. Fortunately, club soda and other bottled waters are fashionable and usually plentiful at parties these days, and offer an alternative to alcohol or soft drinks laden with sugar. If you do indulge at a cocktail party, aim for the more nutritious snacks—cheese and crackers over potato chips, raw vegetables *undipped*, stuffed mushrooms instead of sausages. And skip dinner. At a buffet apply the same choice and control you would at a restaurant.

In every eating-out situation, remember that you are an adult: no one can make you eat anything you don't want to. It's true, and believing it helps.

Eating Sensibly
A Diet for Pregnant Women

As natural a pair of conditions as the world has ever known, pregnancy and breast-feeding nevertheless are still the subjects of heated and contradictory nutritional advice. The reason is obvious: the outcome matters so much that the merest hint of a "new" development leads to dogmatic pronouncements and worried acquiescence on the part of mothers determined to do everything just right.

A case in point is the matter of weight gain. How much is normal and desirable during pregnancy? When childbirth was still very risky for mother and child, and a small infant was easier to deliver, women were urged to restrict weight gain to between 10 and 15 pounds. But studies completed within the last 10 to 15 years have shown that gains by the mother of 20 pounds or more actually increase the infant's chance of survival under modern delivery conditions. Now most obstetricians urge a gain of from 24 to 30 pounds; nearly half of that will be the fetus, placenta, and amniotic fluid which are expelled at delivery; the rest is mainly the calorie bank that the mother will draw on for lactation and increased postpartum activity (see chart at right).

Because women who are significantly under- or overweight at the start of pregnancy stand a greater chance of developing complications, modest compensatory adjustments in weight gain are generally recommended, with underweight women encouraged to gain up to 30 pounds, and overweight women urged to hold weight gain to the average. More than others, pregnant teenagers must "eat for two"—to accommodate their own growth needs as well as that of the fetus. Under no circumstances should pregnancy be viewed as an opportunity to lose weight.

The pregnant woman has three basic and complementary dietary obligations. The first is to consume approximately 80,000 additional food calories during the nine-month period over and above what she needs to sustain her own weight and normal activity. This works out, over nine months, to about 300 extra calories per day, but no more than 150 extra calories a day should be consumed during the first trimester, increasing to 300 per day in the second trimester, and 400 to 450 during the third. The second obligation is to obtain sufficient amounts of selected nutrients needed for fetal development. The increased requirements for specific nutrients are shown on the chart opposite. The third obligation,

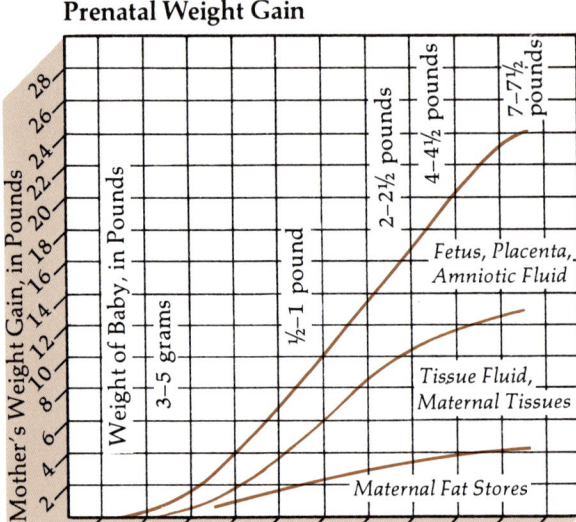

Prenatal Weight Gain

to meet your body's increased need for iron, may have to be met by an iron supplement.

Your body requires liberal intakes of liquids during pregnancy, up to eight 8-ounce glasses in addition to milk. Choose well: fruit and vegetable juice, not soft drinks, which may contain large amounts of caffeine. Cut back on coffee and tea and consult your doctor about alcohol. Recent studies have linked large intakes with fetal damage.

Cigarettes? Throw them out the minute your pregnancy is confirmed. Smoking adversely affects fetal growth and weight gain.

Problems of Pregnancy. One thing the pregnant woman should expect is a change in appetite of some sort. Though not inevitable, such alteration is extremely common. Decreased appetite, whether punctuated by morning sickness or not, is a normal condition. So too are cravings; though science has failed to explain their origin, cravings are quite real and, barring a taste for chalk or laundry starches, quite harmless. Indeed, the majority of minor physical complaints of pregnancy are related to changes in diet. Fortunately, most of them can be alleviated.

• Constipation: increase fiber and bulk in the diet, drink water. Avoid laxatives. Get exercise.

• Hemorrhoids: avoid constipation.

• Heartburn: likelihood increases as fetus grows, putting more pressure on the stomach. Switch to smaller, more frequent meals, avoid a full stomach.

EATING FOR GOOD HEALTH

- Morning sickness: nausea and possible vomiting, usually but not always in the early hours of the day. Nibble dry, salted crackers. Eat small amounts of food every few hours, interspersed with liquids. Report persistent vomiting to your doctor.
- Leg cramps: result from a low-calcium, high-phosphorus imbalance in the blood. A calcium salts supplement *without* phosphorus (prescribed by a doctor) will help, as will stretching exercises.

Diet During Breast-Feeding. The best method of feeding a newborn, breast-feeding, is also a boon to the mother. Barring illness, mother's milk is reliable, plentiful, and always at hand. No preparation is required and no expense is incurred. Finally, in one of nature's more elegant exchanges, lactation steadily uses up the fat stores accumulated during pregnancy at the rate of 100 to 300 calories a day. An additional 500 calories above one's normal intake are needed to produce sufficient milk for infant nursing, but beyond that, the nutritional requirements of nursing mothers differ only slightly from those of pregnant ones (see chart pages 32-33).

The daily need for protein drops from a pregnancy high of 74 grams to approximately 64. Any shortage will be at the expense of the mother, since the milk yield will contain adequate protein even if it has to be drawn from the mother's tissue. Calcium, iron, and vitamin D requirements remain at pregnancy levels, but other vitamin and mineral needs vary between pregnancy and breast-feeding. Most of these additional nutrients will be supplied naturally through the balanced diet recommended for pregnancy, plus an extra 2 cups of whole milk and an extra serving of whole grains.

To maintain milk yield as well as her own health, a lactating woman should drink at least 2 quarts of other liquids a day. Milk volume may be depressed by cigarettes and oral contraceptives, and the former have been identified as potentially toxic to the nursing infant. Remember that breast milk is highly sensitive to contaminants of all sorts: eat only healthy, unadulterated foods while lactating, for your sake and that of your baby.

Nutritional Needs During Pregnancy and Breast-Feeding	Daily Amount	Protein for tissue growth	Calcium and Phosphorus for bones and teeth	Vitamin C	Vitamin D	Iron for blood, cells*	Vitamin A for growth, vision	B Vitamins (thiamin, riboflavin, niacin)	Iodine	Energy
Foods										
Milk (fortified), cheese, yogurt	4-6 cups	40%	100%	10%	100%	—	24%	10%		640
Meat, fish, poultry, liver once a week	4 oz	40%	—	—	—	10%	—	50%		420
Eggs	3-4 week	10%	—	—	—	—	16%	—		80
Vegetables dark, leafy green, deep-yellow, other	1 cup 2 cups	10%	10%	100%	—	—	200%	10%		100
Potato with skin	1 medium	5%	—	40%	—	—	—	13%		75
Citrus or tomato Other fruit	2 2	5%	10%	100%	—	—	16%	1.6%		320
Grains, cereals, legumes	4-5 servings	10%	10%	—	—	30%	—	21%		540
Fats, oils	2 tbsp	—	—	—	—	—	16%	—		200
Salt, iodized	—	—	—	—	—	—	—	—	100%	—
Liquids in addition to a quart of milk	6-8 cups									
Custards, puddings	for energy	10%	14%	—	—	—	9%	2%		200
Folacin: increased need for folacin (for cell growth and protein synthesis) is 400 micrograms.					*30-60 mg supplement is recommended					2,375/ 2,500

Eating Sensibly
Feeding Your Baby

The first two years following birth encompass the most concentrated period of physical growth and arguably the most radical display of individual change to be experienced in a lifetime. The infant emerges from the womb a tiny (however "large") and helpless creature, with limited survival skills—the ability to suck and swallow, to cry for attention—useless, of course, without someone nearby.

By the end of the first year, the infant has become a child; he has tripled in weight and increased his length by 50 percent, is mobile, capable of eating solid food, and is probably saying his first few disconnected words. By the end of the second year, he is a figure to be reckoned with: independent minded, if still largely dependent, the 2-year-old is usually very clear, or at least vocal, about food and other likes and dislikes, is terrifyingly energetic, and virtually unrecognizable as the creature of 24 months earlier.

Up to 6 months of this stupendous transformation can be fueled by mother's milk alone, so complete a form of nourishment does it provide—although supplements of vitamin D, fluoride, and iron are often recommended. Between their sixth and twelfth months, most infants need other foods to supply additional calories and necessary nutrients, but there is no need to stop breast-feeding in the meantime.

What, when, and how much to feed are important questions at this time—not only because of the great surge of growth that takes place but also because it is in this early period that experts believe one's lifetime appetite and attitudes toward eating are set. The likes and dislikes your infant acquires from you will be with him a long time.

Birth to 1 Year. There is no longer any question but that mother's milk is the optimal food for a newborn. Indeed, when a mother cannot or chooses not to breast-feed her baby, her alternative is almost invariably a commercial formula designed to approximate as closely as possible the composition of mother's milk. Exceptions are special formulas for digestive or allergic conditions.

Depending on his size, a newborn baby requires from 275 to 580 food calories a day, equal to about 2½ to 3 ounces of mother's milk (or formula) per pound of body weight per day. Not every baby needs this exact amount, however, and most healthy infants will successfully regulate intake on their own. Furthermore, studies suggest that, left to themselves, babies born slightly underweight or slightly overweight will adjust their intake instinctively, with the result that a small infant will actually often have a higher calorie-to-body-weight ratio than will a large baby.

The number of calories consumed daily per pound of body weight declines from approximately 50 at birth to 45 at one year. During the first three months, when the infant is most often sleeping if he is not eating, fully a third of his calorie intake is used just for growth. Between the ninth and twelfth months, by which point total intake has risen to 800 to 1,200 calories daily, the proportion devoted to growth has slowed to 6 percent, with the remainder spent in increased activity and in the maintenance of a body now greatly increased in size.

The advantages of breast-feeding are both immediate and long-term: mother's milk is more easily digested than formula or cow's milk; it is thought to provide some protection against an array of diseases, particularly common respiratory and gastro-intestinal infections. Moreover, it promotes intimacy between mother and child. (Bottle-fed babies should be held close, as if they were being given the breast.) Because the infant can control intake, there is less chance of overfeeding than when an anxious parent is intent on emptying the bottle. Finally, because the milk in a woman's breast changes from a thin, watery consistency to a richer form as feeding progresses, the infant is able to pause between breasts. If he needs to continue sucking to satisfy his thirst, he can nurse at the second breast for a while, drawing out only the thin fluid, without having to consume more heavy milk than he wants.

Introducing Solid Foods. There is no premium attached to early feeding of solid food to an infant. It is not an accomplishment, like walking or talking, and it should never be forced. Up until the fourth month, even semisolid foods, such as cereal or pureed vegetables, are not readily accepted and will most likely be spit back. Between the fourth and sixth months, a spoon gently inserted between the lips is more likely to be accepted; the ability to swallow nonliquids has become established; and adequate salivary and intestinal enzymes needed for digestion are being produced. By the seventh to ninth months, teeth and chewing movements will be obvious, and you will have no difficulty telling that your baby wants to be biting on something.

A useful rule of thumb is to introduce one new food a week while continuing to breast- or formula-feed. This careful introduction also helps to identify any allergies. Offer small portions, a teaspoon at a time. Don't overwhelm your baby: even at 1 year, his stomach can only hold a cupful of food; yours holds 2 quarts! If he turns away from pureed peas the first time out, wait a few days, then try again. If he still declines, try a different food. Don't make a big fuss or you'll wind up with a problem eater. Be patient. Every child likes *something* good. Experiment until you hit on your little darling's delight.

There's no denying the convenience of commercial baby and junior foods, except that making your own isn't much harder than opening a jar. Homemade baby foods—chopped, pureed, or diced in a food mill, blender, or processor or on a board with a knife—allow you to exercise greater control over your baby's diet, and save money. You should plan menus carefully to avoid extra salt and other additives and allow for baby's higher needs for such nutrients as iron and vitamin D. If you do go in for home-prepared foods, remember to reserve baby's portion before seasoning, use fresh foods as much as possible, and avoid refreezing thawed foods. Babies are much more sensitive to bacteria than you are, so absolute hygiene is essential.

The Second Year. By your child's first birthday, he is ready to start feeding himself. Though not every family's schedule permits, many experts suggest that 1-year-olds join the family at the table. Make sure he has a spoon he can handle and a plate that won't break. Cut his food into bite-sized pieces, mashing vegetables so they can be eaten with a spoon. Close your eyes to all but the most flagrant violations of table manners; those can be learned later. A 1½-year-old is discovering things about food you may have forgotten; he needs to mix and match colors and textures in ways that may make you queasy. Arrange your food the way you like it and let him do the same.

Keep portions small. One or 2 tablespoons of each food should suffice. If he wants more, he'll ask. Don't overstuff your child when he's small: either he'll refuse to eat, or he'll begin to think that being loved means eating too much.

Introducing Solid Food

Solid foods should be introduced in small portions (1 teaspoonful) no oftener than one new food a week for taste adjustment and to detect food allergies. Increase to ¼ cup by one year.

Cereal: iron-fortified dry rice cereal mixed to thin consistency; oat, barley, then wheat and corn cereals can be tried.

Snacks: arrowroot cookies or oven-dried toast for teething and hand-to-mouth reflex.

Fruit: mashed ripe banana or cooked and strained unsweetened apples, peaches, or pears.

Juice: fresh, frozen, or canned citrus juice, diluted at first with equal parts boiled, cooled water. Start in bottle, serve later in cup.

Vegetables: start with mild, dark-green or deep-yellow vegetables pureed. Later serve chopped to promote chewing.

Meat/fish: go from light to dark—chicken, veal, lamb, beef, liver; whitefish such as halibut, cod, flounder, all bones removed.

Dairy products: cottage cheese, yogurt.

Eggs: start with yolk only, well-cooked and mashed. By one year, serve whole egg soft-boiled, poached, etc.

Potatoes, pasta: mashed potato thoroughly cooked, macaroni, or spaghetti.

Finger foods: green beans, toast, cheese.

Desserts: ice cream, yogurt, custard, gelatin.

Menu at 8 to 12 Months

7 A.M.	1 cup milk
9 A.M.	¼ cup fortified cooked cereal
	2-3 tablespoons strained fruit
Midmorning	1 slice dry toast or zwieback
	½ cup orange juice
Noon	1 ounce meat, fish, or chicken
	½ cup mashed vegetables
	2 teaspoons butter
	1 cup milk
	¼ cup cooked, strained fruit or pudding
3 P.M.	Toast or crackers
	4 ounces milk or fruit juice
6 P.M.	2 ounces cottage cheese, cereal, or egg yolk
	½ cup whipped potatoes
	¼ cup cooked, strained fruit or pudding
	1 slice toast
	1 cup milk

Eating Sensibly
What Children Need To Eat

Although the nutritional requirements of children between the ages of 2 and 10 do not shift dramatically from year to year, this period is marked nonetheless by pronounced behavioral quirks and by a most significant change in life-style—that which takes place when the child first goes off to school and is thereby removed from easy parental surveillance.

At issue during these years is the task of teaching your child how to eat well as preparation for a long and healthy life. At 2, he is still very much feeling his way—often quite literally, it will seem—through the world of food and, though hardly unaffected, is both unaware of and unconcerned by the relative nutritional merit of foods you serve him. By the time he is 10, his eating habits, if not his permanent tastes for specific foods, will be firmly established, to be dislodged and replaced later in life only with great difficulty. A sensible goal during this period, therefore, is to develop in your child a basic attitude toward food and nutrition that, in time, will enable him to make proper nutritional decisions for himself. This is the time to instill in him a handful of beliefs about food that will withstand peer pressure, television advertising, and the temptations of fast-food chains. This is not to say that you can, or should, raise a dietary purist; the chances are good, however, that you can raise a responsible eater who values his health.

Because the tremendous rate of growth that characterizes infancy has slowed by the end of the third year, the 3- to 10-year-old needs somewhat less food than the infant in proportion to body weight, approximately 41 to 36 calories per pound. This will vary according to how active your child is, and by sex as well, with boys tending to be taller and heavier than girls into the tenth year.

The high protein needs of infancy also begin to decline. By age 10, the child's requirements for proteins/fats/carbohydrates are at a ratio (15/25–35/50–60) that is nearly the same as that for an adult. With the exception of iron, the need for which fluctuates during childhood (1- to 3-year-olds need 15 milligrams daily, whereas 4- to 10-year-olds need only 10 milligrams), and vitamin C, many of a child's vitamin and mineral requirements can be readily met with three 8-ounce glasses of vitamin D-fortified

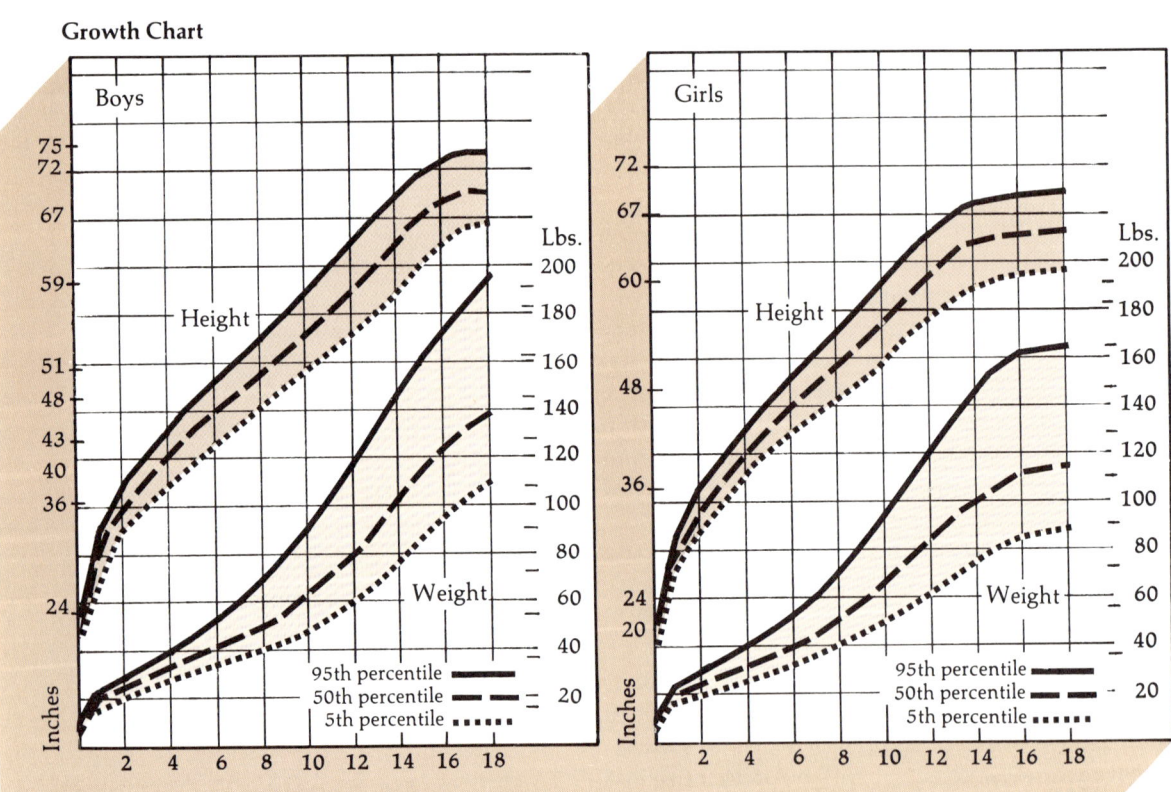

Growth Chart

milk daily (slightly less for children under 4). Since the most common nutrient shortfalls in this age group are calcium, iron, vitamin C, and vitamin A, the consumption of 24 ounces of milk, iron-fortified enriched cereal, and one orange daily will prevent such shortfalls.

From 2 to 3. Although the word "plateau" may seem overly tranquil in connection with a 2- or 3-year-old child, it is a fair description of the eating pattern of most children this age for several reasons. First, at 2 years, a child's actual growth rate has leveled off (see growth chart at left) and he simply needs less food in proportion to his size. Second, a child this age lives in a state of constant excitement, so entranced by the marvels that beckon beyond the family table that he often loses interest in what's on it. Third, his eating perspective, and situation, have changed. At 18 months, he was eating "baby" foods from a "baby" bowl. Now he is working his way through a scaled-down version of the family fare. By comparison to the speed of the others eating dinner, he's going to be a slowpoke.

At 2 or 3, a child's stomach is still very small, and generally is not capable of holding as much food as it needs from meal to meal. Planned snacking (or even minimeals) is a way to fill the gap. Treat snacks as part of the day's food plan, not as forbidden treats or violations, and your child will be less inclined to want to sneak a piece of cake before dinner.

If your child is eating his meals with the rest of the family at age 2 or 3, this is the time to begin developing table manners and personal food control. Make mealtimes quiet and pleasant for everyone, including the youngest member of the family. Eat slowly and encourage him to do so as well. Don't insist that your child "clean his plate"; don't overload it to begin with. Teach him variety by offering it; he won't like everything, but then neither do you. Beware rich sauces and "mystery" foods; children this age want to identify what they eat. Don't let your child ruin your meal: set reasonable rules—no throwing or smearing food, no talking with a full mouth, no shouting—but don't make mealtime an exercise in rigidity. Expect spilled milk, spurned carrots, misjudged appetite. Let your child feed himself at the start of the meal, when enthusiasm is high; if he starts to fade, give him some help, but when he's had enough, let it be.

Caloric Intake of Growing Children			
Age	Weight lb (kg)	Energy Needs (cal)	with range
to 6 mos.	13 (6)	kg×115	kg×(95-145)
6-12 mos.	20 (9)	kg×105	kg×(80-135)
1-3 yrs	29 (13)	1300	(900-1800)
4-6	44 (20)	1700	(1300-2300)
7-10	62 (28)	2400	(1650-3300)
11-14 males	99 (45)	2700	(2000-3700)
females	101 (46)	2200	(1500-3000)
15-18 males	145 (66)	2800	(2100-3900)
females	120 (55)	2100	(1200-3000)

From 4 to 5. Children this age are given to authoritative pronouncements about many matters, so don't be surprised if your 4-year-old suddenly refuses to eat anything orange, or yellow, or brown. Chances are that at some point your child will decide to forego variety with a vengeance. Do your best not to make a huge issue of it while trying to make sure he gets the basic nutrition he needs. Remember that there are many sources for almost every nutrient. If he won't eat fish, forget fish and feed him chicken. He doesn't have to eat fish, even if all his friends do. And if all his friends really do, he probably will too, soon enough. In fact, many of children's food phobias are learned at home. Studies have shown that aversions to certain foods are most frequently picked up from the father and older siblings, without a compensating set of preferences arising from the mother's praise of healthful foods. A child whose father "won't touch" green vegetables, but nevertheless gets a smile from Mommy reasonably infers that there is something to be gained from holding out against spinach. The obvious way to circumvent this pattern is for both parents to side with nutrition, presenting it as a plus, not a painful duty.

From 6 to 10. At about age 6, the child takes a major step into life outside the family and into organized, all-day activities. His energy needs are quite high, both from concentrated mental and physical activity, and because he is continuing to grow rapidly. His mealtime is now set for him by the outside world: if the school bus leaves at 8:00 A.M., he'd better have finished breakfast. If the school lunch hour begins at 12:15, that's when he'll eat—no sooner. This abrupt end to the flexibility of the preschool-

Eating Sensibly
What Children Need To Eat

er makes a good breakfast, always important, critical. Make sure it's a proper meal, and wake your child early enough to eat it. If he is a poor eater of traditional breakfast foods, offer wholesome alternatives: leftover meat and vegetables; cheese on toast; brown-rice pudding with raisins and nuts; unsweetened yogurt with fresh fruit. Don't let him go off to school with an empty stomach; his attention and performance will suffer.

After breakfast, the biggest nutritional issue for school-age children is lunch, the one meal eaten away from home. If the school provides a hot lunch, free or at a price you can afford, and if you judge it to be nutritious and appealing, it's a good bet. Otherwise it's up to you: treat his lunch like an important meal. Send him off with something that is both good for him and that he likes; if he doesn't like it, he'll throw it away or give it to a friend, getting who-knows-what in exchange. Sandwiches are obvious and can be excellent choices, but see the box opposite for additional ideas.

When preparing lunch, add an extra piece of fruit or some carrot sticks for recess, as an alternative to the candy machine. Don't succumb to pleas for ice-cream or candy money; better yet, band together with other parents and have the machines removed.

Trouble Spots. Lifelong problems with overweight often manifest themselves first in early childhood. If your child has not lost his baby fat by the time he is 3, check him against the weight-height chart on page 310 to see whether he exceeds the average weight for his height by more than 10 percent. If he does, consider him overweight, but don't put him on a diet. Stabilize his eating and let him grow into his weight. Take a low-key approach: don't nag, keep him well-fed, but cut back on sweets and fats, and encourage physical activity.

Shopping can also be a problem. Advertisers and marketing geniuses know that children accompany their mothers shopping; that's why they pay to pump their products on cartoon shows and why sugar-coated cereals and desserts are placed within reach of short shoppers. It's hard to battle your 4-year-old and the food industry. Try making an ally of the former. Explain food and its value, and encourage your child to investigate, with your help, advertisers' claims. Give your child a chance to side with you, and then stand firm.

Brownbag Lunches

According to many nutritionists, the second most im portant meal of the day is lunch (breakfast is the mos important meal) and, on the average, one-third of th body's nutritional needs should be provided for b lunch. One of the best ways to make sure that you child gets the proper foods at lunch is to pack c "brownbag" his lunches yourself.

Brownbagging lunch has many positive aspects, a of which can be beneficial to anyone, no matter wh his age. When you pack a lunch, you have control ov what food goes in it, the size of the portions, and th way it is prepared. With a brownbag lunch you als know the food is fresh, good, and as free from undesi able ingredients as possible; many times, it is le expensive than a commercially prepared lunch. If yc plan the weekly menu, you can plan lunches th complement the rest of the daily and weekly meals. fact, you can plan extra portions for dinner to use f the next day's lunch.

For an adult, taking your own lunch also means th you can select the place for eating—a park, outdo concert, or your office desk—and that you have mo free time to do things other than eat. If you are or weight-loss diet, pack a lunch the night before. Aft dinner when your appetite is eased, you will have mo willpower to pack a lunch that fits into your weigh loss plan than if you went out and bought lunch noontime.

What is a good lunch? Those served in schools m follow federal guidelines that, although nutritious, a deliberately broad to allow for the many differences the kitchen capabilities of the schools across the nati and to permit lunches that appeal to the different nee and attitudes of the students. Depending on what served, there can be a great deal of waste. The m popular lunch and the type having the least waste one that consists of juice, a tuna fish or peanut but sandwich on whole-wheat bread, milk, and a piece fruit. With proper selection of ingredients and care preparation, this can be a nutritionally adequate lur for anyone no matter what his age.

As a responsible parent, you should be aware of quality of the lunches served in your child's school he is lucky enough to attend a school with a well-r lunch program that serves nutritious, appetizing me then—aside from choice or economy—there is no n for you to pack his lunches. But, if the lunch progr is not very good, you should get together with the ot parents and do something to make the lunches better. In the meantime, pack your child's lunches rather than let him eat poor fare.

Your plans for good, nutritious lunches, though, can be sabotaged by outside influences. If your child does not like the food, he might not eat it or he might get a less nutritious and more caloric lunch from a vending machine. Some schools avoid this temptation by banning vending machines or by controlling what foods are in them. Other times, students will trade lunches. If all parents banded together and pledged to pack only nutritious lunches, you would be assured that your child eats a good lunch no matter with whom he trades.

To help guarantee that your child will eat the lunch you pack, make the lunch appealing and easy to manage. Try to pack only those foods you know your child will eat. If he refuses to eat sandwiches because of the bread crusts, then cut the crusts off or, better yet, use a cookie cutter to cut out the center area of the bread and use it for the sandwich. Let your child learn about good nutrition by having him pack his lunch with your guidance. Use colorful napkins, plastic utensils, or special straws to make the lunch fun. Use clean, reusable plastic containers with lids to hold foods like salads or coleslaw; use plastic bags for things like raw vegetables, raisins, or dry, unsweetened cereals. Include a surprise in the lunch or even a little love note to make your child feel special. If you want to give him a special treat, make it a nutritious one, such as homemade oatmeal-raisin cookies. Do not take the easy way out by relying on overprocessed, additive-laden, prepackaged convenience foods such as cakes, potato chips, or candies.

Pack the lunch in your child's very own lunch box, one that he has picked out. Make sure the box is cleaned after every use. If you do not use a lunch box, use paper bags bought especially for lunches—do not use bags left over from shopping, which may be contaminated. If necessary, pack a can or bottle opener with the lunch. Don't forget napkins, straws, or any necessary utensils such as plastic spoons, forks, or knives.

Since the lunch will be standing several hours before it is eaten, plan how to keep the foods hot or cold and free from bacteria. If the food is meant to be hot, keep it hot in a sterile, wide-mouthed thermos that is easy to eat out of. If the food is supposed to be cold, keep it cold. If a liquid, you can put it in a clean thermos bottle and pack a straw with it. Remember to thoroughly clean any thermos before using it. To keep other foods cold, pack a freezer gel device with the lunch. You can make your own by filling a clean, plastic margarine tub with water and freezing it. Another idea is to freeze the sandwich; by the time your child is ready to eat, the sandwich will have thawed. To prevent the bread from becoming soggy in freezing, spread butter or margarine thinly on each slice. Frozen sandwiches will keep up to two months when stored at 0° or less. Before freezing them, wrap and label each sandwich. Certain foods like tomato slices, raw vegetables, jam, or hard-boiled egg whites do not freeze well. While making the sandwiches, use tongs or a fork to place meats, poultry, or cheeses into the sandwich and make sure that your hands and all the cutting boards and utensils are clean.

The list below gives suggestions of good, appetizing, and nutritious foods that are suitable for brownbag lunches. Use this list as a guide for the types of foods to pack into a lunch.

Breads. Fortified or enriched white, whole-wheat, rye, pumpernickel, raisin, or pita (pocket) bread; muffins; rolls; thin-sliced breads for weight watchers; bread sticks; crackers.

Sandwich Fillings. Sliced turkey, chicken, well-done roast beef, corned beef, or ham; sliced egg or egg salad; tuna or tuna salad; turkey, chicken, or ham salad; cheese; peanut butter; cottage cheese, plain or with chopped vegetables, fruits, or nuts; meat loaf; a piece of chicken or turkey. Avoid luncheon meats with artificial coloring or additives.

Sandwich Garnishes. Sliced tomatoes, cucumber, or zucchini; lettuce; bean sprouts; pickles; spinach; shredded cabbage; chopped nuts; green pepper.

Side Dishes. Raw or marinated vegetables; salads; coleslaw; celery or carrot sticks; small bags of nuts, seeds, or unsweetened cereals.

Hot Foods. Stew; baked beans; soup, preferably homemade; chili; spaghetti; macaroni and cheese; chop suey; pot roast.

Liquids. Milk; fruit or vegetable juices; lemonade.

Desserts. Yogurt (a frozen container will keep the lunch cool); fresh, dried, canned, or stewed fruits (peel and section the orange for a child with a short lunch period); nutritious cookies such as oatmeal-raisin, peanut butter, or applesauce; date-nut bread or other fruit breads such as banana or cranberry; bran, corn, or whole-wheat muffins; tapioca; custard; gelatin.

Eating Sensibly
The Critical Adolescent Years

Adolescence is a time of extremes and contradictions: a period in which exuberance and lassitude seem to alternate; in which fierce rebelliousness toward parents is often matched by an unquestioning conformity to the attitudes of peers; in which idealism and harshness simultaneously peak. Biologically, sexually, psychologically, mentally, the child is coming of age, and as part of this process is undergoing the greatest spurt of physical growth since infancy. This intense growth usually occurs in a concentrated period of 18 to 24 months sometime between the tenth and fifteenth year in girls, and between the twelfth and sixteenth in boys, and is accompanied in most adolescents by greatly increased social, athletic, and academic activity.

Every adolescent matures according to his own inner clock, some much later than others, but individual body consciousness is at an all-time high throughout this period, with great emphasis on height, weight, attractiveness, and perceived physical maturity. So while it is true that teenagers are hard to control, nutritionally or in any other way, their acute physical awareness at this time does make them susceptible to carefully framed appeals to self-interest, or self-image. A teenager suffering from acne will voluntarily forswear chocolate, ice cream, and even French fries in hopes of finding relief—even though there appears to be no connection between acne and diet (current thinking attributes acne to hormonal imbalances that are initiated at puberty). That same determined teenager can also be persuaded that the rest of his physical and mental development is best served by a healthy diet.

With the exception of pregnancy and breast-feeding for women, total caloric requirements are at an all-time high during adolescence, although per pound of body weight, the caloric requirement has actually declined from childhood. Boys between the ages of 15 and 18 require an average of 20 calories per pound of body weight a day, or as much as 2,900 calories daily for a normal 5'9" 15-year-old weighing 145 pounds—and even more if he is extremely active. Satisfying the appetite of a teenage boy often seems an impossibility, and indeed cannot always be successfully accomplished in the three main meals of the day. Substantial additions may be needed. Given free rein and the money to pay for it, most will assure themselves of the additional calories quite readily; the difficulty, of course, lies in assuring that the food they eat out of your sight is of good quality.

Adolescent girls also have high calorie needs. But women store more of their body weight as fat, and fat uses fewer calories than muscle. Thus, their needs are appreciably lower than boys', about 17 calories per pound of body weight, for a daily average in the range of 1,200 to 3,000 calories, depending on build, height, and degree of physical activity.

The trickiest dietary problem among girls in this age group is maintaining a balanced weight while satisfying nutritional needs. Girls must pack in all the essentials in far fewer calories than boys in order not to put on unwanted pounds. Because girls are exposed as regularly as boys to high-calorie foods of questionable worth, they are particularly vulnerable to becoming overweight and malnourished.

An equally serious problem among girls, although it affects fewer of them, is chronic underweight, most frequently the result of intermittent dieting aimed at ensuring a fashionably reedlike look. For some, a psychologically based preoccupation with thinness veers into a hard-to-reverse, dangerous condition called anorexia nervosa, almost exclusively an affliction of teenage girls, in which the victim, no matter how thin, is convinced that she is overweight and stops eating (see pages 316-317).

For most teenagers, however, the situation is anything but dire. The average adolescent likes to eat, and furthermore is exposed to more new foods than he was as a child. An increased desire for independence may cause sporadic rejection of old family standbys but is likely to be compensated for by fresh suggestions gleaned from the tables of friends. In nutritional matters, the adolescent's adventurous side is well worth cultivating.

The chief task of the parent, then, is to provide wholesome food at home, both at regular mealtimes, and for the inevitable (and for boys, essential) snacking between meals. Adolescents of both sexes should be eating a balanced diet that includes foods from the Basic Four Food Groups every day: three or more servings of meat, fish, or other protein-rich foods, and four or more (depending on current weight and height) servings each of milk or milk equivalents, vegetables and fruits, whole grains and cereals.

The most serious nutritional deficiencies among teenagers are calcium and iron. The calcium shortage is rooted in the sudden availability of soft drinks and their frequent substitution for milk. Not only does milk consumption (which should be a quart a day) drop, but the phosphorus in soft drinks and processed foods reduces the efficiency of calcium absorption by the body. Iron shortages are due to increased demand for the manufacture of blood and tissue in both sexes, and the onset of menstruation in girls. The iron requirement of 18 milligrams daily is at a nonpregnant lifetime high for women and an all-time high for men. Although iron-rich foods—liver, dried fruit, whole grains—should be prominent in the diet, an iron supplement is probably necessary.

The extra calories teenagers need should not come packaged in sugar or grease. Though there is little you can do about what your teenager eats when out of the house, at home you have great power. If you stock the refrigerator with sugar-loaded soft drinks, they will be swiftly consumed; store only milk, tomato juice, and assorted, unsweetened fruit juices, and they will disappear just as quickly. Refuse to keep pretzels, salted peanuts, potato chips, ice

Coping with Fast Food

	Energy	Protein	Carbohydrate	Fat	A	D	C	Thiamin	Riboflavin	Niacin	Calcium	Iron	Sodium
	calories	grams			IU	micrograms	milligrams						
Girls: 17 calories per pound	2,100	46	304	70	4,000	10	60	1.1	1.3	14	1,200	18	2,000 max.
Boys: 20 calories per pound	2,800	56	406	93	5,000	10	60	1.4	1.7	18	1,200	18	2,000 max.
Breakfast													
1 cup enriched cereal	106	2.4	23.6	.4	—	10	—	.25	.03	1.1	11	.8	226
1 cup vitamin D-fortified milk	150	8	11	8	307	2.5	2	.09	.40	.2	291	.1	122
½ cup orange juice	55	1	13	.3	250	—	60	.11	.04	.5	13	.25	1.5
Lunch of Fast Food													
Hamburger with everything	541	25.6	39	31	327	1.0	2	.35	.37	8.2	175	4.3	963
French fries	211	3	25	10.6	52	—	11	.15	.03	2.9	10	.5	112
Apple pie	295	2.2	30	18.3	68	—	3	.02	.03	1.3	12	.6	408
Vanilla shake	324	10.7	52	8	347	1.0	3	.12	.66	.6	361	.2	250
Subtotal: 2 meals	1,682	52.9	193.6	76.6	1,351	14.5	81	1.09	1.56	14.8	873	6.75	2,082.5
Dinner													
¼ broiled chicken	130	23	—	3.8	80	—	—	.05	.19	8.8	9	1.7	66
1 large raw carrot	30	1	7	—	7,930	—	6	.04	.04	.4	27	.5	47
½ cup spinach	20	2.5	3	.3	7,300	—	25	.06	.13	.4	84	2.0	45
Baked potato with skin	145	4	33	.2	—	—	31	.15	.07	2.7	14	1.1	6
Banana	127	1.6	33	.3	270	—	15	.08	.09	1.0	12	1.0	2
1 cup milk	150	8	11	8	307	2.5	2	.09	.40	.2	291	.1	122
Total: 3 meals	2,284	93	280.6	89.2	17,238	17	160	1.56	2.48	28.3	1,310	13.15	2,370.5

Because fast foods are high in protein, fat, and sodium, daily allowances for these nutrients are often met or surpassed after a fast-food lunch. Youngsters will have to make up for lack of carbohydrates, iron, and fiber by eating extra fruit or vegetables. She should forego the pie as unnecessary calories and fat, whereas he will make up for his missing calories with another serving of chicken, 2 slices of whole-wheat bread with butter at breakfast, and a custard or pudding for a snack. Both need iron supplements.

Eating Sensibly
The Critical Adolescent Years

cream, cake, and cookies around, and your hungry teenager will resort to whatever he finds in the refrigerator—leftover vegetables, fresh fruit, etc.

There remains that nagging question of what adolescents eat when they are on their own. The answer is not mysterious—they eat fast food: pizza, hamburgers, hot dogs, "milk" shakes of nondairy origin, French fries, French-fried onion rings, fried chicken, fried fish, and soft drinks by the case. Unless you plan to run blood tests on your teenager to prove otherwise, assume he eats a lot of this kind of food and compensate for it at home with extra vegetables, fruit, and fiber-rich foods. Not all fast food is alike, although most of it is high in calories. To know what you are up against, here are a number of popular items with their calorie count and grams of protein (1), carbohydrate (2), and fat (3).

	Calories	1	2	3
Fish and chips, coleslaw (3-piece dinner)	1,100	55	91	65
Cheeseburger	760	34	51	47
Hot dog with chili	330	14	25	19
French fries	211	3	25	10
Fried chicken, mashed potatoes, coleslaw, roll and butter	1,070	54	74	62
Pizza, half of 15" pie	1,200	83	148	31
Milk shake (freeze)	520	11	89	13

A condition of special concern in adolescence is teenage pregnancy. The under-17-year-old who becomes pregnant bears a heavy burden nutritionally, since her own growth is not yet complete. Pregnant adolescents should be given special dietary attention to ensure that they receive adequate calories and nutrients to protect themselves and provide for their infants. (See pages 306-307 for basic nutritional requirements during pregnancy.)

Another concern is teenage obesity. Adolescence is a period during which the body can accelerate its addition of fat cells. And, if for no other reason, obesity in adolescence should be fought. An estimated one-third of all teenagers are overweight, with girls suffering more than boys. Attempt to motivate your overweight adolescent to take primary responsibility for his eating, and provide all possible support. Do not nag or ridicule; being a teenager and fat is hard enough. If the problem seems beyond family management, seek professional help.

Dangerous Dieting

Betsy Conley, a New York free-lance writer, recounted her brush with anorexia nervosa in *Glamour*.

It began harmlessly enough. I had gained 10 pounds during my freshman year in college and, as summer and a lifeguarding job drew near, I had nightmares about waddling about in a swimsuit. I started my diet in earnest. At first, I was sensible about the foods I ate.

My efforts showed immediately and I enjoyed the scale's indicator inching downward. I became more vigilant and, by the time I finished my exams, I was back to 110 pounds, which is a pretty normal weight for 5 feet 3 inches.

But it was no longer thin enough. My younger sister, Sarah, and I embarked on a dangerous partnership: we kept each other completely honest about what we ate. Our breakfast remained cereal, we rarely ate lunch, and at dinner we would have melon with yogurt while the family ate a hearty casserole.

By the end of the summer, we were each down to 94 pounds. Our tans gave us a deceptively healthy glow and we had new clothes in tiny sizes. We were both high from the lack of food and the absence of fat. I, who had never had much of a bustline, lost it completely and took to going braless.

Back at college, I stuck to my diet, convinced that my sister was gaining on me (which meant losing faster than I was). I picked vegetables from stews and called that a meal. I drank black coffee endlessly to curb my appetite. I slept four or five hours a night, kept awake by caffeine and low-grade starvation. But I was always at breakfast for my sustaining bowl of cereal.

At home on vacations, I would be very cheerful and energetic to waylay any criticism. My mother would hard-boil eggs and write "eat me" on them; I would eat the white of the egg but discard the calorie-laden yolk. My father stopped the dinner conversation one night as he watched Sarah and me sit down with a bowl of yogurt (plain) and some carrot sticks while spaghetti was heaped in front of the rest. He announced abruptly, "After dinner I want to weigh you in upstairs!" I was 89 pounds and Sarah was a strapping 94.

I went to England for my junior year abroad and spent the summer working as a mother's helper. By this time I was unable to look at myself in the mirror and see how thin I was. I thought I was average, that any indulgence would put me on the road to obesity. The family with whom I stayed were concerned b could find no grounds for criticism. I was enthusiastic, helpful, outgoing. The children got along well with me, and I truly believed that I was able to manage at such a weight.

When I went off to an English university in the fall, I still reveled in my thinness. I remember feeling superior: I had such self-control, such willpower. English institutional food was so unappetizing that I didn't have much trouble dieting. I worked at a pub at night and drank an occasional pint of beer—which, more than anything else, probably kept me alive.

But there were moments of misgiving about what I was doing. I was so very hungry in the small hours of the morning that I couldn't sleep: I would imagine that I was in a concentration camp and think of what I would eat when I was released.

I know now that this is typical of a woman near the anorexic threshold: I was obsessed by thoughts of food, but the act of eating disgusted me. My self-image was based solely on how little I could eat.

My parents visited me before I returned to the United States, and I saw the pain written in their eyes at what I looked like—nervous, emaciated, close to 80 pounds.

The turning point came one night when my sister Ann and her husband cooked a delicious steak with the usual array of fresh salad and vegetables, baked potato, and dessert. I couldn't keep any of it down long enough to digest it. I was quick to attribute that episode and others like it to an uncertain stomach from jet lag and diet change. But I knew that wasn't why my stomach rejected it. There simply was no room down there for a normal amount of solid food. My parents resorted to ultimatums, and I did try to eat more in their presence. But I longed for the opening of college and escape from their loving vigilance.

When I had my college physical, I weighed in with a nurse who started the balance on the 100-pound slot. As she had to continue sliding it downward, she began to focus on the body standing on the scale. Then she wrote "84" on the weight line on my form, circled it, and sent me into the doctor's waiting room. I was furious: the nurse had joined the conspiracy against my being slender and beautiful. I considered excusing myself and asking a friend to pose as me.

I entered the doctor's office. His perfunctory glance up from his desk rested on me long enough to change to another, steadier look. I began quickly defending myself. Lots of people lose 30 pounds and don't get fussed over. And besides, so long as I was healthy, why did it matter?

His responses were quick and convincing. Thirty pounds accounted for more than one-quarter of my original weight. My thin hair, he said, was undernourished and might fall out at an unhealthy, not to mention unattractive, pace. My skin was dull. My nerves were constantly on edge.

Then he got to the question I had been most frightened of—when was my last period? I was sufficiently humiliated to answer honestly, "15 months ago." The doctor was horrified that a young adult, a college student, would be so careless and ignorant about such an important function.

The doctor told me I had anorexia nervosa and went on to explain what it was and how I was to combat it. He added that he felt he had caught it in time. He described the hospitalization and intravenous feeding of others whom he had discovered at a later stage. I could avoid that by actively attacking my psychological aversion to food. But no matter what I did, he could not predict what my chances were for bearing a child. That struck home.

I left the office embarrassed, grateful, uncertain, reprieved—I had been given permission to have milk shakes, cookies, and seconds? Could I, without turning into a self-indulgent blimp?

Yes. I hesitantly and unenthusiastically began accepting the ounces that indeed were lurking around every corner. I allowed myself flavored yogurts, meat, and vegetables, sometimes seconds. My stomach did rebel at first, and I would find myself hanging over the toilet in sweating nausea. But the fight was on.

My senior year was marked by consultations and weigh-ins with the college doctor. Irrational fears of obesity drove me to tears in the infirmary, near hysterics in my dorm room. I learned how an anorexic suffers from a lack of positive self-image: the mirror reflected not a clear image but a fat, distorted person. I would retreat on occasion to my old ways, but the doctor taught me to read the scale until I could read myself objectively in the mirror.

I'm one of the lucky ones. I did recover, as much as an anorexic can. I am now 102 pounds and always trying to lose "just a few." I still think I eat too much but I control my worries better. When I look at myself in the mirror I still think I am overweight. And I still don't know whether I can have a child.

Eating Sensibly
The Advancing Years

Three different kinds of changes jeopardize nutritional health among the over-65 population, that large category of citizens (more than 10 percent of the U.S. population) that includes both the vigorous and athletic as well as the extremely debilitated. Most obvious are the physical signs of aging: the slowing or faltering of bodily functions and skills. But perhaps as significant are the psychological and socioeconomic changes that can radically alter the pattern of life itself: retirement, reduced income, estrangement from family, the loss of friends, and the depression and apathy these bring.

Not infrequently, a combination of factors from all three categories make old age a misery, and poor nutrition one of its hallmarks: the housebound elderly living on little money are ill-equipped to shop and cook nutritious meals for themselves. Elderly people living alone, whether poor or affluent, are likely to eat less well, less regularly and, in the end, more expensively, than those who live with another person or in a community. Although food programs such as Meals on Wheels (which delivers a hot meal to elderly persons five or more times a week) are available, individual attention is needed to determine current health status, nutritional needs, and physical or economic bars to self-help. Following is advice for the concerned relative or friend of an elderly person, as well as for someone interested in improving his own eating habits.

The Physical Condition. Anyone familiar with older people has observed that with age, digestive difficulties increase, food preferences narrow, and constipation or diarrhea often become chronic. Yet not one of these conditions is inevitable. Each has a cause, and a cure. On the other hand, some changes observed in older people—we all age at different rates—are unavoidable; these require intelligent adjustments of diet.

Daily caloric needs begin dropping in early adulthood, but decrease sharply, by 8 percent per decade or more, after age 55. Even heavy or obese persons over that age will have reduced appetites and will suffer real gastric distress if that diminishment is not respected. Yet nutritional demands remain high, as is the case with infants and small children, so more nutrients must be packed into fewer calories.

In concert with the lowered metabolism of the elderly, the gastrointestinal system begins to slow: salivary secretion decreases, making chewing and swallowing harder; denture wearers (about half of all over 65) and those who suffer from gum diseases often resort to soft foods, thus depriving their systems of needed bulk and fiber, as well as giving up much of the pleasure of eating. The digestive system's capacity to process fats and protein and absorb vitamin B_{12} and iron is also reduced with aging, and in general operates more slowly in breaking down all foods, tending to result in excess unexpelled residue, which can cause flatulence.

Coping with Reduced Appetite. What kind of diet is suitable for the elderly, then, and just as important, how can it be achieved? A healthy diet for an older person in good health differs very little from that at any other age. However, moderation in portion sizes may be in order, and particular attention is necessary to make sure that the foods chosen are high in the protective nutrients—protein, vitamins, and minerals—since many older people are less active than they were in earlier life. To cope with reduced appetite, the older person might have nutritious snacks in addition to three smaller meals daily. Too much food at one time ignores reduced appetite, involves extra work, and promotes indigestion.

As is true of every other age group, the elderly are best served by a varied diet drawn from the Basic Four Food Groups. Protein needs remain steady through old age, about ⅓ of a gram per pound of body weight, or 44 grams daily for a 120-pound woman, 56 grams for a 154-pound man. Because digestive difficulty is so common, protein can be supplied by soups, small portions of lean meat or fish, eggs, and vegetable proteins.

Carbohydrates are more easily digested, provide needed fiber and nutrients, and are thus superior foods for the elderly. Whole-grain breads and cereals, green and root vegetables, potatoes and enriched pasta are all good choices. Fresh fruit or fruit packed in its own juice is far preferable to pastries and other sweets as a dessert.

Consumption of fats should be restricted to no more than 30-35 percent of total calories daily to prevent gastric stress. The danger of atherosclerosis, linked to fat intake and cholesterol-rich foods, however, appears to be less critical for this age group than the middle-aged—which suggests that elderly persons not already afflicted need not sacrifice such excellent, but high-cholesterol sources of protein as eggs, milk, beef, and liver.

Loss of appetite and depletion of vitamins and minerals in the aged is primarily because of poor diet but is aggravated by therapeutic drugs and laxatives (see pages 38-39). Any person taking medication regularly should be on the alert for side effects and arrange for vitamin supplements if necessary. Calcium deficiency is a major factor in the development of osteoporosis, a reduction of bone mass that frequently leads to bone fractures, particularly of the hip. Adequate consumption of milk or milk products—2 or more glasses a day—will help prevent this and related degenerative bone ailments.

Anemia, because of reduced intake or reduced absorption of a number of nutrients, including iron, is common among the over-65 population. Proper nutrition is the appropriate, and relatively cheap, remedy, if only the need is recognized. Similarly, many chronic and painful kidney conditions, as well as constipation, can be eased simply by drinking water in sufficient amounts—5 to 8 glasses daily.

For the physically handicapped or housebound, assistance in shopping for food, especially perishables, or in food preparation, may be necessary. If you find yourself in need of such help, ask for it from friends, relatives, or from government agencies funded by your taxes. If you are the relative or concerned friend of an aged person or couple living independently, check to see what kinds of meals are being eaten, and how you could be of help. Urge your aged loved one to attend to nutrition and make yourself available to shop, help prepare meals ahead of time, plan menus, seek additional information on reducing use of drugs and vitamins, and so forth. If you want to make gifts of food, make them wholesome—no cookies unless they come with a loaf of whole-wheat bread, a cut of meat, fresh fruit, or vegetables. Better still, invite elderly guests for dinner, or invite yourself over. Nothing stimulates care in preparation of food, not to mention actual appetite, like the prospect of company. Many nutritional ailments are symptomatic not just of poor diet but of poor social contact. One noted and elderly nutritionist advises attending to the loneliness first, then the diet. Eating is a part of life. Those who believe they have a future, and a stake in present health, will make a greater effort to participate in life by caring for themselves through diet.

Meal Planning for the Elderly

Nourishing food and proper eating habits can reverse the downward spiral of depression and apathy, aggravated by decreasing interest in food, that so many elderly persons experience. Here are some nutrition tips, followed by a day's sample menu:

- If dentures and decreased saliva secretion make chewing and swallowing harder, try soft, mashed, chopped, or strained foods; some nutrients may be lost in preparation but more will be properly digested and absorbed.
- Get your essential proteins from stews, hearty broths, flaked fish, or purees of meat, eggs, milk, cereal, and gelatins.
- Relieve intestinal problems with the natural roughage of fruits and vegetables.
- Soften toast or zwieback in milk or soup; it will be more easily digestible than soft breads, which tend to ferment in the system if improperly chewed.
- Avoid fried foods or rich sauces.
- Since warm foods or beverages are more easily digested than cold, start meals with soup or a warm beverage.
- Eat at least three meals a day—small ones are more easily digested—and snack in between.

6 A.M. Tea or coffee or hot milk
8 A.M. Citrus fruit or juice
    Iron-fortified cereal or soft-boiled egg
    Toast and butter or margarine
    Tea, coffee, cocoa, or skim milk
Noon Cream or thick vegetable soup or juice
    Sandwich of meat, fish, egg,
       cheese, or peanut butter
          on whole-wheat bread
    Green vegetable or raw salad
    Stewed fruit, rice pudding,
       or tapioca
3 P.M. Broth, milk, or hot chocolate
    Toast or crackers
6 P.M. Minced chicken, lamb,
       or broiled hamburger
    Potato, baked or mashed, or rice
    Cooked, mashed vegetable,
       green or yellow
    Toast with butter or margarine
    Custard, plain cake, or fruit
    Tea or coffee
10 P.M. Fruit or juice
    Toast, or cheese and crackers

Getting into Shape

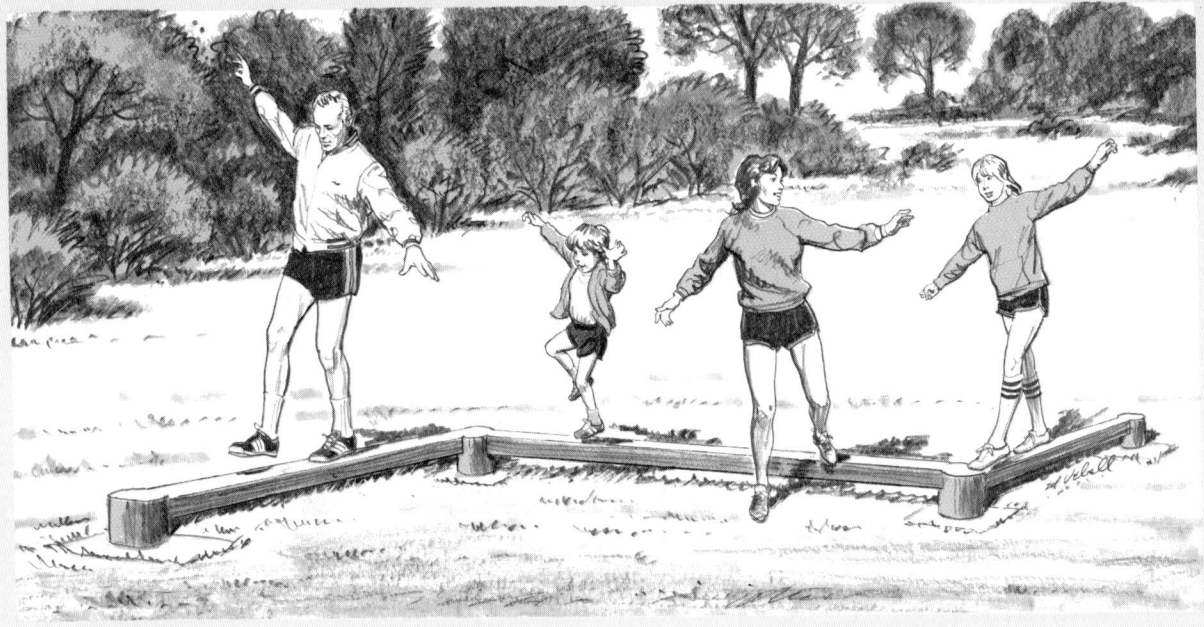

Learning to eat sensibly is only the first step toward achieving and maintaining your ideal weight. You also need exercise.

Recent studies suggest that overweight is more often caused by lack of exercise than by overeating. From age 20 on, most Americans show signs of "creeping obesity," gaining between ½ and 1½ pounds of weight per year, most of it in fat, primarily because they get so little exercise. Our ancestors of only a century ago walked to work; we drive or take a bus. They toiled in the garden; we drive once a week to the supermarket. They danced and played sports for entertainment; we watch television.

A host of modern conveniences deprive us of natural opportunities to use our bodies. We prefer vacuum cleaners to brooms and mops, elevators and escalators to stairs, golf carts to legs, snow blowers to snow shovels. Gas, electric, and oil heat has eliminated the need to chop wood or shovel coal, and today we needn't even exert ourselves by walking across the room to switch channels on the TV set— we can do it by remote control. As a result, we just don't burn up enough calories. Instead, we get fat, flabby, and weak.

Benefits of Exercise. While helping to keep the fat away, regular exercise will improve your health and appearance in other ways, too.

- Studies show that exercisers pay half as much in medical bills each year as do nonexercisers and have only one-third the number of sick days.
- Exercise enables your cardiorespiratory system to function more efficiently as your lungs take in more air and deliver more oxygen to the tissues, and as your heart pumps more blood with each contraction and delivers more oxygen to your muscles.
- Regular aerobic training lowers blood pressure, reducing the chances of suffering a stroke.
- Exercise increases muscle strength.
- If you are under stress or suffer from insomnia, exercise can help bring relief.
- Many researchers are sure that regular exercise slows most symptoms of aging such as fat accumulation, weakened muscles, and reduced balance, flexibility, agility, and reaction time.
- Doctors now prescribe exercise for certain types of depression. Recent studies at Loma Linda University in California indicate that a body hormone, beta-endorphin, secreted in increased amounts during exercise, is a natural euphoric or antidepressant— which may account for "runner's high." Beta-endorphin also increases tolerance of pain, which explains how injured athletes finish the game.
- Exercise will make you look and feel better—an irresistible appeal to your vanity and an unchallengeable argument in favor of exercise.

FITNESS THROUGH EXERCISE

The Components of Fitness. Jogging is a fine exercise, but neither jogging nor any other activity can give you complete *dynamic fitness* (the ability to move freely and live energetically) as compared to *organic fitness* (your size, bone structure and build, age, sex, general health, and any physical handicap). Unlike organic fitness, over which you have little control, you can do something about your dynamic fitness. Dynamic fitness includes five components, and you cannot properly assess your own fitness level without understanding precisely what these five components are.

- *Efficiency and endurance of heart and lungs.* A strong heart that can pump blood to billions of body cells, healthy lungs that can process large quantities of oxygen, and elastic blood vessels are the marks of cardiorespiratory fitness, the most important fitness component.
- *Muscular strength and endurance.* Unused muscles grow weak, stiff, and flabby, whereas those constantly required to perform hard work increase in size and strength.
- *Balance.* Our sense of balance decreases with age unless it is continually reinforced.
- *Flexibility.* Stiff, aching joints and restricted movement are considered early signs of aging, but more frequently they are simply the natural result of inactivity. Stretching exercises—as we know from watching cats—keep the muscles loose and supple and the joints flexible.
- *Coordination and agility.* Most sports require coordinating several parts of the body in a single, agile movement, but if you have not participated in a sport for several years, you probably have not maintained this fitness component.

Whatever your needs—more freshness and endurance for the job, vitality and well-being for getting more out of life, freedom from fatigue or insomnia—exercise can help. On the following pages are presented a selection of the most popular physical activities with assessments of how they contribute to the components of fitness. Some are done alone, some require equipment or opponents, some are seasonal and must be complemented by other activities in the off-season. Some—isometrics—develop and firm up muscles; others—aerobics—improve your cardiorespiratory efficiency. Whichever activity you choose, the hardest exercise is the first move—beginning a physical fitness program.

Exercise Myths

- *Exercise increases appetite.*

Moderate exercise tends to *decrease*, not increase, appetite. Prolonged strenuous exercise does increase appetite, but the added calories are used for energy, not stored as fat.

- *Any exercise benefits the heart.*

Only activity that increases the pulse rate to at least 70 percent of maximum for 20 to 30 minutes and is repeated two to five times a week will do much good.

- *Nonporous (rubber or plastic) warm-up suits help in weight loss.*

Your body maintains a core, or inner, normal temperature during exercise by the evaporation of sweat. Nonporous suits prevent evaporation, forcing the body to sweat more—a condition that may result in dehydration, heat exhaustion, or more serious complications.

- *I'm too old to exercise.*

Anyone of any age or physical condition, even quadraplegics, can benefit from exercise. A moderate exercise program retards the conditions usually associated with aging.

- *I haven't the time.*

Every person is allowed eight hours of "play" per day. Some corporations have discovered the relationship between an employee's fitness and his productivity and are providing facilities and time for exercise during the work day. Even housewives, whose "work is never done," can incorporate fitness activities into their day and may find themselves so invigorated that chores go easier.

- *It takes a marathon to work off a pound.*

True. But if you run half an hour a day, three days a week, you will lose 15 pounds a year. If you walk briskly 30 minutes every day you can lose up to 20 pounds a year.

- *I'm too tired to exercise.*

On the contrary, exercise relieves fatigue, stress, and tensions.

Getting into Shape
Testing Your Dynamic Fitness

Exercise will be more fun and more beneficial if you ask neither too much of yourself nor too little. That's one reason to learn before you start just how fit you are.

The first and most important component of dynamic fitness to measure is cardiorespiratory efficiency. Approximately one in 10 middle-aged American men have "silent" heart disease and might be harmed by overexertion. Anyone might have an unrecognized heart condition, but you should be particularly concerned if:

- You have ever had heart disease before;
- You have the "risk factors" for heart disease—high blood pressure, overweight, a family history of heart disease, diabetes, high blood cholesterol level, or a cigarette-smoking habit;
- You have ever suffered chest pain, shortness of breath, or dizziness following physical activity;
- You are more than 30 years old and have not been physically active for years.

Under any of these circumstances, you should definitely have a doctor's approval before starting an exercise program.

The Exercise Stress Test. If your doctor has any questions about how your heart will react to exercise, he might order an exercise or stress test. While you ride a stationary bicycle or jog on a treadmill, an electrocardiogram records your heart's electrical activity, and additional equipment monitors pulse rate, blood pressure, and other vital signs. As the test progresses, heart rate approaches maximum capacity, and unrecognized cardiac defects now usually (but not always) become obvious.

Although the stress test is useful, it is not infallible. In more than half of the cases in which it indicates heart disease, further tests show there is no defect. More significantly, the test might show no abnormality when coronary heart disease does exist.

No matter what the stress test says, if during a subsequent exercise period you become extremely breathless, trembling, dizzy, nauseous, or suffer chest pain, stop exercising immediately. If the symptoms persist, seek medical help.

Strength, Flexibility, and Balance. To determine your muscle strength and flexibility—two other components of dynamic fitness—take the Kraus-Weber tests shown on page 329.

No doubt you already have a reasonably accurate idea of how well coordinated you are. If you can ride a bicycle, play baseball or tennis, or skip a rope 10 times in succession, then you probably have adequate coordination, balance, and agility. On the other hand, if you cannot maintain your balance on one foot for 30 seconds, cannot jump a rope even twice in a row, and dance with "two left feet," this will reveal the areas of dynamic fitness to which you must pay attention in choosing an exercise.

Choosing Your Exercise Activity. Having determined (by test or by obvious need) which fitness components you want to develop, examine the chart opposite. On it are rated the most popular sports as well as some of the daily activities you now consider chores but which could become an important part of your exercise program.

The benefits of any activity, of course, depend a great deal on how much you put into it. Swimming is top ranked for both cardiorespiratory efficiency and weight loss; but that means swimming, not sunbathing or paddling. Tennis as played by a beginner is mostly calisthenics: practice serving, lunging, bending to pick up balls. Skillful tennis players who keep the ball in play for several sets are developing all the components of dynamic fitness. Golf is about equal to a moderate walk, plus some upper torso muscular exertion.

Prevention Program. Physical fitness has been defined as the ability to meet ordinary and even unusual demands of your daily life safely, effectively, and without undue fatigue—to walk briskly for 10 minutes or climb 3 flights of stairs without discomfort, to lift and carry moderately heavy loads without feeling the strain, to get up suddenly without dizziness, to participate in some physical activity at least an hour a day or intensive exercise for 10 to 15 minutes a day.

Even a moderately active life may meet the daily requirements for adequate exercise: climbing those 3 flights of stairs to get your heart rate up; walking 3 to 4 miles or doing an hour of moderate housework to maintain your ideal weight; lifting a heavy bag of groceries to load your muscles to one-half of their maximum; spending at least 10 minutes per hour on your feet and moving. In short, you must make physical activity a part of your daily routine.

FITNESS THROUGH EXERCISE

Rating Physical Activities

Activity can be graded in terms of oxygen consumption in liters per minute or—of greater interest to most people—in calories spent per kilogram (2.2 pounds) per hour. Of course, rates vary with age, sex, physical condition, environment, degree of competitiveness, skill, and training.

Light Activities. Normal office or housework, shopping; occupations involving light physical work (lab, restaurant, hospital, carpentry); yoga, bowling, golf, canoeing 2½ mph, purposeful walking on level ground 2½-3 mph. Insufficient for weight control or fitness as heart rate seldom exceeds 110 per minute.

Moderate to Heavy Activities. Working as a general laborer, building trades, farming, heavy housework such as scrubbing floors, normal gardening; volleyball, tennis, badminton, walking 4-5 mph, cycling 5-10 mph. All get the sedentary and over-35 into the target zone (page 326). Average people spend 1 hour or less in such activities per day.

Heavy Activities. Skating, climbing stairs, basketball, rowing, swimming, squash, cross-country skiing. Sustained energy expenditure seldom lasts more than 20 minutes, and few get into this range during a normal day. However, farming, lumbering, walking uphill with a heavy load, felling trees result in similar energy output. Very Heavy (over 12 calories/kilogram/hour). Heart rate nears maximum.

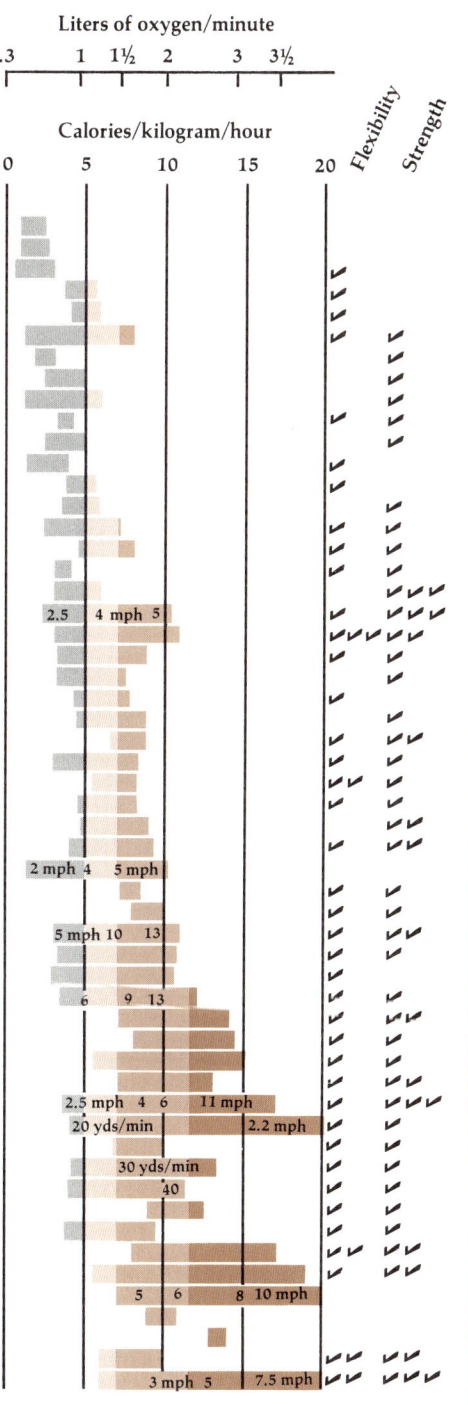

Getting into Shape
What's Best for You

Cardiorespiratory efficiency, strength, flexibility, coordination—all are among the fitness goals set by doctors and physiologists. However, there are other more obvious and tangible goals that often motivate fitness programs. Most people will start *feeling* better as soon as they look better: simply being able to wear one size smaller is enough to lift your spirits and put a spring in your step. Even a modest effort will often tone up atrophied muscles.

There are many excuses for not exercising. None has any validity. Your size, age, and sex will have an obvious influence on the specific kinds of activity that can do you the most good. They do not provide an excuse for *not exercising*.

Body Type. If you've been living a sedentary life, a fitness program will probably do wonders for your physical appearance, removing unwanted flab and building firm tissue. No amount of exercise, however, can change your basic body type. There are three basic body types; although few people fit exclusively into any single category, we all lean toward one.

Ectomorph. Thin, small framed, often tall, slender, delicate, and lanky, the ectomorph can excel in running and jumping sports where the less weight carried the better. He may find swimming strenuous since lacking body fat he must work harder to stay afloat. The ectomorph, if physically fit, has good endurance and agility.

Mesomorph. Of medium or average build, broad shouldered and well muscled, the mesomorph does well in any sport requiring strength, endurance, or agility. Although aesthetically proportioned and athletic in appearance, the mesomorph is not necessarily in better physical condition.

Endomorph. Round and soft with ill-defined muscles and short limbs, the endomorph is compact with good power and strength but often lacking in endurance. With good buoyancy he will do well at swimming but will not excel in running or tennis.

Age. If you are middle-aged or older, do not expect to recapture the physique of your youth. Regular activity, however, can keep a 75-year-old in better condition than a sedentary man half his age. Physiologists have found that active elderly people have better reaction reflexes than younger nonactive people. In skill sports like tennis, a father can often beat his son by relying on neuromuscular speed and strategy. Exercise is as safe for the elderly as for any other age group when caution is used. Conversely, it is never too soon to begin exercise. Studies show that active children tend to become physically healthy adults.

Sex. Gender need not influence your choice of exercise or sports, although in some cases it will affect the degree of excellence you will be able to achieve. Males are taller (see illustration at right), with longer limbs, have broader shoulders and stronger arms, which aid in throwing and hitting skills. But they carry more weight on a higher center of gravity, which can be a disadvantage in upright, endurance sports such as running.

Women have greater body-fat stores, which provide buoyancy, insulation, and energy reserves for swimming and distance running. Women are already bettering the men's Olympic records in swimming and are narrowing the sex gap in distance running. Finally, neither menstrual cycle nor pregnancy need keep a woman from exercising.

Personality. Gregarious, extroverted people need company and will do well in a social, competitive sport like tennis. Romantics and artists will be able to stick with a skill or form sport like swimming, figure skating, or alpine skiing where a technique can be perfected. The type A personality—competitive, aggressive, hostile—however, is warned against competitive or social sports. Type A tensions and drive are better eased in solitary, rhythmical activities such as jogging, swimming, or skating.

Handicaps. For those suffering from arthritis or heart condition, exercise is sometimes recommended by physicians as therapy. Unless their condition is acute, arthritics can find relief in water sports, and many cardiac patients can bring their functional capacity back to normal under an exercise program prescribed by a doctor. Even impaired vision or loss of a limb need not be a deterrent. Although the choice of sports may be somewhat limited for the handicapped person, the ability to perform is not; the handicapped have excelled in many fields. Even temporary handicaps—muscle strains, blisters—need not interfere. Runners with leg problems can switch to swimming or biking.

FITNESS THROUGH EXERCISE

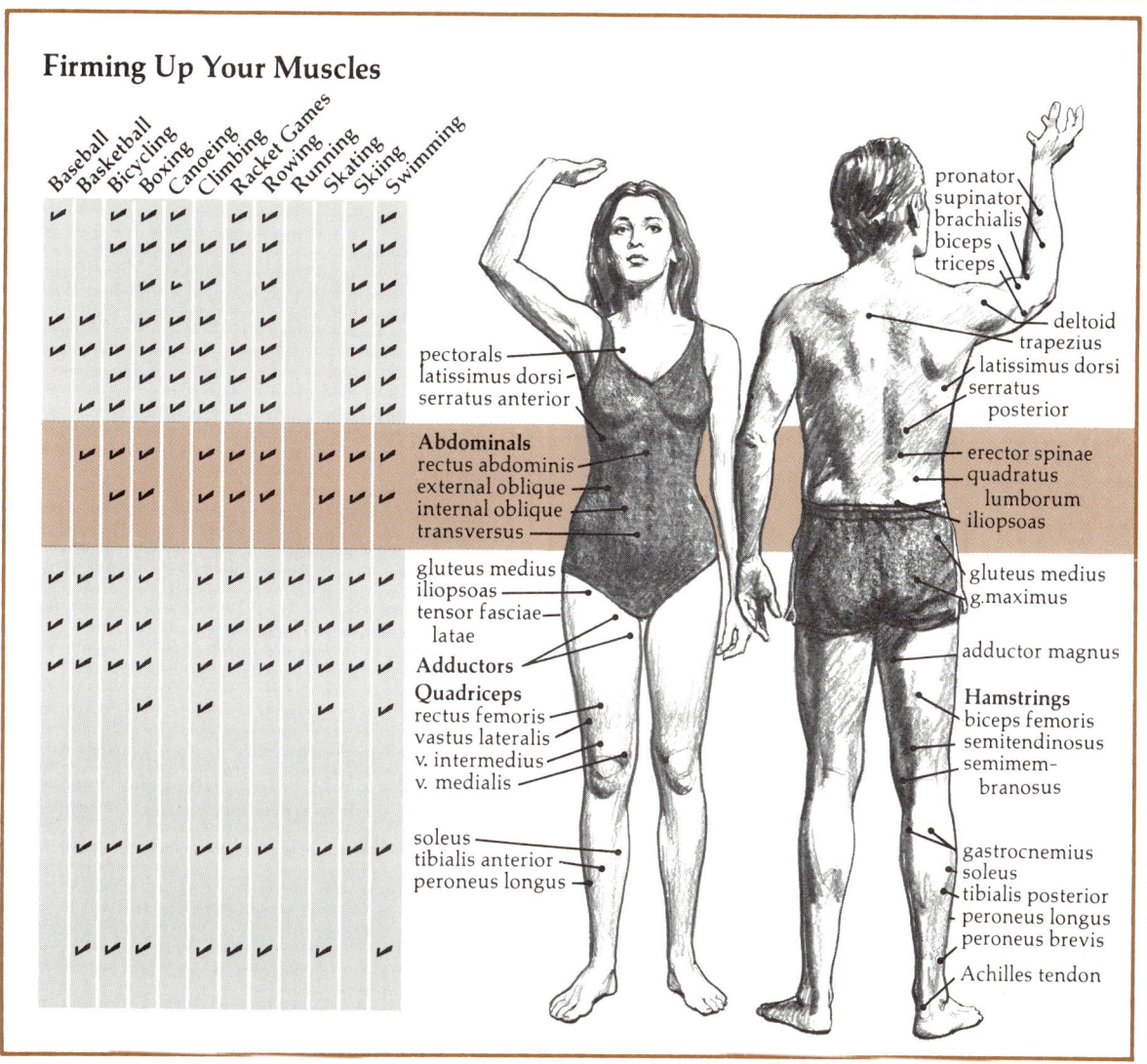

Firming Up Your Muscles

Life-style. Your type of work, where you live, the time of day you wish to devote to exercise, the availability of facilities and partners or opponents, the expense—all these must be taken into account in designing your fitness program.

City dwellers may find facilities for many sports but should examine them first. City tennis courts may be cement, have no nets, or be in constant use for handball. Under such adverse conditions, it is difficult to muster enthusiasm or avoid injury.

In any case, don't take up an exercise "because it's in vogue." Select the exercise you will enjoy, so that you will not easily tire of it.

Set Your Goals—and Stick to Them. Perhaps you already know what your fitness goals are—a thinner waist, more stamina, more grace and coordination on the dance floor. Perhaps you have simply resolved to achieve a higher level of overall fitness. Whatever your goals, get serious about them now; write them out as specifically as you can. Not, "lose weight," but "lose 27 pounds." Not, "build stamina," but "jog 2 miles in 20 minutes." Once you are clear and determined about the goals you wish to accomplish, they will be easier to achieve. And as your fitness improves with training, those early goals will come to seem like child's play to you.

Getting into Shape
The Exercise Routine

Three keys to a successful exercise program are frequency, duration, and intensity. Exercise shouldn't be painful but it should make you sweat. How you achieve that sweat is your decision. Any activity from bouncing on a trampoline to running around the block is acceptable if it brings your heart rate up into the target area (see the chart below and the illustration at right).

Swedish studies have shown that 15-minute periods of intense exercise three times a week and a brisk one-hour daily walk will considerably improve cardiovascular fitness. In general, exercise physiologists recommend 20 to 30 minutes of sustained effort, sufficiently strenuous to maintain a pulse rate in the target area.

Frequency. To gain the greatest benefit from your program, plan to exercise three to five days a week. Three days is typical, with rest days in between. Five days will produce faster results if you are exercising for weight control. Since deconditioning occurs rapidly, you should not go more than three consecutive days without exercising; if you discontinue exercising for five weeks, you will lose almost 50 percent of the fitness you have achieved. After 10 weeks, deconditioning will be total and you will be in the same condition as before you began—though reconditioning should be easier and quicker.

Duration. With time allowed for warm-ups and cool-downs, plus the 20- to 30-minute stimulus period, your exercise should take under an hour.

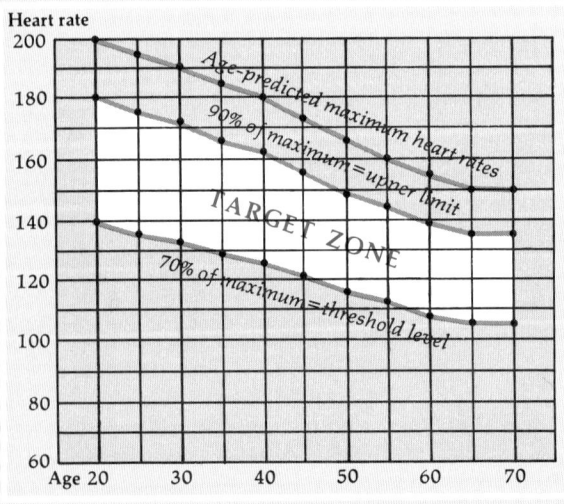

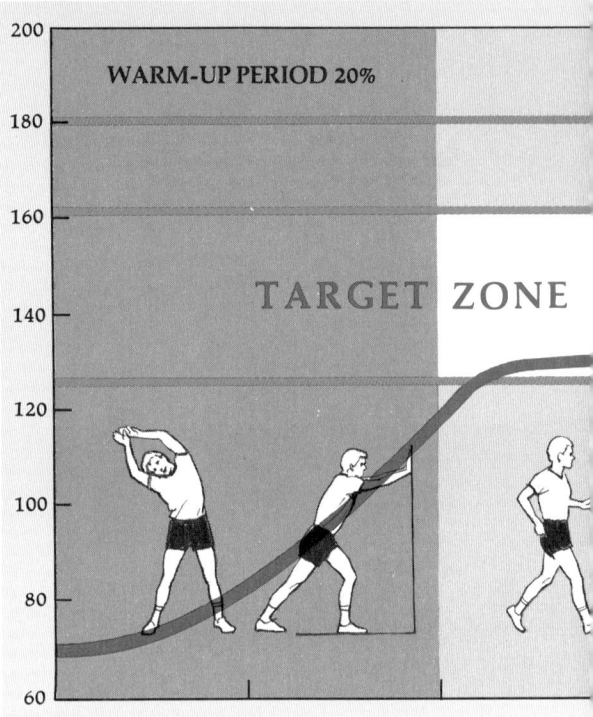

The stimulus time can be broken up into five-minute stints with brief rest periods—as long as the total stimulus period is 20 to 30 minutes. Swimmers doing sprints or walk-joggers are automatically doing this "interval training." With high-intensity training, 10- to 15-minute stimulus periods will produce results.

Intensity. The level of effort—that is, the appropriate amount of stress for your system—depends on your degree of fitness or present work capacity. One determinant is maximum heart rate. The chart at left, below, shows age-predicted maximum rates. These figures hold for most people—plus or minus 10 beats per minute—and work out to 220 minus your age. A more precise figure is obtained from taking an exercise stress test (see page 322).

If you reach and maintain about 70 percent of your maximum, you will be improving your aerobic capacity. This 70 percent training threshold is sufficiently intense but not uncomfortable. For instance, you should be able to converse with a fellow runner at this level. The upper limit, above which no gains can be made, is estimated to be at some 90 percent of maximum heart rate. With training, aero-

FITNESS THROUGH EXERCISE

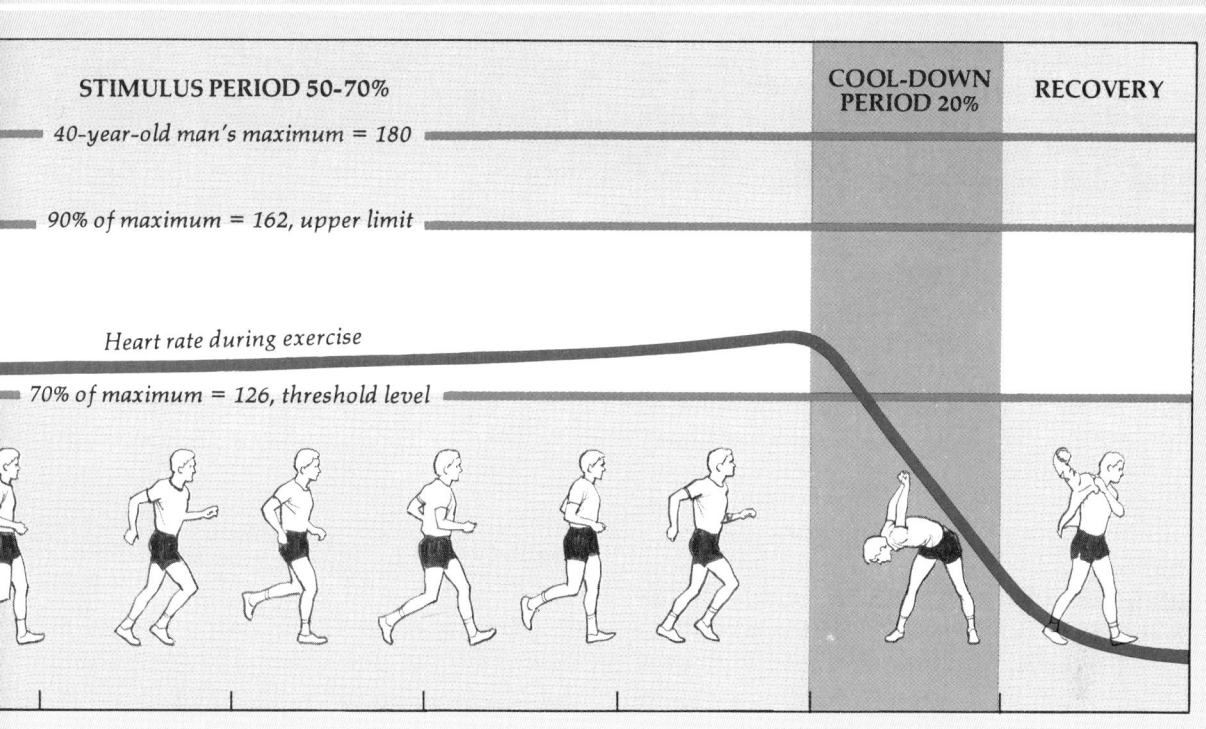

bic capacity improves—as much as 50 percent for sedentary heart patients, but averages between 5 and 25 percent. As you get conditioned, your pulse rate will go down and you will have to work harder to achieve the high heart rates necessary for continued progress in building cardiorespiratory fitness.

Whatever the exercise you have selected, you should follow a definite routine:

Warm-Ups. To exercise when your muscles are stiff is to ask for trouble. Just as you should begin an exercise program slowly, allowing your system to adjust to the new demands being made, so should you begin a daily routine slowly. Many a professional athlete has found himself sidelined by a muscle pull that could have been avoided by a proper warm-up period providing stretching, increased circulation, and higher temperature in the muscles to be exercised.

A sufficient warm-up period lasts several minutes. It starts lightly with some continuous rhythmic activity that gradually increases in intensity until pulse, breathing, and body temperature are elevated—but not into the target zone. When the muscles have been warmed, then do some easy stretching and bending exercises to limber up muscles, loosen tendons, ligaments, and joints. Some activities have a built-in warm-up period: cyclists can start slowly on level ground, runners can jog slowly.

At the end of the warm-up period, pulse should reach 60 to 65 percent of threshold. (Pulse rate can be taken by placing the fingertips on the radial artery inside the top of the wrist or on the carotid artery in the neck under the corner of the jaw between the big neck muscle and the windpipe. Count the beats for 10 seconds and multiply by six.)

Target Zone Activity. As shown in the illustration above, the period of sustained exercise should last 20 to 30 minutes.

Cool-Downs. If exercise is stopped abruptly, blood tends to pool in the enlarged veins of the active muscles, reducing blood supply to the heart and brain. Some people may experience dizziness or chest pains, or even nausea if blood flow is restricted to the heart or intestinal system. A cool-down period of mild jogging keeps the leg muscles moving, massaging the veins and pumping the blood back to the heart. Cool-downs should be relaxed. At the end of a running period, for instance, walk for five minutes and repeat the beginning stretching exercises for another five minutes.

Getting into Shape
Calisthenics for Conditioning

The ancient Greeks, who idealized the human form, coined the word *calisthenics*, or "beautiful strength," to describe the system of exercise that gave them both muscular development and gracefulness. However, calisthenics is much more than jumping jacks, sit-ups, and other similar exercises that many people find boring. All light gymnastics, including yoga and even ballet exercises, are actually calisthenics.

If inconvenience has kept you from exercising regularly, calisthenics can be the answer to your dilemma, for you can do them anywhere at any time, wearing anything (or nothing), and with no more equipment than the furniture in your home—and even that isn't necessary.

There are hundreds of calisthenics exercises—of which we show here only a few representative examples, not as an instruction manual but rather as an introduction to the subject. Calisthenics can help you improve all components of fitness: flexibility, balance and agility, muscle strength and endurance—even cardiorespiratory fitness, *if* you exercise rapidly and long enough to keep your pulse in the target zone (see page 326) for at least 20 minutes.

Even if you use other exercise for your basic fitness program, calisthenics should be part of the warm-up and cool-down periods. Remember to choose calisthenics that flex and loosen the muscles involved in your major activity. Calisthenics can also relieve or prevent most cases of lower back pain, some sleeping problems, and certain types of tension—all by loosening tight muscles.

Caution: avoid quick, jerky movements in calisthenics; don't bob, hold. Do not force a movement

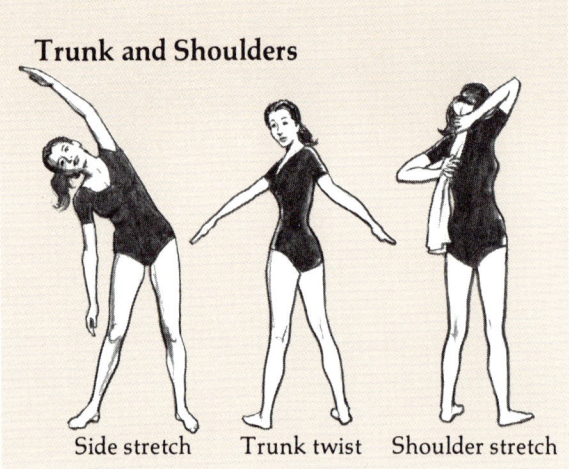

Trunk and Shoulders

Side stretch   Trunk twist   Shoulder stretch

beyond mild discomfort. Concentrate on gracefulness and body control. Extend yourself.

Trunk and Shoulders. While there is no such thing as spot reducing, or eliminating fat from a specific body area, you *can* shape and tone individual muscle groups through calisthenics. Stretching and twisting the trunk (shown above) help flatten the stomach, shape the waist, and provide the flexibility needed for graceful movement. The goal of the shoulder stretch is to clasp your fingers behind your back, but try it first with a towel. The shoulder stretch helps prevent or correct the sedentary syndrome known as "secretary's slump."

Hips, Thighs, and Buttocks. This area of your body can be toned and strengthened through exercises such as those shown opposite: leg and knee lifts,

Posture Tips

Correct body alignment while standing, sitting, or lifting can help prevent back pain. Balance weight evenly, keep head and chest up. Use the large leg muscles, not the back, in lifting; keep the back rounded and support it by resting one hand on knee. For prolonged standing work, have counters and sinks at proper height and rest hips against counter to take load off back.

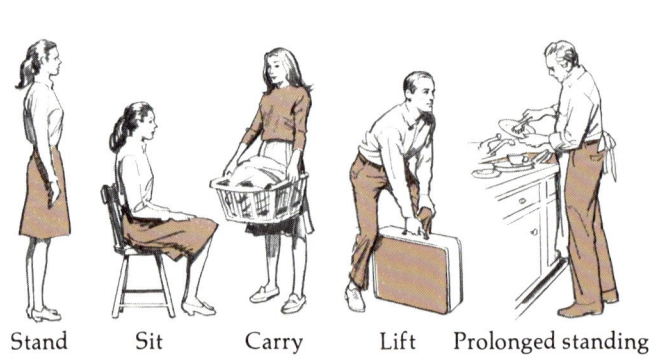

Stand   Sit   Carry   Lift   Prolonged standing

FITNESS THROUGH EXERCISE

knee and trunk rolls, buttocks lift, sit-ups, and flutter kicks. All these exercises involve your body's largest muscle mass, part of the antigravity group that enables you to maintain an upright stance—thus, their importance to posture.

Abdomen. Sit-ups and other reclining exercises that involve lifting the legs or torso are also good abdominal conditioners as long as the back is kept slightly rounded and the knees are bent to prevent lower back strain. For sit-ups, clasping your hands behind your head makes the abdominal muscles do more work. Twisting the torso so that your right elbow touches your left knee (and vice versa) is even more beneficial.

Strength. Calisthenics are used for the Kraus-Weber tests of strength and flexibility (see below). Designed to test the key muscle groups in your body, these exercises will reveal whether you have the necessary strength to handle your own body weight and the flexibility to match your height. If you can perform all six, you meet the minimum level of muscular fitness.

Note: it is permissible to bend your knees in order to touch the floor—and perhaps desirable, to avoid back strain.

Hips, Thighs, Buttocks, and Abdomen

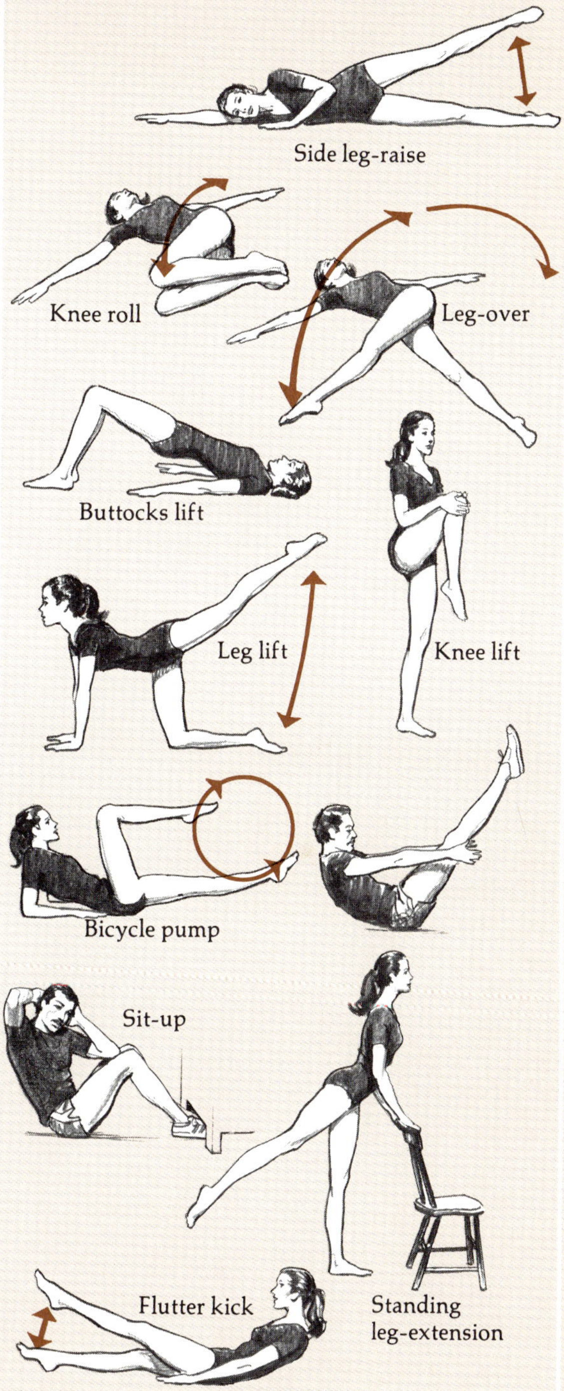

Kraus-Weber Tests

All lifts 10 inches and hold for 10 seconds

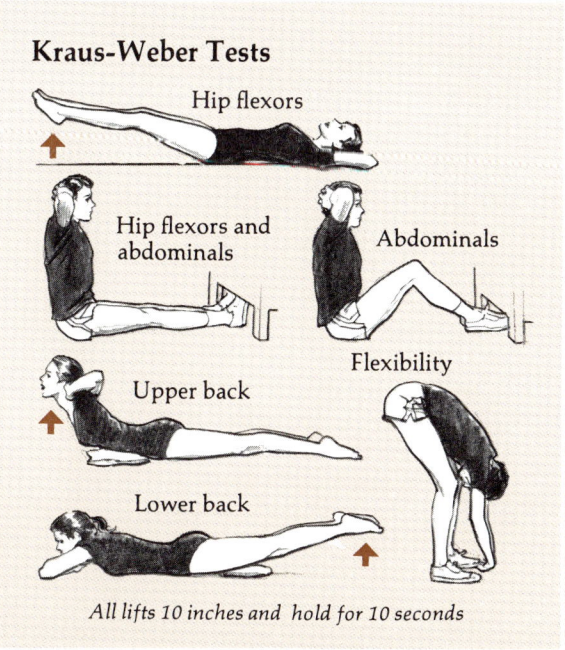

Getting into Shape
Calisthenics Therapy

Calisthenics—training the body to be controlled, coordinated, and strong—is the basis for more than simple spot toning or building strength. Calisthenics is also used to prevent pain, heighten awareness, express vitality, and even for self-defense.

Tension. Our modern civilization has presented us with a paradox: it has eliminated most of the daily physical activities we need for fitness and at the same time has increased the tensions that can best be released by physical activity. Our bodies are underexercised but we are overstimulated, easily frustrated by situations beyond our control—by noise, pollution, overcrowding. The tension and stress of our daily lives too often lead to tight muscles, pain, even physical or mental impairment. Who has not felt muscles in the neck, shoulders, and back tighten under emotional strain? Exercises that stretch these muscles can have a dramatic relaxing effect. Perform the exercises shown at right slowly, holding and stretching each position until you actually feel the muscles relaxing. Headaches caused by tense neck muscles may also be cured by exercise.

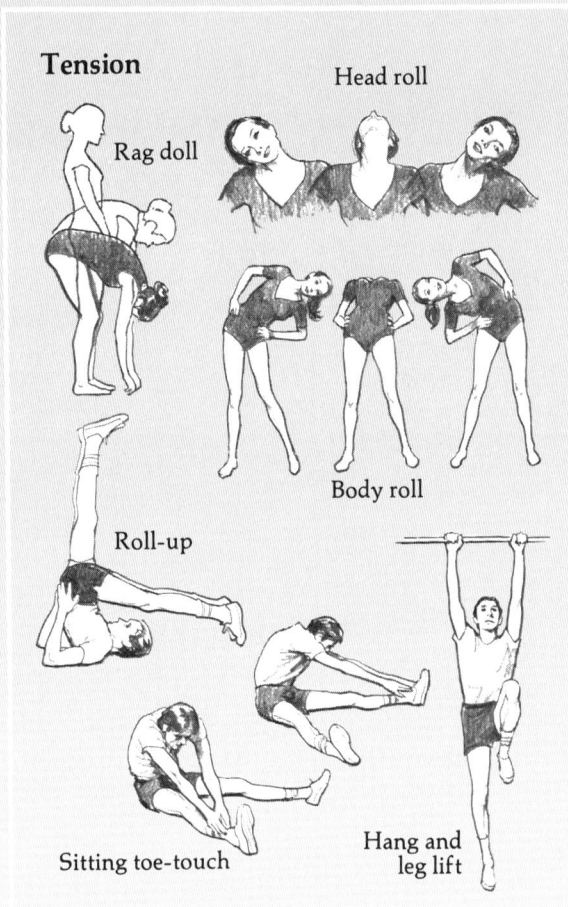

Tension — Rag doll, Head roll, Body roll, Roll-up, Sitting toe-touch, Hang and leg lift

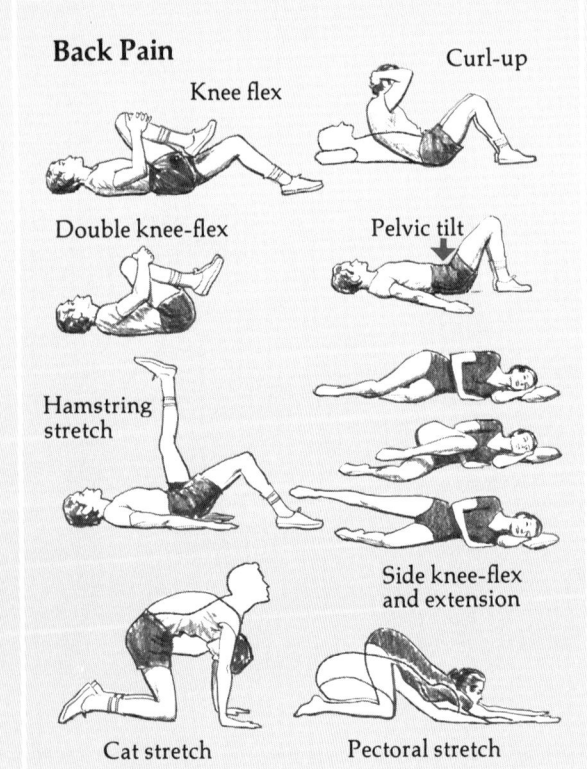

Back Pain — Knee flex, Curl-up, Double knee-flex, Pelvic tilt, Hamstring stretch, Side knee-flex and extension, Cat stretch, Pectoral stretch

Back Pain. Some researchers believe that more than 80 percent of all back-pain cases are caused by underexercise combined with stress and strain and have successfully treated such problems with calisthenics. If you failed one or more of the Kraus-Weber tests (page 329) you probably have or will have back pain. Those very same Kraus-Weber exercises, plus the lifting exercises on the same page, can be used to strengthen back and abdominal muscles and hip flexors. And since back pain is also called "tension syndrome," tension relievers (above) also help loosen up tight back muscles. Corrective exercises to stretch muscles that are too short or too stiff include all the tension relievers above as well as those at left. Hip rotation exercises (knee roll and leg-over, page 329) loosen vertebrae. Doctors also recommend swimming for back-pain sufferers because the horizontal position and support of the water relieve strain on vertebrae.

The Joy of Movement

Yoga. In recent years, physiologists have begun taking yoga exercises seriously. Derived from the ancient Hindu discipline, yoga does not offer cardiorespiratory conditioning, but offers perhaps the best of all flexibility exercises and contributes significantly to strength and balance. Salutations to the Sun (right) is a yoga routine that should be performed in a measured, continuous movement flowing from one position to the next. Whereas back exercises treat symptoms of pain from tension, yoga practitioners claim it will banish tension itself by both mental and physical stretching and limbering exercises.

The Eastern world has long been conscious of the relation between exercise and health. The yoga diet could set an example for weight-conscious Americans: fill half the stomach with food, a quarter with water, and keep a quarter empty.

Dance. Graceful calisthenics movements done rapidly to music can be a total conditioner, if the pace is fast enough and maintained long enough. An evening of polka or disco dancing provides a thorough—and enjoyable—workout. Many classical ballet positions can be recognized on these pages; ballet dancers are among the world's best athletes.

Yoga

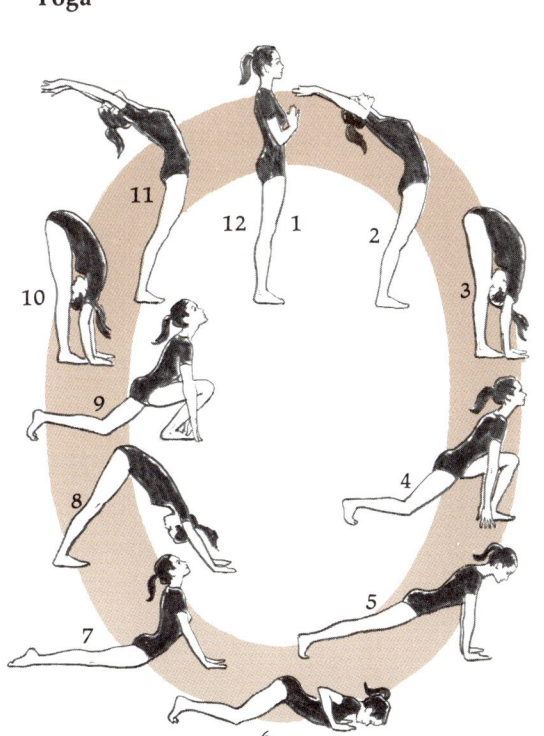

Dance Aerobics

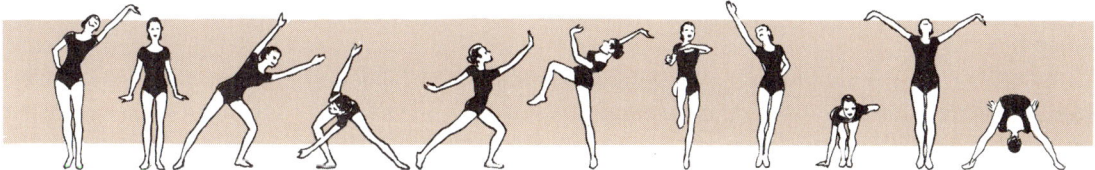

T'ai chi ch'üan

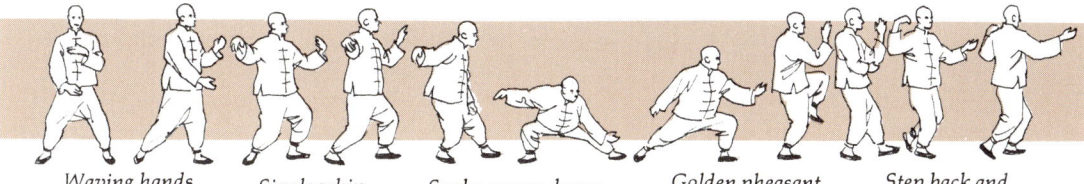

Waving hands like clouds *Single whip* *Snake creeps down* *Golden pheasant stands on one leg* *Step back and repulse monkey*

T'ai chi ch'üan. The graceful, choreographed movements of the ancient Chinese martial art T'ai chi ch'üan are practiced slowly in sequence as an art form. It takes years of concentration to achieve perfection—the controlled energy of a finely tuned body. When performed in self-defense, such calisthenics can be deadly. Perfect balance, weight evenly distributed, with knees in a semicrouch (first position) is the defense position from which—as in fencing—one is able to attack or withdraw and counterattack.

Getting into Shape
Resistance Training

If your exercise goal is to define and build muscles, to give shape and tone to a flabby body, resistance training can produce visible results in a relatively short time. Such a program allows you to concentrate on problem areas and need take no more than a few minutes a day.

How Muscles Work. To do its work, a muscle contracts. There are three kinds of contractions: concentric, in which the muscle shortens, as in lifting a weight against gravity; eccentric, in which the muscle is lengthened, as when the external resistance overcomes the muscle and it lowers the weight; isometric contraction, in which there is no change in the length of the muscle because the object is immovable.

There are three main methods of building muscle strength and endurance: progressive resistance, isometrics, and isokinetics.

Progressive Resistance. Though similar to weight lifting, a competitive sport, progressive resistance (right, above) develops muscular strength and endurance by progressively increasing the overload so that the muscle is forced through a series of compensatory adaptations. For strength and size of muscle you lift progressively greater weights with fewer repetitions. For endurance and definition of muscle you lift a lighter weight (say, 5 or 10 pounds) with more repetitions. If done rapidly enough this method can even be used as a fitness exercise. A muscle trained by lifting weights is limited to the specific training movement, and little of the developed strength is transferable to other kinds of movements.

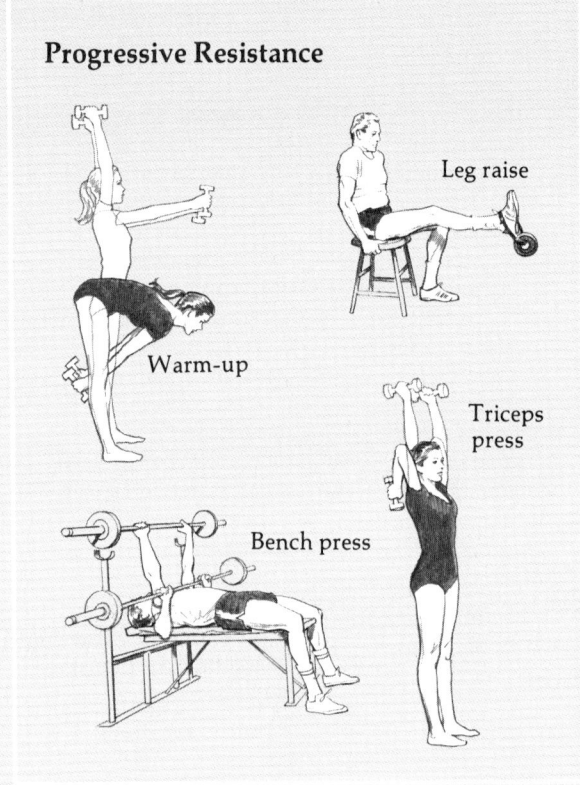

Progressive Resistance — Warm-up, Leg raise, Triceps press, Bench press

Isometrics. The isometric method has one advantage: it is brief. You can only exert maximum force against an immovable object for a second, and partial force for 6 seconds. There are plenty of immovable objects around and, as shown below, there are a variety of ways of unobtrusively working out for brief periods in home or office. However, because so

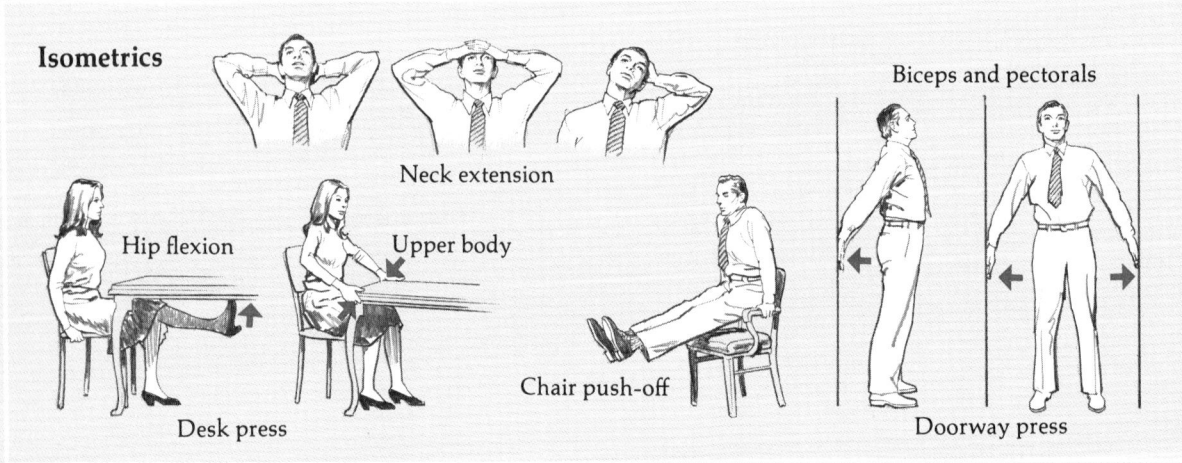

Isometrics — Hip flexion, Neck extension, Upper body, Chair push-off, Biceps and pectorals, Desk press, Doorway press

FITNESS THROUGH EXERCISE

Isokinetics

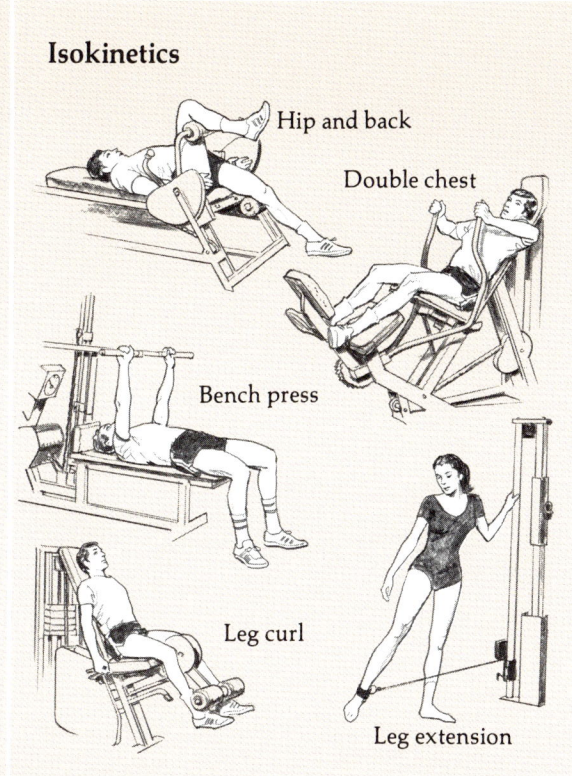

many muscles and muscle patterns are involved in the sequence of a specific movement, the isometrically trained muscle is limited to the same angle of the joint and position of the body during the training period. The muscle may be defined but its use is limited. Finally, it is difficult to measure the amount of pressure and therefore it is difficult, if not impossible, to judge improvement.

Isokinetics. For full muscle development through the complete range of movement, the best training is provided by isokinetics. In this resistance training method a mechanical device maintains a constant load as you speed up muscular contraction so that the muscles are forced to work all the way, meeting effort at any point along the movement. Such machines are now popular at many health clubs and training centers and have been devised to work out all the body's major muscle groups.

Hazards. A lack of flexibility due to one-sided development is the condition known as being muscle-bound. To avoid this, go through the full range of every movement, raise and lower all the way, and for every movement do a contrary flexibility exercise. There is a greater hazard to those who may have cardiovascular disease or varicose veins. In the intense effort of lifting a heavy weight, the breath is held, locking pressure into the chest. This prevents blood from returning to the heart, veins in the neck are extended, and blood pressure can drop to dangerously low levels.

Should You Join a Health Club?

There are both advantages and disadvantages, which you should take into consideration.

Motivation. The new friends you will meet and the group participation are strong incentives to keep at it. So is your membership fee: "I don't like exercising, but I *hate* wasting money," explained one woman.

Instructors. Many clubs have a trained staff to guide you into a fitness program that assures a training effect without exhausting—and discouraging—you.

Equipment. Membership in a health club usually means access to thousands of dollars' worth of training equipment that you would never be able to afford otherwise.

Facilities. Some health clubs offer a variety of facilities, such as pools, jogging areas, tennis and racketball courts, sauna, and such.

Pitfalls. Be sure you understand exactly what you are getting for your money. Some clubs charge a hefty fee for use of the pool, courts, and other facilities, in addition to the average $300 to $400 annual membership fee. (YMCAs are sometimes lower; weight-loss spas often considerably higher.)

Find out how many days a week you may use the facilities. If you are restricted to less than four, reconsider joining.

Before enrolling, visit the club at the time of day you will be using the facilities. You may discover that the management has oversold memberships and there are waiting lines at each piece of equipment.

Check on the qualifications of the program supervisors. While they need have no degrees after their names, each should have solid experience in appraising fitness levels and designing safe, effective programs.

Getting into Shape
Aerobic Conditioning

Although the visible benefits of exercise—a finely tuned body, well-defined muscles, graceful and flexible movement—are primary goals for many, the core of any program should be some conditioning of the less visible but more vital heart and lungs. Aerobic conditioning will give you a visible glow of health as well as the energy and alertness to do more at home, in school, or on the job. It will add more productive hours to your day and can even help retard the aging process.

Frequent and sustained rhythmical activity can bring about a stronger heart, higher heart volume, lower heart rate and blood pressure, stronger respiratory muscles, a more efficient oxygen delivery system, increased endurance and energy for less effort—and burn off pounds in the bargain.

Fueling the Muscles. There are two systems by which the muscles are supplied with energy: for brief, intense efforts like sprints, weight lifting, or blocking the line, the energy comes from glucose and fuel stores in the muscles themselves. As no oxygen is necessary, this short-term fueling is called anaerobic—airless. When the effort is extended beyond a few minutes, the immediate fuel reserves become exhausted, and the body switches to a new system, which demands oxygen for burning the fuel. This sustained exercise is called aerobic—needing oxygen.

Cardiorespiratory System. The organs that must work harder to process and supply this increased demand for oxygen are the heart and lungs, the cardiorespiratory system. Frequent and regular aerobic exercise thus conditions the heart muscle and increases its capacity, and makes the respiratory system more efficient. Moreover, the increased demand for fuel helps burn off all that energy potential that most of us carry around as fat. Fortunately, most natural activities, if done with sustained effort, become aerobic. A half hour of brisk walking, jogging or running 4 miles, a pleasant afternoon spent biking or cross-country skiing, paddling a canoe or pulling the sweeps on a slender shell, swimming refreshing laps in the pool on a hot day—all are equally beneficial and enjoyable. These, the most popular lifetime sports for many Americans, are also the best aerobic exercises, as will be demonstrated on the following pages.

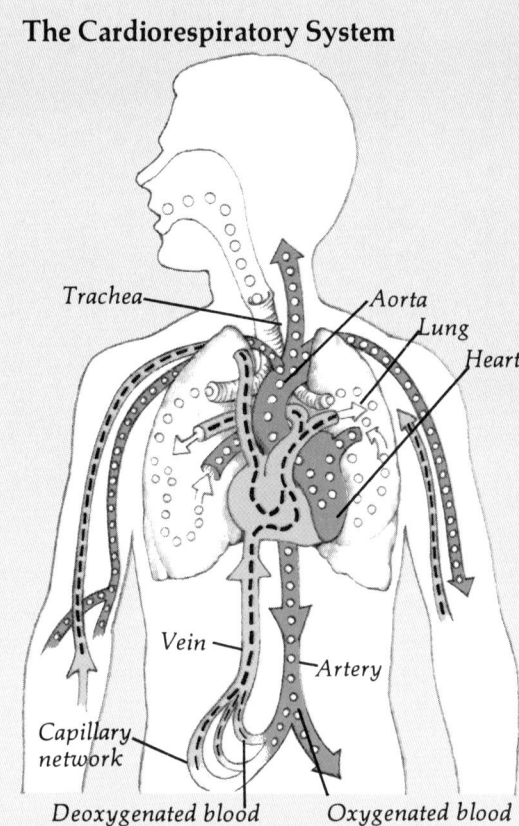

The Cardiorespiratory System

Deep, rapid breathing increases air supply to the lungs, where oxygen enters the bloodstream. Heart rate increases to speed oxygenated blood (o o o o) via the aorta and arteries to active muscles. In the network of capillaries (small blood vessels) oxygen is exchanged for waste products. Deoxygenated blood (- - -) passes to veins under low pressure. Muscle contractions assist the return of blood to the heart, which pumps blood back through the lungs for aeration (addition of fresh oxygen) and recirculation.

Walking. Consider an exercise that takes no learning, no special equipment, no special season, and is easy, convenient, useful, painless, and provides aerobic fitness, strength, and endurance. This ideal exercise is, of course, walking. A brisk half-hour walk a day can burn off 20 pounds in a year while getting and keeping you in shape. Walking is also therapeutic and inspirational—you work out your problems, reduce tension, and you may even come up with some profitable thoughts, as did the poet Robert Burns who composed one of his most popular songs during an evening walk. President Harry Truman was well known for the pace he set puffing secret servicemen and reporters during his brisk constitutional strolls.

Walk with purpose. To keep up your pace, pick a destination, step out with long strides, swing legs from hips, point toes straight ahead. Swing your arms, walk tall. Wear comfortable shoes.

Set a goal of up to 4 miles an hour and work up to it, increasing first distance then intensity. Build walking into your daily routine: get off the bus a few stops early; walk to the supermarket if you are only picking up a few items; walk up and down stairs instead of taking an elevator or escalator.

Stair Climbing. Tops in burning calories and providing cardiorespiratory fitness, stair climbing is not generally thought of as an exercise. Stairs are available in homes and offices, but normally we try to avoid unnecessary trips. With a positive action program you can make that flight or two of stairs beneficial—carry packages up one at a time, go back down for the next. While going down is called negative exercise, it works a new set of muscles and is equally valuable. Gradually increase the number of trips per day, including consecutive climbs, and in a few months, 12 trips will seem easy. A sedentary executive who can climb 3 flights in half a minute (2 steps at a time is even better) and does that 10 times a day has a fully adequate cardiorespiratory fitness program spending only 5 minutes a day.

Breaking Away. Climbing gets you up, walking gets you out. With congested city traffic moving at 3 miles per hour, you could beat the bus downtown while saving wear, tear, and a fare. When you can walk 2 miles in half an hour, your conditioning is good. Maintaining the cadence and lengthening the distance to 4 miles puts you in top shape. To increase fitness you can either add hills (keep your cadence up, just shorten your stride) or break into jogging—America's favorite fitness program.

Weston the Walker

The life of Edward Payson Weston, a frail young American who became what the *San Francisco Examiner* called "the greatest hiker in the history of mankind," is a dramatic testimonial to the benefits of walking. Weston's incredible walking feats between the ages of 22 and 74 set record after record amid ovations on both sides of the Atlantic. His dedication blessed him with a vigorous and youthful body even in his advanced old age. Evidently, he hit upon the secrets of aerobics long before this method of achieving physical fitness was known and studied.

In 1861, the 22-year-old Weston walked from Boston to Washington in 10½ days on a bet. But it was his walk from Portland, Maine, to Chicago—1,326 miles in less than 30 days—that made him an overnight sensation at the age of 28. Thereafter, he continued to bring sports fans to their feet, keep bettors and reporters busy, and astonish medical doctors with his stamina. During the next two decades he won top prizes at long-distance walking races in New York and London, where he beat off walking champions of Europe and won the prestigious Astley Belt by covering 550 miles in 142 hours.

At age 67, Weston walked the 100 miles between Philadelphia and New York City in less than 24 hours. Thirty prominent doctors performed thorough tests on him an hour after his arrival and found "the same elasticity of muscles, the same even breathing, the alertness of the eyes" that other doctors had reported when he was a young man. Next year, as if to accentuate the doctors' findings, Weston repeated his Portland-to-Chicago trek of 40 years earlier—but adding 19 miles and slashing 29 hours from his record.

At age 69 the self-labeled "propagandist for pedestrianism" walked from San Francisco to Los Angeles in 10 days; at 70, New York to San Francisco in 105 days, returning the next year in 77 days; and at 74, New York to Minneapolis in 51 days—"to prove a man my age can enjoy long-distance hikes." Hour after hour, day after day, week after week, Weston walked with his relaxed, rhythmic, and swift stride. He died in 1929 at the age of 90.

Getting into Shape
Running for Health

Today, about 31 million adult Americans have discovered the joy of jogging and running. A *Publishers Weekly* survey lists some 50 books on the subject now in print, some best-sellers. Every town in the country seems to have its neighborhood joggers.

Although many people use the terms "jogging" and "running" interchangeably, the National Jogging Association defines jogging as "a run done at a comfortable pace primarily for exercise and recreation," whereas running is usually faster and geared toward competition. Many runners actually start out jogging for fitness and, after building skill and endurance, go on to compete.

Yet, jogging is not for everyone. Those with a compulsion to compete and excel are likely to push too hard, quickly becoming discouraged and possibly injuring themselves. Others might find it boring, and some might have physical problems that make jogging unwise. Only your doctor can determine if you can physically handle a progressive jogging regimen, but you yourself must decide whether or not you are mentally suited for jogging.

The Right Equipment. One reason that jogging is so popular is that equipment is minimal: you can jog in your high school gym suit (if it still fits), bermuda shorts, old work slacks, even swim trunks—any clothing that fits loosely and comfortably and breathes so that air can continuously evaporate sweat. It is dangerous to jog in plastic or rubber suits that overheat your body.

The only item you will have to purchase for jogging is proper shoes. The right ones will wear up to a thousand miles and remain comfortable for each of the 1¼ million steps you will take covering that distance. Your local sporting goods store is likely to have dozens of running shoes available. Knowing what to look for will help narrow the selection.

A long-wearing shoe should have a reinforced toe guard so that, when you drag your toe or stumble, the shoe will not be scuffed or torn. The heel should be topped with a collar to prevent ankle chafing. At least a minimal arch support will help to absorb the impact when your foot strikes the ground with a force equal to about three times your weight.

Many experts recommend that the heel be elevated to prevent damage to the Achilles tendon. Some joggers do not agree, however. They argue that flexibility exercises keep the tendon loose, and elevated heels cause a jarring stride. In any case, there should be additional shock absorbing material in the heel. The shoe should also include a cup support or reinforced construction behind and at the sides of your heels to guard against ankle and foot strain.

Avoid shoes with uppers that do not breathe or that will be damaged by the moisture from sweating, rain, or wet grass. Nylon and leather are both acceptable; nylon dries faster, but leather adapts readily to the shape of your foot while still offering firm support. Examine the shoe not so much for style as for flexibility and durable construction.

Since feet enlarge slightly as the day progresses, it is best to try on shoes at the time of day that you will use them—and wear sweat socks. Try on both shoes. A foot measurement by the salesperson is the place to start, but remember that shoe sizes vary significantly with manufacturers. Look for room in the toes, with your longest toe a thumbwidth from the front of the shoe. The heel should fit snugly—too much slippage will cause blisters.

Where, When. Your local park is probably an ideal jogging area, for the grass and dirt paths are resilient and absorb the force that might otherwise injure ankles and knees. Parks also provide space, scenery, and usually other joggers, an advantage for those who feel nervous or conspicuous when jogging alone. The major disadvantages are "Keep Off the Grass" signs and stray dogs.

In many communities, high school cinder tracks are available to local residents. They have the advantage of being level and measured so that you can gauge speed and distance precisely. While some

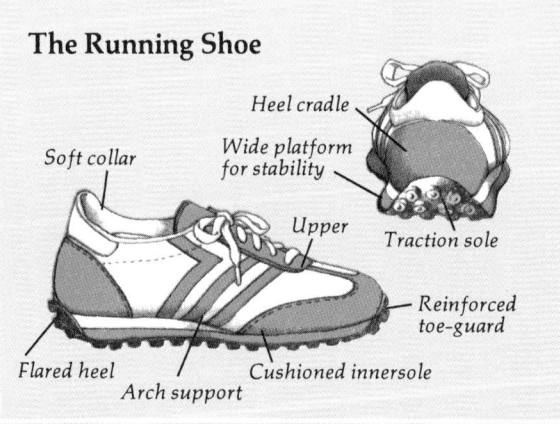

The Running Shoe

Heel cradle
Soft collar
Wide platform for stability
Upper
Traction sole
Reinforced toe-guard
Flared heel
Cushioned innersole
Arch support

A Word of Caution

Dr. Albert J. Ryan, the editor of *Physician and Sportsmedicine* magazine, estimates that running can result in as many as 50 types of injury. However, a commonsense approach can go a long way toward eliminating most jogging injuries, from blisters to fractured bones. Jogging ailments usually result from:

• *Overexertion.* If you have chronic bone and muscle soreness and continual fatigue, you are overexerting. Slow down, skip a few days, begin again at a slower pace.

• *Tight Muscles.* A thorough warm-up program (see pages 326-327) is the key to avoiding injuries caused by tight and unyielding muscles.

• *Bad Technique.* Most running injuries occur from the knee down and can be caused by a poor running style. Such injuries can also result from a structural defect in the knee or foot. Podiatrists and orthopedists trained in sports medicine can diagnose and treat many of these conditions.

• *Improper Foot Gear.* A survey among serious and competitive runners showed that one in five had suffered from chondromalacia ("runner's knee") or from Achilles tendonitis. One in 10 had developed shin splints, foot fractures, heel spurs (bony outgrowths), and breaks, strains, and bruises. In most cases, foot specialists determined that the injuries resulted from ill-fitting or incorrectly designed shoes.

---

people prefer track jogging, others find it boring. You might try jogging on a track once a week in order to measure your progress.

If you choose to jog on neighborhood streets, try to select ones that are paved with asphalt, which is more resilient than concrete. Select an area where traffic is light and jog on the left side of the road so that you can see oncoming cars and move out of their path if necessary. Avoid jogging at night. Although some people do so, wearing reflective clothing, the hazards outweigh the benefits.

Veteran runners are not discouraged by the weather and often enjoy running in the rain. On hot days, it cools them off, and when the temperature is below 55°F they wear light rain jackets to prevent chilling. However, heat and humidity can be dangerous if you stop listening to your body and push yourself to heat exhaustion and heat stroke.

Many runners wear only a sweatshirt over a T-shirt and jogging shorts unless the temperature is below freezing. Although you will want to keep your torso warm, your legs will generate a great deal of heat once you begin exercising. Jim Fixx, in his *Complete Book of Running*, advises sweat pants only in weather below 20°F. Other essentials for cold-weather jogging are gloves and a cap to prevent heat loss through your head.

Cold-weather jogging can be invigorating and more pleasant than warm weather activity, since your body needn't work as hard to dissipate heat. No evidence exists to support the concern that inhaling cold air harms the lungs or is dangerous in any way. If jogging in the rain or cold is not your idea of fun and fitness, look for an indoor track.

The ideal time to jog is the one that works best for you, as long as it is at least two or three hours after your last meal. Running before eating assures that your previous meal has been digested and actually helps curb appetite, enhancing the weight-reducing effect of exercise.

To Get Started. Most jogging programs recommend that you begin by alternating short periods of jogging (about 30 seconds) with brisk walking (1 minute). You may prefer very slow, sustained jogging, since it is not a great deal more strenuous than a fast walk. In either case, the goal is *not* speed, but LSD—long, slow distance.

Aim eventually to cover 1½ to 2½ miles in 20 to 30 minutes. At no time should you exert to the point of breathlessness, dizziness, or nausea. If you are jogging and these conditions develop, slow to a walk. If you are walking and your pulse rate is not in the target zone and your body tells you that you are doing no work, begin slow jogging. You will quickly grow sensitive to the degree of stress that produces a conditioning effect without causing discomfort, and as the weeks progress you will notice the need to increase your pace and/or distance to reach the conditioning level.

Getting into Shape
The Fitness Trail

A decade ago most Americans had not even heard of a *parcours* (French for "course" or "circuit"). Even today, relatively few Americans have used these combination jogging trails and exercise stations, though close to 1,000 have been built in the United States.

The first parcours was built near Zurich, Switzerland, in 1968, following a program used by Swiss foresters. Today's typical parcours covers one or two miles, along which are posted from 10 to 20 activity stations. At these stations are equipment and signs directing the exerciser to perform a specific activity: sit-ups, chin-ups, balance-beam walking, ring swings, etc. Both instructions and equipment provide for different levels of ability and suggest repetition requirements for degrees of fitness. Those finishing the route can be sure they have accomplished a full-fledged physical workout, which is the goal of the exercise trail concept.

On a well-designed parcours, the sequence of exercises is carefully designed, starting with warm-ups (1-4 at right). The more strenuous tasks (5-19) taper off to cool-down activities (20-22). You can bike, walk briskly, or preferably jog between the exercise stations.

Exercise trails are planned to enhance all the components of physical fitness: cardiorespiratory capacity, strength, endurance, balance, agility, and coordination. If your community does not yet have a parcours, you can improvise one in your own backyard or take advantage of playground equipment at your neighborhood school.

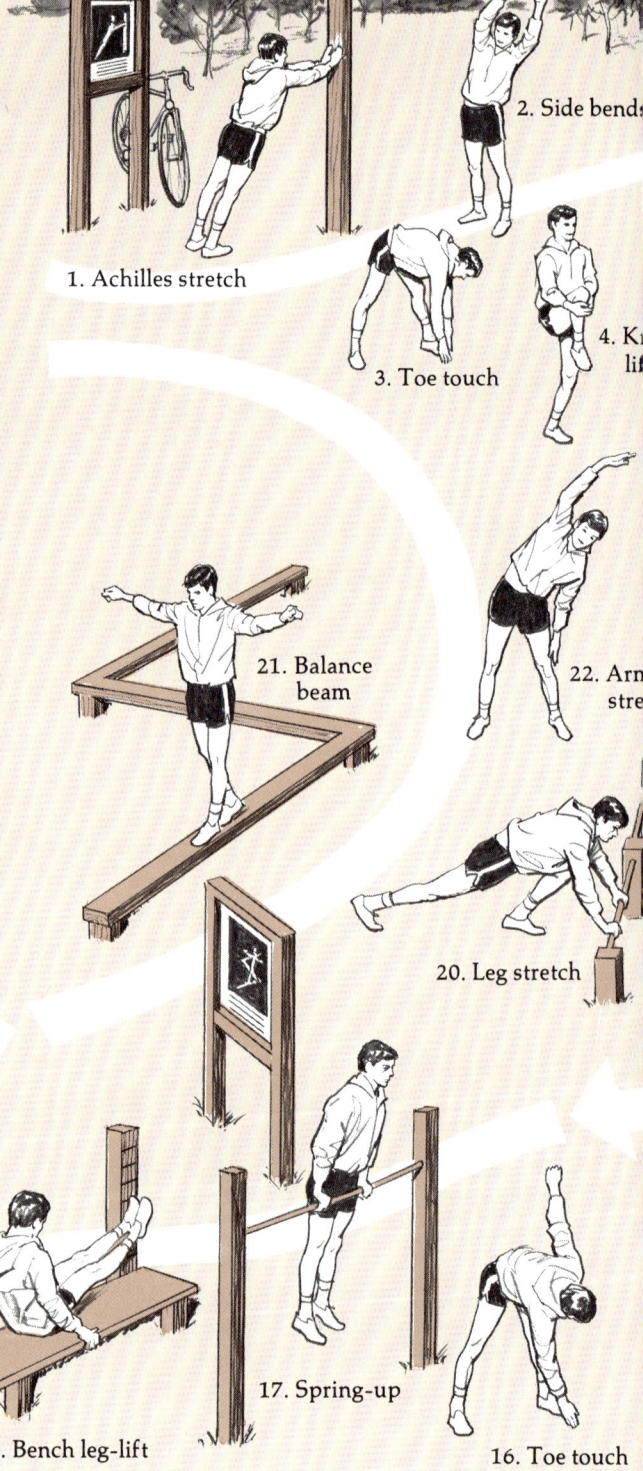

FITNESS THROUGH EXERCISE

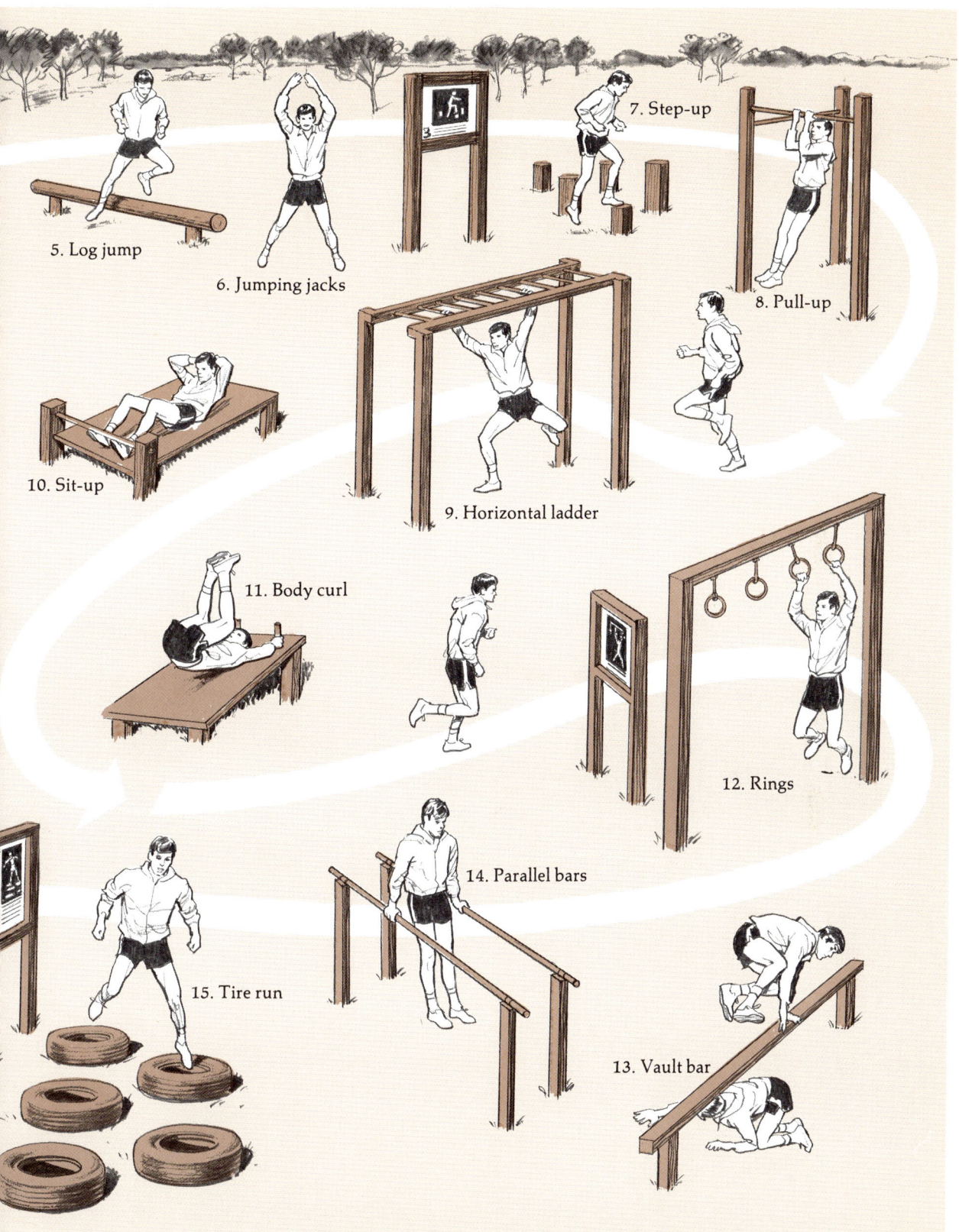

Getting into Shape
Touring Sports

Bicycling

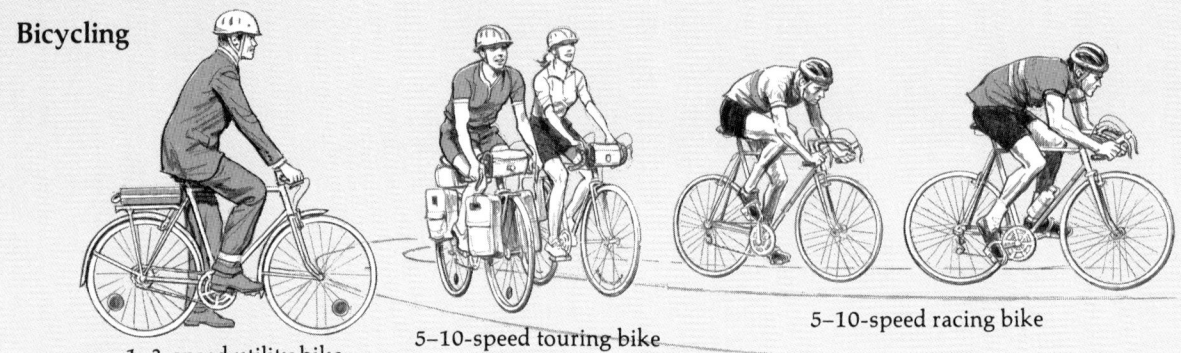

1-3-speed utility bike
5-10-speed touring bike
5-10-speed racing bike

Your exercise program can include relaxing and carefree traveling about the countryside—in such touring sports as bicycling, cross-country skiing, and boating (see page 343.)

Bicycling. For the past century, bicycling has enjoyed recurrent upsurges in popularity. There are now more than 100 million bikes in the United States; half a million are used for commuting. It is a handy vehicle for quick trips to the supermarket, family outings, short commutes, or camping.

Once mastered, bicycling is a skill never forgotten. Most of us learn to ride a bicycle at about age 6; people have been known to cycle into their 90s. Cycling is also used to keep in shape for other sports; speed skater Eric Heiden trained by cycling and was a champion in both sports.

You can cycle slowly around the block or try to set records on a cross-country race. If cycling is to be a part of your fitness program, set yourself goals: distance, speed, longer or steeper grades.

Selecting Your Bicycle. If you are thinking of buying a bicycle for fun or fitness, pick out one that will suit your needs, either a sturdy 1- or 3-speed utility bike, or a 10-speed lightweight touring or racing model. The utility bike usually has a single-speed coaster brake and is designed to be ridden upright, which is comfortable for short distances on the flat and does make you more visible. The wheels are wider and heavier, which makes for a slow but stable and comfortable ride.

The more expensive 10-speed bike has dropped handlebars, hand brakes, and a wide range of gear ratios to maintain a regular and effective rate of pedaling on different grades. It is designed to be ridden in an aerodynamic position with the crouched body offering the least wind resistance and putting the center of effort on the pedal for efficient power. The height of the handlebars can be adjusted for riding comfort and better visibility (higher) or sprint power (lower.) The extension of the handlebars can be adjusted to your arm length or to lower your center of gravity. The hooked shape of the handlebars offers a variety of hand positions. Shifting positions alleviates the fatigue of long-distance rides and allows for different traffic or grade conditions.

The utility bike seat is usually the wide-sprung saddle, good on short trips, but its width restricts leg power and can cause chafing over long distances. The 10-speed bike has a longer, narrower saddle for less restricted leg movement. Plastic saddles are cheap and comfortable, but are impervious to moisture and air, causing rashes and blisters. Leather saddles must be broken in by oiling and kneading.

Fitting the Bike to You. Since most bicycle injuries (other than a fall) come from poorly adjusted equipment or improper riding techniques, it is important to buy the right size frame and adjust the seat, handlebars, and pedals to your needs. If the top tube of the frame (on a man's bike) is ¾ to 1 inch below your crotch when straddling it in bare feet, the bike is a good fit. Adjust the seat until, with pedal cranks in a vertical position, one heel is flat on the lower pedal with the leg in a straight position. As you will be pedaling with the balls of your feet, the heel measure allows for a slight flex in the knee.

A common cycling ailment is numb hands or fingers resulting from road shock transmitted through the handlebars to the ulnar nerve in the hand. Wear padded gloves, pad your handlebars, change hand positions frequently, raise the handlebars to move your weight back, or reduce air pressure in the front tire to absorb some of the shock. Avoid loose clothes which might get tangled in the gears or spokes; roll up your pant legs or use clips. And wear a helmet, even for recreational biking—it can make the difference between a minor spill and serious injury.

Cross-Country Skiing. Nordic, or cross-country, skiing, unsurpassed as an aerobic exercise, enhances other fitness components as well. Improved balance, agility, strength, and coordination are all part of the benefits package for the serious cross-country skier. Yet, unlike jogging, skiing is not merely an exercise. Long a common method of winter transportation in northern European countries, cross-country skiing has become popular in the United States only in recent years. Many people with no particular interest in fitness find a cross-country ski outing exhilarating. Others use their skis as a convenient means of travel. For fitness, fun, and practicality, you can't find a better winter exercise than cross-country skiing which, as shown in the illustrations below, is nothing more than an exaggerated form of walking.

Preparation. Skiing requires strong muscles, and that means five or six weeks of conditioning before the ski season begins. In addition to jogging or brisk walking, concentrate on strengthening the abdomen (sit-ups, knees bent), arms (push-ups, chin-ups, bench presses, etc., but canoeing or kayaking are more fun), and legs (summer cycling prepares you for winter skiing).

Equipment. Cross-country skiing is an inexpensive sport compared to downhill, or Alpine, skiing. The skis, which vary widely in price and quality, are the most costly item. Before buying skis, borrow or rent some to see what suits you best. A ski held vertically at your side should reach the wrist of your arm extended above your head. Ask the dealer for guidance in selecting the proper ski flexibility and width for your weight and local snow conditions.

You will also need a set of durable metal or fiberglass poles that fit snugly under your armpits. The pole tip should have a slight forward curve for easy release from the snow.

Finally, you must have ski boots that are designed for use with the particular type of skis and bindings that you purchase. Ski boots should be tried on while you are wearing the pair or two of socks that you will use while actually skiing.

Several layers of loose-fitting clothing, such as light wool sweaters and shirts, are better than a single heavy jacket because they provide more space for trapping air and preserving body heat. Also, as your body warms with exercise, you can remove just enough clothing to keep comfortable. Thermal underwear and loose trousers kept snug around the lower leg (knickers and knicker socks are recommended) should be sufficient to keep your legs warm. Some skiers use one-piece suits to keep out wind and snow, but these alone are not warm enough in cold weather unless you are skiing at racing speed.

Gaiters, which fit over the tops of your boots at the ankles, will help keep snow from getting inside your boots. You can also buy boot-gloves, which are worn over boots to keep your feet warm and dry.

Lined gloves and a hat with ear protectors or a ski mask are also essential to prevent frostbite. Sunglasses or goggles protect against snow blindness.

A daypack, while optional, is a handy addition to the cross-country skier's equipment list. It is a small knapsack in which he can carry snacks, first aid essentials, compass and maps, skin cream, ski wax, matches, and extra clothing (especially dry socks and a weatherproof shell). Don't ski alone unless the trail is patrolled at the end of each day.

Cross-Country Skiing

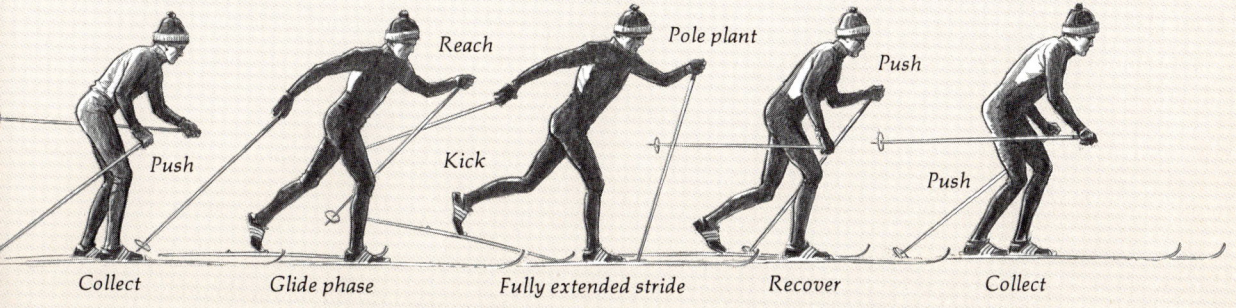

Getting into Shape
Swimming

One reason swimming is so popular a sport, even among those who use it for aerobic conditioning, is that it is a comparatively painless form of exercise. On a hot summer day, the water dissipates body heat; in the winter, heated indoor pools are a comforting alternative to outdoor activity. Swimming is a particularly good exercise for those who are otherwise restricted in movement because of age, disease, or injury. Babies introduced to water at age 2 months demonstrate no fear. For the elderly, swimming is an easy and restful way of maintaining fitness. Even people with back problems, arthritis, and minor aches and pains find they can exercise vigorously yet comfortably in the water. With no solid resistance to body movement, the swimmer is spared the trauma of such rhythmical gravity sports as running.

Variety of Strokes. There are four competitive strokes and two resting or survival strokes:

The *crawl*, or freestyle, relies on the upper body, back, shoulders, and arms and hands for power. The flutter kick, which supplies only 20 percent of propulsion, essentially keeps the hips up and the body horizontal in the water, thus reducing drag. The fastest competitive stroke, the crawl is also the best long-distance stroke because of the efficiency of its smooth, effortless motion.

The *back crawl* is an equally vigorous stroke but somewhat easier to perform because you do not have to synchronize your breathing. The same flutter kick (though, of course, reversed) achieves power on the upstroke and provides body stabilization. Since you see where you have been, not where you are going, memorize marks on the ceiling or side of the pool to alert yourself to the end of the lane.

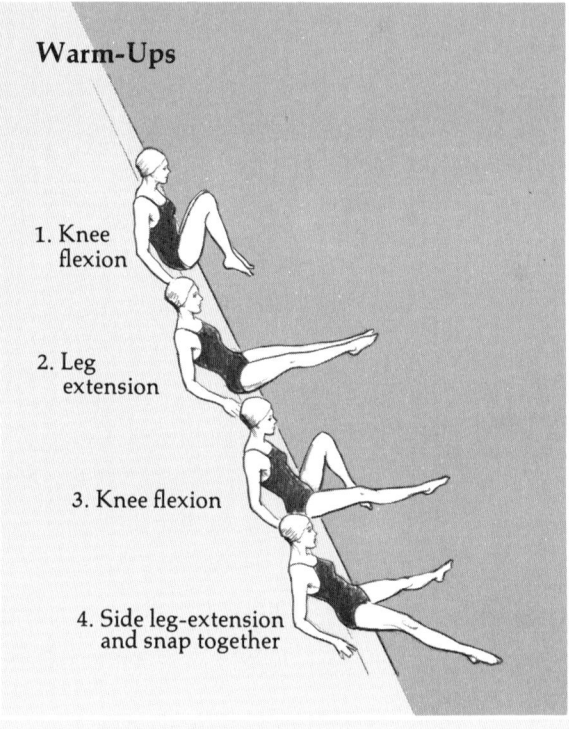

Warm-Ups

1. Knee flexion
2. Leg extension
3. Knee flexion
4. Side leg-extension and snap together

The *breaststroke* builds chest and leg muscles (with its vigorous frog kick) but makes low energy demands because the motions are more natural. A competitive stroke, it is also a good utility stroke for distance and perhaps most popular for recreational swimming. Since it lifts you out of the water, it is a good stroke for rough seas or lifesaving.

The *butterfly*, a development of the breaststroke, is rarely maintained for long periods because it requires a great deal of energy and places great demands on the arm and shoulder muscles as the upper

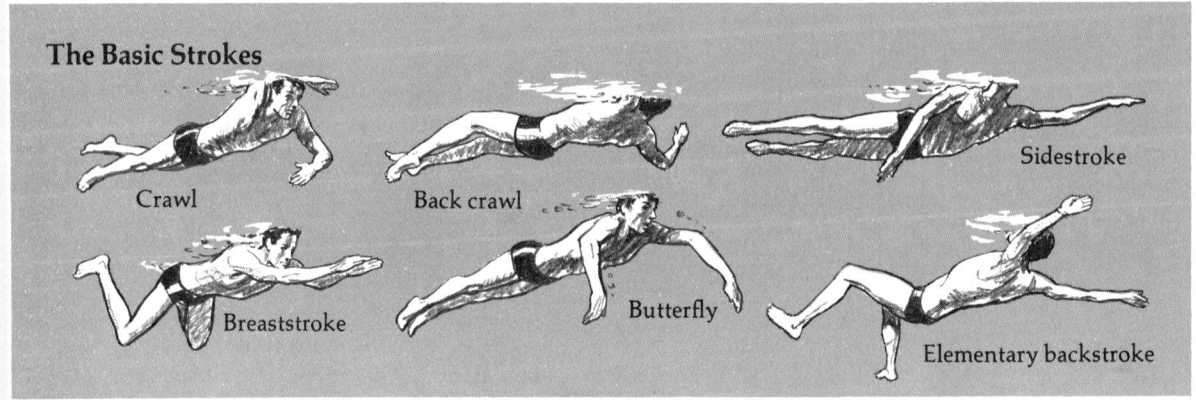

The Basic Strokes

Crawl — Back crawl — Sidestroke
Breaststroke — Butterfly — Elementary backstroke

body is lifted out of the water for each stroke. A fast sprint stroke, the butterfly is too exhausting for beginners. The dolphin, or fishtail, kick is the most powerful kick and gives abdomen, hips, thighs, and ankles as good a workout as the chest, arms, and shoulders get from the arm stroke.

The *sidestroke*, the most popular resting stroke, achieves propulsion about equally from arms and legs. Because you can see either ahead or behind and can keep the upper arm free for carrying something, it is a stroke used by lifeguards or anyone with a burden. The sidestroke is also used for cool-downs.

The *elementary backstroke* is another good utility stroke, easy to learn and not demanding. However, these last two strokes do not offer a wide range of motion and you should learn one or two of the competitive strokes to provide yourself with some speed in the water and to exercise more muscles.

Proper Form. Swimming calls for a correct body position and skilled arm and leg movements coordinated with proper breathing techniques. The body should be high in the water with shoulders slightly higher than legs. Maintain a long, clean line for least resistance. Follow through on arm strokes for full power. Kick from the hips.

The more level you hold your head in the water, the more horizontal your body remains and the less drag. Many people object to putting their faces into the water because the chlorine in public pools irritates their eyes. Properly fitted goggles will help prevent chlorine problems as well as eye infection from microorganisms in ponds, rivers, and lakes.

Like any exercise routine, swimming should be preceded by warm-ups, which can be poolside practice for swimming skills such as kicks (opposite, above). Cool-downs can be a few laps of slow swimming to bring your heart rate down.

Caution. Always enter the water slowly to accustom your cardiovascular system to the change of environment and temperature; never jump into unfamiliar waters.

Cramps, usually occurring in calf or foot, are sudden contractions of muscle fibers due to fatigue, cold water, tight muscles, or dietary problems. Flex and extend foot or toes and knead vigorously. To avoid stomach cramps, do not eat for at least two hours before swimming.

Exercise Afloat

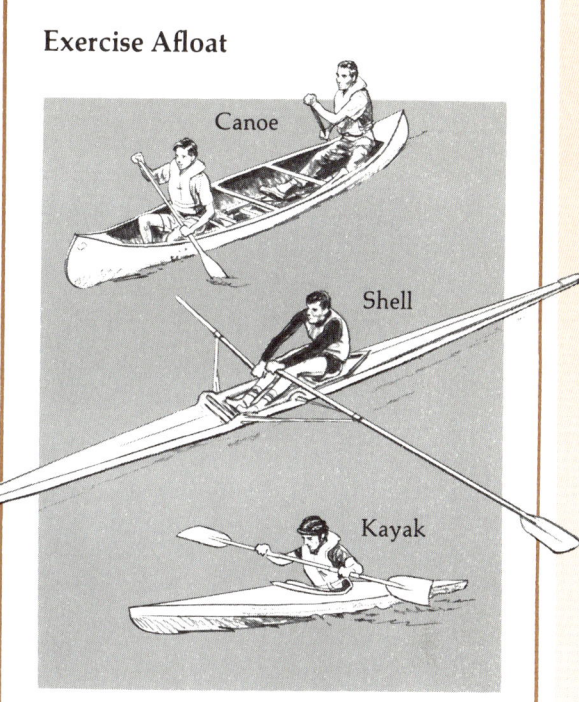

Working out in a small boat is certainly one of the most pleasurable ways to get in shape. There is none of the traffic, noise, or air pollution of city streets, none of the trauma of jogging. Canoeing or rowing not only provide excellent opportunities to improve physical fitness, they can be combined with fishing and camping to achieve relaxation and tranquility.

The *canoe*, as the Indians taught us, is an extremely useful and versatile boat, one that can hold two people and their camping gear and can be portaged (carried overland) for exploring or seeking better fishing waters. It is, of course, the arms and shoulders that get the workout—other than in portaging.

For more strenuous exercise, you might want to graduate from a rowboat to the *shell*, a finely designed craft that is second only to the bicycle in utilizing manpower for transportation. Rowing a shell helps condition the entire body.

The *kayak* calls for powerful upper body muscles, conditioned reflexes, cardiorespiratory efficiency, and even some acrobatic skills. A sensitive craft, the kayak rights itself as easily as it turns over; a proficient kayaker barely misses a stroke during a 360-degree roll-over.

Getting into Shape
Aquaexercises

If the pool is too small or too crowded for lap swimming, you might consider an aquaexercise program. Even people who are not good swimmers or those with a physical limitation can benefit from such activities.

The greater resistance of water will hasten warm-up, and increase muscle strength during calisthenics such as the toe touch and side straddle-hop (right). Stretching and twisting exercises include bounding with arm stretch, leg swing, and such gutter-holding drills as the leg cross (far right).

You can practice your swimming strokes in shallow water. The standing crawl (right, center panel) will help perfect the efficiency of your arm and hand motions; the frog kick used in the breaststroke can be practiced while holding on to the gutter. Later, separate arm and leg movements can be coordinated with each other and with proper breathing.

Aquaexercises can also be used for strengthening muscles: the wall push-away will help tone thighs, shoulders, and abdomen; the knees up and leg twist will tighten abdominal muscles at the same time legs and hips are worked; the wall push-up (far right) builds arm muscles and gets you out of the pool at the same time.

Bobbing and Sculling. Unsurpassed for cardiorespiratory conditioning, high bobbing (right) is one expert's choice if you have only five minutes for a fitness program. Starting from a treading position in water 1 to 3 feet over your head, execute a frog kick and bring your arms sharply down to your sides. As you rise above the surface, inhale. Exhale as your body sinks to the bottom. A second explosive bob is powered by a leg thrust as your upstretched arms execute a breaststroke.

Sculling, using flat hands as directional and power paddles, is used for maneuvering or lifting the body, as in treading water (far right). Deep-water calisthenics and turning maneuvers (bottom right) contribute to flexibility, strength, and circulation.

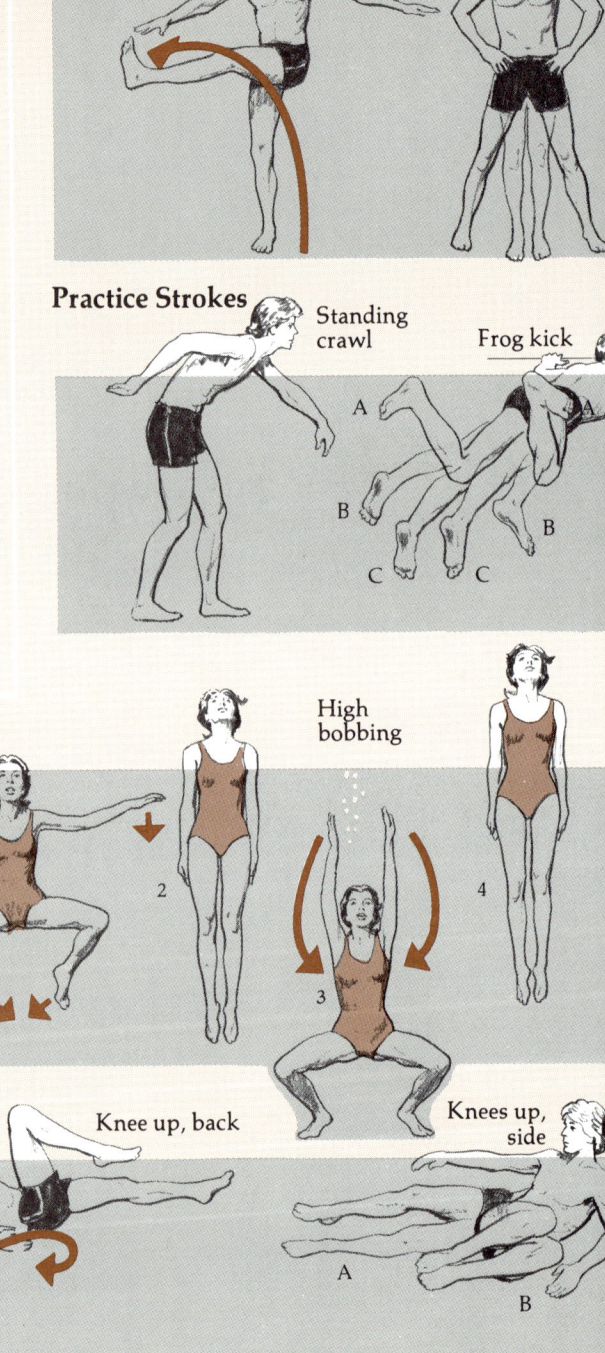

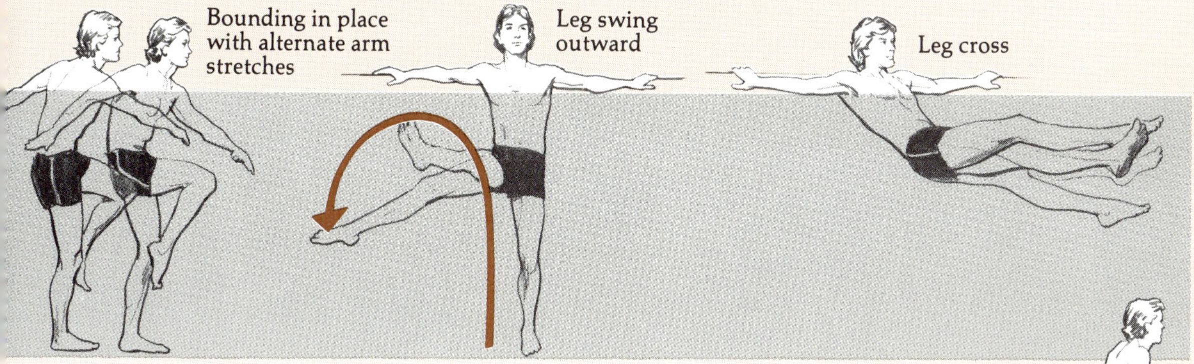

FITNESS THROUGH EXERCISE

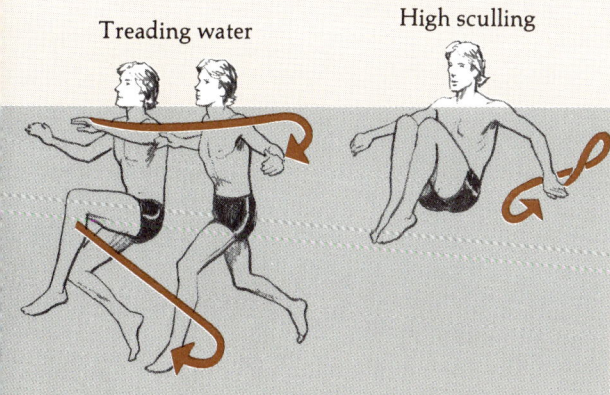

Muscle Tone

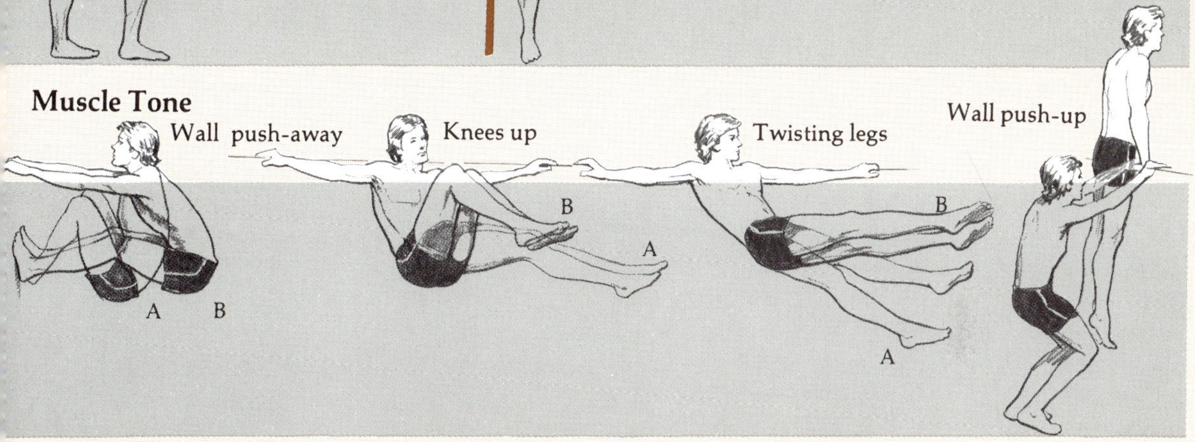

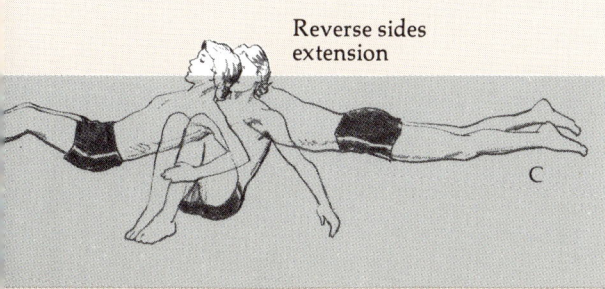

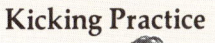

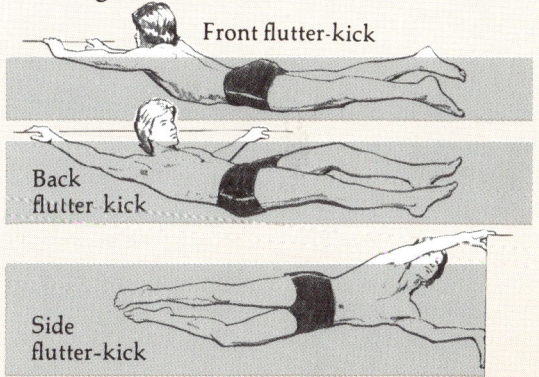

Kicking Practice

Kicking helps keep the body on a horizontal plane, reducing drag, but does not contribute significantly to propulsion. Kicking as an exercise, however, is a good conditioner of the abdominal and thigh muscles. Use thighs, back, and abdominal muscles to move the entire leg from the hip—not only good swimming form but also a fine cardiorespiratory exercise. As shown above, the flutter-kick at poolside can be performed on front, back, or side.

Getting into Shape
Court and Field

If you are bored by solitary fitness activities such as jogging and swimming, you might find excitement, variety, and challenge in court and field sports. Immediate rewards include mastery of new skills, the building of a strong, supple body, and the exhilaration of competition—you may be one of those people who need the incentive of scoring to undertake an exercise program.

Unfortunately, there are limitations to the conditioning benefits of court and field sports. To be aerobically beneficial, an exercise activity must be sufficiently taxing to raise your pulse to the target area (see page 326) and keep it there for 20 minutes. Only the most demanding court sports, squash and handball, require you to sustain a pace that can produce aerobic conditioning. Although a game of volleyball may offer no more aerobic conditioning than a brisk walk, it does increase the other components of dynamic fitness—agility, balance, coordination, and flexibility.

Such energetic field sports as football, however, fail to provide aerobic conditioning. Why, then, are football and basketball players among our best-conditioned athletes? The answer might well help you, too, to reach a superior fitness level. Athletes don't play sports to condition—they condition in order to play sports. If you can find a sport that really excites you, one that you really want to excel in, you will probably have motivation to undertake additional exercise and the concentrated practice to build the necessary strength and cardiorespiratory endurance required to be a superior player.

Nonetheless, opportunities for exercise in court and field sports are limited. You will have to find a partner or join a team, as well as locate an available facility. Many companies, social clubs, and churches have softball, touch football, and volleyball teams, as do YMCAs and YWCAs. Your local parks commission will probably have a list of sandlot clubs that use its facilities, and perhaps you can join one of these groups. In any case, outdoor sports are seasonal and can be rained out. Indoor sports require special facilities, which usually means membership in a health or athletic club. The cost of membership is a worthwhile investment only if it assures you of exercise that you would otherwise not get.

Aerobic Endurance. Although few group sports offer the aerobic benefit of jogging or swimming, the

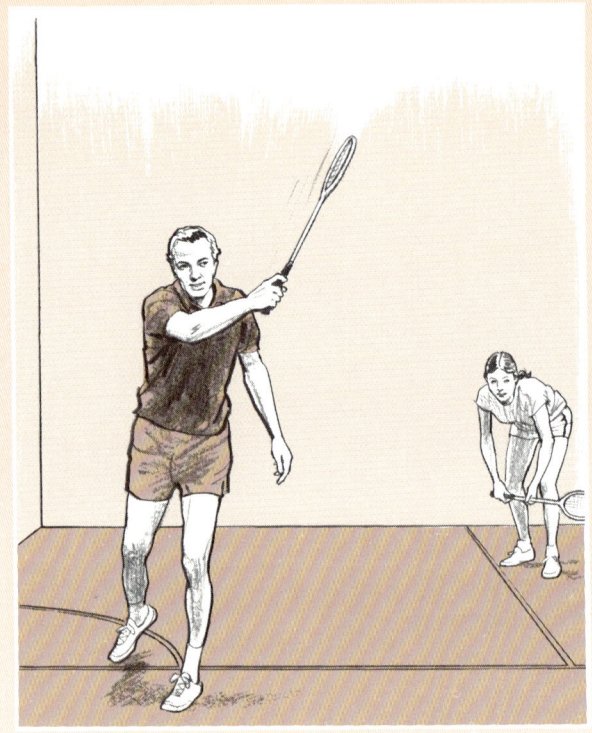

best are those requiring continuous activity or sustained periods of energy output. The fewer the players, the more workout each derives. Thus, two-man handball and squash are rated with cross-country skiing, swimming, and running a 6-minute mile on the basis of oxygen uptake, a useful measurement of aerobic benefit. These two also rank at the top among group sports for general conditioning, possibly because the small size of the court requires the player to use a greater range of movements to maneuver into position. It is slightly smaller than half a tennis court, but the game is much faster as the wall cuts the travel distance and waiting time in half. Squash offers a total body workout and burns up as many calories as running.

Field games such as soccer and field hockey require more running but less upper-body work. Play is related to the length of the field—all are about 300 feet long. However, both soccer and field hockey have separate positions for attack and defense (forwards and backs), so that a single player's field of activity is somewhat reduced. Nonetheless, during the course of a game, a player may run the equivalent of the 100-yard dash several times over in a combination of power sprints and sustained running.

Volleyball

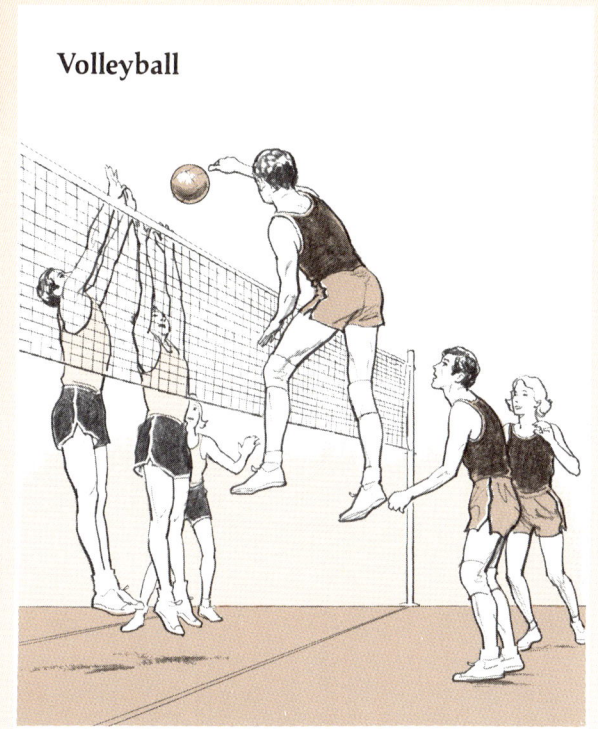

Frisbee

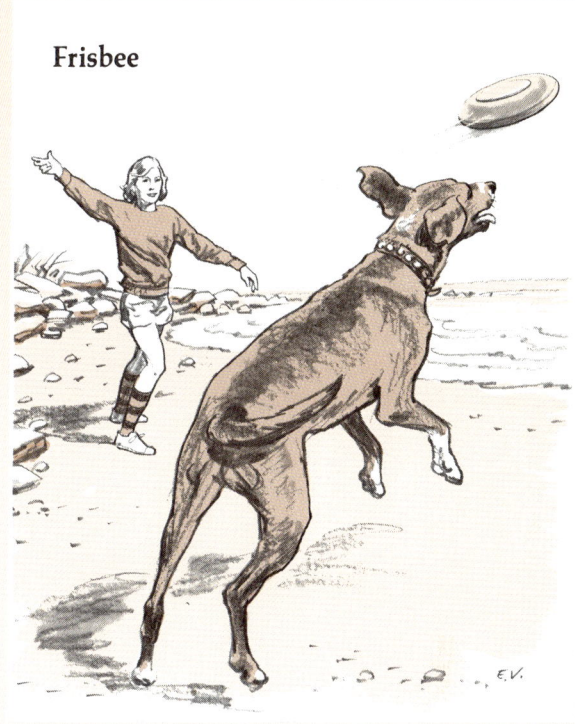

Sustained Power Sports. In sports like tennis, badminton, and volleyball, where brief bursts of activity are followed by longer recovery periods, the muscles are fueled anaerobically—without air. The oxygen uptake and caloric expenditure of these sports is only half that of squash but equal to that of brisk walking, downhill skiing, or cycling. Playing 3 to 4 sets of tennis 2 or 3 times a week can be a lifetime fitness program; age is not necessarily a drawback. The distances to be run in tennis and badminton are short, and rest periods can be frequent. But if played "cooperatively" for sustained rallies, rather than competitively, the game can be fast and aerobically demanding. Tennis is a sport that benefits both fitness and skill.

Soccer, with 11 players on a 130-yard field, provides more running than volleyball (6 to 12 players on a 30-foot side), but the latter is easier to learn and can be set up anywhere with any number of players. Fast-break, full-court basketball rates even higher than tennis for cardiorespiratory fitness and general well-being. Shooting baskets in the backyard develops skill and limbers muscles but won't give you the aerobic conditioning provided by the bursts of activity in a full-court game.

Minimal Exertion. Baseball, long America's favorite sport, offers a minimum of aerobic conditioning. The pitcher gets the most sustained workout, with the catcher perhaps second. The base runner gets his exercise in short sprints but then stands around waiting for his next turn at bat so that his workout is actually limited.

Golf and bowling, the sole source of physical activity for many men and women, have little to recommend them as fitness programs. It would take over 2 hours of golf to produce the same conditioning effect as a brisk, hour walk. Bowlers burn up a few more calories but receive no aerobic benefit.

Still, any activity, even frisbee throwing, is a great improvement over a totally sedentary life-style. In fact, an hour of vigorous frisbee throwing might be quite an effective conditioner. Most people need a partner, but dogs make good frisbee retrievers, and more accomplished practitioners learn to throw the frisbee so that it returns to them like a boomerang—thus they become both pitcher and catcher.

The point is that any sport, if it gets your body moving, offers at least some benefits. And, if you make up your mind to improve at the sport, you might be able to increase your overall fitness as well.

Getting into Shape
Adding Variety to Exercise

What can a swimmer do when he finds no heated pool in winter, or a skiier when there is no snow? Must a tennis player sit by the television when the tennis court is covered with ice? How can a canoeist strengthen his legs, or a jogger his arms? Can a person keep fit when sidelined by injury or sickness? The answer to all these questions is: variety in your physical activities.

Pursuing more than one sport or exercise offers not just challenge and adventure; it also serves more important purposes. An athlete who specializes in a particular sport may use a combination of activities to condition himself for his major pursuit. A player of a seasonal sport can in the off-season substitute an alternate sport or exercise to keep the same muscles in working shape. Muscles in our bodies work in opposite or antagonistic groups, but most sports develop only certain groups of muscles while neglecting the opposite groups. This may result in a lopsided physique, even injury to the neglected muscles. A person who day in and day out concentrates on a single sport or exercise may also suffer from sheer boredom. All these situations indicate that variety in our physical activities is not only desirable, but often essential.

Combining Activities. Most professional and serious amateur athletes combine their speciality with some other activities to improve skill, stamina, strength, and fitness. Some football players, for instance, take up ballet for flexibility. Baseball players as a rule do rigorous calisthenics during the baseball season. The classic example is the boxer's workout for total body training. He runs for cardiorespiratory endurance and weight control, skips rope for balance and agility, hits the speedbag to improve timing and coordination, and works on a punching bag to develop strength (below, left).

Alternating Activities. To keep in shape during the gaps between seasonal sports, athletes seek off-season substitutes that involve similar skills or use the same muscle groups. Tennis players often play squash or badminton in winter. The different pace and form of these games may not improve their tennis skill, but they keep their muscles and reflexes in top condition. Racing cyclists switch to speed skating in winter, for the same muscles that thrust pedals around also propel the body forward on ice. The reverse is also true: some Olympic skaters are also successful competitors in bicycle racing. To

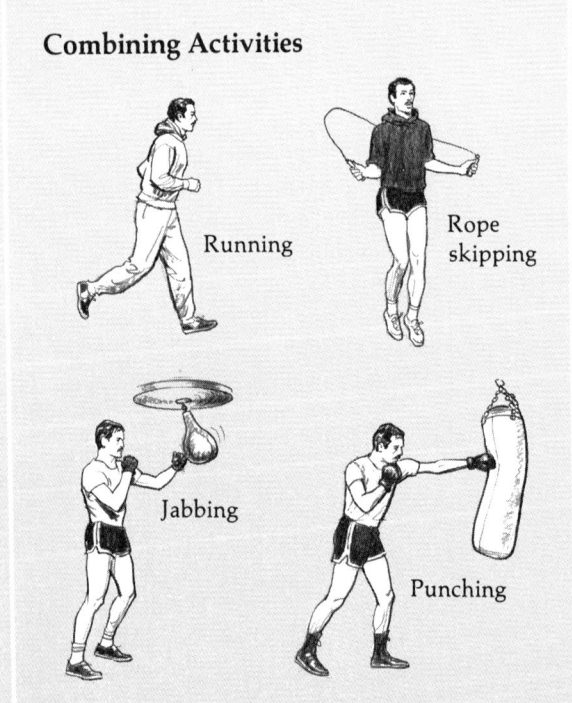

Combining Activities

Running

Rope skipping

Jabbing

Punching

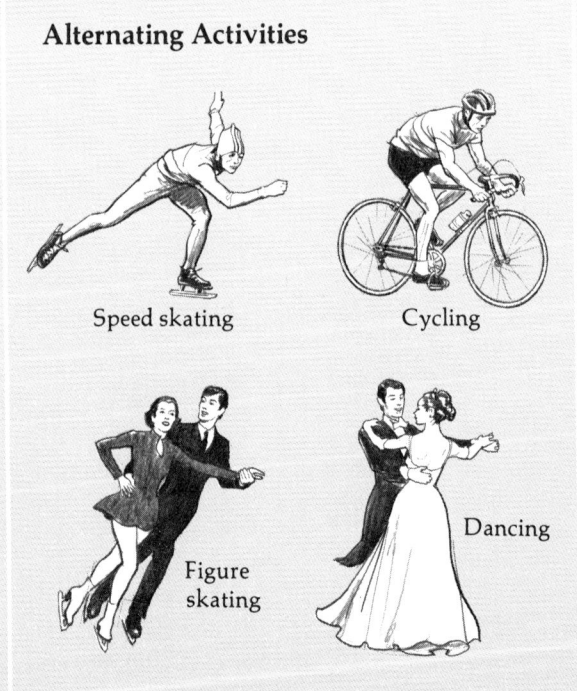

Alternating Activities

Speed skating

Cycling

Figure skating

Dancing

FITNESS THROUGH EXERCISE

perfect their coordination and balance, figure skaters engage in ballroom and modern dancing in the off-season (opposite pages, below right).

Complementary Activities. Sports such as jogging, golf, and canoeing tend to develop certain muscles but leave others underdeveloped. Injury can result if the imbalance between working muscles and their weak antagonists is too great. Exercise physiologists thus recommend that athletes and exercisers engage in what is called "reciprocal training"—to develop the neglected muscle groups—with complementary activities. The jogger, for instance, can lift weights to build up his inelastic shin or pretibial muscles, or run backwards to strengthen his quadricipital, pretibial, hip flexor, and abdominal muscles, and to balance his overdeveloped hamstring, gluteal, plantarflexor, and back muscles. Since canoeing is an upper-body sport, a canoe enthusiast should engage in some complementary activities such as portaging (carrying a canoe overland) or mountaineering. Backstroke swimming that requires the legs to kick forward against water resistance is another form of reciprocal training for a jogger or runner and develops the upper body.

Variety for Total Fitness. Whether an active sportsman or a cardiac patient, one should first analyze the kind of activities in which he is already engaged, then tailor additional sports or exercises for a total, balanced fitness. An office worker in our sedentary society may be extremely busy at his work, but his upper body does far more physical work then his lower. As a result, the larger, more important hip and thigh muscles are usually neglected. A person with a heart condition should, with the help of his physician, do exercises for his leg muscles, which help to pump blood back to his heart, while avoiding doing only arm exercises or sports. To shape up the lower body muscles, which contribute heavily to cardiovascular fitness, choose from skating, dancing, swimming, or any sport or exercise that offers a wide range of leg movements: extension, flexion, and rotation. The lunge embodies all these leg movements but also is a total body conditioner because it usually includes an arm thrust. The lunge is found in such diverse activities as the warm-up exercise used by all athletes, fencing, badminton and tennis, yoga exercises and the ancient Chinese martial art of T'ai chi ch'üan, baseball, skating, and even dancing (some of which are shown below).

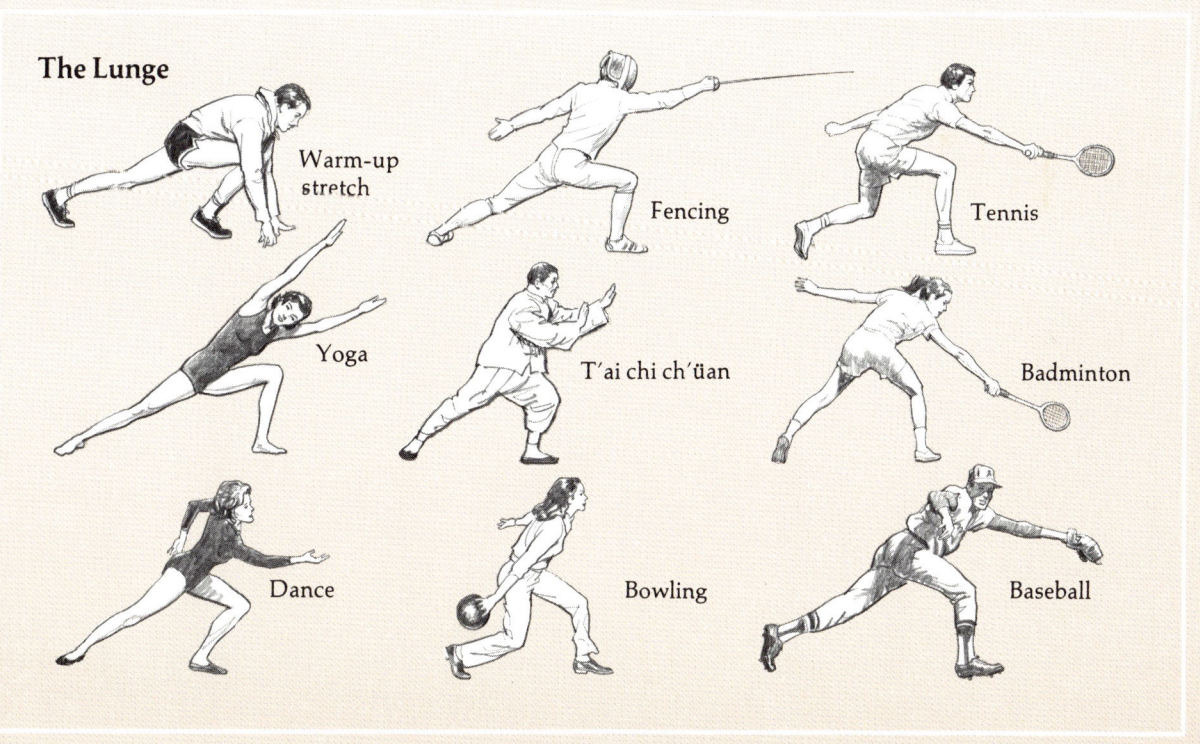

The Lunge — Warm-up stretch, Fencing, Tennis, Yoga, T'ai chi ch'üan, Badminton, Dance, Bowling, Baseball

Getting into Shape
Exercise in Your Daily Routine

Many people feel they have neither the time nor the inclination to pursue a formal exercise program. Whether such an attitude is justified is not important, so long as they maintain a high level of fitness simply by weaving physical activities into their daily schedule. House and yard work are in reality a sort of hidden exercise and can have the same beneficial effects on the body as formal exercise or sport.

Reaping the benefits of such hidden exercise, however, requires a different kind of thinking than most of us are used to. As pointed out earlier, our sedentary lives and labor-saving gadgets are making many of us lethargic and flabby. If we are as concerned about this as we should be, yet have no opportunity or inclination to engage in regular exercises or sports, we should deliberately make of our daily activities a physical fitness program.

Household chores are understandably not as interesting as ball games and other sports, but they are perhaps no more boring than calisthenics and gymnastics. Furthermore, they serve a practical purpose. The floor gets scrubbed, the rug vacuumed, the lawn mowed, or the vegetable garden planted.

Work in and around the house involves a surprising amount of physical activity. Compared to the more rugged chores of our grandparents, the work load in our modern homes could still be quite heavy for us, because our physical work capacity is comparatively lower than that of our forebears. Thus—within safe limits—if we engage in house work that burns off a large number of calories and improves our cardiorespiratory fitness, the result of such hidden exercises is fitness.

House Work and Sports. Physiologists report that vacuuming or mopping the floor use up the same number of calories per hour as gymnastics or playing croquet. Pushing a lawn mower or cleaning windows is about equal in effort to playing volleyball or badminton. Light carpentry, house painting, gardening, or leaf raking gives one the same benefits as tennis or baseball. The more strenuous snow shoveling or wood chopping is about the same as swimming the crawl. Stair-climbing is among the most vigorous of home activities, as its equivalent ranges from jogging to running or cross-country skiing at 8 mph. Even the seemingly effortless walk downstairs is equal to leisurely skating.

By checking the heart rate while performing such physical activities, one can gauge the relative cardiorespiratory benefits available from particular activities. The following lists what a housewife, with a resting heart rate of 70, goes through in a segment of a typical morning:

Time	Activities	Heart Rate
8:00 A.M.	Dish washing, tidying living room, walking around	70-90
8:15 A.M.	Storing pots and pans in lower cupboards and food in upper ones	90-120
8:25 A.M.	Hanging up children's clothes, putting away toys and books, carrying vacuum cleaner upstairs, vacuuming upstairs rooms	120-140
8:50 A.M.	Carrying vacuum cleaner downstairs, vacuuming stairs and downstairs rooms	140-160
9:05 A.M.	Polishing dining room table, scrubbing bathroom floor	150
9:30 A.M.	Sitting down briefly, then stretching out on the rug for a two-minute rest	120-80

Stretching out horizontally can be a cool-down exercise. It causes the blood to be pumped from the exercised muscles back to the heart and intestines, thus normalizing the heart rate.

Commuter's Exercise. The woman's husband also incorporates a fitness scheme into his daily routine by cycling to the suburban railroad station, walking from the city station to his office, and using the stairs instead of the elevator to reach his third-floor office. At home, he disengages his television remote-control, and walks upstairs to use the phone instead of the downstairs extension. In the backyard, he mows the lawn, rakes leaves, shovels snow, and splits and stacks firewood.

These home activities bring the couple more relaxation during their leisure hours, and less boredom, which they used to dispel with calorie-rich snacks between meals. More than that—they now have the satisfaction and pride of improving their home through their own labor. Tension headaches and occasional insomnia disappear as they discover a new enthusiasm for life.

Creative Fitness. By analyzing your personal habits and your own fitness goals, you can program your daily activities at home, in the office, and in between so that they become exercises or sports. Of course, vacations are golden opportunities for fitness activities. Make good use of swimming, hiking, and other sport facilities in resorts and wilderness areas. Sightseeing in cities can be done through walking and cycling, instead of viewing everything from a tour bus. The key is to think movement, as Dr. Joseph S. Rechtschaffen advises: "Don't sit when you can stand. Don't stand when you can walk. Don't walk if you can run. Move."

Here are some sample suggestions for turning routine activities into fitness exercises:

Bathing. Stretch, reach, and towel with exaggerated, vigorous movements.

Dressing. Use shoulder stretch to button or zip up at the back. Practice balance and coordination while putting on trousers and shoes.

Putting articles away. Climb and reach, or do knee bends while storing articles in cupboards.

Dusting, waxing, and polishing. Use rapid, sweeping movements to rhythmic music. Cluster aerobic chores to keep heart rate up longer.

Shopping. Carry bags in from the car or upstairs individually.

Laundry. Try scrubbing and wringing by hand. Hang clothes on the line outside with stretching and bending movements.

Climbing stairs. Do two steps at a time to heighten aerobic benefits.

Exercise and Longevity. Regular physical activity throughout life contributes significantly to health and fitness, and retards the aging process. To put it another way, exercise promotes longevity. A fitness and weight-control program belatedly begun in middle age can still minimize or offset degenerative diseases such as arthritis, high blood pressure, and coronary heart disease, which once were considered unavoidable in the later years. For the elderly, it has been demonstrated, a 10-year fitness program not only will improve general fitness but also can elevate mental awareness and outlook. Even among the elderly who suffer from some disability, regular physical activity improves alertness and gives a sense of independence and usefulness. It is never too late to exercise.

Fitness Begins Early

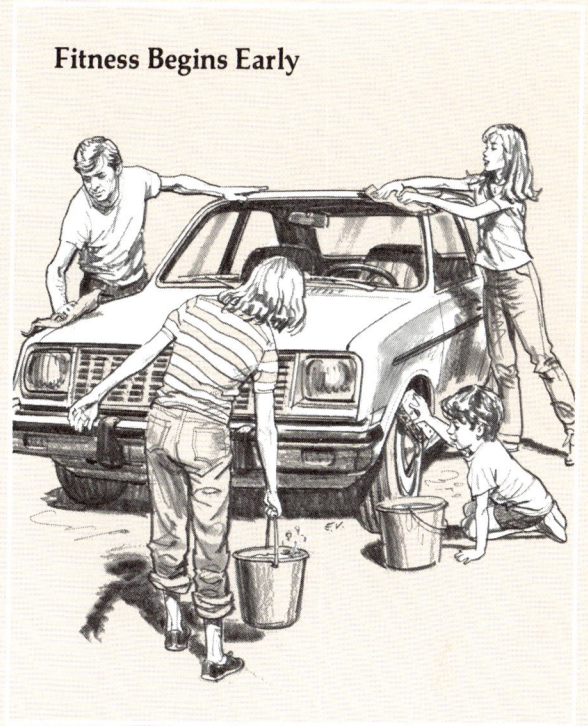

Active Children. A popular myth is that children get all the exercise they need. In reality, many do not. Studies show that a majority of American youngsters lack adequate flexibility, muscular strength, and cardiorespiratory endurance. Sedentary parents tend to bring up sedentary offspring. Television and video games are drawing an ever increasing number of American children away from the playground.

It is therefore desirable that children be given good opportunities to play games and sports, and to share house and yard work. Only 10 or 15 minutes a day of rope skipping, trampolining, raking, or sweeping provides adequate aerobic fitness. As much as possible, parents ought to participate, not merely supervise. Weekends are the best time for family fitness activities. Playing ball or frisbee, taking short hikes, and doing simple calisthenics are all within easy reach. Small children like grown-up tasks. Parents should assign and supervise some household chores to children as their hidden exercises. Lethargic children grow up to be flabby adults, but active ones carry over to their maturity the quick reflexes, balance, coordination, and grace acquired in the early years. It is never too soon to exercise.

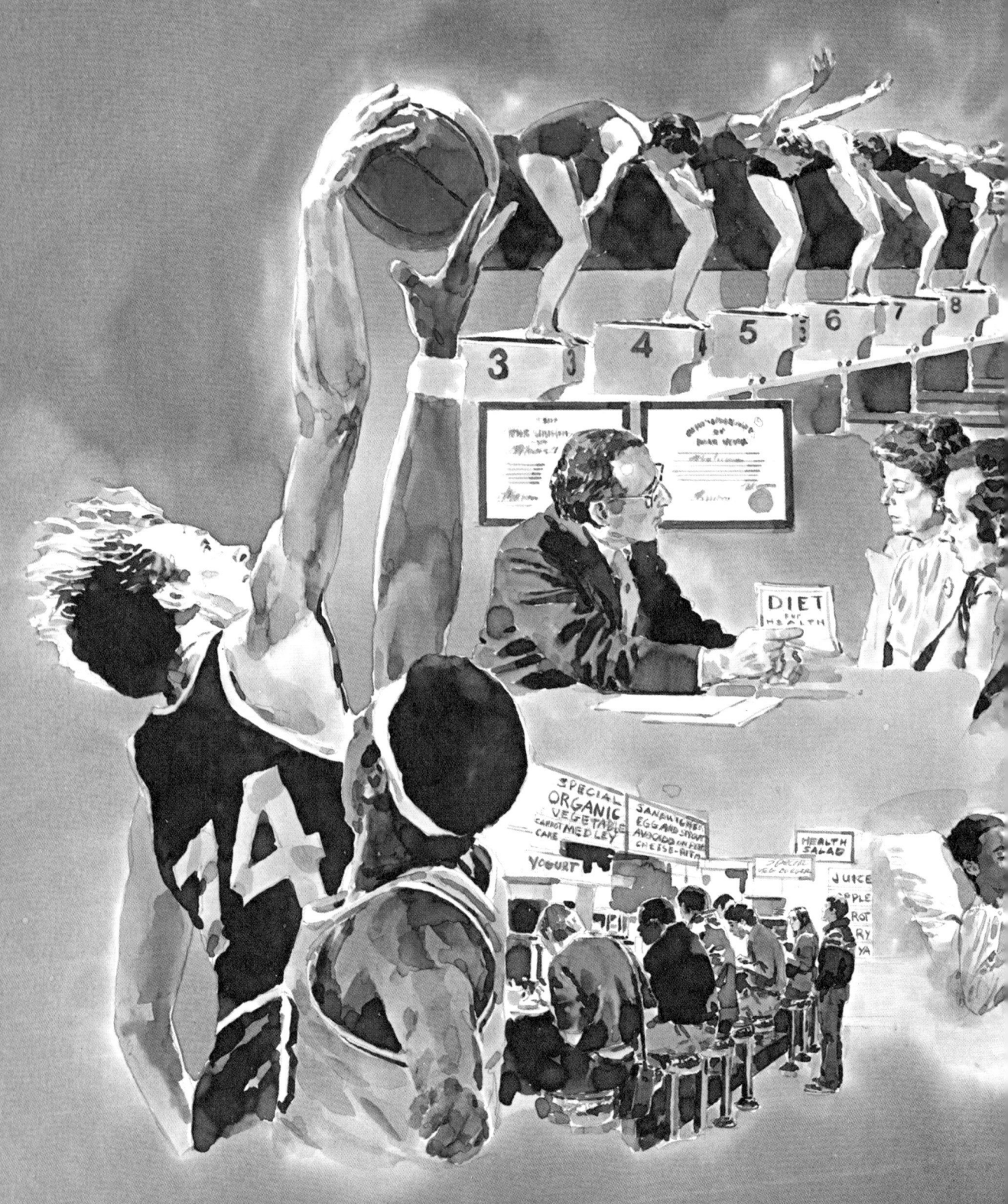

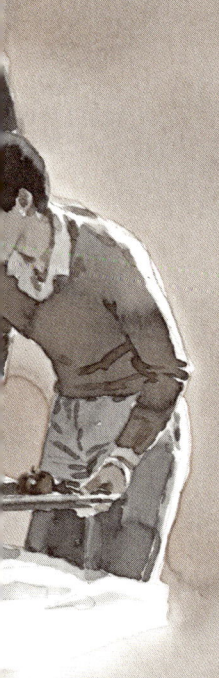

4. SPECIAL DIETS FOR SPECIAL NEEDS

Food for convalescence and common ailments: cold, fever, sore throat, diarrhea, constipation. How to detect food allergies and what to do about food intolerance. Coping with sodium-, sugar-, and fat-controlled diets. What to feed picky eaters, vegetarians, or your family athlete.

Food and Health/
  Nutrition Obstacles 354
Dealing with Common
  Ailments 358
  Liquid Diets 359
  Soft Diet 361
  Bland Diet 362
    The Ulcer Mystery 363
  High-Fiber Diets 365
    Fiber on a Scale of 0 to 6 .. 367
Detecting Food Allergies/
  Elimination Diets 368
    Related Food Allergies ... 370
Food Intolerance/Lactose-
  Restricted Diet 371
Gluten-Restricted Diet 372

Coping with Dietary
  Limitations 374
    Food Exchange Plan 375
  Sodium-Controlled Diets ... 376
    The No-Extra-Salt Diet .. 378
  Sugar-Controlled Diets 381
    The Dessert Dilemma 383
  Fat-Controlled Diets 384
    Diet and Cancer 386
Self-Imposed Food Restrictions/
  Picky Eaters 388
  Vegetarian Diets 390
    Sample Vegetarian Meals . 394
  The Athlete's Diet 395
    The Supercompensation
    Diet 397

Food and Health / Nutrition Obstacles

Most of us, most of the time, have the same nutrition needs as the next person: a variety of foods, chosen in balance, eaten in moderation. But some of us have special needs that are not so easily met. We may have to restrict certain foods because of a health problem, or we may wish to do so because of personal preference or, for various reasons, we may not be physically able to eat foods prepared in the normal way. This concluding section of EAT BETTER, LIVE BETTER is for those who have special needs themselves or do the cooking for others who do. The information will be helpful in meeting the dietary needs of a vegetarian friend, a diabetic child, or a mother-in-law who has been told to go easy on salt—without sacrificing the elegance of a dinner party or the joy of birthday celebrations.

The aim of meeting people's special needs is to keep them getting what all people need under any circumstances—adequate nutrition. There is nothing magic about softness or blandness, and nothing essentially evil about sugar, salt, or meat. Softness is helpful because soft foods are easy to chew and swallow, so that a person who is feeling weak or has a sore throat can nevertheless manage to eat enough to meet his needs until eating becomes easier. A diabetic needs neither more nor less sugar than anybody else, but he cannot utilize sugar as well as other people can. His diet must be adjusted to meet his requirements in other ways, primarily by substituting carbohydrates that are broken down more slowly into the necessary sugars. If somebody chooses a vegetarian diet, the concern is to provide adequate nutrition despite the lack of complete sources of amino acids, which the body requires to maintain its own proteins. Special diets are simply ways of getting around special obstacles to good nutrition.

Any infectious illness, from the common cold to much more serious ailments, is an obstacle to nutrition. The body is challenged to perform at an accelerated pace and in unusual ways to raise its internal temperature, destroy microorganisms, repair damaged tissue, replace ruined cells, and create novel products such as the agents of immunity. This stress, like that of running a race or writing a book, must be supported by the full gamut of nutrients. But, unlike the runner or the writer, the sick person usually does not feel hungry. When your mother used to say, "Eat it, it will help you get better," she was quite right. Without food, a sick person's body in effect robs Peter to pay Paul—takes nutrients from *this* tissue to manufacture *that* product, lowers the level of *this* function to divert energy toward *that* encounter.

Lack of appetite comes up again and again in this section of the book not only as an obstacle to adequate nutrition during a long bout with the flu, but when someone must permanently bear with the tastelessness of a low-salt diet or the boredom of a soft one. For this reason, special recipes and tips have been included that will add interest to some of the diets on these pages. These recipes can also usually help you to save money. Dietetic products now available in markets or specialty food stores, while convenient, are often quite expensive. Homemade ones are cheaper and can even taste better.

You will not find the details of therapeutic diets here. These must be given by a doctor after careful diagnosis of a person's condition, with a thorough knowledge of his medical history and attention to his individual needs. Our purpose, rather, is to give some background in layman's terms and help you in managing such a diet once your doctor has suggested or prescribed it. If someone in your family must avoid wheat products, what unfamiliar terms among ingredients on labels should you be aware of? If a bland or light diet is prescribed, does that mean you cannot season with pepper or have butter on your toast? And with any special need, even if it is simply feeding a child with a sore throat, how can that be done nicely, easily, and without disrupting everybody else?

Food Notions: True or False?

Throughout history, people have considered that they can eat their way out of illness as well as into it. Green apples bring on belly aches; chicken broth—and warm milk, prunes, or any of thousands of other traditional nostrums—can cure the ache or some other common ailment. Many popular notions about therapeutic diets have the ring of common sense, yet are not true. Within the last generation, the following beliefs, for example, have been widely held: since acne is associated with oily skin, avoiding oily foods like chocolate and potato chips results in improvement. Since bones may become brittle in old age through loss of calcium (a condition called osteoporosis), a diet high in calcium prevents brittleness. Since ulcers are exacerbated by "strong" substances such as coffee and alcohol, a bland diet hastens recovery.

Such beliefs are arrived at through analogy rather than through investigation. Oily food does not necessarily bear any relation to oily skin. Calcium in the diet is not necessarily used for remineralizing bone. Foods that look bland, feel bland, and taste bland are not necessarily bland in physiological action. In fact, diet is no longer considered a crucial factor in acne or ulcers.

A few similarly intuitive notions have resulted in serious consequences. In the mistaken belief that milk neutralizes stomach acid during its entire time in the stomach, ulcer patients were once kept on a diet that included enormous amounts of milk and cream—but little else. Those who did not "cheat" eventually risked malnutrition.

Trial and error has, on the other hand, produced popular remedies that really do work, although it has taken science to elucidate the reasons. Buttermilk and yogurt were used to treat thrush (now called oral candidiasis), a fungus infection of the mouth, before the invention of fungicides. Fresh limes were used to treat scurvy in sailors, as cod liver oil was used to treat rickets in children, before science had stumbled upon vitamins or understood deficiency diseases. Generations of people sipped warm milk at bedtime to make them sleepy without having an accurate idea of how the remedy worked.

Now doctors understand the mechanisms by which these and other old remedies have therapeutic value. Foods can be therapeutic in several ways: by providing a nutrient in a form a sick person can use; by providing an unusually high level of a nutrient in which a person is deficient; by providing a drug or a substance that stimulates a specific physiological action; and, finally, by changing the ecology within the body. Chicken broth is a classic example of the first remedy. While it is by no means loaded with nutrients, clear chicken broth is easy for a sick person to swallow and digest, so that the fat and protein it contains provide at least a short-term source of nourishment that is better than nothing at all. Fish livers, used in making cod liver oil, contain lots of vitamin D; citrus fruits contain large amounts of vitamin C. Scientists have only recently discovered the reason why milk is helpful at bedtime: milk contains an amino acid that causes the brain to release a mildly tranquilizing substance that encourages drowsiness. The buttermilk treatment for a candidiasis infection is a good example of the third therapeutic mechanism: changing internal ecology. The mouth is home to an everyday population of both fungi and bacteria that, because they are competitors, tend to keep one another's numbers in check. Mouth bacteria may be killed off (a course of antibiotics is frequently the cause) leaving a runaway population of candidiasis fungi. Yogurt and buttermilk contain bacteria that can restore the balance, putting the candidiasis fungus back in its place.

What To Eat, What To Avoid

Most therapeutic diets emphasize less what a person is supposed to eat than what he is not supposed to eat. Food avoidance, like food as a remedy, is also an old treatment idea that has now come to be better understood. Again, what once appeared to be obvious often has turned out to be wrong. Celiac disease, in which bowel movements are extremely fatty, used to be treated by scrupulous avoidance of fat—to no avail. The illness is now known to be caused by an intolerance to gluten, and the food to be avoided is wheat.

Today the traditional prescription of food as medicine has been largely abandoned by the medical profession in favor of more convenient forms of drugs and supplements. Also, in this way the doctor is assured that the patient is actually getting what he needs. The person with iron-deficiency anemia who used to have to swallow huge amounts of cooked and raw liver can now recover on little pills. Other kinds of therapeutic diets, however, have not been replaced and continue to be important in the treatment of many conditions. Some restrict amounts of certain foods or eliminate them altogether. Restriction and elimination diets are used when a food is actually injurious to a person; he is allergic to it or his body cannot tolerate it. Other diets control amounts of substances such as sodium, protein, sugar, and fat that everybody needs and that cannot be eliminated. Controlled diets are used to adjust the amounts or proportions of such substances upward or downward, depending on a person's specific needs.

The special needs that most people have to cope with most often are common ailments with symp-

Food and Health
Nutrition Obstacles

toms such as sore throat, fever, or nausea. For these and other symptoms, the form in which food is prepared is adjusted to a person's needs, so that it is served in liquid form to a child with tonsillitis, in an easily digested form to a person recovering from abdominal surgery, and in a bulky, fibrous form to a person who is chronically constipated.

Check with Your Doctor

Some of the diets here may be used without a doctor's continuing supervision. A bland diet, for example, can be followed for a few days to help a person recover from intestinal upset, or a high-fiber diet can be used permanently to regulate bowel function. Where continuing medical supervision is not crucial, you can use the information to help you plan meals, including sample menus. However, you should never prescribe even these diets to yourself or others. Prescription requires diagnosis—for instance, of an underlying condition as opposed to a common tummy ache—that only a professional can make. There is no way to know, without medical diagnosis, whether the person who has a fever with a cold and who might ordinarily be safe on a liquid diet also has diabetes, is hypertense, or is allergic to eggs, so that the liquid diet here is not safe for him. Always check with your doctor first before you go on any special diet.

Other diets require not only medical prescription, but continuing medical supervision. The information about these diets in this section is mostly general, and not sufficient for meal planning. Although you may wish to reduce salt, sugar, or fat in your diet, and may get some good ideas for how to do that from reading those pages, they are really intended for people who have been told by their doctors to reduce salt because they have hypertension, saturated fats because they have atherosclerosis, or sugar because they have diabetes. These conditions are typified by individual and complicating factors that must be taken into consideration when planning the diet. Our intention is only to make the planning easier, the food tastier.

For long-term or permanent changes in diet, your doctor may send you to a nutritionist (or you may want to ask him to recommend one), a medically or scientifically trained person who will help you make a detailed diet plan based on your physician's diet prescription. You can find out whether there is a board-certified nutritionist in your area by writing to the American Board of Nutrition, 9650 Rockville Pike, Bethesda, Maryland 20014.

Your doctor may also refer you to a registered dietitian, a person who has studied dietetics or nutrition at an accredited college or university and has had several years of intership or a master's degree in the field. Such a person should be a member of the American Dietetic Association. Be sure to check the credentials carefully, for this is a field rife with charlatans. You can recognize a nonqualified person by one or more of the following characteristics: phony degrees from institutions you've never heard of; claims of quick or miracle cures; prescription of megadoses of vitamins, minerals, or other food supplements; claims that "natural" vitamins are more effective than "synthetic" ones; attempts to sell you something you wouldn't ordinarily buy.

Doctors and families alike have found that mere prescription of a diet does not guarantee that a patient will follow it. People are attached to their accustomed ways of eating and find change—particularly restrictive change—hard to accept. It does not help that diets as conceived by dietitians give no inkling as to how the daily dole of chicken might translate into a creamy fricassee, a colorful stir-fried chicken with red peppers, or a spicy Indian curry laced with ginger. With your doctor's permission, there is probably room to individualize a diet according to your traditions or in a spirit of adventure.

Even with flexibility, ingenuity, and help, some diets create a challenge to menu planning. Since sheer tedium and difficulty have been still other reasons why patients resist their doctors' best advice, dietitians have come up with a simplified method for figuring out what to eat for breakfast, lunch, and supper without constantly referring to typewritten sheets. It is called the exchange method, and has been adapted here to serve several special diets, including a weight-loss plan.

People often wonder if the same diet that is used therapeutically after someone becomes ill would also work to prevent the illness were it adopted earlier in life, or would reverse the course of events if it were instituted before the condition had advanced too far. The answer is, we do not know.

The biochemistry of the body is enormously complicated, and the subtle effects of one food or another can take circuitous pathways. Even when a pathway can be traced, and the biochemistry understood, the relationship between chemical effects and disease processes often remains mysterious. More confusing still, effects vary greatly from one individual to another, within one environment or another, and also differ according to a person's age, life-style, and temperament. Researchers are studying the question of how diet relates to preventing and reversing the course of disease processes by experimenting on animals in the laboratory, by comparing populations through statistical means, and by recording in detail the nutritional and medical status of many hundreds of individuals over the entire course of their lives in hopes that predictable patterns may yield clues.

You may read of the effects of cholesterol on laboratory animals, or the effects of exercise on the residents of Framingham, Massachusetts, or the differences between the rates of coronary artery disease in Japan and in America. The way such articles are written lead the reader to believe that, at last, an answer has been found. Unfortunately, other studies—and other articles—reach conflicting conclusions. For example, a study of the Seventh-Day Adventists, whose diet is high in vegetable fiber and low in animal fats, indicates that this regimen reduces a person's chance of developing a variety of bowel diseases, including cancer of the colon. But another study concentrates on Mormons, who also show a low rate of cancer of the colon; yet their diet is not low in animal fats or very high in vegetable fiber. Still another study traces the incidence of bowel disease in Japanese before and after they emigrate to the United States. In Japan, they have a low rate of bowel disease and a diet similar to that of the Seventh-Day Adventists, yet here their risk of bowel disease relates more closely with the typical American one. Is the reason dietary, or are there other factors as yet unrecognized? The matter is still one of opinion, not of fact.

It is wise to be skeptical of any exaggerated or overpositive claim that what you eat can prevent, reverse, or cure a specific condition. Most such claims are nonsense; many are merely hypotheses that have yet to be tested according to the rigorous standards science requires. Indeed, if you were to follow all the advice the latest news suggests, you would become too confused to eat at all.

Beyond following an adequate and varied diet, it is impossible to guarantee that any special adjustment of fiber, fat, and so on will result in better health. Nonetheless, from what is known about populations that traditionally eat more fiber and carbohydrates, but less sugar, salt, fat, and protein than Americans do, you can be certain that nutrition itself will not suffer. The emotional advantages of taking extra good care of yourself and of your family in sickness and in health may be immeasurable.

Herbal Remedies

Nostalgia for the old-fashioned herb garden, the appeal of the "natural," and a lore as long as human history combine to perpetuate an often dangerous faith in herbal remedies.

The plants themselves are not to blame. Many of our most valuable drugs are derived from plants: licorice root yields a drug that speeds the healing of ulcers; rauwolfia, a compound to control high blood pressure; curare, a muscle relaxant used in surgery; and foxglove, the digitalis used to treat heart disease. Digitalis alone is taken daily by 3 million Americans, and can be given full credit for keeping them alive.

The trouble is that to use plant products in their natural form—bark, seeds, leaves—requires immense knowledge. Unprocessed plant materials contain risky impurities that can cause harmful side effects. Dosage is tricky. The difference between a therapeutic and a toxic dose may be small. Active ingredients vary in strength depending on where the plant was grown, when it was picked, and what the weather had been. Combinations of herbal medicines, like the combination of alcohol and tranquilizers, can have unexpected and dangerous outcomes.

In previous generations, housewives who had command of the use of scores of plants had access to a large body of oral knowledge accumulated and passed down over many generations. Recognized herbalists, such as Navajo medicine men, are able to prepare and prescribe medications derived from 200 plants, but only after years of training—as long or longer than college and medical school combined. You would not entrust your health to an amateur doctor; you should not entrust your health to an amateur herbalist either.

Dealing with Common Ailments

Nature's medicine for all common ailments, from the common cold to convalescense, is a dose of time. There is no specific remedy for the flu or mononucleosis; they must simply run their course. The time it takes to convalesce from an acute illness or from surgery is even harder to guess, and can drag on for many weeks. Meanwhile, the family has on its hands a member who feels ill, acts restless, and is disinterested—even in meals.

Should you worry? Can a sick person get along for a while without eating normally? The body has sufficient stores of nutrients to get along for a few days without adequate nutrition. Usually nutritional needs are no different during an illness than they are in health. However, running a fever uses up extra calories to produce the extra heat, so the old advice to "starve a fever" is not wise because a fever depletes the body's reserve of nutrients.

More worrisome than food needs is the body's water requirement during illness. Without sufficient water the body becomes dehydrated. Dehydration is a particularly likely complication to feverish illnesses and to bouts of vomiting and diarrhea, especially in children. To be sure the sick person does get enough to drink, offer liquids every hour or two, and keep drinks varied—from fruit juices diluted with water to soup.

The easiest way to feed a sick member of the family is to serve exactly what everyone else is having. Of course, there are circumstances under which you will not be able to offer food prepared the normal way. The patient's throat may be so sore he just can't swallow solid food, or he may have dental problems that interfere with chewing. Ordinary meals may add to abdominal discomfort after surgery or prolong diarrhea. Your doctor may advise a liquid diet, a soft diet, or a bland diet. These are used separately or one after the other to provide the best nutrition under the circumstances until the patient can again enjoy regular family meals.

Food for the Common Cold

Noted food writer Mimi Sheraton published the following tips in The New York Times.

In our home, the recommendation to feed a cold is still considered gospel. The only real problem is to choose food or drink that is appealing enough to stand up to the classic symptoms of the cold: a stuffy, aching head, the congested nasal passages that knock out the sense of smell and so the sense of taste, and the general hot-cold malaise that tends to make ordinary food seem uninteresting.

I make marvelous soups for members of my family who fall ill. But when I am sick, I have had to rely on dreary canned substitutions, there being no one on the premises who knows how to make real soup. In defense, I now freeze portion-size containers of homemade beef and chicken stock, broths to build on when colds arrive unexpectedly. That way, I can add beaten eggs to make egg-drop soup, or add pastina, dried split peas, or barley for more body; turn beef broth into Spanish garlic soup; or simply add a dash of lemon juice or Madeira.

Freshly squeezed lemon juice frozen in ice-cube trays allows a head start toward preparing hot and cold lemonade and leads to far better results than frozen concentrates. Also, when coolness seems in order, I rely on sour lemon or grapefruit sherbet or cold grapefruit juice, freshly made or thawed from homemade frozen cubes.

As the most extreme cold symptoms have faded away, the enemy in food becomes blandness, and I long for sharp, strong flavors that not only take effect on a numbed palate but also clear up some of a cold's symptoms, if only temporarily. My favorite liquid then is Chinese hot and sour soup. If it has enough Sichuan chile oil, I will breathe clearly for at least an hour.

Cool relief comes by way of gazpacho fired with Tabasco sauce and heady with minced raw scallions. Even a simple mix of tomato juice and beef bouillon simmered together with a dash of crushed, dried, red Italian peppers has an immediate and beneficent effect.

But of all the edible cures I have found for the common cold, few work as well as pickled herring, garnished with rings of thinly sliced, raw Bermuda onion. An added bonus is the thirst that forces me to drink the fluids doctors prescribe.

If it is true that not even the most inviting menu could make me wish to catch a cold, at least I know that if one catches me, I am prepared to make the most of it.

Liquid Diets

A liquid diet can be used whenever a person is not up to more than sipping his food. This may be during the most miserable days of the flu, when a sore throat makes swallowing painful, after dental surgery, or simply when solid foods are unappetizing. Liquid means any food that is really watery, such as milk or broth, any food that becomes a liquid as it warms, such as gelatin or ice cream, and any food that can be made runny, such as thinned cooked cereal or pureed vegetables. Custards and cornstarch puddings are also included among liquids because their solid aspects are negligible as far as digestion is concerned.

Doctors may prescribe a clear liquid diet or a full liquid diet. Clear means the liquid has no residue; it is transparent. Gelatin is a clear liquid and so are broth and fruit ices, but milk, ice cream, and thickened soups are not. Clear liquids are usually used when vomiting is a problem; for example, after a concussion, following anesthesia, or during an intestinal illness. Sipped often and in small quantities, clear liquids leave the stomach promptly and are absorbed quickly—thus, it is hoped, before they can come up again. (When even very small amounts of clear liquids still cause vomiting, try giving the patient cracked ice cubes to suck on.)

Clear liquids are almost entirely devoid of nourishment. Because of this, a clear liquid diet is a temporary measure to be replaced as soon as possible with a full liquid diet complete with nourishing soups, milk drinks, thinned cereals, and eggs. Even a full liquid diet is hard to bring up to normal nutritional standards, and so is rarely used for longer than a week or two.

Clear Liquid Diet: Permitted Foods
  Clear bouillon, broth, consomme,
    or jellied soups
  Carbonated beverages
  Plain gelatin desserts
  Juices: apple, cranberry, grape, strained
    orange or grapefruit; lemonade
  Tea, coffee, if tolerated

Full Liquid Diet: Permitted Foods
To the above foods add the following:
  Milk, cream, yogurt
  Milkshakes, cocoa
  Strained cream soups (meat, fish, vegetable)
  Meat-based soups with rice, noodles, pureed
    meat, or pureed vegetables
  Baked custard
  Milk puddings (cornstarch or rennet)
  Ice cream or sherbet (no nuts or fruits)
  Refined cooked cereals (cream of rice or
    wheat); strained oatmeal; infant cereals
  Tomato or blended vegetable juices
  Cooked vegetables or fruit, strained or
    pureed in a blender
  Applesauce
  Eggnog with raw eggs or dried egg powder

Although a full liquid diet can be nourishing, ingenuity is required because a steady diet of liquid foods is so boring the patient may not eat enough to provide adequate nourishment. You can sneak extra nourishment into soups by thickening them with cream, egg yolk, pureed vegetables, or pureed chicken. Serve soup with a spoonful of sour cream, perhaps, or, at the last minute, stir an egg into the steaming hot bowl of soup to slightly poach, and serve while the egg is still semisoft. When the patient is able to manage more solid stuff, you can add small quantities of rice, pasta, or croutons to make a soup both more nourishing and more interesting.

Eggnogs are the time-honored way of getting the most nourishment into the smallest package. To avoid boredom, try adding a variety of flavorings to the basic eggnog recipe.

BASIC EGGNOG

3 cups milk
4 eggs
½ cup sugar
1½ teaspoons vanilla
⅛ teaspoon salt
¼ teaspoon nutmeg

MAKES FOUR SERVINGS

1. Place all ingredients in blender container and blend until thoroughly combined. Or beat with an egg beater.
2. Store, covered, in refrigerator.

Variations. Add any of the following to one serving of the basic mixture:
  2-3 tablespoons chocolate syrup
  2 tablespoons chocolate syrup plus 1 teaspoon
    instant coffee powder
  ⅓ cup orange juice
  3-4 tablespoons maple syrup
  2 tablespoons malted milk powder
  Garnish top of eggnog with cinnamon,
    nutmeg, or instant cocoa mix

Dealing with Common Ailments
Liquid Diets

Milk Toast and Other Pleasures

When you were sick and very young, do you remember the rich comfort of milk toast? The steam of hot broth, the drowsy lassitude that came over you after a cup of hot tea laced with lemon, honey, and perhaps even a whiff of whiskey? Somehow, being sick with grown-up ills lacks the nostalgic pleasure of childhood ills when a sore throat was almost worth the luxury of sick-bed fare. We cannot recapture that pleasure, but we can give it to our children in their turn. There is nothing to making milk toast. Scald milk. Toast bread; butter it. Put the buttered toast into a bowl and sprinkle it with sugar. Pour the hot milk over.

Less nostalgic but nevertheless effective in sparking a sick child's interest in food—and creating his future nostalgia—are a number of pleasures that appeal to sick children with dull appetites. The pleasures are reminiscent of traditional preludes to adult dinners: flavorful, pretty drinks, plus tidbits of tasty food. Pink eggnogs, for example, are more appealing than plain ones. Use grenadine syrup for the raspberry color and sweeter flavor. Add a lemon slice to any beverage, even ginger ale. Preschool-age children who have long since given up baby bottles can nevertheless enjoy chocolate milk from a bottle again—just for fun. If that doesn't appeal to your child (or to you) a plastic bendable straw might, or maybe tiny drinks poured from a measuring pitcher into a jigger.

Just as pink drinks are better than plain ones, toast cut into fancy shapes is more interesting than the usual triangles or rectangles. Use cookie cutters, the smaller the better. In fact, anything you can do to make food finger-sized is helpful; coping with utensils can be tedious to young children, the more so when they are sick. Paper frills, still sold in supermarkets, turn the wings from a roast chicken into a finger feast (cut off the wing tip and divide the wing into two pieces at the joint). Serve cheese cubes on toothpicks, and if you are making meatballs for the rest of the family, make some tiny ones too, to be eaten by hand or on picks. Another toothpick-sized favorite is cocktail frankfurters, which can be dipped in catsup or, more interestingly, in a mixture of honey, soy sauce, and mustard. Cooked carrot slices are also good this way.

Dips usually reserved for cocktail parties delight children, especially if there is intrinsic interest in the dipper itself. Try fish-shaped crackers, ruffle-cut carrot slices, or popcorn. The dip can be dairy based—sour cream or cream cheese—with whatever flavorings your child would like, or hard-boiled egg yolk mashed with mayonnaise, lemon juice, and paprika; or even sardines mashed with catsup and mayonnaise.

Hearty spaghetti or macaroni dishes are not at all appealing to a sick child, but there are diminutive pastas that are. Alphabets are an old standby; less familiar is pastina, shaped like a star and no bigger than a pinhead. These could be served hot with a pat of butter melting over the surface, or moistened with hot chicken broth. Pastina and alphabets slide easily down a sore throat. In keeping with the suggestion to offer foods in an interesting way that is also easy to cope with, serve miniature pastas in a tea cup with a small spoon.

Make surprises out of ordinary fare. Float a few alphabet noodles or strips of bean curd in broth. Serve peas in an egg cup. Use an ice cream scoop to serve mashed potatoes, and trim the balls with parsley trees.

Bland desserts like tapioca pudding or custard can be brightened up with a bit of currant jelly or with colorful sprinkles. Caramel sauce improves custard too. Heat a half-cup of sugar in a pan, stirring until the sugar melts and turns a toasty brown. Add boiling water slowly and cautiously, still stirring, until the caramel is a thin syrup.

If you make gelatin with somewhat less water than the package calls for, the consistency will be firm enough so that it can be cut into cubes and eaten with the fingers. Let it set in a pie plate instead of a bowl for easy cutting. You could distribute grapes in the gelatin too, so that each cube contains one. More straightforward is applesauce with whipped cream. Strained applesauce for infants can be more tasty than other commercial applesauce; the whipped cream adds nourishment. This dessert can be served straight from the jar with the whipped cream piled on top.

One last idea would be annoying to a busy parent, but might be enjoyed by other children in the family: string doughnut-shaped breakfast cereal onto hat elastic to make the young patient between-meal snacks of stretchable, edible necklaces.

Soft Diet

The soft diet consists of foods that are easy to chew and swallow. For example, skin is removed from chicken and the membranes from orange sections so that the meat and fruit will be easy to manage.

When a soft diet is prescribed in a hospital, anything hard to digest is not allowed. That includes the usual offenders—fried foods, the cabbage family, and onions—and even soft melon, since it leaves a fibrous residue. In fact, anything with a strong flavor may be excluded. Mustard may be prohibited, and there will be no garlicky salad dressing, no turnips, and no Gorgonzola cheese. The diet is used as a transition from liquid to normal foods for patients who are recovering from surgery or suffering prolonged debilitating illness, so every precaution is taken, including the possibility that strong flavor and difficult digestion go hand in hand.

You will not usually have occasion to use the soft diet at home. It is so similar to the bland diet, differing mainly in paying more attention to the physical softness of the food, that you can use the bland diet on page 364 as a transition between liquid and normal meals and also when ease of digestion is to be considered. However, your doctor may prescribe a soft diet, or you may find it necessary to feed a person who is temporarily or permanently unable to chew or swallow more demanding foods.

Just how soft food must be depends on the patient's needs. A teenager with mononucleosis may have such a sore throat that he is not able to endure anything harder than oatmeal or applesauce for weeks. On the other hand, a grandmother with denture problems may be able to eat roast chicken, providing she gets the softest portions. Soft fish, such as sole or whitefish, is easier to manage than swordfish, and poaching or steaming fish gets rid of the problem of the crust formed during broiling or pan frying.

What's Allowed, What Isn't

Any meat, poultry, or fish is allowed on a soft diet as long as it is either naturally tender or can be made easy to chew through special preparation. Remove skin and gristle. Stew tough cuts until they fall apart, or serve tough cuts ground as patties or incorporated into dishes that call for finely diced or slivered meat. Bacon will be easy to chew if it is cooked until very crisp.

No raw vegetables are allowed. That means no salad greens, but a cooked vegetable salad would be fine, and avocados, sometimes listed under fruit, are also allowed. Cook vegetables past the crisp stage in any case, and if food must be very soft, continue cooking until the vegetable can be mashed with a fork. Squash and peas lend themselves better to mashing than beets or mushrooms, but beets could be grated as for borscht, and mushrooms could be chopped fine. Avoid potato skins and don't bother with corn unless you want to puree it for a cream of corn soup, the only way it would be allowed.

In the hospital version of this diet, only bananas and citrus fruits—membranes removed—are allowed raw. This is because other soft fruits such as ripe peaches, plums, and melons leave an undigested fibrous residue. If your doctor agrees that digestion is not an issue, such fruits can be eaten provided they are truly ripe and carefully peeled. You probably won't want to bother peeling grapes. Cooked or canned fruits, including applesauce, are fine.

The soft diet prohibits all berries, and also figs, because their seeds can be a problem. Dried fruits are too hard to chew, and the same goes for candied fruits, nuts, and coconut. You'll be surprised at how often some of these prohibited items crop up in ordinary foods: nut toppings on cookies, orange rinds in marmalade, raisins in bread, sesame or poppy seeds on sandwich buns, strawberries in strawberry ice cream. Watch out for coarse or whole grains and bran in breads, cereals, or crackers. Stick to refined wheat or rye products.

In the hospital, one might not be able to tell the difference between a flavorless diet and ordinary hospital fare. At home, especially if the person is elderly or debilitated and must eat soft foods permanently, the soft diet as specified in hospital dietitians' manuals may be so lacking in flavor that too little is eaten to provide nourishment. Starting with small amounts, and after consulting your doctor, use the seasonings the patient is accustomed to; allow strong-tasting cheeses and cold cuts, as well as strong-tasting vegetables such as broccoli and turnips. Other appetizing ideas for soft foods include many dishes the whole family can enjoy: quiches made with finely chopped cooked vegetables and meats; highly seasoned but soft foods such as chicken liver pâté, spinach pie, chili con carne, pasta with meat or sausage sauce; hearty soups such as Scotch broth, fish chowder, and minestrone.

Dealing with Common Ailments
Bland Diet

A bland diet (sometimes called a light diet) eliminates foods that might be irritating to the digestive tract. Stomach and intestines can be irritated in various ways. Some foods, such as nuts, whole grains, and raw fruit are mechanically irritating; their fibers and husks scrape and rub. Others are chemically irritating because they stimulate spurts of stomach acid. Meat extracts, caffeine-containing drinks such as coffee, tea, and cola, as well as alcohol, are all acid stimulators. Foods can be physiologically irritating by causing gas, as cabbage often does, by being difficult to digest, like fried foods, or by causing particularly bulky bowel movements. A soft-cooked egg, a bland-looking food, may be restricted in a bland diet because, even though it is not fibrous like bran, much of its bulk is not digested, leaving a large residue in the bowel. Finally, food can be thermally irritating—either steamy hot or icy cold—so that it further irritates the sore lining of an inflamed stomach. In addition to mechanical, chemical, physiological, and thermal blandness, the bland diet tastes bland.

The bland diet is prescribed to patients who are recovering from abdominal surgery, and a similar, very low residue diet may be prescribed during flare-ups of such chronic intestinal conditions as diverticulitis and ulcerative colitis. The idea is to give the flaccid or inflamed intestinal tract, from the stomach to the bowel, the least possible work to do and the least irritating environment in which to do it so that, with rest, the system can recover normal function. The same principle makes the bland diet useful during the bouts of common diarrhea everybody suffers from time to time. The bland diet can be used as a transition from liquids to ordinary meals as a person recuperates from any common ailment.

Even minor abdominal surgery is enough of a shock to the digestive system to make intestinal action sluggish or even to bring it to a temporary halt. The muscles become slack, peristaltic action is slowed. Not only is less food digested, but it takes an abnormally long time to get from one end to the other. As a result, intestinal bacteria have a heyday. With more food to eat and a longer time in which to eat it, they multiply rapidly, releasing large amounts of their gassy by-products. The patient experiences bloating, flatulence, and often a good deal of pain from the distention.

Although it may not be possible to avoid discomfort altogether, sticking to foods that are easily digested and avoiding ones that are known to cause gas at least keep distention to a minimum.

Diverticulitis is an acute, infected episode of an underlying condition in which pouches (diverticula) have formed in the wall of the lower bowel. When food material becomes trapped in these pouches, bacteria may multiply, causing the episode of infection. Ulcerative colitis is also an infection of the lower digestive tract, often acute and very painful. The bland diet is not a cure for either of these chronic conditions, but its lack of harshness and bulk is sometimes prescribed to alleviate symptoms.

Common diarrhea is associated most often with a virus infection that causes the mucous membrane within the bowel to become inflamed and irritated. Instead of absorbing water from food material, the usual final step in forming feces, the mucous membrane leaks water into the bowel. The result is runny, frequent bowel movements. Again, the bland diet is not a cure but a palliative.

Avoiding Irritants

The largest category of foods not allowed in the bland diet are those that are mechanically irritating. They include many of the hard-to-chew foods forbidden in the soft diet, plus a few more. The problem of fibrous residue knocks out every raw fruit and vegetable except bananas and avocados. Peach ice cream is not allowed because the fruit in ice cream is not cooked. Olives and pickles are also considered raw vegetables, and so is chopped parsley garnish. Fruits are allowed if they are canned or stewed (without skins) and have no seeds. That leaves out berries. All coarse and whole-grain products are excluded from the diet too.

Because they are associated with the digestion problems of some people, many cooked vegetables may be excluded, leaving perhaps only asparagus, beets, carrots, peas, spinach, squash, green beans, wax beans, tomatoes (skinned), and mushrooms. Dried beans aren't usually allowed. In certain forms of the diet, tomatoes must be seeded before cooking or strained after cooking.

When the bulk of bowel movements is at issue, as it may be with diarrhea, there may also be restriction of perfectly smooth and nongas-producing foods such as milk, potatoes, Swiss cheese, and soft-boiled eggs because of the large residue that still remains after digestion. On the other hand, high residue may be helpful for constipation (see page 365).

People are often confused about the instruction to avoid fried foods. Does that mean a hamburger should be broiled, not pan fried? Is sautéeing in a little butter or margarine considered frying? What commercial products, besides the obvious French-fried potatoes, are fried? And what is it about frying that causes indigestion?

The indigestion is purely a matter of fat—too much of it. Frying in deep fat is the worst cooking method for a fat indigestion problem because a large quantity of fat is absorbed by the food as it fries. Pan frying a hamburger, on the other hand, will remove some of the fat from the meat and will be equivalent to broiling provided you have not added any fat to the pan and that you drain the patties of liquid fat before you serve them. Sautéeing requires judgment. If you wish to sauté a fillet of fish in a pat of melted butter or margarine, and that amount of fat is allowed in the diet, the method itself is not intrinsically harmful. But if to you sautéeing means drowning food in butter, and that amount of fat is not allowed in your diet, of course you should not do it. Finally, if a diet says "no fried foods," you can assume that means not only deep-fried no-nos like doughnuts and potato chips but also greasy pastries, pie crusts, and croissants.

Avoiding chemical irritants is straightforward in one respect: substances like caffeine, alcohol, and meat extracts prohibited in the bland diet are known stimulators of stomach acid. But if your doctor has prescribed a detailed bland diet, you may find the particular version also prohibits a discouraging number of flavorings that are suspected of being either chemical or physiological irritants. These may include garlic, vinegar, catsup, mint, horseradish, Worchestershire sauce, Tabasco, pepper, and nearly every spice.

Even more confusing, bland diets vary so that on one set of instructions cocoa, cinnamon, allspice, mint, mace, and caraway seeds are allowed, but on another version mint and caraway seeds are not allowed, and even molasses is forbidden, leaving only paprika—and plain vanilla. The reason is that, in a medical sense, there is no single "bland diet" but rather many diets that are bland in certain respects. The details of each are geared to a patient's particular needs. For example, the few caraway seeds on a crust of rye bread are unlikely to bother a 10-year-

The Ulcer Mystery

For many years, common sense dictated that since ulcers occur in the presence of excess stomach acid, foods that neutralize acid should be eaten by ulcer patients, whereas those that aggravate the condition should be avoided. Unfortunately, the picture turned out to be not nearly so simple.

Some people produce excess stomach acid without developing ulcers. Of those who do develop ulcers, some suffer pain from the aggravating effects of such foods as Brussels sprouts and hot peppers, but others are not bothered by these foods at all. Milk, which neutralizes acid when it first reaches the stomach, has a long-term effect quite the opposite: it stimulates acid later in the digestive process. In fact, there seems little agreement on any basically dietary approach, much less for such extremes as the once-popular "white diet" that prescribed veal instead of beef, white grains like rice in preference to dark grains, and potentially dangerous proportions of dairy products in the belief that pale color and insipid flavor was intrinsically nonirritating to the stomach.

The greatest mystery of all is the declining incidence of ulcers in America—and everywhere else in the Western world. In 1975 statistics showed that 3,955,000 people suffered from ulcers, but by 1980 the figure had declined to 3,615,000—a drop of more than 10 percent.

These days, ulcers are treated mostly through medication, including large amounts of antacids. Dietary treatment includes avoidance of substances that particularly stimulate the production of acid—caffeine, alcohol, and meat extracts—and elimination of particles that might conceivably get stuck in an open ulcer, such as berry seeds and bran. Perhaps equally important, patients are also advised to eat frequent meals or snacks, a tactic that seems to alleviate attacks of pain.

Dealing with Common Ailments
Bland Diet

old who has just had a hernia repair, but those same few seeds could actually get stuck in a pouch of intestine in the patient suffering from diverticulitis, contributing to his problem. Thus there is a great difference between a bland diet prescribed by your doctor for a diagnosed condition and eating bland foods for a few days while recovering from "what's going around." You should certainly do as your doctor says in the former case, but you may please yourself somewhat more if it is merely the latter case.

There is no evidence, for example, that rough particles irritate the normal intestine if they have been well-chewed. Gas producing foods do so only in some people. Hot peppers produce a burning sensation, and can hurt ordinary skin, but they seem not to damage mucous membrane. Some doctors have claimed that the relaxing effects of a little wine during dinner offsets any stomach-irritating effects of the alcohol.

A Question of Choice

With your doctor's permission, you may want to be somewhat flexible about following a bland diet if you are using it for a common ailment. The benefit of flexibility is that food will be more tasty, and therefore more appetizing. Anyone who has to subsist on a bland diet for even just one week will certainly appreciate a little variety at meals.

Some suggestions for modification are: restrict rather than eliminate disallowed foods, and add tasty seasonings, albeit with caution. As the days go by, move gradually toward a normal diet as the patient tolerates it. The plan that follows is just such a sequence, beginning with a good deal of restriction in stage 1 and easing gradually toward normal meals by stage 3.

Stage 1
- Sliced banana
- Rusk or melba toast
- Hot, sweetened skim milk sprinkled with nutmeg
- Poached egg on toast
- Cocoa made with skim milk
- Steamed chicken breast
- Rice cooked in saffron-seasoned broth
- Hot mulled cider

Stage 2
- Milk toast made with skim milk
- Applesauce
- Hot bouillon
- Jelly omelette
- Banana milkshake made with skim milk
- Fish and potato chowder made with skim milk
- Soda crackers, water biscuits, or matzohs
- Lemonade or ginger ale

Stage 3
- Cream of rice or plain boiled rice sprinkled with cinnamon and sugar
- Baked apple (no skin)
- Weak tea
- Tuna fish (packed in water) served on boiled noodles moistened with broth
- Cold skim milk or soda
- Broiled hamburger (round or top sirloin)
- Boiled new potatoes
- Steamed asparagus seasoned with lemon juice
- Canned pears with ladyfingers
- Any beverage

People who suffer frequent attacks of indigestion or heartburn often put themselves permanently on a bland diet to alleviate the discomfort they experience after meals, or because their doctor suggests it. More important than blandness in general is specific avoidance of a few substances and adherence to a few rules.

- Avoid caffeine-containing beverages (tea, coffee, cola drinks).
- Avoid smoking.
- Avoid meat extracts (bouillon cubes, concentrated canned broths, canned gravies).
- Eat or drink acid-containing foods (pickles, tomato juice, oranges). Drink mildly alcoholic beverages (wine, beer, diluted drinks) during meals only. Avoid strong alcoholic drinks entirely.
- Test your individual tolerance for foods known to cause indigestion and heartburn (sauerkraut, hot dogs, raw onions, beans, citrus juices, ice cream) by trying a small amount of one food at a time, then waiting to see if it has a bad effect. Avoid any that cause discomfort.
- Arrange for long, relaxed mealtimes (no food on the run; no arguments during dinner).
- Eat slowly, chew thoroughly.
- Do not eat very large meals; do not lie down until several hours after a meal.
- Do not go too long between meals.
- Be sure you are getting adequate nutrition.

High-Fiber Diets

Fiber consists of the indigestible skins, seeds, shreds, and coatings of vegetables, fruits, and grains. Because these materials remain undigested, they increase the bulk and coarsen the texture of bowel movements. Such bowel movements also hold more water. The effect of a high-fiber diet when eaten over a period of time is to regulate bowel function in several ways. If the time it takes for food to travel the length of the large bowel is unusually brief, the time will be increased; and if the time is unusually long, it will be decreased. Both overly loose and overly compressed bowel movements will tend to change toward a normal volume and consistency. Because of these changes, the straining pressures of the bowel will also be moderated.

Under the name of roughage, doctors and grandmothers have been advising high-fiber diets to relieve constipation for many decades. High fiber is nothing new. What is new is the claims made for it, which include prevention of coronary artery disease, diabetes, cancer of the colon, appendicitis, and even tooth decay. Many of these claims have merit (see Constipation Complications at right).

Some claims are largely based on epidemiological studies. Among people who eat a diet high in fiber and low in both animal fats and refined sugars, the incidence of several diseases is lower than among people who partake of the typical American diet, which is low in fiber and high in animal fat and refined sugar. Recently, researchers have hypothesized that these two diets may each result in somewhat different environmental conditions within the bowel. Waste products from bacteria-digested fiber differ both in kind and quantity, bringing about a change in the local biochemistry of the bowel, the outcome of which might be related to disease processes. At any rate, the differences in diet are more complicated and subtle than sheer bulk of fiber.

Besides its efficacy for relieving constipation, doctors may also prescribe a high-fiber diet for the two bowel conditions known as diverticulosis and irritable bowel syndrome. These conditions are typified by either hard, small, infrequent bowel movements, or loose, large, frequent ones—or both alternating. Because fibrous residue tends to regulate bowel function, both diarrhea and constipation may be relieved.

"High" is usually taken to mean from 5 to 6 grams of nondigestible fiber per day. In terms of food, that is about 2 apples (including skins), or ¼ cup of 100

Constipation Complications

Constipation is not only one of the commonest of common ailments, it is also behind a host of less common—but sometimes troublesome—health problems.

Constant straining to push out hard bowel movements increases pressure within the bowel, and so does the accumulation of hard, large masses of fecal material that may result from infrequent bowel movements. The extra pressure interferes with normal blood circulation upward from veins in the lower part of the body. Veins in the legs may bulge out and become what are known as varicose veins. Veins in the rectum may bulge outward to become what are known as hemorrhoids.

Sheer straining can have other outcomes. The stomach can be pushed upward so that it protrudes somewhat above the diaphragm. Often there are no symptoms from this condition, called hiatus hernia, but it can lead to chronic heartburn. At the other end of the digestive tract, straining can push out the wall of the lower bowel so that it forms the pouches (diverticula) of diverticulosis (see accompanying text). Again, the condition may or may not lead to symptoms.

In the chronically constipated person, fecal material may become so dry it forms into tiny stonelike bits. Such feces become stuck in diverticula, and also in the cavity of the pouchlike appendix. Once a pouch is stopped up by fecal matter, bacteria multiply, and infection—appendicitis or diverticulitis—occurs.

Before launching on any new diet to alleviate constipation, you should find out if you are really constipated. Many people think they are constipated because they usually have a bowel movement only once every two or three days; some think they should have more than one bowel movement every day. People vary, however, in what is normal for them. Daily regularity may not be normal for everybody. Check with your doctor to see if your bowel function really involves smaller, harder feces or greater straining than is good for you. Occasional constipation such as that caused by unfamiliar diet, schedule, and surroundings while traveling should not concern you.

Dealing with Common Ailments
High-Fiber Diets

percent bran cereal, or 2 to 3 slices of whole-wheat bread. (For a list of high-fiber foods see page 19.) But no optimal level of fiber has been found, and exact measurement is not possible because of variations both in an individual's ability to digest and in the food products themselves. Corn kernels of any sort may go through a child's system quite unchanged, whereas in adults, young corn may be completely digested, while older kernels are only partially digested. Therefore the idea of a high-fiber diet is to increase the amount of fiber rather than to achieve any ideal level of fiber.

People who increase their intake of fiber rapidly may experience unpleasant side effects, including both flatulence and diarrhea. There are two ways to plan for a gradual increase of fiber to avoid side effects. The bran method maintains your normal diet, but adds gradually increasing amounts of bran (the outer coating of wheat) sprinkled on cereal or mixed into beverages and sauces over a period of weeks. Start with the addition of 1 tablespoon of bran each day for the first week, add a second tablespoon each day for the following week, building up to a comfortable level (perhaps 6 tablespoons) at the same gradual rate of increase over the next month. Because water is absorbed by the colon as well as the bran, be sure to drink up to 8 to 10 glasses of water or other liquids daily.

The second method calls for a gradual evolution of your basic diet from whatever it normally has been to a total of about 5 grams of fiber per day, or whatever regulates bowel function for you. Plan to add about 1 gram to your daily menu for the first week, 2 grams the following week, and so on.

The Seventh-Day Adventists recommend a diet high in vegetable fiber and low in animal fats. (Their high-fiber diet plan is presented on the opposite page.) They suggest eating 2 or 3 servings per day of the highest fiber groups: vegetables such as artichokes, broccoli, peas, corn on the cob, and dried beans; cereals such as shredded wheat; whole-wheat bread, rye crackers, or bran muffins; fruits such as blackberries, figs, and unpeeled apples. Of the food groups that contain less fiber, they suggest somewhat fewer servings, with only occasional indulgence in low- or no-fiber foods. You would have to take a total of 12 servings from various high-fiber groups, plus 4 tablespoons of unprocessed bran, each day to meet both nutritional requirements and high-fiber standards.

The same problem is experienced by those who switch to a vegetarian diet (page 390), and in fact the two diets are quite similar. You may want to compromise in the following ways: substitute winter squash, bulgur wheat, or a dried-bean dish for potatoes, pasta, or rice several times a week. Change from low-fiber breakfast cereals like cornflakes to high-fiber granola or 100 percent bran cereals. Prefer apples or pears (both with skins) and oranges to plums, bananas, and melons. Serve corn on the cob, peas, and broccoli more often than soft vegetables like asparagus and beets. Dried fruits, sunflower seeds, and nuts can be used as snacks.

The bran method may be preferable for the elderly who eat little and often have difficulty chewing. An excellent way to add bran is to include it in muffins and pancakes. Each muffin in the following recipe contains 1½ tablespoons of bran.

BASIC BUTTERMILK BRAN MUFFINS

1¾ cups all-purpose or whole-wheat flour
1¾ cups bran
2 tablespoons sugar
1½ teaspoons baking soda
2 cups buttermilk
1 egg, beaten
½ cup unsweetened molasses (blackstrap)
3 tablespoons melted butter or margarine

MAKES EIGHTEEN TO TWENTY MUFFINS
1. Combine the flour, bran, sugar, and baking soda in a large bowl.
2. Beat together the buttermilk, egg, molasses, and butter or margarine.
3. Add the liquid mixture to the dry ingredients in the bowl and stir together only enough to moisten.
4. Fill greased muffin tins two-thirds full and bake for about 25 minutes in a 350-degree oven.

The dry ingredients in this recipe can be kept as a mix to use at your convenience. Quadruple the quantities and store in a tightly closed tin or jar. When you wish to make muffins, measure out 3½ cups of the dry mixture and proceed with the recipe. For variety, you can fold in 1 cup of chopped nuts, raisins, dates, or candied orange rind just before baking, or you can add 2 tablespoons of grated orange rind to the dry mixture just before you add the liquid. A half cup of mashed, ripe bananas stirred into the finished batter gives you banana muffins.

Fiber on a Scale of 0 to 6

Most people can easily fulfill moderate needs for fiber in the diet just by eating fresh fruit or bran cereal or whole-wheat bread each day. However, when a person is told to eat a high-fiber diet, the choices can be difficult. Where will all that fiber come from? The Seventh-Day Adventist Dietetic Association has devised the following plan for a high-fiber diet which groups foods according to their fiber content—beginning with Group 0, which is nearly fiber free, to Group 6, highest in fiber. The idea is to limit servings of low-fiber foods (Groups 0-2) and eat most foods from Groups 3-6.

Group 0: Residue free; limit use.
Cereal beverages
Bouillon, broth
Margarine, butter, vegetable oil
Whipped cream, nondairy creamer
Eggs
Meat, poultry, fish
Fruit juices, clear
Seasonings

Group 1: Minimal fiber; limit use.
Flour, white; jelly, plain
Bread, plain white, cornbread, French bread
Crackers, plain white, no seeds
Pasta; rice, white, refined
Cereals, plain, cooked, refined
Oatmeal, instant, quick cooking
Fruit juices, nectars
Vegetable juices, strained
Texturized vegetable protein entrées

Group 2: Low in fiber; may use some.
Rice, brown
Cereals, most cold
Applesauce, avocado, banana, cantaloupe
Plums, canned
Asparagus tips, canned; beets, cooked
Lettuce, butterhead, red leaf
Tomato, peeled, canned
Oatmeal, rolled oats, old fashioned
Cornmeal cereal; pancakes, plain

Group 3: Use at least 2 servings.
Fruit, most canned, cooked, peeled, fresh ½ cup or 1 medium; strawberries, fresh, 10 large
Vegetables, most canned or cooked without peel or seeds, ½ cup
Cucumber, ¼ medium
Turnips, fresh, ¼ cup
Tomato, fresh, peeled, 2 small
Peanut butter, 2 tbsp, smooth
Lettuce, iceberg, romaine, endive, 2 cups
Split peas, cooked, 1 cup

Group 4: Use at least 5 servings.
Cereals, with dried fruits or nuts, ½ cup
Beans, green or wax
Raisins, 8 tbsp
Oranges, fresh, 1 medium
Figs, fresh, 2 small
Dates, 4
Prunes, 6 large
Potato, white with peel, 2½" diameter
Beet greens, ½ cup
Pumpkin, canned; winter squash, ½ cup
Beans, pinto, brown, ½ cup
Popcorn, 3 cups

Group 5: Use at least 2 servings.
Flour, bread, or crackers, all whole wheat or rye, 4 tbsp, 2 slices, 6 crackers
Corn, 4" ear or ½ cup
Broccoli, 1 stalk
Parsnips, ½ large
Peas, green, ½ cup
Beans, white, soy, lentils, kidney, ½ cup
Nuts, Brazil, 4 medium; cashews, 16; pecan halves, 12; filberts, 4; pistachio, 30
Pear, 1 large
Cereal, shredded wheat, 1 large biscuit

Group 6: Use at least 3 servings.
Cereals, bran, ¼ cup
Bran, unprocessed, 4 tbsp
Bran muffins
Raspberries, blackberries, fresh, ⅓ cup; canned, ¼ cup
Figs, dried, 2 small
Persimmon, fresh, 1 medium
Currants, dried, ¼ cup
Apple, fresh, 1 large
Artichoke, cooked, edible portion
Garbanzos (chick-peas), ½ cup
Sunflower seeds, ½ oz

Detecting Food Allergies/Elimination Diets

Allergic reactions occur when the body attacks and attempts to rid itself of a foreign substance, usually a protein. Chemicals produced by the body during the attack are responsible for allergic symptoms. The attack—often mild at first and severe only subsequently—may be occasioned when the offending substance touches the skin, as with poison ivy, or the mucous membranes of eyes and the respiratory system, as in hay fever and asthma. The reaction may also be caused by eating the substance.

Symptoms are not determined by the way in which the allergen is contacted. Food allergies may result in symptoms of many kinds. The person who eats a food he is allergic to may cough, wheeze, or get a stuffy nose. He may develop a headache or feel dizzy, complain of cramps and bellyache, vomit or get diarrhea, or simply belch often. A classic symptom of food allergy is hives—patches of red, swollen, itching skin—but rashes and eczema are common too. Allergic symptoms are so varied that mild food allergies may be mistaken for a prolonged cold, dry skin—or not even noticed. In fact, mere dislike for a certain food may indicate a food allergy. Doctors have found that discomfort following the eating of a particular food is registered, perhaps at a subconscious level, as an aversion to that food.

Inherited Tendencies

Food allergies are common in infants as they are introduced to cow's milk and solid foods. These early allergies tend to fade away after the age of 6. However, food allergies can begin at any age and actually are more common in adulthood than in childhood. The tendency to develop an allergy runs in families. For example, parents who have hay fever or any other sort of allergy may have a child with eczema or any other sort of allergy.

The most common allergy-causing foods are:

Wheat	Chocolate	Tomatoes
Milk	Corn	Chicken
Eggs	Nuts	Pork
Seafood	Strawberries	

Reactions can also be to "hidden" ingredients such as the corn oil in baby's formula or the mold in cheese. Small quantities of a food may not cause a reaction, whereas a normal or a large amount will, so that if a child is allergic to chocolate he may be able to eat a chocolate chip cookie but can't gobble up those chocolate bars he collects on Halloween. There are a few foods that almost never cause allergic symptoms. They are:

Rice	Peaches	Artichokes
Lamb	Pears	Sesame oil
Gelatin	Carrots	
Apples	Lettuce	

Once a doctor suspects a food allergy, he may suggest one or more tactics for identifying which food (or foods) is the culprit. Skin-patch tests, so useful for tracking down other sorts of allergens, are not very accurate for food allergies and are only used as confirmation with other methods of diagnosis. The food diary is more helpful. A food diary is a detailed record kept by the patient of all food and medication taken daily over a period of weeks. The patient also notes the times of allergic symptoms in an effort to associate the onset of an allergic reaction with a specific food eaten. But allergic reactions may occur anywhere from 20 minutes to a day after the food is eaten, so a food diary by itself is often not sufficient either.

Another method to track down the offending food is called simple elimination and challenge. First, those foods that are notorious for causing reactions (see preceding list) are eliminated from the diet. If symptoms subside during the three weeks the patient adheres to the diet, he is challenged with each of the foods in turn—in small amounts and at 10-day intervals—to see which of the foods causes the reaction to flare up again. That food can then be avoided in the future.

The most accurate, but also the most demanding tactic for identifying foods a patient is allergic to is called sequenced elimination. The method entails scrupulous adherence to one or more diets over a period of several months.

Each of the diets allows only foods that rarely cause trouble, and each of the diets in the sequence is more restricted than the one before. Diet 1, for example, may eliminate all cereals and dairy products but allow a good selection of fruits, vegetables, and meats. If the patient still has symptoms on that diet, the next elimination diet may restrict him to two kinds of meat, six vegetables, and no fruits at all. By the time a patient whose symptoms still persist must follow the last diet, his eating is very

The Chocolate Headache

People get headaches for many reasons—a sinus infection, a hangover, tension—but some pains in the head are caused by foods in the stomach. Allergic headaches may be the mild sort that are often accompanied by a stuffy nose or a feeling of pressure in the sinuses. Or they may be pounding headaches that make you really want to get away from it all. At the worst, food allergy can cause migraine, a particularly painful type of headache that usually affects only one side of the head and may be accompanied by dizziness, nausea, and oversensitivity to light and sound.

Notorious headache foods include wine, nuts—and chocolate. Some people can diagnose their chocolate headache easily. They eat a chocolate bar and within 20 minutes they begin to feel stuffed up and headachy. In other cases, the headache is not so easily connected with what was consumed. A new white wine may contain smaller quantities of allergenic products than an aged, red Bordeaux, with other wines, including sherries, vermouths, cordials, and brandies, falling in between. The same is true of nuts. So a person may have white wine with salted almonds for cocktails one night and feel fine, but be felled with a splitting headache after an apparently similar cocktail menu of sherry and cashews.

Certainly, if you are the sort of person who gets frequent headaches, you should ask your doctor about the possibility of a food allergy before you assume that you are a tense, grouchy person.

---

restricted indeed. One version calls for lamb, potatoes, peas, carrots, and pearl tapioca—every day for three weeks!

Some aspects of sequenced elimination diets may seem irrational. Why pearl tapioca specifically when minute tapioca would be so much easier? The answer indicates just how detailed this procedure is. Minute tapioca contains citric acid, one of the suspected substances eliminated at this phase of the plan. Because of such detail, the number of substances and foods the person is *not* allowed to eat is far too long to bother printing. Sequenced elimination diets list only what the patient is allowed to eat. Needless to say, the whole procedure is for naught if the patient does not follow it assiduously.

Luckily, many people with a suspected food allergy do not have to go through the entire course of sequenced elimination. The foods they are allergic to are most likely to be among those eliminated in the first phase, when the choice of foods is reasonably large. But even if symptoms subside early, reintroduction of each eliminated substance is done very gradually, waiting each time to see whether there is a reaction before reintroducing the next food to the diet.

When an allergen is identified through reintroduction, close relatives of that food may be suspect too. A child allergic to peanuts, a legume, will often be allergic to other legumes, such as beans and peas, but not allergic to true nuts such as cashews or walnuts. The groups of foods listed in the chart on the following page show some of these food-family relationships. A person allergic to one food in a family is likely to be allergic to some or all of the other foods in that group.

The usual treatment of a food allergy is simply to avoid the food. This is not difficult for a single, seasonal food such as strawberries. But avoidance may be more complicated than that—or more tricky. People who are allergic to fish, for example, may get a reaction from licking labels that have been spread with an adhesive derived from fish. People who are allergic to nuts may have to watch out for walnut oil and coconut oil, and if they are allergic to peanuts and beans too, many other oils derived from legumes will have to be eliminated, leaving limited choice for cooking and salad dressings. When a person is allergic to a really common ingredient, such as eggs, milk, or wheat, labels on every sort of commercial food product must be scrutinized carefully to determine what it contains. Egg, milk, and wheat derivatives are found in many foods, from candy bars to canned soups. Because allergens may be hard to recognize under their various aliases—and also because there may be many allergens involved or there may be obscure additives or ingredients that manufacturers are not legally required to disclose—allergists must tailor particular diets for their pa-

Food Allergies
Elimination Diets

tients and offer specific instruction in their use.

Desensitization to a food allergen is possible, but is important only when the food is a nutritional staple such as milk or wheat. Under a doctor's supervision, the patient takes minute quantities of the allergen at prescribed intervals. The substance is sneaked in, so to speak, in amounts so small the body's defenses are not alerted. In time, as amounts are increased very gradually, the patient may become able to eat normal quantities without provoking a reaction.

Food allergies often subside or disappear over time without treatment, especially if the reaction was originally mild. Your doctor may suggest trying a small amount of the food once or twice a year to check for a reaction. If the reaction was originally severe, such trials are not advisable unless under the doctor's close supervision.

Infant Allergies

Foods to which babies most frequently become allergic are cow's milk, eggs (especially the whites), citrus juice (if it contains oils from the skin and seeds), and wheat. Since the tendency to allergy is inherited, allergy-prone families should be sure to consult their doctor about introducing cow's milk and solid foods to their baby. Some doctors prefer to delay introduction of eggs, orange juice, and baby cereals that contain wheat until the baby is over six months old. Since cow's milk is so frequently a problem, most doctors recommend breast-feeding in the early months.

Once a baby is suspected of having a food allergy, he is often put on what is called a basic trial diet made up of foods that seldom cause a reaction. Usually the diet is rice cereal and strained carrots, peaches, pears, and lamb, plus a vitamin supplement.

For babies sensitive to cow's milk, substitutes include goat's milk, soy milk (but this is also a common allergen), or a meat-base formula, particularly lamb. Meat-base formula is liked by babies and is nutritionally adequate, being similar in composition to the breast milk they are accustomed to drinking.

Related Food Allergies

Apple	Apple, pear, quince
Blueberry	Blueberry, huckleberry, cranberry
Citrus	Orange, lemon, grapefruit, lime, tangerine, kumquat, citron
Rose	Strawberry, raspberry, blackberry, boysenberry
Plum	Plum, cherry, peach, apricot, nectarine, almond
Melon (gourd)	Watermelon, cucumber, cantaloupe, pumpkin, squash, other melons
Potato	Potato, tomato, eggplant, green pepper, red pepper (including chilies, paprika, cayenne; but not black and white peppers); chili powder
Parsley	Carrot, parsnip, celery, parsley, anise, dill, fennel, celery seed, cumin, coriander, caraway
Mustard	Mustard, turnip, radish, horseradish, watercress, cabbage, sauerkraut, Chinese cabbage, broccoli, cauliflower, Brussels sprouts, collards, kale, kohlrabi, rutabaga
Aster	Lettuce, chicory, endive, escarole, artichoke, dandelion, sunflower seeds, tarragon
Beet	Beet, spinach, chard
Laurel	Avocado, cinnamon, bay leaves
Buckwheat	Buckwheat, rhubarb, garden sorrel
Onion	Onion, garlic, asparagus, chives, leeks, sarsaparilla
Pea	Peanuts, peas, beans, licorice (also acacia and tragacanth, which are sometimes used as food additives)
Ginger	Ginger, cardamom, turmeric (which are ingredients of curry powder)
Grass	Wheat, corn, rice, oats, barley, rye, wild rice, millet, bamboo sprouts (cane, as in cane sugar, and sorghum, as in sorghum molasses)
Chocolate	Chocolate, cocoa, cola
Mallow	Cottonseed, okra
Fungus	Mushrooms, yeast, molds, antibiotics
Walnut	Walnut, black walnut, pecan
Cashew	Cashew, pistachio, mango
Myrtle	Allspice, guava, clove, pimiento
Palm	Coconut, date
Crustacean	Crab, lobster, shrimp
Mollusk	Oyster, clam, mussel, snail (escargot), squid, octopus, abalone
Bird	Chicken, turkey, duck, goose, guinea fowl, Rock Cornish game hen, pigeon, quail, pheasant, eggs
Fish	Fish of all kinds, including tuna, sardine, catfish, trout, and crappie

SPECIAL DIETS FOR SPECIAL NEEDS

Food Intolerance/Lactose-Restricted Diet

Food intolerance is often confused with food allergy because abdominal symptoms such as bellyache and diarrhea may be similar. With a food allergy the body's defense system against a foreign substance is responsible for symptoms, whereas with intolerance the body's lack of an enzyme to digest the substance or the inability of the intestine to absorb it is responsible for symptoms.

The two substances to which intolerance is most common are lactose, the major sugar in milk, and gluten, a protein in wheat. Gluten intolerance is relatively rare, affecting only 1 in 1,500 people in this country. Lactose intolerance is quite common. In fact, it has been estimated that from 70 to 90 percent of most peoples in the world have some difficulty with milk sugar digestion.

The Trouble with Milk

The milk sugar lactose is found in every kind of milk, whether from a cow, goat, or human. Babies produce an enzyme called lactase to digest lactose. But mammals normally produce less and less lactase after weaning and as they grow to adulthood, and this is true of many humans also. The milk sugar can no longer be completely digested. Instead, the sugar remaining in the intestine provides extra nourishment for bacterial colonies, and their by-products in turn cause reactions that contribute to unpleasant symptoms ranging from mild distention and bellyache to severe cramps and diarrhea.

Lactose intolerance is common among those of African, Asian, American Indian, or Mediterranean descent. It is rare among those of Caucasian (Central or Northern European) descent. Children who claim to dislike milk may have developed the aversion unconsciously as a result of the discomfort that follows drinking milk. Therefore, you should suspect lactose intolerance if a child avoids drinking milk or if any person complains of discomfort after having milk, ice cream, or cream cheese. Your doctor can diagnose the condition by a blood test following the drinking of a lactose solution.

A person's lactase deficiency is seldom so severe that he must eliminate all lactose from his diet. He may be able to enjoy an ice cream cone, but not be able to drink a full glass of milk without feeling the effects later. Also, fermented milk products, such as buttermilk, sour cream, yogurt, cottage cheese, acidophilus milk, and aged cheeses may not affect him because most of the milk sugar has already been digested by the fermenting bacteria. Therefore, milk products are restricted rather than eliminated. A severely restricted or even lactose-free diet is seldom required. When it is, medical supervision is needed because the diet supplies inadequate calcium.

Since many lactase-deficient people can tolerate up to a half-cup of milk or its equivalent, the following equivalents should help menu planning.

Dairy products with amount of lactose equivalent to that in ½ cup milk.

Milk: whole, low fat, skim, buttermilk, ½ cup
Condensed milk, 2 tablespoons
Evaporated milk, ¼ cup
Processed cheese food or cheese spread, 3 ounces
Cream: half-and-half, whipped, sour, ½ cup
Yogurt, ½ cup
Ice cream, ½ cup

The following foods contain small amounts of lactose and are generally well tolerated.

Butter
Cottage cheese
Soft cheeses (cream cheese, Neufchatel)
Aged cheese (Swiss, American, and others)
Commercial foods processed with small amounts of milk, milk products, milk solids, or lactose

For those who experience discomfort even after the small amounts of lactose found in breads or breakfast cereals, label reading will be necessary. Whey and malt indicate a milk product that contains lactose. Lactalbumin, lactate, lactic acid, and calcium compounds do not contain lactose.

Watch out for unlikely products that may contain milk solids. Frankfurters and cold cuts are two examples. A completely lactose-free diet even lists molasses, chocolate, chewing gum, and orange-flavored Kool-Aid under foods to avoid (lactose is used as a sweetener in these and other products). If your doctor prescribes a severely restricted diet, you may wish to write to selected manufacturers for a list of the lactose-free products made by that company. Soybean products, from soy milk to bean cheeses, can be a great help in filling the nutritional gap left when dairy products are very restricted. Your doctor may advise such a strategy, especially with growing children. Calcium, riboflavin, and vitamin D supplements are prescribed in cases where children's diets contain less than the equivalent of 3 cups of milk per day.

Food Intolerance
Gluten-Restricted Diet

Gluten is a protein found in large quantities in certain grains, including wheat, rye, barley, and oats, and in much smaller amounts in many other foods. People who cannot tolerate gluten are not deficient in the proper enzyme for its digestion, as are people who cannot tolerate lactose. Rather, their intestinal lining is sensitive to a portion of the gluten protein and fails to absorb it. The most obvious symptom of gluten intolerance is large, greasy, smelly bowel movements.

For a long time, there seemed to be several disorders that shared the same symptom. The condition was called celiac disease in children, nontropical sprue and ideopathic steatorrhea in adults. It is now thought that all three conditions are probably the same disorder, which has been renamed primary malabsorption syndrome. The condition appears to be hereditary and affects about 1 in 1,500 people in this country (it is far more common in Ireland and England). Symptoms vary in severity from mild diarrhea to serious debilitation unless treated. Intolerance is also variable. Some gluten intolerant people are not able to cope with even minute amounts of gluten, whereas others can eat a slice or two of bread each day.

The treatment for gluten intolerance is dietary. Gluten is restricted by eliminating all grains except corn and rice (which are low in gluten). Baking, thickening, and breading is done with flours, meals, and starches derived from corn, rice, soybeans, potatoes, or tapioca. Most of these products are available where specialty foods are sold.

Unfortunately, the disallowed grains are ubiquitous ingredients in all sorts of food. Malt (sprouted barley or other grain) is used in cereal beverages, so malted-milk powders and diet drinks are not allowed. Malt is also an ingredient of beer and ale. Wheat flours are used to thicken commercial sauces, gravies, soups, puddings, ice cream, mayonnaise, and even salad dressing. Wheat flours and breadcrumbs are used as binders and fillers in meat loaf, sausages, frankfurters, and cold cuts. Many commercial candies contain grain products; so do most cheese spreads and many brands of instant coffee. Since manufacturers are not required to list gluten as an ingredient on labels, even pickles and bottled horseradish are suspect unless the manufacturer has verified that they are gluten free, or unless they appear on special brand-name product lists supplied by your doctor.

Some of the terms that might appear on labels, and that mean gluten is present, include:

wheat, rye, barley, oats	malt
wheat flour	malted milk
enriched wheat flour	hydrolyzed vegetable protein
wheat starch	plain vegetable protein
cake meal	starch
rye flour	hydrolyzed plant protein
oat flour	modified food starch
rolled oats	cereal
flour	millet
graham	

A number of companies make gluten-free products. For a list, write to the American Celiac Society, 45 Gifford Avenue, Jersey City, New Jersey 07304.

The Origin of Tolerance

Because a lessened ability to digest milk sugar in adulthood is normal both in humans and other animals, the question is not why there is intolerance but why anyone past infancy should tolerate lactose at all. Why do some groups of people continue to produce babylike levels of lactase all their lives?

The answer may lie in the nutritional history of each people over thousands of years. Those groups who never had to rely on dairy products of any kind did not develop lactose tolerance. That includes most African and some Asian peoples, whose adult levels of lactase are properly mature—and low. Those groups who depended on low-lactose dairy products such as yogurt and aged cheese developed sufficient tolerance to cope with small amounts of dairy foods. That is true of most Mediterranean and some Asian peoples whose diet included fermented, but not fresh, dairy products. Finally, those who depended on fresh milk and cream in addition to fermented products developed the unusual ability to maintain high levels of lactase even in adulthood. Before modern refrigeration, that was possible only in cool climates where souring could be prevented. Today, most Central and Northern European peoples are lactose-tolerant.

Less Food for Stones

In the United States, about 1 in 1,000 adults suffer from stones that form in the kidney or bladder. From 70 to 90 percent of these stones are made up primarily of calcium, and in about half these cases the urine is found to be unusually high in calcium. The calcium remains undissolved and comes together as the crystals that form the stones. Acidic urine helps to redissolve crystals, but often the urine of patients plagued by stones is alkaline.

Using common sense, doctors have put such urinary stone patients on a dietary regime that has three goals: to dissolve more calcium by drinking lots of fluids, to prevent calcium crystals from forming by restricting foods to those that make urine more acidic, and to decrease the amount of calcium by limiting calcium-containing foods.

Although stones occur with greater frequency in people who drink large quantities of milk (several quarts a day), for many patients there is no relationship between how much calcium is eaten and how much calcium appears in the urine. Also, calcium stones may form even when calcium levels in urine are normal. Therefore, a calcium-restricted diet is prescribed to selected patients who may benefit from it.

The Recommended Dietary Allowance for calcium is 1,200 milligrams for children up to 18, and 800 for adults. Calcium intake can be cut to 600 milligrams a day by eliminating all milk, cheese, ice cream, custards, and cream soups as well as calcium-containing greens such as collards, dandelions, and beet greens. Canned sardines and canned salmon are not allowed either because the bones in them contain large amounts of calcium.

A less restricted diet may allow up to 600 milligrams of calcium in the form of 2 cups of milk, 3 ounces of cheese, or 3 cups of ice cream—hardly a sacrifice.

Much of the world does not grow quantities of such gluten-rich grains as wheat and barley. Therefore, there are interesting cuisines to turn to that can supply carbohydrates and other nutritional needs through allowed grains and starches. Hispanic cuisines, including Mexican and Puerto Rican, emphasize corn meal and corn flour, delicate, starchy yams, and a member of the banana family called plantain that is used as a starchy vegetable. In addition, they have tasty rice and bean dishes. Both Chinese and Japanese people use rice as their staple grain. In these cuisines soups and sauces are thickened with cornstarch, tapioca, or water-chestnut starch; cookies, candies, and other confections are made from rice flour and soybean paste; and deep-fried meats and vegetables are coated in a delicate cornstarch batter. It would certainly be worthwhile to take some Hispanic and Oriental cookbooks out of your local library to try some of the tasty, low-gluten alternatives for which these cuisines are known. You and your family will be delighted.

When planning meals, emphasize gluten-restricted dishes that everyone will like. That way, special cooking is avoided, and the person who is gluten intolerant does not have to feel put out or left out. For example, here are some excellent suggestions to add variety to Sunday breakfasts.

- Eggs and bacon with grits (a corn cereal also called hominy) served with butter, salt, and freshly ground black pepper
- Potato pancakes served with applesauce
- Cold boiled rice sprinkled with currants and served with cream and brown sugar
- Cinnamon toast or French toast made with homemade gluten-free bread, and broiled ham
- Pan fried or baked cornbread served hot with melted butter and maple syrup
- Corn fritters dusted with confectioners' sugar

Snack foods are no problem. Corn chips, popcorn, and potato chips are all allowed, and so are the variously shaped and flavored corn and rice breakfast cereals—not to mention lots of healthier snack fare. Morning toast and sandwiches might be the biggest sacrifice were it not for the fact that you can get gluten-free wheat flour to make your own bread dough. Or you can substitute 1⅓ cups soy flour for 1 cup of wheat flour in recipes. Don't expect success on the first try, but with a little practice you can make even hotdog and hamburger rolls.

Coping with Dietary Limitations

Many Americans today are concerned that their diets include too much fat, sugar, and salt. They have read that overconsumption of salt is implicated in high blood pressure; that unusual levels of certain kinds of fat are involved in coronary heart disease; and that high levels of both fat and sugar are a probable factor in diabetes. These three conditions together affect close to 50 million adult Americans and constitute leading causes of premature death in this country. But an exaggerated concern is not justified; the evidence linking these diseases to diet is inconclusive.

Common as it may be for a doctor to suggest that a patient control the amounts of fat, sugar, or salt in his diet, that is rarely his first advice. More likely, he will have noted another, underlying condition long before the middle-aged symptoms that warn of impending disease. That condition is obesity. Up to 85 percent of the adults who develop diabetes are obese at the time of onset, and so are many patients who develop high blood pressure. There is little medical justification for controlling the proportions of fat, sugar, or salt in your diet if you remain fat. So when a doctor suspects that you are a candidate for such diet-related diseases, he will often suggest merely that you get your weight down. Maintaining normal weight alone may well allow you to continue to eat the proportions of animal fat, refined sugar, and table salt that you have always enjoyed.

That is the good news. The bad news is that there is only one intelligent way to lose weight: consume fewer calories. Water, bananas, unusual proportions of protein or carbohydrates—all these fad diets are ineffective and sometimes risky (see pages 282-292). Yet cutting down on calories is essentially a boring method for losing weight; it will never make the best-seller lists. To relieve boredom and engage your own ingenuity in the struggle against overweight, learn the ins and outs of a diet method called an exchange plan. Used without creativity, an exchange plan at least makes menu planning easier. Used with panache, it can make the whole routine a foxy game of food finagling.

This is the way a weight-loss exchange plan works. Food is divided into six exchange groups: milk, protein, vegetable, fruit, fat/oil, and bread/grain/starchy vegetables. Each group is a list of foods, specified by serving size, that are identical in the amounts of calories they contain per serving. In the protein group, for example, 1 ounce of fresh lean meat, or 5 clams, or ½ ounce Roquefort cheese, or 2 teaspoons of peanut butter each contain 60 calories. You are allowed a specified number of servings (called exchanges) in each group each day, depending on your calorie needs as determined by your doctor. So long as you stick with the right number of exchanges in each group, you need not worry about nutrition—that is built into the plan—or about calories.

Now comes the creativity. Perhaps you have been suffering through repetitive yogurt lunches (or perhaps you refuse to). Yogurt, you will find, is a milk exchange that you may take in the form of whole milk if you wish. That whole milk might be used to turn a dull dinner into luscious oyster stew. Oyster crackers to go with the stew? No problem. You are allowed 20 oyster crackers as one bread exchange—the equivalent of a piece of toast. Getting back to lunch, now that you don't have to eat yogurt you may think you will have to suffer instead with spinach salad dressed with lemon juice. But no, there is no rule against salad dressing in this exchange plan, nor are fatty avocados forbidden. If you want to indulge in an avocado salad dressed with vinaigrette that day, all you have to do is forego gravy—which doesn't go well with oyster stew anyway—or refuse nibbles of peanuts with cocktails. About that cocktail, it is allowed as a starch exchange—occasionally.

The choices go on and on. You do not have to give up cream in your coffee or even sour cream and a baked potato so long as you acknowledge that you thereby use up one of your fat exchanges and one of your starch exchanges. Happily, you are even allowed a sugar exchange dole of jam or syrup every day. The cleverest dieter will realize that since the 75 calories in a sugar exchange is without nutritional value, those calories could be traded in for a second helping of spaghetti.

The creative knack will not come all at once. Probably the best approach is to choose your least favorite group—the milk exchanges perhaps—and see if you can find ways of using them that are more interesting than a straight glass of milk. Next, learn your way around with the other small exchange groups, the fats and the proteins. Finally, take on the great challenge: carbohydrates. Goodbye parsnips—hello pancakes!

Food Exchange Plan

Each of the following food groups contains foods of similar nutritional quality. Foods in one group may be substituted or alternated with any other food in the same group, keeping in mind the serving size. *Caution:* limit pastries, cakes, pies, candy, ice cream, fried foods, cream sauces and soups, alcohol.

Milk Group *(80 cal per serving)*
Whole milk ½ cup
Skim milk 1 cup
1% milk ¾ cup
Buttermilk (skim) 1 cup
Evaporated whole milk ¼ cup
Yogurt, low fat, plain ¾ cup
Yogurt, low fat, fruit ⅓ cup
Nonfat dry milk powder ⅓ cup

Protein Group *(60 cal per serving)*
Beef, pork, lamb, veal, lean, trimmed cuts 1 oz
Poultry, without skin 1 oz
Fish, all kinds fresh or frozen 1 oz
Fish, canned ¼ cup
Crab, lobster ¼ cup
Clams, oysters, shrimps, scallops 5 of each or 1 oz
Organ meats 1 oz
Cottage cheese, regular ¼ cup
Cottage cheese, low fat ½ cup
American process cheese ½ oz
Cheddar or Swiss cheese ½ oz
Roquefort or blue cheese ½ oz
Egg 1
Peanut butter 2 tsp
Frankfurter (8-9 to a pound) ½
Lunch meats, lean roast beef, boiled ham, chicken or turkey 1 oz (if other, ½ oz)

Bread, Grain, Starchy Vegetable Group *(70 cal per serving)*
Bread, white, French/Italian, whole wheat, rye, pumpernickel, raisin 1 slice each; corn 2" × 2" × 1" piece
Bagel, biscuit ½
English, corn, plain muffin ½
Hard roll ½ or 3" diameter
Hamburger, frankfurter roll ½
Tortilla (6" diameter) 1
Barley (cooked) ½ cup
Breadcrumbs 3 tbsp
Ready-to-eat cereal ¾ cup
Cooked cereal ½ cup
Rice, grits, spaghetti, noodles, macaroni (cooked) ½ cup
Cornmeal 2 tbsp
Flour 2½ tbsp
Wheat germ ¼ cup
Crackers, matzoh 4" × 6" ½, saltines 6, Graham 2, oyster 20
Popcorn (homemade) 1½ cups
Pretzels 3⅛" × 1⅛" 25
Rye wafers 2" × 3½" 3
Beans, peas, lentils (dried, cooked) ½ cup
Bean, pea soup ¼ cup
Canned soup (not creamed) 1 cup
Corn ⅓ cup
Corn on cob 1 small
Lima beans ½ cup
Parsnips ⅔ cup
Peas, green ½ cup
Potato, white 1 small
Potato, mashed ½ cup
Pumpkin ¾ cup
Squash, acorn, butternut, winter ½ cup
Yam ½ cup
Pancake (4" diameter) 1
Waffle (7" diameter) ⅓

Note: *Occasionally* one of these items may be substituted for one serving: 3 oz *dry* wine; 6 oz beer; 1 oz rye, scotch, gin, etc.

Vegetable Group *(25 cal per serving)*
(except as noted, ½ cup cooked or ¾ cup raw)
Artichoke, Asparagus,
Bean sprouts, Beets, Broccoli,
Brussels sprouts, Cabbage,
Carrots, Cauliflower, Celery,
Chicory 1 cup,
Chinese cabbage 1 cup,
Cucumbers, Eggplant,
Endive 1 cup, Escarole 1 cup,
Green pepper, Greens (beet, chard, collards, dandelion, kale, mustard, spinach, turnip), Lettuce 1 cup,
Mushrooms, Okra, Onions,
Parsley 1 cup, Radishes 1 cup,
Rutabaga, Sauerkraut, String beans,
Squash, summer, Tomatoes,
Watercress 1 cup, Zucchini

Fruit Group *(40 cal per serving)*
(all unsweetened)
Apple ½ medium
Apple juice ⅓ cup
Applesauce ½ cup
Apricots, fresh 2 medium
Apricots, dried 4 halves
Banana ½ small
Berries, blackberries, blueberries, raspberries ½ cup each, strawberries ¾ cup
Cherries 10 large
Cranberry juice ¼ cup
Dates 2 Figs, dried 1
Grapes 12 Grape juice ¼ cup
Grapefruit ½ medium
Grapefruit juice ½ cup
Mango ½ small
Melons, cantaloupe ¼ small, honeydew ⅛ medium, watermelon 1 cup
Nectarine 1 large
Orange ½ medium
Orange juice ½ cup
Papaya ¾ cup
Peach 1 medium
Pear ½ medium
Pineapple ½ cup
Pineapple juice ⅓ cup
Plums, prunes 2 medium
Prune juice ¼ cup
Raisins 2 tbsp
Tangerine 1 medium

Fat/Oil Group *(45 cal per serving)*
Butter, lard, hydrogenated shortening, vegetable oil, margarine 1 tsp
"Low-calorie" margarine 2 tsp
Salad dressing, mayonnaise 1 tsp
Salt pork ¾" cube
Gravy 1 tbsp
Sour cream 2 tbsp
Heavy cream 1 tbsp
Half-and-half 2 tbsp
Bacon (crisp) 1 strip
Avocado (4" diameter) ⅛
Nuts 1 tbsp
Olives 5 small

Coping with Dietary Limitations
Sodium-Controlled Diets

The probability that you or a member of your family will be put on a sodium-controlled diet at some point in your life is quite high. The reason is that there are so many and such common conditions for which less sodium is considered beneficial. Heart conditions, kidney disease, and hypertension—high blood pressure—are the more serious of those conditions. In addition, some degree of sodium control is often advised during pregnancy for patients taking some steroid medications, and even for women who suffer from premenstrual tension.

About a third of the sodium we consume occurs naturally in food, but the rest of it we add either in processing foods or in our own kitchens and dining rooms via the saltshaker. Table salt, or sodium chloride, is 40 percent sodium. The average American consumes at least 2 teaspoons of table salt each day, or nearly 4,000 milligrams of sodium. The body needs only 200 milligrams of sodium or less per day to function properly. That is the amount of sodium in about $\frac{1}{10}$ teaspoon of table salt.

Only hospitalized, very seriously ill patients would be put on a diet that kept sodium as low as twice the minimum requirement, or about 500 milligrams. Some people with a heart condition or hypertension have to cope with a restriction as severe as 1,000 milligrams of sodium per day—quite a demanding task for the meal planner, shopper, and cook. More often, however, sodium is restricted to between 2,000 and 3,500 milligrams per day, a level that is not nearly so hard to reach. Perhaps most frequently of all, a person is simply advised by his doctor to "cut down on salt," without either a specific goal in milligrams or a demanding strategy for sodium reduction. Whatever the degree of restriction, high blood pressure—or the avoidance of it—is the usual reason.

It has been estimated that 35.5 million Americans have high blood pressure, and of these about 90 percent have what is called essential hypertension, the type of high blood pressure that often responds to the lowering of sodium. Restricting sodium decreases blood pressure through a rather complicated mechanism having to do with how fluids move among cells and tissues, exerting pressure from within the blood vessels or balancing that pressure from without. When a person is found to have essential hypertension (through the simple procedure of a blood pressure test—that pumped-up cuff around the arm), the doctor almost always prescribes a change in diet as the primary course of treatment, with or without medication. Sodium will be reduced to some degree, depending on the severity of the person's condition; and if he is above his ideal weight, his diet will also limit the number of calories.

For mild hypertension, the No-Extra-Salt Diet (see page 378) or a similar list of instructions is generally prescribed. But for moderate or severe hypertension, or when there are other factors to be considered, instructions will probably be more complicated and may be in the form of an exchange plan (see page 375). The doctor may think it necessary to restrict cholesterol as well as sodium, for example, or may add potassium-containing foods to replace potassium that is lost with the use of some medications. You will have to consider the suggestions that follow in context with the diet your doctor prescribes for your unique needs.

To eat without the amount of salt you are accustomed to is to suffer, at least for a while. For one sufferer, famed gourmet Craig Claiborne, having to give up salt became a challenge for restructuring the eating habits of a lifetime. Refusing to give up the enjoyment of food, he banned salt from the kitchen and dining table, but launched into a cooking adventure that culminated in a triumph of brightly seasoned fresh foods.

Fresh Herbs All Year

Herbs fresh from the garden—or the windowsill—have far more distinctive flavors than the dried versions, and they can be used in larger quantities without unpleasant taste or texture. The most useful homegrown herbs are parsley, chives, mint, basil, sage, thyme, oregano, dill, marjoram, and tarragon. All of these are available either as seed or as young plants sold in garden centers during the spring. Harder to get, but worth the search, are rosemary and bay leaf, both of which make large, handsome houseplants (sage does too).

Indoors, all herbs require is plenty of sun and frequent pinching to keep the plants compact. None likes frequent watering, and their food needs are not voracious. Should a plant give up the ghost, replacing it is usually cheaper than buying a bottle of basil.

Tricks of the Trade

Nobody is perfect, and no diet is without its loopholes. Given the less than perfect patient who dreams of ways around restrictions and the loopholes that do exist in sodium-restricted diets, cleverness can pay off.

An exchange plan, for example, may allow the patient 2 milk exchanges a day, which might be taken as 2 glasses of milk—more than most adults are interested in—or 3 tablespoons of Parmesan cheese—enough for the whole family! No other aged or ripened cheeses are listed. Looking at the list on page 49, Parmesan cheese is much higher in sodium content per ounce than Brie, Camembert, Cheddar, mozzarella, Swiss, or blue cheese. The person who knows the tricks of the trade will weigh out the Parmesan, and then exchange it for its weight (or more) of ripe Brie or biting Cheddar.

Again, although an exchange plan might allow 2 units of salted fat, such as butter or margarine, it does not mention that the simple substitution of sweet butter allows you to sneak an extra 232 milligrams of sodium into some other sort of food. Two pats of sweet butter will buy you 8 black olives or more than a dozen potato chips! Or, the salt you save by opting for those same two unsalted pats could be traded in instead for catsup (52 milligrams per teaspoon), Worcestershire sauce (84 milligrams per teaspoon), or prepared mustard (57 milligrams per teaspoon). Those are all forbidden items on most sodium-restricted diets you see, but they are forbidden only because of their sodium content, not because the members of the medical profession bear any particular grudge against condiments.

Most lists and plans unequivocally prohibit bacon and yet allow bread. The average slice of bacon, however, contains an average of from 70 to 103 milligrams of sodium (depending on which list you read), whereas white bread averages 120 milligrams a slice. Give up 2 slices of toast, treat yourself to 2 slices of bacon.

To really learn such tricks of the trade, of course, you need extensive information about the sodium content of foods as well as your doctor's permission to exercise flexibility. A helpful publication is the U.S. Department of Agriculture's *The Sodium Content of Your Food*, available from the Consumer Nutrition Center, USDA, Federal Building, 6505 Belcrest Road, Hyattsville, Maryland 20782. Ask for Home and Garden Bulletin number 233. For a list of cookbooks and other useful information, write to the High Blood Pressure Information Center, 120/80 National Institutes of Health, Bethesda, Maryland 20205.

The list on page 49 gives you an idea of how much foods vary in their sodium content. But it is wise to always check with your doctor in case there are other dietary restrictions besides sodium to consider.

He says, "I know for a certainty that I taste natural flavors in greater depth.... It may take as long as four months before you notice a decided alteration in your taste buds and appreciation of flavors, but it does occur."

Why freshness and seasoning are crucial becomes obvious when you study the No-Extra-Salt Diet. Besides having to curtail the use of table salt severely, sodium-high condiments are not allowed. You cannot even get away with a gherkin. You will be even more dismayed if you are given an extensive list of additional foods forbidden because they contain naturally high sodium levels or because they are processed with sodium compounds. In the milk group, chocolate milk and malted milk may be prohibited. Among vegetables, tasty ones like artichokes, turnips, and mustard greens may be forbidden because, though unsalted, they are naturally higher in sodium than most vegetables. Dried fruit is often not allowed because it is processed with sodium sulfate. The forbidden bread and cereal list may be truly formidable: anything with baking soda or baking powder in it may not be allowed (both are sodium compounds), and quick-cooking or enriched cereals may not be allowed because they too are processed with a sodium-containing wetting agent. Anything that contains monosodium glutamate—MSG—is also prohibited. That includes just about any Chinese food unless you cook it yourself—without soy sauce, of course.

In fact, reading the labels on many kinds of processed foods will reveal sodium compounds:

Coping with Dietary Limitations
Sodium-Controlled Diets

sodium nitrate, sodium nitrite, sodium propionate, sodium alginate, and others. Claims such as "no salt added" or "low salt" do not guarantee low sodium. Unless the exact words used are "low-sodium dietetic," you must scrutinize the ingredients list. Even then you will have to trust your prohibited lists because there is as yet no law that forces manufacturers to list the sodium content of foods.

The No-Extra-Salt Diet

1. Do not add any salt to food at the table.
2. Limit salt used in cooking to ¼ teaspoon per pound of meat, and ⅛ teaspoon per serving of potatoes, vegetables, and cooked cereals.
3. Avoid the following foods:

Salt-cured meats; salted, canned, or processed meats, fish, and poultry; bacon; ham; dried beef; corned beef; salt pork; frankfurters; cold cuts; sausages; sardines; salted cheese and cheese foods; commercial casserole mixes; frozen dinners.

Sauerkraut; pickled vegetables; olives.

Commercially frozen vegetables and vegetable mixes with sauces.

Canned soups; dried soup mixes; broth; bouillon.

Commercially prepared salted salad dressings (except mayonnaise and mayonnaise-type dressings); commercial gravy and gravy mixes.

Salted snack foods; salted crackers; salted popcorn; pretzels; potato chips; corn chips; salted nuts and salted peanuts.

Cultured buttermilk; cocoa mixes; cocktail beverage mixes; club soda.

Seasoning salts; seasoning mixes; meat tenderizer; monosodium glutamate (MSG); soy sauce; bottled meat and barbecue sauce; catsup; prepared mustard; prepared horseradish.

4. Limit the following foods:

Organ meats (such as liver, heart, kidney); shellfish (such as shrimp, clams, lobster); and peanut butter to 2 servings per week.

Tomato-juice or vegetable-juice cocktail to ½ cup per day.

The reassuring thing to note about the No-Extra-Salt Diet and the more restrictive plans is that most high-sodium foods are processed in some way, from old-fashioned salt-cured hams and briny pickles to newfangled snack concoctions. That still leaves, as Craig Claiborne emphasizes in his low-sodium cookbook, *Craig Claiborne's Gourmet Diet*, most of nature's fresh meats, fish, poultry, vegetables, fruits, grains, and herbs, as well as butter the way it comes from the cow—sweet, not salted.

The following menus rely on fresh foods and fresh seasonings. Broth used in cooking, or bread to accompany meals, could be either commercial, low-sodium dietetic products or homemade without salt.

Breakfast	Honeydew melon sprinkled with fresh lime juice
	Irish oatmeal served with sweet cream and brown sugar
	Eggs scrambled with chopped fresh chives
	Tea or coffee
Lunch	Three-decker club sandwich with tomato, lettuce, and sliced chicken, seasoned with salt-free mayonnaise, freshly ground black pepper, and fresh basil
	Iced tea, coffee, or lemonade
Dinner	Hamburger, preseasoned with garlic put through a garlic press, and crushed green peppercorns (charcoal broil if possible)
	or
	Striped bass or red snapper, steamed in white wine with fresh ginger and green onions
	Asparagus or broccoli with simple vinaigrette (see recipe page 245, omit the salt)
	Bulgur wheat cooked in broth
	Wine, beer, or milk

The most lenient diet may allow ¼ teaspoon of table salt, which can be measured out each day into your personal saltshaker and used on whatever food on your day's menu you feel would be most enhanced. On a moderately restricted diet, the few fresh foods naturally high in sodium—chicken livers, mussels, spinach—may be allowed occasionally, and their strong flavors will be welcome. The strictest diet substitutes dialyzed low-sodium dairy products for regular ones and allows no high-sodium foods ever, much less any additional salt.

Whether your diet is lenient, moderate, or strict, you might wish to search out cuisines with an unusual complement of seasonings, such as Indian or North African, both of which use spices in abundance; and also those that offer novel combinations to please the palate. Russian cuisine combines preserved fruits with meat, for example. You can often double, triple, or even quadruple the seasonings called for in standard American recipes. We are known for a rather bland approach to food, so that the typically Americanized Italian recipe can use far more oregano, basil, or parsley than is called for. Favor snappy seasonings: cayenne pepper, green peppercorns, fresh ginger, fresh garlic, lime and lemon juice, various vinegars. Use fresh herbs whenever possible (see page 376 and also Herbs and Spices, pages 176-179). Grill meats over charcoal for extra flavor, or braise with very little liquid (try wine), lots of onions, garlic, and soup vegetables. The cooked-down sauces of nouvelle cuisine should come in handy here. Try for interesting textures too. Whole oats are chewy, whereas rolled oats are merely mushy. Cooked vegetables should be crisp instead of soft. Serve a greater number of items per meal so that there are as many different tastes as possible. Finally, expand your repertoire of condiments and relishes, all of which can be made without salt. Here are several you will find easy to make.

Salsa Fria

Salsa fria is a Mexican relish of fresh raw vegetables. Use it with hamburgers, chili, or on meat sandwiches.

2 pounds tomatoes, peeled, seeded, and chopped
1 Italian green pepper, chopped
1 large onion, chopped
1 clove garlic, pressed
1 teaspoon pepper
1 teaspoon crushed red pepper, or to taste
2 tablespoons fresh lemon juice
1 tablespoon olive oil

MAKES ONE PINT

1. Mix all the ingredients together in a large bowl.
2. Chill for several hours, then drain in a large strainer before serving.

Whole Tomato Chutney

This chutney is bright red, sweet, gingery, and chewy. The hotness depends on how much cayenne you use. It goes as well with roast meats and poultry as it does with Indian dishes. (If fresh ginger root is unavailable, you can substitute ½ teaspoon powdered ginger.)

1 pound-12-ounce can whole tomatoes, drained
6-8 cloves garlic, peeled and finely chopped
2-inch-long piece of fresh ginger root, peeled and finely chopped
1½ cups granulated sugar
⅛-½ teaspoon cayenne pepper
2 tablespoons golden raisins (optional)
2 tablespoons blanched slivered almonds (optional)
1½ cups wine vinegar

MAKES ABOUT ONE PINT

1. Place all the ingredients except the optional raisins and almonds in a heavy 4-quart saucepan.
2. Bring to a boil. Lower heat and simmer gently, uncovered, for about 1½ to 2 hours or until the liquid is syrupy.
3. Stir only occasionally at the beginning; toward the end stir frequently.
4. Add raisins and almonds at the very end, and simmer for 5 more minutes.
5. Remove from heat and let cool. Syrup should thicken to about the consistency of honey.

Marinated Carrot Relish

This tangy relish is good with any food that goes well with pickles or pickle relish such as meat loaf or grilled chicken or fish.

1 cup cooked carrots cut in julienne strips
Cider vinegar
⅛ teaspoon ground cayenne pepper, or to taste

1. Place the carrot strips in a small bowl and pour enough cider vinegar over them to cover.
2. Set aside to marinate for 3 to 6 hours.
3. Drain in a strainer and then mix ground cayenne pepper into the carrots, to taste.

Coping with Dietary Limitations
Sodium-Controlled Diets

BALLPARK MUSTARD

¼ cup mustard seeds
6 tablespoons dry mustard
1 tablespoon turmeric
1 teaspoon dried tarragon
1¼ cups boiling water
½ cup tarragon vinegar
½ cup dry white wine
1 tablespoon vegetable oil or peanut oil
¼ cup sugar
½ cup finely chopped onion
2 teaspoons finely minced garlic
¼ teaspoon ground allspice
¼ teaspoon ground cinnamon
¼ teaspoon ground cloves

MAKES ABOUT ONE AND ONE-HALF CUPS

1. Combine the mustard seeds, mustard, turmeric, tarragon, and water in a small bowl and let stand 1 hour.
2. Combine the vinegar, wine, oil, sugar, onion, garlic, allspice, cinnamon, and cloves in a saucepan.
3. Bring to a boil and simmer 5 minutes.
4. Pour the mustard and vinegar mixtures into the container of a blender and blend for about 2 minutes.
5. Scrape the mixture into the top of a double boiler and cook, stirring, for about 5 minutes. The cooled mustard can be sealed in jars and stored in the refrigerator.

OVERNIGHT PICKLES

Although pickles made without salt are never quite as crunchy as the usual product, these are very close, provided you choose your cucumbers carefully. Avoid those that are waxed because the flavors cannot easily penetrate the wax coating.

4 very firm, medium-size pickling cucumbers, scrubbed and thinly sliced
3 teaspoons whole pickling spices
2 teaspoons honey (or more if sweeter pickles are preferred)
2 teaspoons fresh dill, finely chopped
6 tablespoons white vinegar
2 tablespoons red wine vinegar
⅛ teaspoon cayenne pepper, or more to taste

MAKES ABOUT ONE PINT

1. Place the sliced cucumbers in a bowl.
2. Combine the remaining ingredients in a saucepan, bring to a boil and simmer for 1 minute.
3. Pour the hot mixture over the cucumbers and let stand for about an hour, or until the cucumbers have become slightly limp.
4. Empty the cucumbers and juice into a jar, cover and let chill in the refrigerator overnight.

The pickles can be safely stored in the refrigerator for several months. This same recipe can be used for pickling beets. Cook, peel, and slice 6 medium beets, and mix with a few thin slices of Bermuda onion if you wish. Continue as for cucumbers, leaving out the dill.

Salty Water

Water that contains more than 10 milligrams of sodium per cup may have to be included in your day's sodium tally, or it may not be allowed at all. To find out the sodium level in the public water supply, call your public health department, local water company, or local heart association. If you have a private water supply, such as a well, ask the public health department how to go about obtaining an analysis of its sodium content.

Water softeners add sodium to the water. Either do not use a water softener, or have it hooked up only to the hot-water system. That way you can use the cold tap water for both drinking and cooking.

When there is no way to get around a high-sodium water supply, you will have to buy distilled water both to drink and to use in cooking. Bottled spring water cannot substitute because it, too, may be high in sodium.

Besides these recipes, many cookbooks have recipes for catsup, mayonnaise, and various dressings that can be made for the person on a sodium-controlled diet merely by leaving out the salt. You might also be interested in *Better Than Storebought*, a cookbook written by Helen Witty and Elizabeth Colchie. It contains recipes for all sorts of foods forbidden on sodium-restricted diets, including meat extracts and bouillon cubes that are made without salt and many other commercial-like products such as prepared horseradish, cream cheese, peanut butter, liverwurst, and chili powder that can be made by leaving out the salt called for in the recipe. Dill pickles, alas, will not crisp without brine, but for flavorful brineless pickles try the recipe at left.

Sugar-Controlled Diets

Two disorders, hypoglycemia and diabetes, are often treated by controlling the amount of sugar in the diet. Both disorders involve abnormalities in glucose metabolism. Insulin, a hormone produced in the pancreas, facilitates the transport of glucose—blood sugar—into the body cells, thus providing energy for normal body functions. When converted into fats, glucose can be stored or excreted as the body requires. The amount of insulin in the bloodstream controls the amount of circulating glucose. When there is too little insulin, glucose accumulates in the bloodstream to damaging levels. When there is too much insulin, glucose levels drop to less than the body requires for ongoing energy needs.

In the person who has hypoglycemia, consumption of sugar triggers too sharp a rise in insulin. The insulin surge depletes glucose drastically, causing weakness, dizziness, faintness, and nausea. In diabetes, the pancreas does not produce adequate amounts of insulin. Glucose levels rise too high, yet because there is not enough insulin to convert glucose to usable forms, the body cannot easily meet its energy needs. Other routes to energy production are resorted to, and damage to blood vessels and serious chemical imbalances may result.

Although you may have heard quite a few people claim they suffer from hypoglycemia, it is actually a rare disorder. When the body detects a drop in glucose, it activates a general alarm: a surge of adrenalin. It is the adrenalin that is responsible for the symptoms of hypoglycemia. Most of the people who get those typical attacks of weakness and palpitations are instead suffering from anxiety. Anxiety attacks, however, also occasion a surge of adrenalin resulting in identical symptoms. There is no way for a doctor (or yourself) to differentiate between hypoglycemia and anxiety attacks by judging symptoms alone. Diagnosis can be accomplished only by a rather lengthy test. After fasting, the patient is given a measured amount of a glucose solution, then samples of blood are taken at 30-minute intervals over the next five hours. In the healthy person, the amount of glucose will peak in the first hour, then decline gradually to a point slightly below normal; in the hypoglycemic patient the already low glucose level will rise briefly, then drop to well below the norm. If such a low is reached and the symptoms are relieved by glucose, diagnosis is almost certain. Diet is similar to that for diabetes. Of course, it goes without saying that chronic anxiety over a long period is also a disorder, and should be treated.

There are two kinds of diabetes, one that begins in childhood and is usually severe, and another that begins in adulthood (sometimes hypoglycemia is a precursor) and ranges from very mild to severe. Many diabetics can be treated by diet alone. Some

Traveling on a Special Diet

For anyone on a demanding diet—and that includes any strict version of salt-, sugar-, or fat-controlled diets—traveling presents special difficulties. Snack foods are anathema, yet snacks are the common fare at roadside stops. Most restaurants are not prepared to cater to special needs. Airlines alone provide an impressive range of meals tailored to passengers' needs and preferences. Most require that you order 24 hours in advance.

For low-sodium dieters, here are some ways to get around salty restaurant foods. Scan the menu for cooked-to-order foods such as grilled or sautéed meats and fish. These can be ordered unsalted. Salads are salt free if eaten with oil and vinegar or lemon juice instead of prepared dressings. Baked potatoes are also salt free. Pasta with oil and garlic has very little salt. Vegetarian, health food, and nouvelle cuisine restaurants tend to salt food less than others.

For those on diets that control fats, sugars, carbohydrates, or overall number of calories, exchange lists (see page 375) offer the best guide to ordering from a restaurant menu.

When driving for long distances, take snacks that conform with your diet. A little picnic basket packed with the following snacks would be suitable for people on fat-controlled, sugar-controlled, and leniently salt-controlled diets:

Dried pork bits, unflavored rice crackers, cherry tomatoes, unsweetened dates, shelled walnuts, yogurt with raspberries

The only snack that needs cooking are the pork bits. Use pork loin, trimmed of all fat. Cut into ½-inch cubes and spread on cookie sheet. Season with pepper (and with salt if allowed). Bake in a 200-degree oven, turning occasionally until the cubes are dry and chewy—about 2 hours.

Coping with Dietary Limitations
Sugar-Controlled Diets

must receive insulin as well as attend carefully to diet. Children may be treated by medication alone; they are growing rapidly and their total caloric needs are not easy to meet when their sugar intake is too severely restricted. In contrast with the varying approaches to treating diabetes, people with hypoglycemia are treated only through diet.

Adult onset diabetes occurs most frequently in people whose diet is high in both fats and sugars, and who are obese. Although other factors such as inheritance play a role, the biggest contributors are too many calories in general, and too much sugar and fat in particular. Fat interferes with the ability of insulin to maintain blood sugar at normal levels. Therefore, the dietary principles are:

• Reduce caloric intake to achieve and maintain ideal weight.

• Decrease amounts of sugars such as sucrose, dextrose, and others (see page 196) that are rapidly absorbed and converted to glucose within the body.

• Increase the amounts of complex carbohydrates such as bread and potatoes that are absorbed over a longer period of time and converted to glucose more slowly within the body.

• Adjust the amounts of other foods such as fats and proteins as necessary to stay within the calorie limits of the diet.

In addition, sugar-controlled diets often call for a timing element that is not usual in other diets. Complex carbohydrates are eaten at intervals, as an afternoon or bedtime snack as well as at regular mealtimes, so that glucose production remains steady rather than fluctuates up and down. Even more specific timing is required when a person is also receiving insulin. The timing is tailored to the form of medication—whether oral or by injection—and to the dosage so that, depending on the doctor's exact instructions, the person may be eating specified portions of certain foods at certain times of the day in relation to the medication schedule. Often the "rules" must be worked out over a period of time to suit the patient's individual reactions.

Usually all "quick" sugars—including honey and sweetened fruit juices as well as cake, jam, and syrup—are forbidden. Carbohydrates may amount to half the day's allowance of calories. Since a frequent cause of premature death in diabetics is artery disease leading to heart attack, it is sensible that those who must control sugar intake eat prudently in other ways as well. For that reason, salt, saturated fats, and cholesterol may be limited too.

A diabetic diet is almost always presented as an exchange plan (see page 375). The exchange groups are about the same as in a weight-loss exchange plan, but in addition to each item in a group being equivalent in calories, items are also equivalent in the number of grams of protein, carbohydrate, and fat per serving. Serving sizes are specified, and the individual patient is told how many servings from each of the exchange lists he may have each day.

The American Diabetic Association explains how to use the concept of an exchange plan to decide whether you can allow yourself various processed foods that are probably not listed specifically on your prescribed plan. The technique uses information listed on the nutrition information panel of many processed foods. For example, the top portion of the panel on a package of brown-and-serve dinner rolls may give the following information:

Nutrition Information per Serving

Serving size	1 roll
Calories	120
Protein	2 grams
Carbohydrate	15 grams
Fat	5 grams

In order to decide whether you can use the dinner roll in your exchange plan, you need to know the protein, carbohydrate, and fat value per serving for each of the exchange groups.

	Protein	Carbohydrate	Fat
Milk exchange (low fat)	8 grams	12 grams	(trace)
Bread exchange	2 grams	15 grams	(trace)
Vegetable exchange	2 grams	5 grams	(trace)
Fruit exchange	(trace)	10 grams	(trace)
Meat exchange (low fat)	7 grams	(trace)	3 grams
Fat exchange	(trace)	(trace)	5 grams

Comparing the amounts of protein and carbohydrate in the dinner roll and in a bread exchange, they are exactly equivalent; the roll, however, contains an additional 5 grams of fat. If you wish to have a dinner roll, then, you would have to count it as one bread exchange plus one fat exchange.

What if the label on the dinner roll stated that it had 20 grams of carbohydrate? You might then

SPECIAL DIETS FOR SPECIAL NEEDS

The Dessert Dilemma

For families in which dinner has always been topped off by dessert, the evening meal may feel unfinished, the appetite unsatisfied, without a little something sweet. Letting everybody else have cake while the diabetic has a fruit exchange is not a happy solution. A better approach is to experiment with sugar-free desserts for everyone.

Begin with a common European dessert tradition: fruit and cheese. Try a ripe, juicy pear eaten with a tangy wedge of Camembert or, to prolong the eating, green grapes with cubes of sharp Cheddar. Walnuts and raisins are a wonderful fruit/nut combination; another good one is dates stuffed with blanched almonds. Dried apple rings all by themselves have the advantage of a satisfying chewiness, and the same is true of fresh coconut.

Many fruits freeze well. The American Diabetic Association suggests strawberries, blueberries, peaches, and melons in particular. They recommend freezing the fruits first spread out on a cookie sheet covered with waxed paper so the fruits are not touching one another. After they are hard (about four hours) scoop them into plastic bags. Frozen in this way, the fruits remain separate and can be shaken out of the bag in whatever quantities you wish without thawing the rest of the package. Serve thawed melon balls with lime juice or with chopped mint; berries are tasty served with sweet or sour cream.

Canning without sugar is also a possibility. Artificial sweeteners are not advisable, but you can use apple, pineapple, cranberry, or orange juice as the liquid called for in the recipe. Unsweetened applesauce, cooked with the red skins for a fine pink color, is very tasty.

Sometimes the richness of a dessert is as much a part of its appeal as its sweetness. Homemade ice cream, thick with cream and eggs, is incomparably smoother and richer than any commercial product. The sweetness of peaches or strawberries is sufficient—just leave out the sugar called for in the recipe if you are adding them to ice cream.

A good baked custard—again particularly if enriched with egg yolk and heavy cream—can be served with crushed pineapple; or a boiled custard could be poured over fresh peaches. Both can be made without sugar. There is even a way to make fruit-juice custard. Mix together 4 beaten egg yolks with 1 cup of fruit juice (a combination of apple and pineapple would be good). Bake as you would ordinary cup custard. Make a fruit soufflé with the 4 egg whites. Beat them until stiff, fold in ⅔ cup of a fruit puree (banana, plum, peach, or a combination of fruits), add a squeeze of lemon, and bake at 400 degrees for about 18 minutes.

Holiday times may be the hardest times for the dessert lover who is no longer allowed sweets. Starting with Valentine's Day, Coeur à la Crème is a rich dessert molded in a heart shape from cream, cream cheese, and cottage cheese, and served with fresh raspberries briefly stewed in their own juice, or frozen raspberries.

Halloween is even easier: there is a generous variety of Nature's autumn desserts, including nuts in their shells, golden raisins, and, perhaps, the surprise of a pomegranate. For Thanksgiving, a sweet-potato pie is naturally sweeter than a pumpkin pie, but do increase the amounts of spices somewhat. Christmas, of course, summons up those "visions of sugarplums"—an old-fashioned confection that can be replaced by fresh pineapple, dates, Temple oranges, and nectarines amid the fragrance of bayberry candles and balsam boughs and coupled with hot mulled cider.

consider giving up a vegetable exchange (5 grams of carbohydrate) as well as the bread exchange and the fat exchange in order to munch that roll. On the other hand, the roll may not be worth what could amount to a nice baked potato, butter, and a serving of fresh asparagus.

The total number of exchanges allowed in each group per day will vary with the number of calories your doctor recommends. A person on a 2,000 calorie plan might be allowed, for example, 8 meat exchanges, 7 fat exchanges, 3 nonfat milk exchanges, 9 bread exchanges, 4 fruit exchanges, and 2 vegetable exchanges each day. If 200 more calories were allowed, the person could add another bread, meat, fruit, and milk exchange. The total exchanges should be divided rather evenly between three or four meals a day. You will be happy to know that dill pickles, clam broth, and vinegar are "free."

Coping with Dietary Limitations
Fat-Controlled Diets

Americans eat astonishing amounts of animal fats and die of coronary artery disease at an astonishing rate. That does not prove that our diet is the cause of the disease; the relationship between dietary fat and coronary artery disease has so far defied elucidation. What is known, however, suggests that cutting down on our consumption of certain kinds of fats is at least prudent.

Coronary artery disease is marked by fatty deposits on the inside walls of the coronary artery which gradually impede the flow of blood to the heart and predispose a person to heart attack. The same condition in other arteries is implicated in stroke. When a person has extensive fatty deposits within the arteries, he is often also found to have high levels of a lipid (a type of fat) called cholesterol circulating in his blood, and possibly abnormal levels of other lipids as well. A diet that controls the kinds and amounts of fats eaten reduces the level of circulating cholesterol. So does a life of strenuous exercise, a reduction in the amount of refined sugar in the diet, and—most important of all—achieving and maintaining optimal weight. There is statistical evidence that a full regimen of exercise, maintenance of ideal weight, and carefully controlled diet for a period of from 5 to 10 years offers some protection against coronary attacks for some people.

Doctors differ in how they approach the subject of heart attack prevention through diet. Most doctors agree that a first step is to achieve and maintain optimal weight. Once obesity is no longer a factor, cholesterol levels may return to normal regardless of kinds and amounts of fat in the diet. For some people, cholesterol levels remain high even after optimal weight is achieved—or is high even if they have never been obese—and for these patients a fat-controlled diet may be recommended, possibly along with an exercise program (see pages 320-351). Some doctors take a middle road no matter which category a patient falls into: a fat-controlled diet cannot hurt, and it may help.

The original preventive diet for potential heart attack victims was published in a 1952 book *Reduce and Stay Reduced* by Dr. Norman Jolliffe (see page 291). Called the Prudent diet, it is in line with recommendations of the American Heart Association. Your doctor may prescribe a similar diet, though it will no doubt differ in detail and be specific to your condition. There are many conditions in which cholesterol and other lipids are present in excessive amounts and must be brought under control. As always follow your doctor's instructions; however, for comparison, you may want to know that the Prudent diet seeks to:

• Change the ratio of fats to complex carbohydrates so that at least half the total calories come from starches, such as grains and starchy vegetables.

• Change the ratio of saturated to unsaturated fats to tip the balance in favor of unsaturated fats.

• Reduce the amount of cholesterol.

In addition, the American Heart Association also advises the following dietary changes:

• Control the total number of calories.

• Change the ratio of simple sugars to complex carbohydrates so that starch is increased while sugar (sucrose in particular) is decreased.

• Reduce the amount of sodium by cutting down on table salt (see pages 376-380).

The various shifts required to achieve these objectives amount to a fundamental change in typical American eating habits. People committed to change eat only 6 ounces of meat a day, trim off visible fat and skin, and avoid fatty meats such as sausages and bacon and even ordinary hamburger. They eat much larger quantities of fruits and vegetables, which contain no cholesterol and are low in fat, salt, and calories in general. To cut down on cholesterol, prudent dieters eat no

Low-Fat Diet

Persons suffering from disorders of the gallbladder, usually gall stones, may be put on a diet in which every kind of fat and oil is severely restricted. Fat stimulates the release of bile, an enzyme that digests fat, from the gallbladder. Restricting fat intake minimizes stimulation and so gives the gallbladder a rest. The strategy may help prevent painful spasms of the bile duct too.

Severe restriction is usually temporary while the condition is being diagnosed and, if surgery is performed, during recovery. For chronic gallbladder conditions in which surgery is not warranted, the doctor may prescribe a low-fat diet, but it would be difficult if not impossible to follow one in which fat is avoided altogether.

SPECIAL DIETS FOR SPECIAL NEEDS

Choosing the Right Fat

The American Heart Association recommends that of the total fat in your diet, the ratio of saturated, monounsaturated, and polyunsaturated fats be no more than 1 to 1 to 1. That means it would be best if about one-third of the total fat you eat each day were polyunsaturated. No matter how carefully you trim meat, it will contain some fat—and all saturated. But by carefully reading the nutrition information panel on the processed oils and fats you do have control over, you can figure out which ones are closest to the prudent ideal.

The list below ranks the popular fats and oils from those with the highest proportion of unsaturated fatty acids to those with the highest proportion of saturated fatty acids.

> Safflower oil
> Sunflower oil
> Soybean oil
> Corn oil
> Cottonseed oil
> Sesame oil
> Tub margarine, liquid safflower oil
> Mayonnaise
> Tub margarine, liquid corn oil
> Peanut butter
> Stick margarine, liquid corn oil
> Olive oil
> Vegetable shortening, hydrogenated
> Peanut oil
> Tub or stick margarine, hydrogenated or hardened fat
> Lard
> Butterfat
> Coconut oil

According to this list, corn oil would be a better choice than peanut oil for frying, and mayonnaise would be a better sandwich spread than stick margarine.

more than 4 servings per week of high-cholesterol foods such as eggs, and they further reduce cholesterol by avoiding whole milk and whole-milk products, including ice cream, most cheeses, and butter. In order to have enough fat for cooking, they substitute cooking oils and margarine low in saturated fat and high in mono- and polyunsaturated fat for butter, lard, or hydrogenated (hardened) vegetable shortening. Avoiding sweet or fatty breads, cereals, flour products such as Danish pastry, or snack foods such as corn chips further cuts down on cholesterol and calories. In addition, prudence dictates that the person committed to change ban the saltshaker from the dining table.

Some of these changes present real obstacles. Butter is basic to some cuisines, cheeses provide the essential flavor for many dishes, cream gives a richness impossible to reproduce with other substances. But that is not true of the most sweeping change of all: the reversal in the proportion of meats to vegetables and grains. Exploring cuisines already geared to less meat and few dairy products is also the route to surmounting other obstacles.

Oriental cuisines are sparing of animal fats and meat and favor large quantities of vegetables and rice. Nouvelle cuisine uses small portions of meat but quantities of vegetables and relies on light sauces thickened without the help of flour and butter. Vegetarian cuisine (see pages 390-394) includes hearty vegetable and grain dishes that satisfactorily take the place of meat. Grain, pasta, and bean dishes from many parts of the world contain little or no meat. These classics include North African couscous, Middle Eastern bulgur, Mexican chili, and Italian pastas and risottos. The choices are, indeed, so intriguing that the following suggestions could constitute the menu of a restaurant that might be called The Prudent Place.

Vegetarian dishes Ratatouille (zucchini, eggplant, and tomatoes with garlic)
Stuffed vegetable platter (mushrooms, squash, tomato with herbs)
Indian fritters (deep-fried with corn, yams, and parsnips, with dipping sauce)

The above are served with garlic bread and a side order of fresh pot cheese.

Bean and grain dishes Pinto-bean chili with cubes of top round
Garlic black beans with pork strips and pimientos

The above are served with sliced tomatoes and your choice of cornbread or Boston brown bread.

Coping with Dietary Limitations
Fat-Controlled Diets

Couscous with lamb and chick-peas, spiced with cinnamon
Shrimp pilaf
Spinach tortellini with fresh, herbed tomato sauce

The above are served with spinach salad.

Stir-fried dishes Diced beef with broccoli and black mushrooms
Chicken with six vegetables
Hot, spicy pork bits with crisp-fried green beans

The above are all seasoned with garlic and ginger and served with boiled rice.

Because even these tasty dishes represent a rather drastic adjustment from the meat and gravy meals so many of us are accustomed to, shifting to a low-fat diet might be easier if it is done gradually. First, do the obvious: change cooking oils to favor a higher proportion of polyunsaturated fats, and trim all meat carefully to cut down on saturated fat and cholesterol. Avoiding whole milk is not difficult for most adults, and cutting down on cheese may not be a great sacrifice either.

Next, determine to set aside one or two nights a week for experimenting with new menus. You will surely hit on some that please the whole family as much as roasts and grills. Start serving desserts as celebrations only—a good report card, a new job, a birthday—and perhaps for Sunday dinner. Gradually shift away from fatty, sweet snacks toward fruits, raw vegetables with cottage-cheese dips made from skim milk, a small baked potato, or a chunk of hearty cornbread. Begin to serve two vegetables with meals so that you can cut down on meat portions, and don't be wary of the large helpings of starchy foods that may have worried you in the past. So long as you are controlling the total quantity of fats in the family's diet, increased starch will not raise total calories.

Those who have made these changes—and come to appreciate new tastes and textures as much as potentially better health—have found that it takes about two years to prune their eating habits down to the proportions of fat, salt, and sugar called for in the Prudent diet. Unless your doctor feels there is a particular urgency in your case, you have time to change at a rate that is comfortable for your family.

Diet and Cancer

Americans may eventually have the option of adopting a diet that could reduce their chances of getting cancer by as much as one-third. That was the startling, if tentative and qualified, conclusion of a report, "Diet, Nutrition, and Cancer," issued in June 1982 by a committee of the National Research Council (NRC). The study had been commissioned by the National Cancer Institute.

"The evidence is increasingly impressive that what we eat does affect our chances of getting cancer, especially particular kinds of cancer," stated the committee chairman, Clifford Grobstein of the University of California, San Diego. "That is . . . good news because it means that by controlling what we eat we may prevent such diet-sensitive cancers."

According to some estimates, as much as 90 percent of all cancer in humans has been attributed to environmental factors, including diet. One recent study suggested that dietary modification would have the greatest effect on the incidence of cancers of the stomach and large bowel and, to a lesser extent, on cancers of the breast and lung. Such evidence as this led the NRC panel to propose that most major-site cancers "are influenced by dietary patterns." Nonetheless, cautioned Grobstein, the committee was not yet prepared to say how much the incidence of particular cancers might be reduced by dietary alteration. "Certainly we have no ideal cancer-preventing diet to announce." Indeed, the committee report stated, "It is not now possible, and may never be possible, to specify a diet that would protect everyone against all forms of cancer." However, the committee did conclude that it was possible "to formulate interim dietary guidelines that are both consistent with good nutritional practices and likely to reduce the risk of cancer." The guidelines are similar to the Dietary Goals issued in 1977 by the U.S. Senate's Select Committee on Nutrition and Human Needs (see Foreword, pages 5-6) and the Dietary Guidelines of 1980, prepared by the U.S. Departments of Agriculture and Health and Human Services (see pages 96-97).

The "interim dietary guidelines" for reducing the risk of cancer are four in number:

1. Reduce the consumption of both saturated and unsaturated fats from the present level of approximately 40 percent to 30 percent of total calories. Fat has probably been studied more thoroughly than any other dietary factor and has been linked most frequently to disease. Moreover, the committee found that, of all the dietary components it studied, the evidence was "most suggestive for a causal relationship between fat intake and the occurence of cancer"—especially cancer of the colon and breast. Data could be used to justify an even greater reduction in the percentage of fat in the diet, but the committee judged the one-quarter reduction in fat consumption to be "a moderate and practical target."

The report did not indicate that saturated fat was any more likely to cause cancer than unsaturated fat, nor did it make any recommendation about cholesterol—though both saturated fat and cholesterol have been mentioned as possible contributing factors to cardiovascular disease.

2. **Include fruits, vegetables, and whole-grain cereal products in the daily diet.** Although others have urged an increase in the consumption of fruits and vegetables, the NRC committee specifically recommended those rich in vitamin C and betacarotene, the precursor of vitamin A. These include apricots, peaches, cantaloupe, watermelon, strawberries, citrus fruits, and broccoli, spinach, kale, escarole, Romaine lettuce, parsley, peppers, cabbage, white and sweet potatoes, acorn and butternut squash, Brussels sprouts, and carrots. Consumption of such vegetables of the mustard family as cabbage, broccoli, cauliflower, kale, and Brussels sprouts has been linked to a reduced incidence of gastric and colon and rectal cancer.

This recommendation applies only to foods—not to dietary supplements of individual nutrients. The committee was "unable to predict the health effects of high and potentially toxic doses of isolated nutrients consumed in the form of supplements."

3. **Keep the consumption of food preserved by salt curing, salt pickling, and smoking, to a minimum.** In countries where such foods are frequently consumed—China, Japan, and Iceland—there is a higher incidence of cancer of the esophagus and the stomach. To adhere to this dietary guideline, Americans should cut back on sausages, smoked fish and ham, bacon, and hot dogs. However, the evidence linking charcoal-broiled food to cancer has not been sufficiently assessed to draw any conclusions.

4. **Alcoholic beverages should be consumed only in moderation.** Heavy drinking, especially in combination with cigarette smoking, has been associated with an increased risk of cancer of the upper gastrointestinal and respiratory tracts, as well as with other adverse health effects.

The NRC committee was unable to reach a firm conclusion about protein, though some studies suggest an association between high levels of dietary protein and increased cancer risk. (In general, Americans consume more protein than is required.) The committee was likewise unable to endorse the protective effects of fiber against cancer, although it recommended high-fiber, whole-grain cereal products. The fiber in whole-wheat was judged "most likely" to be protective.

Another topic discussed in the report was food additives. In the United States, nearly 3,000 substances are added to foods during processing, the committee noted; an additional 12,000 chemicals, classified as indirect or unintentional additives, have been detected in some foods. Those few food additives that have been tested and found to be carcinogenic in animals have all been banned from use in the food supply, with the exception of saccharin. The committee did not find convincing evidence that food additives contribute significantly to the overall risk of cancer in humans. Nor were environmental factors such as exposure to pesticides and industrial chemicals judged to make a major contribution to cancer risk.

Cigarette smoking is the cause of 25 percent of cancer deaths in the United States—a link first proposed 20 years ago. If the public had been persuaded to stop smoking then, the NRC committee claims, these deaths would not now be occurring.

"The public is now asking about the causes of cancers that are not associated with smoking. What are these causes, and how can these cancers be avoided," the committee noted in its executive summary to the report. "Unfortunately, it is not yet possible to make firm scientific pronouncements about the association between diet and cancer. We are in an interim stage of knowledge. . . . Therefore, in the judgment of the committee, it is now the time to offer some interim guidelines on diet and cancer." Americans once more are being asked to modify their dietary habits for the sake of good health. The advice is bound to be provocative and controversial.

Self-Imposed Food Restrictions/Picky Eaters

Many families who do their best to plan balanced meals feel defeated because a member of the family refuses to eat most of what is prepared. Young children are notoriously faddish about food; it is not unusual for a toddler to eat almost nothing but tuna fish for several weeks, whereas a school-age child may turn down all vegetables except carrots and corn for many months. A teenager may become vegetarian overnight, suddenly spurning the roast that is the main feature of the meal to the rest of the family. Adolescence is also prime time for fad diets, especially among girls (see page 314). These days still another kind of self-imposed food restriction has posed a challenge to the cook: the family athlete—runner, cross-country skier, or tennis player—who has his own ideas about how meals should be planned to suit his special needs.

The fact that these are all self-imposed food restrictions may make you worry all the more about nutritional implications. After all, the doctor has not ordered such special diets. Shouldn't you worry about the health of a "poor eater"? Can a teenager really get enough protein from a vegetarian diet? Are steak and eggs a proper breakfast for a would-be marathoner? And how in the world are menus to be planned and meals prepared to satisfy everybody's special needs when all their needs differ?

A first step to managing the range of self-imposed food restrictions that may crop up in the family is to understand both the bases for such choices and the nutritional problems they can entail.

Developing Food Prejudices

Food dislikes generally begin in infancy and tend to become more widespread as the baby grows into childhood. Babies are sensitive to the textures of solid foods first introduced to their diet. They may, for example, reject strained beets because their rough texture is harder to manage than velvety strained foods such as applesauce and oatmeal. Over the next few years, parents may discover their children are developing eating patterns distinctly different from their own. Strong flavors that adults enjoy, including asparagus, turnips, cheese, chicken livers, and clams, are heartily disliked by their offspring. In general, the children may eat fewer vegetables and more meat, starch, and sweets than the grown-ups of the family eat.

There is probably a physiological basis for both these differences. Children's sense of smell is keen; what is a heady aroma to us may be unpleasantly strong to them. They are so active and growing so fast that only a rather high proportion of carbohydrates can satisfy their calorie needs (the childhood "sweet tooth" often disappears rather abruptly in adolescence). Their stomachs are small—too small to hold large enough quantities of vegetables and grains to meet their protein requirements. Meat supplies a compact source of protein to match their limited capacity.

Occasionally food idiosyncrasies during childhood prove to have a medical basis. Some children who hate fish or will not touch tomatoes are found to be allergic to just the foods they dislike. The abdominal discomfort they experience after eating the offending food works as a subliminal warning to avoid that food in the future (see page 368). Similarly, a strong aversion to milk often indicates that the child's digestive system is unable to digest milk sugar (see page 371).

There are also powerful emotional reasons behind some of the self-imposed food restrictions of childhood. Many 2-year-olds, as they struggle to become toilet trained and to be clean in general, develop a

Changes in Appetite

Sudden changes in a person's appetite can be a sign that something is physically or emotionally wrong. Loss of appetite may signal an illness before more obvious symptoms appear. The way a person eats is also a sensitive indicator of his emotional well-being. People who become depressed may have too little interest in life to bother much with eating. Those who become lonely, whether through loss of a loved one or for other reasons, may eat in an attempt to relieve the sensation of emptiness. Anorexia nervosa (see pages 316-317) is often preceded by extreme avoidance of carbohydrates and severe dieting. Although you should not be overly alarmed at transient idiosyncrasies in eating habits, any obvious change in overall appetite, whether toward eating more than or less than is usual for that person, should alert you to the possibility of an underlying problem.

distaste for foods that are "messy," like stews or meat with gravy, and for foods that are "smelly," like ripened cheese. As children become aware that the meat they eat was originally an animal they like—a lamb or a chicken—a few develop transient aversions to meat. Some children will not eat beans, peas, or fruit that contain seeds for fear these foods will grow inside them the way the bean they plant in nursery school grows into a vine. Perhaps fortunately for the family food budget, many children find lobsters and crabs too scary to eat—especially after seeing a live lobster plunged into boiling water.

Few of the food idiosyncrasies of childhood carry over into adulthood. So long as no great issue is made of them as they arise and the family in general enjoys a wide range of foods, nutrition is rarely compromised. Although this book suggests balancing meals on a day-to-day basis, that is for the convenience of the planner. The body does not require that each meal be balanced, or even that each day's food meet the total requirement, so long as balance is achieved over longer periods of several days or a week. Experiments have shown that when children are given free access to a large variety of foods over a period of weeks, they choose in a way that looks faddish over the short run but which meets their nutritional needs over longer periods of time. For example, they may eat nothing but bread and peanut butter for days, but then shift to fruit and potatoes, cheese or tuna fish, or carrot sticks, apparently as their bodies require the particular nutrients each food offers. Although few parents would wish to institute such an experiment, they can feel relieved that doctors simply do not see cases of childhood malnutrition caused by finickiness.

Preparing special foods for the fussy eater or limiting family menus to the few foods the picky child will eat is sure to annoy the rest of the family. On the other hand, forcing the poor eater to clean his plate—or even to try every food—is sure to make the whole problem worse (see below). The wisest solution seems to be this: offer the child unlimited access during mealtimes to favorite, but nutritious, substitutes such as peanut butter, apples, carrot sticks, American cheese, or hard-boiled eggs to which he can help himself if nothing else on the table appeals to him. Try to keep foods looking simple and clean; serve gravies and sauces separately if possible. When serving foods the child will accept, serve unusually small portions with plenty of space between the various kinds of food. The poor eater may even prefer one kind of food at a time on his plate. Offer second helpings, but do not press more food on the finicky child in any way.

Eating Disorders

Struggles over food and the use of food as emotional coinage during childhood may lead to real eating disorders, including both food aversions and food indulgences.

During infancy, feeding a baby on a rigid schedule or in set amounts rather than as he expresses hunger may discourage first his motivation to make his hunger known, and then his capacity to be aware of hunger sensations. A frequent finding in eating disorders is that the person denies ever feeling hungry, regardless of whether he is overeating or undereating.

Another sort of problem may arise during the toddler years. Dealing with frustration, boredom, anger, pain, and anxiety by offering cookies or other snacks undermines a child's ability to deal with his feelings more directly, and may establish a lifelong pattern of self-solace through eating.

Failure to accept a child's tastes in food anytime during childhood leads to trouble. Nagging, shaming, and forcing has caused many a child to hold food in his cheek until he can get rid of it, or hide it in his napkin. Under such pressure, some children even gag or vomit. Pleasure the child might have had in mealtimes is undermined; snacking between meals may become the preferred alternative.

Adolescence is a particularly vulnerable period. An excessive atmosphere of struggle, especially when carried out at the dinner table or over food-related issues, is fertile ground for the development of rebellious forms of food faddism. On the whole, families might consider whether the preferences and restrictions a child chooses for himself are not healthier in the long run than the repercussions of struggle.

Self-Imposed Food Restrictions
Vegetarian Diets

Many vegetarians are edged toward their ultimate choice of diet by what amounts to a food aversion: a reluctance to eat meat. Although the aversion may stem from a specific objection to killing animals for food, a general impulse toward a benevolent way of life often characterizes the vegetarian choice. Thus vegetarians may be opposed to the use of pesticides, adhere to the energy-saving principles of organic gardening, hold firm beliefs about the special benefits of such natural products as ginseng root and herb teas, or shun any "artificial" ingredients.

To the vegetarian, the restrictions he places on himself express commitment to a healthy, natural, and simplified way of life. To the family that does not share his commitment, life is by no means simple—especially for the cook. Not only must the special needs of the vegetarian member of the family be respected, but care is required to provide a nutritionally adequate diet.

There are three types of vegetarian diet. The lacto-ovo diet includes milk and eggs, a practice justified because these are animal products, not the animals themselves. The lacto diet eschews eggs (they are viewed as potential animals) but still allows milk. The pure vegetarian diet, sometimes called the vegan diet, consists only of fruits, nuts, seeds, grains, and vegetables.

There are two other variations on vegetarianism that should be mentioned, the first because it presents no problems at all, the second because it can be a nutritional disaster. A few vegetarians, perhaps illogically, include fish in their diet. Since fish is as concentrated a source of quality protein as meat, this diet is nutritionally no different from one that includes beef and chicken. The various Zen macrobiotic diets are another story. The Zen regimen calls for a person to work his way gradually through a sequence of diets, each more restricted than the one before, in an attempt to reach the "ideal" of a diet made up exclusively of grains. The latter stages of the regimen are so deficient in nutrients that they can lead to serious, even fatal illness.

Vegetarian diets in general have certain advantages over the typical American diet. They are usually lower in calories and in saturated fats and refined sugars in particular. Because of the large amounts of vegetables, fruits, and whole grains, they are automatically high in fiber content.

Lacto-ovo, lacto, and vegan vegetarian diets can all provide adequate nutrition if the contribution of the various food groups is well understood and if the person eats according to that understanding. A basic consideration is the total amount of protein. The Recommended Dietary Allowance for, say, a 154-pound adult is only 56 grams. This total is not difficult to obtain if milk products or eggs or both are included in the vegetarian diet. Protein in milk and eggs is more efficiently used than that in meats and fish, so a little goes a long way.

That 56-gram level is somewhat more difficult to obtain on a pure vegetarian diet. Total protein needs can be met efficiently only if legumes (peas, beans, peanuts) are a daily staple. Soybeans contain the highest percentage of protein among all vegetable foods. One cup of cooked soybeans contains about 20 grams of protein (more than one-third the RDA) or about the same amount as you would get from 3 hot dogs or a ¼-pound hamburger or 2 large glasses of milk or 3 eggs or 3 ounces of cheese.

There is a problem with bean sources of protein. Some people—children especially—have trouble digesting daily doses of beans large enough to meet their protein requirements. There is an additional concern with any individual who is unable to eat very large meals. Without sufficient calories to meet energy needs, body proteins are consumed regardless of how much protein is in the diet. Children kept on pure vegetarian diets seem unable to eat the sheer bulk of vegetable foods necessary to supply enough carbohydrates, enough protein, or both. They are typically undersized compared to their nonvegetarian peers, and clinical malnutrition has also been reported. The nutritional demands of pregnancy and lactation pose similar problems.

Beyond the sheer quantity of protein, the vegetarian must also consider whether the proteins he is consuming have the proper balance of amino acids. The advantage of animal protein, whether from an animal's milk, eggs, or flesh, is that it is made up of about the same proportions of amino acids humans require to build their own proteins. That is not so of plants. You can consider both milk and eggs as complete sources of all the amino acids you need, but each group of plants has its own strengths and weaknesses as far as amino acids are concerned.

The four essential amino acids that are in short supply in the vegetable kingdom are lysine, isoleucine, methionine, and tryptophan. They are distrib-

SPECIAL DIETS FOR SPECIAL NEEDS

Our Daily Beans

Beans provide a substantial proportion of the protein in a vegetarian's diet, but unless the entire family is vegetarian, coming up with daily bean dishes requires considerable foresight and effort. Except for lentils and split peas, dried beans take an hour or more to cook even if you have remembered to soak them beforehand. Canned beans are an acceptable substitute on occasion, but that canned flavor lingers and they are decidedly mushy.

A simple alternative is frozen beans. Cook garbanzos or navy, Great Northern, kidney, pinto, or black beans until they are just tender. You don't have to taste the beans often to determine their degree of doneness. Pluck a bean from the water and blow on it. If the translucent outer skin cracks and peels, the bean is done or almost so. Rinse the cooked beans under cold water and drain well in a colander. Freeze individual portions in ziplock freezer bags or small freezer containers.

With a stock of several kinds of frozen beans on hand, you will have a great deal of flexibility in menu planning (or if you haven't planned, a last-minute way to get that protein in). Sprinkle a handful of garbanzos into the vegetarian's salad or make an individual bean salad. Navy or Great Northern beans are delicious with oil, lemon juice, garlic, and chopped parsley. Pintos and kidney beans are especially tasty with a mayonnaise dressing. Beans can be added to many soups without compromising the flavor. Black beans would be good in cream of tomato soup; garbanzos would work in a mushroom and barley chowder.

You might also want to pull together quick, hot bean dishes from the freezer selection. Heat pinto beans in crushed, canned tomatoes; add cumin seeds and oregano for a distinctive flavor. With the addition of chili peppers and garlic, this dish becomes a vegetarian chili. Recook black beans with a little oil and water and fresh, crushed garlic; garnish with thinly sliced scallions. Fresh ginger root, peeled and finely chopped, goes particularly well with black beans. Another quick, hot bean dish is navy beans reheated in a little sour cream and generously sprinkled with coarsely ground black pepper and chopped chives.

For those nights when any extra effort is too much, you might want to keep on hand containers of frozen hummus, a chick-pea paste that can be used as a dip or spread. Cook the beans until they are quite soft. Drain and mash them together with about one-third the quantity of tahini (sesame seed paste), and lemon juice, salt, and pressed garlic to taste. Add water until the mixture has a light, velvety texture. Freeze in the smallest size containers so that the hummus can be thawed quickly. Used as a spread on whole-grain bread, hummus will help to complete the protein for any meal. It can also be used as a dip with any number of raw vegetables.

---

uted among the major plant-food groups and milk and eggs as follows:

	Weaknesses	Strengths
Legumes	Tryptophan, methionine	Lysine, isoleucine
Grains	Lysine, isoleucine	Tryptophan, methionine
Seeds and nuts	Lysine, isoleucine	Tryptophan, methionine
Other vegetables	Isoleucine, methionine	Tryptophan, lysine
Eggs	None	Tryptophan, lysine, methionine
Milk products	None	Lysine

Amino acids must be balanced at each meal if they are to be usable in building human proteins. It does no good to have lysine-deficient grains for lunch and try to make up the missing lysine by having beans for dinner. Such complementary amino acids must be included in the same meal (although not necessarily in the same dish). For that reason, the vegetarian has to learn to combine certain foods as a matter of course. You do not need elaborate calculations to do this. Just remember the following principles.

• Combine eggs or dairy products with any vegetable protein.
• Combine legumes (dried peas, beans, peanuts) with grains (rice, wheat, corn).
• Combine legumes with seeds (sesame seeds, sunflower seeds) and nuts (cashews, almonds).

Traditional combinations of vegetable proteins with milk, eggs, or both are so ordinary as to be

Self-Imposed Food Restrictions
Vegetarian Diets

commonplace: for breakfast, oatmeal with milk, French toast, or pancakes; for lunch, potato salad (the egg is in the mayonnaise), an egg salad, or a cheese sandwich; for supper, macaroni and cheese, Chinese fried rice, mashed potatoes made with milk, spinach salad with hard-boiled egg, eggplant Parmesan, cream of vegetable soup, or any vegetable or potato served au gratin. For dessert, there is rice pudding. You can even count strawberry shortcake with whipped cream as a balanced source of amino acids. (See also The Powerful Proteins, pages 24-29.)

If the vegetarian is a vegan (no milk, no eggs), there are of course fewer choices, but, interestingly, many traditional cuisines have developed just the right combinations of foods to balance

What To Do with Tofu

Tofu, or soybean curd, is made by pressing soaked, ground soybeans to obtain a milky fluid which is then treated with a coagulant to form it into curds. The curds are pressed into blocks and sold fresh. Once available only in Oriental markets, tofu can now increasingly be found in the produce section of supermarkets. Tofu and other soybean products are also discussed on page 163.

Many vegetarians rely on tofu for its high protein content and prize it for its versatility, pleasant consistency, and mild, creamy flavor. The uninitiated, however, may be nonplussed by what looks and feels like a cake of white custard. What, the uninitiated may ask, does one do with tofu?

Traditionally, tofu is prepared in one of three ways: by blanching, stir-frying, or deep-frying. Blanching improves the flavor and texture of tofu, and is the technique used to prepare it for serving cold. Cut the block into six slices. Place the slices in a large strainer and lower them into boiling water for half a minute. Drain and cool. The slices may be added to a salad or they may be served the Oriental way: mix together equal quantities of soy sauce and peanut oil; pour the mixture over the tofu slices and, if you wish, season with pepper and slivered scallions.

The next simplest way to prepare tofu is to stir-fry it. Cut three blocks into 1-inch cubes. Cut a scallion stalk into 1-inch pieces. Heat about ¼ cup peanut oil in a wok and stir-fry the scallion pieces until they are translucent. Add the tofu gently and tilt the pan this way and that so that the hot oil heats them through (tofu is too fragile for vigorous stir-frying). When hot, season with soy sauce and serve immediately.

If this basic stir-fry method is too soft and bland for your taste, you can make a more toothsome dish by adding slivered mushrooms or snow peas along with the scallions. A sharper flavor is obtained by sprinkling the finished dish with a few drops of hot sesame oil or by adding a tablespoon of fermented black beans. The beans should be soaked in hot water for a few minutes, then drained, mashed, and cooked briefly in the oil before the vegetables are added. Since beans already taste salty, be especially sparing with the soy sauce.

The third basic way to prepare tofu is to deep-fry it. Cut the blocks into 1-inch cubes and blot them dry with paper towels. Heat oil for deep-frying. Lower the cubes a few at a time into the hot oil and fry until puffy, crisp, and golden. You can serve the deep-fried cubes sprinkled with salt, add them at the last minute to any other stir-fried dish, or eat them with a dipping sauce. An excellent dip is made by combining 1 tablespoon soy sauce, 1 tablespoon peanut butter, and 2 tablespoons peanut oil. A more piquant dip might include a few drops of sesame oil or ½ teaspoon hot sauce.

Those who have trouble handling tofu because of its fragile texture or those who wish a less custardy, more chewable product might want to press the curd before using it in any of the above ways. Wrap each block in cheesecloth. Place the wrapped blocks next to one another between two boards (bread boards are fine). Put them on the drain portion of the kitchen counter, and weight the top board with heavy cans or books. Leave for six hours or until a good deal of moisture has run out and the cakes feel firm to the touch. You will find that pressed tofu can be cubed or slivered without falling apart; the texture is slightly chewy.

In addition to traditional Oriental cooking techniques, tofu has been adapted to Western recipes that include everything from tofu mayonnaise to tofu quiche. The *Book of Tofu* by William Shurtleff and Akiko Aoyagi contains 250 recipes using tofu.

amino acids. For example, Mexicans combine corn-based tacos, tortillas, and enchiladas with beans, and also eat rice with beans. In the Middle East, pita bread is stuffed with a chick-pea fritter known as felafel. Another Middle Eastern favorite is hummus, a knowing combination of chick-peas (a legume) with tahini (a paste made from sesame seeds). In India, rice or bread is frequently eaten with dal—bean stew made with lentils or other legumes. The American tradition that best meets the grain with legumes requirement is, of course, the peanut butter sandwich.

Besides these classics, you may want to try some more outlandish combinations just to assure variety. An easy one is macaroni enriched with soy flour. Tofu—or soybean curd—can be sprinkled with sesame seeds to achieve amino acid balance, and sesame meal can be added to any bean soup. Meat analogs—the height of the food processor's art—come in handy too. They mimic everything from breakfast sausage to baloney and are often fortified to assure complete protein nutrition. The U.S. Food and Drug Administration is presently developing guidelines that will require meat analogs to provide nutrient levels equivalent to the meats they replace, but at the moment only careful label reading will inform you of the nutrition you are getting.

Vitamins and minerals should also concern the vegetarian. Lacto vegetarians have an advantage, since fortified milk products contain just the vitamins and minerals vegetables are short on: calcium, riboflavin, and vitamins A, D, and B_{12}. If eggs are included too, they are a primary source of iron. Even with eggs and milk, however, vegetarians should eat a large variety of plant foods. Each plant group provides somewhat different nutrients. You will be able to avoid the need for vitamin and mineral supplements by choosing your daily menu according to the charts on pages 52-93.

Pure vegetarians have to be particularly careful about their choice of foods. Vitamin B_{12} is found only in foods of animal origin. Deficiency in this essential nutrient may go unnoticed for many years, but the ultimate effects, including anemia and central nervous system damage, are profound and may be irreversible. B_{12} can be obtained by tablet, or through B_{12}-fortified soy milk or nutritional yeast. Other yeast products—brewer's yeast, baker's yeast, and live yeast cakes—have almost none of this vitamin.

Getting enough calcium without milk products presents difficulties to the pure vegetarian too. The tables beginning on page 84 indicate which vegetables, such as some of the greens, broccoli, and okra, contain significant amounts of calcium. Many of the same vegetables are good sources of riboflavin. Blackstrap molasses is another calcium source, as are almonds and most dried fruits. Vitamin D should be no problem to anyone who exposes his skin to sunlight on a regular basis, but if necessary it can also be obtained through vitamin D-fortified margarine.

When these various concerns about total calories, total protein, and balanced amino acids, vitamins, and minerals are translated into daily menu plans, you can see that to be a successful vegetarian, you must be a hearty eater. Jane Brody, personal health columnist of the *The New York Times* tells us just how much. Looking just at calories, Brody says, a nonvegetarian man might eat a 1,500 calorie dinner made up of a 6-ounce steak, a potato with butter, a half-cup serving of carrots, salad with blue cheese dressing, and a slice of apple pie. For a pure vegetarian to get down as few as 900 calories, he has to eat a cup of brown rice with lentils, a large baked potato with margarine, a full cup of carrots and peas, a lettuce and tomato salad with dressing, and for dessert, a fruit salad made with a whole banana, a whole apple, a whole orange, 2 tablespoons of raisins, and half a dozen walnuts. He will leave the table stuffed, and still 600 calories behind the steak eater.

The menus on the next page, based in part on plans devised by the New York City Department of Health's Bureau of Nutrition, supply from 2,200 up to 2,800 calories per day—an indication of the amount of food that must be consumed in order to get adequate nutrition on vegetarian diets.

Most of the items on these menus present no special problems for the cook. Breakfast foods are staple products in all three vegetarian diets. Lunch foods are mostly staples but include some bean and pasta dishes. The day's complement of vegetables is balanced between the various categories no differently than is recommended for an ordinary diet except that quantities would be larger for the vegetarian in general, and the vegan in particular might require more mustard greens and spinach (for calcium and iron) than the family is accustomed to. The real challenge is the dinner entree for lacto-ovo

Self-Imposed Food Restrictions
Vegetarian Diets

and lacto vegetarians, and both the lunch and the dinner entrée for vegans, who must rely particularly heavily on beans.

Some families will settle for one bean supper a week, and perhaps a pasta meal as well. In summer, they might bear the strain of bread and salad for dinner. But unless your family is unusually fond of split peas and macaroni, that leaves many main meals for which the vegetarian needs a special entrée. The box on page 391 suggests freezing small containers of beans to use in last-minute dishes. There are three other alternatives. The first, but the most expensive, is to keep commercially prepared vegetarian products on hand. The second is to cook vegetarian entrées in quantity and store in individual portions in the freezer. The last, and perhaps the best alternative, is to help the vegetarian learn to cook dishes for his special needs—all by himself.

Sample Vegetarian Meals

LACTO-OVO			
Breakfast	**Lunch**	**Dinner**	**Snacks**
½ grapefruit 1 oz cheese 2 slices whole-grain or enriched toast 1 pat margarine ½ c skim milk	1 c Haitian black beans* and rice Mixed green salad ½ c cottage cheese 1 tbsp salad dressing 1 slice whole-grain or enriched bread 1 pat margarine Wedge of cantaloupe	Italian casserole* ½ baked acorn squash ½ c coleslaw 1 tsp mayonnaise 1 slice whole-grain or enriched bread 1 pat margarine Indian pudding*	¼ c sunflower seeds ½ c milk ¾ c bulgur ¼ c raisins Pear

LACTO			
Breakfast	**Lunch**	**Dinner**	**Snacks**
1 orange ¼ c cottage cheese 2 slices whole-grain or enriched toast 1 pat margarine ½ c skim milk	1 c black bean soup* Sesame crackers Tomato and cucumber salad 1 tbsp salad dressing Baked apple* ½ c skim milk	Fresh fruit cup Eggplant Parmesan* ½ c collard greens 1 slice whole-grain or enriched bread 2 pats margarine ½ c junket	1 slice part-skim cheese 4-6 whole-grain crackers 2 prunes ¼ c roasted soybeans 1 whole-grain or enriched roll ½ c buttermilk

VEGAN			
Breakfast	**Lunch**	**Dinner**	**Snacks**
1 orange 1 c bulgur with 1 tbsp brewer's yeast 1 slice wheat-soy toast 1 tbsp honey	2 c split pea soup 2 slices whole-grain or enriched bread 2 tbsp peanut butter 1 tbsp honey Fruit sunflower-seed salad: ½ medium apple ½ medium banana ¼ c sunflower seeds 1 lettuce leaf	Vegetable paella* 1 c collards Pear	¼ c shelled almonds 1 peach ¼ c raisins

*See recipe index beginning on page 411.

The Athlete's Diet

No, steak and eggs are not the best breakfast for an athlete before the big event. Nor do gelatin, vitamin B supplements, vitamin E, wheat-germ oil, or bee pollen have any known effect—except a psychological one—on athletic peformance. If Mom is training for the marathon and Johnny is determined to make it to the soccer sectionals, the family will have to turn a deaf ear to these and many other myths about what athletes should eat to win.

Faddism in athletes' diets has been traced back to the 5th century B.C. in Greece. Until that time, Greek athletes had raced and wrestled on a diet that included mostly grains, figs, and cheese, with very modest amounts of meat. In those days, there were no weight categories for wrestlers, so that any extra brawn a wrestler could put on was decidedly to his advantage. With that extra brawn in mind, Dromeus of Stymphalus, an Olympic long-distance runner and trainer, invented the wrestler's meat diet—and it has been around ever since.

The idea of a high-protein diet for those who lead a strenuous life is based on a simplistic notion: that meat is needed to replace the protein "lost" through muscle work. Work does not, however, damage muscle proteins; strenuous activity does not involve increased consumption of proteins. Sound nutrition for the athlete is the same as sound nutrition for the accountant.

Naturally, the more active a person is, the greater his need for calories. The chart on page 323 compares the calorie expenditure of people participating in various sports and other physical activities. Although the chart is interesting, athletes will rarely need to refer to it to gauge their caloric needs. Unlike sedentary people whose bodies seem to lose the ability to signal their actual caloric needs, those who live a strenuous life tend to assess their energy needs accurately. No one has to tell a football player to eat more during preseason practice than he ate during the lazy summer days. His appetite tells him. So long as his diet is nutritionally sound, increased consumption alone will meet his special needs in proportion to the requirement of his activity. That rule applies not only to protein requirements, which may increase transiently during rapid muscle buildup or the adolescent growth spurt, but also to the vitamins and minerals generously available in a balanced diet.

The ordinary, underactive American already exceeds the Recommended Dietary Allowance of protein by a good deal. Athletic training diets frequently advise two or three times that allowance. Such a high-protein diet poses several difficulties. First, the waste products of protein metabolism can only be excreted through urination. The more such wastes the kidneys must handle, the more fluid they must draw from other body tissues. Athletes are ill-advised to follow any regimen that tends to draw off fluids at the expense of muscles. The second difficulty is that a diet high in protein tends also to be high in fat. Several careful studies in which the athletic performance of people kept on various diets was compared have shown that high-fat diets are detrimental, especially to endurance.

In short, the proper diet for an athlete is the Prudent diet, which is increasingly suggested as a wise choice for most other people, too. The details of the Prudent diet are explained on page 291, but briefly, the plan cuts fats down to 30 to 35 percent of the total caloric intake and limits proteins to a modest 12 to 15 percent. Since carbohydrates are increased accordingly to at least half the total calories, one could call this a high-carbohydrate diet.

This news will not be welcomed by many athletes. The stress of training, the high hopes, the very mystique of sports seem to call for something more special in how or what athletes should eat. Fortunately, that is quite so. What is special is how and what athletes participating in an endurance sport calling for prolonged aero-

Coffee or Beer?

Trainers frequently ban all alcohol and all stimulants from the training table, but in fact researchers have not found evidence that a cup of coffee or a glass of beer during training has any long-term adverse effect. Before the event, however, there is good reason to avoid both alcohol and stimulants. Even small quantities of alcohol affect coordination and timing. While the caffeine in tea, coffee, and cola drinks is stimulating and may improve performance for a while, many people experience a letdown three or four hours later. A cup of coffee at that last meal three hours before the contest is not a good idea. During very long events, periodic sips of sweetened tea is a helpful way to keep energy levels high.

Self-Imposed Food Restrictions
The Athlete's Diet

bic activity should eat in the days and hours preceding the event itself.

You still won't get that traditional breakfast of steak and eggs, but you can indulge in a scientifically developed technique called carbohydrate loading. To understand how the technique works, you need to know how muscles work. What factors limit the muscles' ability to work? Or, to put the question another way, how do muscles become exhausted?

There are two factors that lead to muscle fatigue: running out of fuel and building up excess waste products in the muscle tissue. Like all body tissues, muscles obtain their energy by burning glucose. They obtain glucose from various sources, depending on the nature of the activity. During light exercise—a leisurely bike ride or an everyday fitness regimen—glucose is supplied as needed from the breakdown of fat and from glycogen, a fuel substance stored in the muscles and in the liver. As exercise becomes more strenuous and continues for more than 15 minutes, as in long-distance cycling or running, muscles draw increasingly on their own store of glycogen. When that is used up, the muscles run out of energy; the athlete feels exhausted. The factor that limits endurance is the amount of glycogen stored in the muscles.

The mechanism that causes exhaustion after brief, very intense effort such as a sprint or weight lifting is quite different. During such extreme effort, muscles do their work without using oxygen. Waste products build up very rapidly. The waste products, mostly lactic acid, cause exhaustion long before glycogen stores are depleted. Special dietary regimens other than a good balanced diet cannot improve performance for brief, intensive athletic events. Carbohydrate loading can nevertheless be useful if one considers that a track meet, for example, may call for many such spurts of effort.

Glycogen is most efficiently replenished through carbohydrate metabolism. Logic indicates that loading up with carbohydrates prior to prolonged, strenuous effort should help muscles to replenish depleted glycogen and store up maximum amounts of fuel for the event. This has proven to be true in practice as well as in theory.

Carbohydrate loading does not mean stuffing on starchy foods on a day-to-day basis, nor does it mean hyping up on sweets just before the big game. For activities of relatively short duration, increasing the percentage of carbohydrate in the diet two days prior to the event would be enough to increase glycogen stores. The athlete should taper off on rigorous training during the first day and rest the second. This tapering off of exercise followed by complete rest relieves the drain on glycogen stores and gives muscles a chance to restock to the maximum level. Increasing the percentage of carbohydrates in the diet is most easily done by adjusting second helpings. If you would normally have second helpings of everything, have no seconds of chicken but double your second helping of potatoes. If you would usually have two eggs and two slices of toast, make it one egg and three slices of toast.

A more extreme procedure is glycogen supercompensation. As outlined in *Exercise Physiology* by McArdle, Katch, and Katch, this two-stage plan involves a week of dietary modification and training prior to the event (see opposite).

It is also a good idea to avoid any foods that might cause intestinal discomfort or the disaster of needing to defecate during a marathon. Consider, for example, avoiding beans, fried foods, and gas-producing vegetables as well as high-fiber foods (see page 367) that cause bulky bowel movements.

The last meal should be no less than three hours before the event to allow adequate time for digestion. Undigested food not only feels heavy, but active intestines compete with active muscles for the body's blood and oxygen supply. Other than the timing, the meal can be the same type of high-

Sugar Feedings

At intervals during prolonged, exhausting contests, cyclists, runners, and swimmers may want a quick dose of energy in the form of sugar. The contestant should not, however, take a spoonful of honey, munch a sugar lump, or pop a glucose pill. All such forms of sugar make the intestines draw fluid from the body to aid in digestion and absorption. Since the endurance athlete wants to avoid dehydration in his muscle tissue, any loss of water beyond the unavoidable loss through sweating is no help. Sweetened tea with lemon avoids this problem and still provides the needed sugar feeding.

carbohydrate, low-fat meal of the last two days.

If the weather is very warm, or if you know from experience that you will be sweating profusely, you might wish to take some extra salt—though salt tablets are dangerous and not recommended. Exercise in itself does not deplete the body of salt, but sweating does. Unless 5 to 10 pounds are lost through sweat, you need not replace salt. If you do lose that much, one good technique is to drink bouillon three hours before the event.

Proper hydration is essential to an athlete in regulating wastes, body temperature, blood pressure, and oxygen supply. But do not wait to drink until you are thirsty. You need to down 1 quart of water for every 1,000 calories consumed. For the athlete that can be 3 to 6 quarts each day. Drink 3 or more glasses of water—or fruit juice, skim milk, clear broth—three hours before the event, and take another 2 glasses an hour and a half later, or even up to 15 minutes before the event. Continue to drink 2 glasses of water every hour during an extended event.

The aim of the athlete's diet is to leave your innards empty of wastes, your muscles full of energy, and yourself in shape to do your very best.

The Supercompensation Diet

To deplete glycogen stores in his muscles, the athlete performs a rigorous workout of specific muscles in the first day of Stage One. For the next three days he trains only moderately and eats a low-carbohydrate diet to further deplete glycogen stores. This diet allows approximately 100 grams (400 calories) of carbohydrate. Physical exertion may be difficult because of weakness, and care should be taken to prevent injury or infection during this stage.

In Stage Two, the final two-to-three days before the event, he increases carbohydrate intake to 400 to 625 grams (1,600 to 2,500 calories) per day with a normal amount of protein and fat.

Periodic shifts from one dietary extreme to another can be hazardous. Unbalanced diets can lead to deficiencies of vitamins and minerals and may require supplementation. The regimen of supercompensation should be followed very infrequently and only under close medical supervision. For most sports competition, a normal diet of 50 to 60 percent carbohydrate provides adequate glycogen reserves without the hazards of dietary modification.

Stage 1 Depletion	Stage 2 Carbohydrate Loading
Breakfast ½ cup fruit juice 2 eggs 1 slice whole-wheat toast 1 glass whole milk	**Breakfast** 1 cup fruit juice Hot or cold cereal 1 to 2 muffins 1 tbsp butter Coffee (cream/sugar)
Lunch 6-oz hamburger 2 slices bread salad 1 tbsp mayonnaise and Salad dressing 1 glass whole milk	**Lunch** 2–3-oz hamburger with bun 1 cup juice 1 orange 1 tbsp mayonnaise Pie or cake
Snack 1 cup yogurt	**Snack** 1 cup yogurt, fruit or cookies
Dinner 2 to 3 pieces chicken, fried 1 baked potato with sour cream ½ cup vegetable Iced tea (no sugar) 2 tbsp butter	**Dinner** 1–1½ pieces chicken, baked 1 baked potato with sour cream 1 cup vegetable ½ cup sweetened pineapple Iced tea (sugar) 1 tbsp butter
Snack 1 glass whole milk	**Snack** 1 glass chocolate milk with 4 cookies

Bibliography

About Nutrition. Seventh Day Adventist Dietetic Association, Nashville, Tenn., Southern Publishing Association, 1971, 1974.

Angier, Bradford, *Feasting Free on Wild Edibles.* Harrisburg, Pa., Stackpole Books, 1969.

Arlin, Marian Thompson, *The Science of Nutrition.* New York, Macmillan Publishing Co., Inc., 1972.

Bayrd, Edwin, *The Thin Game.* New York, Newsweek Books, 1978.

Berkeley Food Co-op Food Book, Helen Block, ed. Palo Alto, Calif., Bull Publishing Company, 1980.

Berland, Theodore, *Diets '81.* Skokie, Ill., Consumer Guide, 1981.

Block, Zenas, *It's All on the Label.* Boston, Mass., Little, Brown & Co., 1981.

Bottomley, H.W., *Allergy, Its Treatment and Care.* New York, Funk and Wagnalls, 1968.

Brackett, Babette, and Lash, Maryann, *The Wild Gourmet.* Boston, Mass., David R. Godine, 1975.

Brewster, Letitia, and Jacobson, Michael F., *The Changing American Diet.* Washington, D.C., Center for Science in the Public Interest, 1978.

Brody, Jane E., *Jane Brody's Nutrition Book.* New York, W.W. Norton & Company, 1981.

Bronfen, Nan, *Nutrition for a Better Life.* Santa Barbara, Calif., Capra Press, 1980.

Brown, Joe Giese, *The Good Food Compendium.* Garden City, N.Y., Dolphin Books, Doubleday & Co., Inc. 1981.

Burkitt, Denis, *Eat Right—To Keep Healthy and Enjoy Life More.* New York, Arco, 1979.

Burton, Benjamin T., *Human Nutrition,* Formerly *The Heinz Handbook of Nutrition,* 3rd edition (published for the H.J. Heinz Company). New York, Blakiston Publication, McGraw-Hill Book Co., 1959, rev. 1976.

The Buying Guide for Fresh Fruits, Vegetables, Herbs, and Nuts. Educational Department, Blue Goose, Inc., Hagerstown, Md., 1980.

Clayton, Jr., Bernard, *The Complete Book of Breads.* New York, Simon & Schuster, 1973.

Cooking Without Your Salt Shaker. American Heart Association, 7320 Greenville Ave., Dallas, Texas, 75231, 1978.

Corbin, Cheryl, *Nutrition; A Preventive Medicine Institute/Strang Clinic Health Action Plan.* New York, Holt, Rinehart and Winston, 1980.

Deutsch, Ronald M., *Realities of Nutrition.* Palo Alto, Calif., Bull Publishing Company, 1976.

Diet Manual, 7th edition. The Mount Sinai Hospital of New York, 1975.

Dietary Goals for the United States—Supplemental Views. Prepared for the staff of the Select Committee on Nutrition and Human Needs, U.S.Senate, Washington, D.C., 1977.

Doyle, Rodger P., and Redding, James L., *The Complete Food Handbook.* New York, Grove Press Inc., 1978.

Feeding Guide, A Nutritional Guide for the Maturing Infant. Health Learning Systems, Inc., Evansville, Ind., Mead Johnson & Co.,

Fleck, Henrietta, M.D., *Introduction to Nutrition,* 3rd edition. New York, Macmillian Publishing Co., Inc. 1976.

Food. Science and Education Administration, Human Nutrition Center, USDA, Washington, D.C., 1979.

Garrett, Blanche Pownall, *A Taste of the Wild.* Toronto, Canada, James Lorimer & Company, 1975.

Goldbeck, Nikki and David, *The Supermarket Handbook.* New York, Harper & Row, Publishers, 1973.

Hall, Alan, *The Wild Food Trailguide.* New York, Holt, Rinehart and Winston, 1973, 1975.

Harris, Robert S., and Karmas, Endel, *Nutritional Evaluation of Food Processing,* 2nd edition. Westport, Conn., Avi Publishing Co., 1975.

The Harvard Medical School Health Letter Book, G. Timothy Johnson, M.D., and Stephen E. Goldfinger, M.D., eds. Cambridge, Mass., Harvard University Press, 1981.

Herbert, Victor, and Barrett, Stephen, *Vitamins and "Health" Foods: The Great American Hustle.* Philadelphia, Pa., George F. Stickley Company, 1981.

How to Grow Herbs. Editors of Sunset Books and Sunset Magazine. Menlo Park, Calif., Lane Books, 1975.

Ideas for Better Eating. Science and Education Administration, Human Nutrition, USDA, Washington, D.C., 1981.

Jacobson, Michael, *Nutrition Scoreboard.* New York, Avon Books, 1974, 1975.

Krause, Marie V., and Mahan, L. Kathleen, *Food, Nutrition and Diet Therapy.* Philadelphia, Pa., W.B. Saunders Company, 1979.

Lappe, Frances Moore, *Diet for a Small Planet,* rev. ed. New York, Ballantine Books, division of Random House, 1978.

Kutsky, Roman J., *Handbook of Vitamins, Minerals and Hormones,* 2nd edition. New York, Van Nostrand Reinhold Company, 1981.

Mayer, Jean, *A Diet for Living.* New York, Pocket Books, 1975.

Mayer, Jean, *Human Nutrition.* Springfield, Ill., Charles C. Thomas, Publisher, 1972.

Mayo Clinic Diet Manual, A Handbook of Dietary Practices, 5th edition. By the dietetic staffs of the Clinic, Rochester Methodist Hospital and St. Mary's Hospital. Philadelphia, Pa., W.B. Saunders Company, 1981.

McCay, Clive M., and McCay, Jeanette B., *The Cornell Bread Book.* New York, Dover Publications, 1980.

McGraw-Hill Encyclopedia of Food, Agriculture & Nutrition, Daniel N. Lapedes, ed. New York, McGraw-Hill Book Co., 1977.

Modern Nutrition in Health and Disease, 6th edition, Robert S. Goodhart and Maurice E. Shils, eds. Philadelphia, Pa., Lea and Febiger, 1980.

Nutritive Value of Foods. Home and Garden Bulletin No. 72, USDA, Washington, D.C., 1981.

Nutritive Value of American Foods in Common Units. Agriculture Handbook No. 456. Agricultural Research Service, USDA, Washington, D.C., Nov. 1975.

Obesity in America, George Bray, ed. DHEW Public Health Service, National Institutes of Health, NIH publication No. 80-359, GPO Washington, D.C., 20402, Rep. 1980.

Owen, Millie, *A Cook's Guide to Growing Herbs, Greens, and Aromatics.* New York, Alfred A. Knopf, 1978.

Pennington, Jean A.T., and Church, Helen Nicols, *Bowes and Church's Food Values of Portions Commonly Used.* Philadelphia, Pa., J.B.Lippincott Company, 1980.

Perkins, Wilma Lord, *The Fanny Farmer Cookbook,* 11th edition. Boston, Mass., Little, Brown & Co., 1965.

Rechtschaffen, Joseph S., and Carola, Robert, *Dr. Rechtschaffen's Diet for Lifetime Weight Control and Better Health.* New York, Random House, 1980.

Recommended Dietary Allowances, 9th rev. ed. National Academy of Sciences, Washington, D.C., 1980.

The Rodale Herb Book, William H. Hylton, ed. Emmaus, Pa., Rodale Press Book Division, 1974.

Rombauer, Irma, and Becker, Marion Rombauer, *Joy of Cooking.* Indianapolis, Ind., Bobbs-Merrill Company, Inc., 1931, 1976.

Root, Waverley, *Food.* New York, Simon & Schuster, 1980.

Runyan, Thora J., *Nutrition for Today.* New York, Harper and Row, Publishers, 1976.

Saunders, Charles Francis, *Edible and Useful Wild Plants of the United States and Canada.* New York, Dover Publications, 1948.

Shurtleff, William, and Aoyagi, Akiko, *The Book of Tofu,* rev. ed. New York, Ballantine Books, 1979.

The Sodium Content of Your Food. Science and Education Administration in cooperation with Northeast Cooperative Extension Services, Washington, D.C., Home and Garden Bulletin No. 233, USDA, 1980.

Tannahill, Reay, *Food in History.* New York, Stein and Day, 1974.

Townsend, Doris McFerran, *The Cook's Companion.* New York, a Rutledge Book, Crown Publishers, 1978.

Van Brunt, Elizabeth R. and others, *Handbook on Herbs.* Brooklyn, N.Y., Brooklyn Botanic Garden, 1958-1980.

Exercise

Adult Physical Fitness, A Program for Men and Women Prepared by the President's Council on Physical Fitness. U.S. Government, Printing Office, Catalog No. PR 35.8:P56/AD9, 1979.

Astrand, Per-Olof, and Rodahl, Kaare, *Textbook of Work Physiology*, 2nd edition. New York, McGraw Hill Book Co., 1970, 1977.

Caldwell, John, *Cross-Country Skiing Today.* Brattleboro, Vt., Stephen Greene Press, 1977.

The Complete Book of Body Maintenance. Oliver Gillie and Derrik Mercer, eds. New York, W.W. Norton & Company, 1979.

Katz, Jane, with Bruning, Nancy, *Swimming for Total Fitness, A Progressive Aerobic Program.* Garden City, N.Y., Dolphin Books, Doubleday, 1981.

Marino, John, May, L., and Bennett, *John Marino's Bicycling Book.* Los Angeles, Calif., J.P. Tarcher, Inc., 1981; dist. by Houghton Mifflin, Boston, Mass.

McArdle, William D., Katch, Frank I., Katch, Victor L., *Exercise Physiology, Energy, Nutrition, and Human Performance.* Philadelphia, Pa., Lea and Febiger, 1981.

Kauz, Herman, *Tai Chi Handbook, Exercise Meditation and Self-Defense.* Garden City, N.Y., Dolphin Books, Doubleday, 1974.

Zohman, Lenor R., Kattus, Albert A., and Softness, Donald G., *The Cardiologists' Guide to Fitness and Health Through Exercise.* New York, Simon and Schuster, 1979.

Periodicals

Consumer Reports. Consumers Union of the United States, Inc., Mt.Vernon, N.Y.

FDA Consumer. Food and Drug Administration, Rockville, Md. Available through Superintendent of Documents, Government Printing Office, Washington, D.C.

The Harvard Medical School Health Letter. Department of Continuing Education, Harvard Medical School, Cambridge, Mass.

Nutrition and Health. Institute of Human Nutrition, Columbia University College of Physicians and Surgeons, New York, N.Y.

Nutrition & the M.D. PM Incorporated, Van Nuys, Calif.

Nutrition Action. Center for Science in the Public Interest, Washington, D.C.

Note: The U.S. Department of Agriculture issues a number of useful, reasonably priced publications. To obtain a list of those currently available, write to each of the following: USDA/AMS Publications Office, Room 2638 South, Washington, D.C. 20250; and USDA/FSIS, Publications Office, Room 1163 South, Washington, D.C., 20250

Acknowledgments
The editors are grateful to the following people for their generous assistance.

John Caldwell, Putney, Vt.

Emil Corwin and members of the Public Affairs staff, Food and Drug Administration, Washington, D.C.

Frances Cronin, M.D., and members of the Human Nutrition Information Service, U.S. Department of Agriculture, Washington, D.C.

Doris Erickson, Consumer Consultant, Cooperative Extension of Nassau County, U.S. Department of Agriculture, Plainview, N.Y.

William Heird, M.D., Associate Professor, College of Physicians and Surgeons of Columbia University, New York, N.Y.

Frank Hepburn and members of the Nutrient Data Research Group, Consumer Nutrition Center, U.S. Department of Agriculture, Hyattsville, Md.

Michael Jacobson, PhD., Executive Director, Center for Science in the Public Interest, Washington, D.C.

Thomas H. Jukes, M.D., Department of Biophysics and Medical Physics, University of California, Berkeley, Calif.

Gary H. Lincoff, New York, N.Y.

Maine Department of Marine Resources, Augusta, Me.

Mary Mead, R.D., M.Ed., Frances Stern Nutrition Center, Boston, Mass.

Ralph E. Miller, M.D., Lexington, Ky.

National Livestock and Meat Board Staff, Chicago, Ill.

National Oceanic and Atmospheric Administration, U.S. Department of Commerce, Washington, D.C.

Madeline Nelson, Health and Physical Education Director, Crozier, Va.

Joyce A. Nettleton, D.S., R.D., Massachusetts Nutrition Resource Center, Boston, Mass.

Richard Rivlin, M.D., Memorial Sloan-Kettering Cancer Center, New York, N.Y.

C Lavett Smith, PhD., American Museum of Natural History, New York, N.Y.

Mary Lou Tenney, Extension Associate, Division of Nutritional Sciences, Cornell University, Ithaca, N.Y.

Illustration Credits

Ann Brewster, 115, 117, 119,

Roy Coombs, 108, 109, 110, 111, 112, 114, 115, 117, 118,

Howard S. Friedman, 125, 126, 128, 130, 133, 153, 160, 166, 167,

Nancy Halliday, 137,

Victor Kalin, 112, 122, 123, 130,

Ted Lewin, 2-3, 8-9, 94-95, 280-281, 352-353

Harriet Pertchik, 97, 98-99, 100-101, 102-103, 104-105, 108, 109, 110, 111, 112, 113, 114, 115, 116, 117, 118, 119, 121, 122, 123, 143, 145, 147, 149,

Charles Pickard, 152,

Josephine Ranken, 108, 109, 111, 113, 117, 118, 119, 120, 121, 122, 123,

John Rignall, 155, 156-157, 158, 159,

Faith Shannon, 124, 125, 126, 127, 128, 129, 131, 132, 133, 134, 135,

Ray Skibinski, 11, 165, 169, 177, 180-181, 334, 336,

Ed Vebell, 320, 325, 326-327, 328, 329, 330, 331, 332, 333, 338-339, 340, 341, 342, 343, 344-345, 346, 347, 348, 349, 351,

Norman Weaver, 137, 139, 141

Credits

Grateful acknowledgment is made for permission to excerpt or adapt featured material from the following works.

p. 19 From Anderson, James W., *Plant Fiber in Foods.* HCF Diabetes Foundation, Lexington, Ky., 1980. **pp. 23, 191,** After Table VI (pp. 158-67) and Table I (p. 151) From *Food Values of Portions Commonly Used,* 13th ed. revised by Helen Nichols Church, B.S. and Jean A.T. Pennington, Ph.D, R.D. Harper & Row, Publishers, Inc. **pp.26-27** From "Vegetarianism." Consumer Reports Magazine, June 1980. **pp. 32-33** From *Recommended Dietary Allowances,* 9th rev. ed., 1980. National Academy of Sciences, Washington, D.C. 20418. **pp.36-37** From "Guide to the Vitamins." *The New York Times,* May 30, 1979, and *Vitamin Facts* used by permission of National Dairy Council. **pp. 99, 101, 103, 105** From "New American Eating Guide," Copyright © 1979, Center for Science in the Public Interest, Washington, D.C. 20009; **pp. 120, 129** From "Food Scorecard," Copyright © 1974, 1980, Center for Science in the Public Interest, Washington, D.C. 20009 **p. 185** From "Nutrition Action," August, 1981 © 1981 Center for Science in the Public Interest, Washington, D.C. 20009; **pp. 202-03, 205** From *Money, Menus, and Meals,* Publication 5275, Division of Agricultural Sciences, University of California. **p. 215** From Table 17.7, page 539, in *Nutritional Evaluation of Food Processing,* Robert S. Harris, Ph.D. and Endel Karmas, Ph.D., eds. Copyright © 1975 by the AVI Publishing Company, Inc., Westport, Conn. **p. 216** From *The Joy of Cooking,* copyright © 1931, 1936, 1941, 1942, 1946, 1951, 1952, 1953, 1962, 1963, 1964, 1975, by Irma S. Rombauer/Marion Rombauer Becker. Used with permission of the publisher, the Bobbs-Merrill Company, Inc. **p. 291** From "Rating the Diets," by Theodore Berland. Consumer Guide Magazine Health Bimonthly May 1981, vol. 304. All rights reserved under international and Pan American copyright conventions. Copyright © 1981 Publications International, Ltd. **p. 292** From *The Prudent Diet,* by Norman Jolliffe, M.D. Copyright © 1952, 1957, 1963 by Simon & Schuster, Inc. renewed © 1980 by Lillian Jolliffe. Reprinted by permission of Julian Messner, a Simon & Schuster division of Gulf & Western Corporation. **pp. 294-95** From *The Story of Weight Watchers,* as told to Joan Rattner Heilman. Copyright © 1970, 1975, 1979 by W/W Twentyfirst Corporation. Used by permission of The New American Library, Inc. **p. 300-01** From *Jane Brody's Nutrition Book,* with the permission of W.W. Norton & Company, Inc. Copyright © 1981 by Jane E. Brody. **pp. 316-17** From "My Sister and I Tried to Out-Diet Each Other With Some Scary Results," by Betsy Conley. Courtesy *Glamour.* Copyright © 1979 by The Condé Nast Publications Inc. **p. 358** From "Cold Comforts a Cook's Elixirs for Winter Ills," by Mimi Sheraton. © 1981/79 by The New York Times Company. Reprinted by permission. **pp. 370, 378** From *Mayo Clinic Diet Manual,* Cecilia M. Pemberton, R.D. and Clifford F. Gastineau, M.D., Ph.D., eds. © 1981 by the Mayo Foundation. Copyright 1949, 1954, 1961 and 1971 by W.B. Saunders Company. **p. 397** From *Exercise Physiology,* by William D. McArdle, Frank I. Katch, and Victor L. Katch. Copyright © 1981 by Lea & Febinger.

Grateful acknowledgment is made for permission to use and adapt recipes from the following sources.

Elizabeth Alston "Parsley Soup," "Scallion Cheese Maltex," "Austrian Curd Cake," and "Rutabaga Pancakes" from *The Best of Natural Eating Around the World,* by Elizabeth Alston. Copyright © 1973 by Elizabeth Alston. All rights reserved. **American Heart Association Northeast Ohio** "Peppered Roast Beef," "Tomato Crown Fish," "Pork Sausage Patties," "Bread Dressing," reproduced, with permission, from *Cooking Without Your Salt Shaker.* Copyright © 1978 by the American Heart Association, Northeast Ohio Affiliate, Inc. **Arbor House** "Green Rice," "Roast Chicken," "Broccoli Harlequin," "Braised Jerusalem Artichokes" from *The Maurice Moore-Betty Cooking School Book of Fine Cooking,* by Maurice Moore-Betty. Copyright © 1973. Reprinted with permission of Arbor Publishing Co. **Atheneum Publishers, Division of Scribner Book Co.** "Bean Sprout Salad" from *Chinese Cooking for the American Kitchen.* Copyright © 1976 by Karen Lee. New York: Atheneum, 1976. Reprinted with the permission of Atheneum Publishers; "Poule au Pot," "Gratin of Spinach and Hard-Boiled Eggs," "Gratin of Chick-Peas with Spinach," from Richard Olney, *Simple French Food.* Copyright © 1974 by Richard Olney New York: Atheneum, 1974. Reprinted with the permission of Atheneum Publishers; "Leftover Chicken Salad," "Roasted Ceci (Chickpeas)," "Grated Beets and Greens," "Lettuce & Asparagus Stew," from Judith Olney, *Summer Food.* Copyright © 1978 by Judith Olney New York: Atheneum, 1978. Reprinted with the permission of Atheneum Publishers. **Autumn Press, Inc.** "Squash and Onions," "Mustard Greens and Onions," "Baked Apples," from *The Book of Whole Meals,* by Annemarie Colbin. By permission of the publisher, Autumn Press, Brookline, Mass. **Basic Books, Inc., Publishers** "Pasta Marinara" and "Pasta e Fagioli II," reprinted from *Noodles Galore* by Merry White. Copyright © 1976 by Basic Books, Inc. By permission of Basic Books, Inc., Publishers, New York. **Mitchell Beazley Publishers Ltd.** "Lentils with Liver and Yogurt," and "Roast Lamb and Beans," recipes as above from *Future Food* by Colin Tudge, published in the United States by Harmony Books, One Park Avenue, New York, N.Y. 10016, and also *Future Cook* by Colin Tudge (the title in Britain) published by Mitchell Beazley, Artists House, 14 Manette Street, London W1V 5LB. **Irena Chalmers Cookbooks, Inc.** "Casserole of Spring Garden Vegetables," from *Casserole Creations* by Irena Chalmers; "Rumanian Chicken Stew" and "Veal Stew" from *Cooking in Clay,* by Irena Chalmers; "Chicken with Citrus Fruits" and "Wrapped Fish" from *Healthy Gourmet,* by Irena Chalmers; "Bulgur Wheat, Sautéed with Yogurt," "Zucchini and Dill," and "Stir-Fried Watercress with Carrots," from *Irena Chalmers Cookbook* by Irena Chalmers; "Chicken and Vegetables in Aspic," from *Ramekins,* by Irena Chalmers. "Melon & Ginger," "Peas," and "Cabbage" from *Salt Free Cookery,* by Irena Kirschman; "Ricotta Cheese Souffles," and "Carrot, Celery, and Egg Salad" from *Fine Fresh Food—Fast,* by Michele Urvater. "Crisp-Fried Turkey Breast," and "Roast Chicken with Canadian Bacon and Cottage Cheese," from *The Confident Cook* by Irena Chalmers. **Elizabeth Schneider Colchie** "Kasha and Red Peppers," from *The March Hare Comes to Dinner,* by Elizabeth Schneider Colchie. Copyright 1982 by Elizabeth Schneider Colchie from *Ready When You Are: Made Ahead-Meals for Entertaining,* published by Crown. **Collier Associates** "Farina Dumplings," and "White Beans in Olive Oil," from *The Eastern European Cookbook,* by Kay Shaw Nelson. Permission to reprint granted by Collier Associates representative of Kay Shaw Nelson. **Lisa Cosman** "Breakfast Broccoli," "Sautéed Liver Dredged in Wheat Germ," and "Steamed New Potatoes Dressed in Broth," from *Whole Food Cookery.* Copyright 1981 by Lisa Cosman. **Delacorte Press** "Goulash Soup," "Barley Casserole," and "Red Cabbage," excerpted from the book *Clancy's Oven Cookery,* by John Clancy and Frances Field. Copyright © 1976 by John Clancy and Frances Field. Reprinted by permission of Delacorte Press/Eleanor Friede. **Doubleday & Co., Inc.** "Roast Pineapple" from *The Art of American Indian Cooking,* by Yeffe Kimball and Jean Anderson. Copyright © 1965 by Yeffe Kimball and Jean Anderson. Reprinted by permission of Doubleday & Company, Inc.; "Scandinavian Dry-Baked Flounder," and "Bombay-Style Flounder" from *Cooking Fish and Shellfish,* by Ruth A. Spear. Copyright © 1980 by Ruth A. Spear. Reprinted by permission of Doubleday and Company, Inc.; "Baked Cherry Tomatoes," "Spliced Carrots," "Brussels Sprouts with Water Chestnuts," and "Grated Zucchini" from *New York Entertains,* by The Junior League of the City of New York. Copyright © 1974 by The Junior League of New York, Inc. Reprinted by permission of Doubleday & Company, Inc. "Hoppin' John" from *Spoonbread and Strawberry Wine,* by Norma Jean and Carole Darden. Copyright © 1978 by Norma Jean and Carole Darden. Reprinted by permission of Doubleday and Company, Inc. **M. Evans & Co., Inc.** "Fennel Salad," and "Cream of Vegetables" from *The Regional Italian Kitchen,* by Nika Hazelton. Copyright © 1978 by Nika Hazelton. Reprintd by permission of the publisher, M. Evans and Company, Inc., New York, N.Y. 10017. **The Fanny Farmer Cookbook** "Herbed Barbecue Sauce" from *The Fanny Farmer Cookbook,* revised by Wilma Lord Perkins. Copyright © 1959, 1965 by Dexter and Wilma Lord Perkins. Used by permission. **Jonathan Rudé Fields** "S'Chee" from *Michael Field's Cooking School.* Published by Holt, Rinehart and Winston, New York; "Baked Kale," reprinted from *Kitchen Bouquets,* by Bert Greene. © 1979, with the permission of Contemporary Books, Inc., Chicago. **Harcourt Brace Jovanovich Inc.** "Baked Carrots and Apples," and "Crisp Shredded Turnips," from *Let's Cook It Right,* by Adelle Davis. Copyright © 1947, 1962 by Harcourt Brace Jovanovich, Inc.; renewed 1975 by Frank Vernon Sieglinger. Reprinted by permission of the publisher. **Harper & Row, Publishers, Inc.** "Pancake and Waffle Mix," from *Better Than Store-Bought,* by Helen Witty and Elizabeth Schneider Colchie. Copyright © by Helen Witty and Elizabeth Schneider Colchie. Reprinted by permission of Harper & Row, Publishers, Inc. "Halibut Salad with Dill," and "Kasha Stuffing," in *From My Mother's Kitchen,* by Mimi Sheraton. Copyright © 1979 by Mimi Sheraton. Reprinted by permission of Harper & Row, Publishers, Inc.; "Peanuts-Go-Lightly Dip," "Indian Kedgeree," "Boston Baked Beans," and "Kidney Beans with Red Cabbage and Apples," from Peta Lyn Farwagi, *Full of Beans.* New York: Harper & Row, 1978, by Peta Lyn Farwagi. Reprinted by permission of the publisher; "Buttermilk Gazpacho," "Oatmeal-Banana Muffins," and "Tarragon-Buttermilk Dressing," from *Half a Can of Tomato Paste and Other Culinary Dilemmas,* by Jean Anderson and Ruth Buchan. Copyright © 1980 by Jean Anderson and Ruth Buchan. Reprinted by permission of Harper & Row,

Publishers, Inc. "Lemon Lamb Roast," and "Lamb a la Grecque en Brochette," from The International Slim *Gourmet Cookbook*, by Barbara Gibbons. Copyright © 1978 by Barbara Gibbons. Reprinted by permission of Harper & Row, Publishers, Inc.; "Eggplant Parmesan," "Italian Soybean-Grains Casserole," "Vegetable Paella," "Black Bean Soup," and "Kasha Pie," from *The Vegetarian Feast*, by Martha Rose Shulman. Copyright © 1979 by Martha Rose Shulman. Reprinted by permission of Harper & Row, Publishers, Inc. **Holt, Rinehart and Winston** "Broiled Tomato Halves" from *Cooking with Michael Field*, edited by Joan Scobey. Copyright © 1971 by Frances Field. Copyright © 1972 by Frances Field and Nelson Doubleday, Inc. Copyright © 1978 by the Estate of Frances Field. Reprinted by permission of Holt, Rinehart and Winston, Publishers; "Mussels," "Bluefish," and "Mustard Sauce" from *John Clancy's Fish Cookery*, by John Clancy and Beatrice Saunders. Copyright © 1979 by John Clancy and Beatrice Saunders. Reprinted by permission of Holt, Rinehart and Winston, Publishers. **Houghton Mifflin Company** "Crumbs for Three Chickens," from *Diet Against Disease*, by Frances Tenenbaum and Alice A. Martin. Copyright © 1980 by Frances Tenenbaum and Alice A. Martin. Reprinted by permission of Houghton Mifflin Company; "Ginger Pears," "Fruit Snowball," and "Rhubarb Compote," from *Woman's Day Low-Calorie Dessert Cookbook*, by Carol Cutler. Copyright © 1980 by CBS Consumer Publications, a Division of CBS, Inc. Reprinted by permission of the publisher, Houghton Mifflin Company. **Alfred A. Knopf, Inc.** "Corn Pone," from *The Taste of Country Cooking*, by Edna Lewis. Copyright © 1976 by Edna Lewis. Reprinted by permission of Alfred A. Knopf, Inc.; "Pizza Rustica," "Basic Shortcrust Pastry," and "Simple Vinaigrette Sauce," from *The Vegetarian Epicure*, by Anna Thomas. Copyright © 1972 by Anna Thomas. Reprinted by permission of Alfred A. Knopf, Inc. "Quick Pickled Peppers," from *The Vegetarian Epicure, Book Two*, by Anna Thomas, illustrated by Julie Maas. Copyright © 1978 by Anna Thomas and Julie Maas. Reprinted by permission of Alfred A. Knopf, Inc.; "Gingered Eggplant Salad," "Marinated Leeks," "Rice Salad Vinaigrette," "Potato Salad Tzapanos," from *The Vegetarian Epicure, Book Two*, by Anna Thomas. Copyright © 1978 by Anna Thomas and Julie Maas. Reprinted by permission of Alfred A. Knopf, Inc. **Little, Brown and Co.** "Basic Pot Roast of Beef," and "Shoulder Lamb Chops Braised with Onions and Peppers," from *James Beard's American Cookery*, by James Beard. Copyright © 1972 by James Beard. By permission of Little, Brown and Company in association with the Atlantic Monthly Press; "Garbure," "Ham Steak Baked in Milk," and "Gado Gado," from *Cooking in a Small Kitchen*, by Arthur Schwartz. Copyright © 1979 by Arthur Schwartz. By permission of Little, Brown and Company. **McGraw-Hill Book Company** "Spinach Creamed with Peaches Instead of Cream," and "Pike (or other whole fish) Baked on a Bed of Aromatic Vegetables," from *Revolutionizing French Cooking*, by Roy Andries de Groot. Reprinted by permission of McGraw-Hill Book Company. **David McKay Co., Inc.** "Marinated Garbanzos," "Tomato Bouillon," "Spanish Chicken," "Colache," and "Five-Minute Soup," reprinted with permission from the book, *The American Heart Association Cookbook*, by Mary Winston and Ruthe Eshleman. Copyright © 1979. Published by David McKay Co., Inc. **William Morrow & Co., Inc.** "Tandoori (Indian Barbecued) Chicken," "Roasted Onions (Bhone Piaz)," "Grated Cucumber Relish," "Onion and Roasted Tomato Relish," in *Classic Indian Cooking*, by Julie Sahni. Copyright © 1980 by Julie Sahni. By permission of William Morrow & Co., Inc., "Cold Vegetable Sauce for Grilled Beef," in *Michel Guerard's Cuisine Minceur*, by Michel Guerard. English translation copyright © 1976 by William Morrow and Company, Inc. "Chicken with Wine Vinegar," in *LaVarenne's Paris Kitchen*, by Anne Willan. Copyright © 1981 by LaVarenne U.S.A. Inc. By permission of William Morrow & Co., Inc.; "Stuffed Chicken Breasts," "Fruited Bulgur," "Pears with Gorgonzola," "Red Plum Compote" in *Pure and Simple*, by Marian Burros. Copyright © 1978 by Marian Fox Burros. By permission of William Morrow & Co., Inc. **Nilgiri Press** "Lasagna al Forno," "Chard and Cheese Pie," "Broccoli Dressing," "Homemade Ketchup," and "Oatmeal Pancakes," reprinted by permission from *Laurel's Kitchen: A Handbook for Vegetarian Cookery and Nutrition*, by Laurel Robertson, Carol Flinders, and Bronwen Godfrey. Copyright 1976 by Nilgiri Press, Petaluma, CA. 94954 **Perigee Books** "Broiled Hamburgers," reprinted by permission of Coward, McCann & Geoghegan, Inc. from *The Gaylord Hauser Cook Book*, by Gaylord Hauser. Copyright 1946 by Gaylord Hauser. **G.P. Putnam's Sons** "Roast Oregon Turkey with Sausage Dressing," "Dirty Rice," "Green Bean Casserole," and "Turnip-Potato Puree," reprinted by permission of G.P. Putnam's Sons from *The New York Times Heritage Cook Book*, by Jean Hewitt. Copyright © 1972 by The New York Times Company; "Yankee Bean Chowder," "Crisp Rutabaga Salad," "Pork Chops with Spinach," reprinted by permission of G.P. Putnam's Sons from *The New York Times New England Heritage Cook Book*, by Jean Hewitt. Copyright © 1977 by The New York Times Company; "Black-Eyed Pea Soup," "Florida Keys Red Snapper," and "Assorted Greens," reprinted by permission of G.P. Putnam's Sons from *The New York Times Southern Heritage Cook Book*, by Jean Hewitt. Copyright © 1976 by The New York Times Company. **Random House, Inc.** "Country Captain," "Curry Marinade," "Grilled Chicken Steaks," "Simple Grape Stuffing" from *The Complete Chicken*, by Carl Jerome. Copyright © 1978 by Carl Jerome. Reprinted by permission of Random House, Inc.; "Louisiana Sweet-Potato Salad," "Mushroom, Egg, Barley Casserole," "Pueblo Cauliflower with Pumpkin Seeds," from *American Food: The Gastronomic Story*, by Evan Jones. Copyright © 1974, 1975, 1981 by Evan Jones and Judith B. Jones. Reprinted by permission of Random House, Inc.; "Pureed Celeriac," "Poached Fresh Peaches with Fresh Raspberry Sauce," "Indian Pudding," from *Cooking with Helen McCully Beside You*, by Helen McCully. Copyright © 1970 by Helen McCully. Reprinted by permission of Random House, Inc.; "Boeuf Mironton (Boiled Beef Baked in Vinegar and Caper Sauce)" and "Soupe de Pecheurs (Rich Fish Soup)," from *The Cuisine of the Sun*, by Mireille Johnston. Copyright © 1976 by Mireille Johnston. Reprinted by permission of Random House, Inc.; "Sherried Mixed Fruit" and "Linguine or Spaghetti with Broccoli," from *Dr. Rechtschaffen's Diet for Lifetime Weight Control and Better Health, with Original Recipes by Anne Seranne*, by Joseph S. Rechtschaffen, M.D., and Robert Carola. Copyright © 1980 by Joseph S. Rechtschaffen, M.D., and Robert Carola. Reprinted by permission of Random House, Inc.; "Beets with Tuna" and "Spaghetti Matriciana Style" (Spaghetti alla Matriciana), from *Italian Family Cooking*, by Edward Giobbi. Copyright © 1971 by Edward Giobbi. Reprinted by permission of Random House, Inc.; ' **Rodale Press, Inc.** "Israeli Carrot Salad," "Mediterranean Ratatouille," "Vegetarian Nut Patties," and "Assorted Fruit with Honey-Lime Dressing," reprinted from *Managing Your Personal Food Supply*. Copyright © 1977 by Rodale Press, Inc. Permission granted by Rodale Press, Inc., Emmaus, PA 18049; "Polenta Cheese Squares" and "Melon Cooler," reprinted from *The Rodale Cookbook*. Copyright © 1973 by Rodale Press, Inc. Permission granted by Rodale Press, Inc. Emmaus, PA. **John Schaffner Literary Agency** "Spring Pea Soup" and "Broiled Chicken Breasts with Lime Juice," from *The Too Hot To Cook Book*, by Miriam Ungerer. Copyright © 1966 by Miriam Ungerer. All rights reserved. **Shambala Publications** "Fresh Fruit Cake" and "Tassajara Granola," reprinted by special arrangement with Shambala Publications, Inc. 1920 13th Street, Boulder, CO. 80302. From *The Tassajara Bread Book*, by Edward Espe Brown. Copyright © 1970 by the Chief Priest, Zen Center, San Francisco. **Simon & Schuster, Inc.** "Caldo Gallego," "Haitian Black Beans," "Mrs. Dross's Acorn Squash," "Italian Carrot Torte" from *Cooking with Vegetables*, by Alex D. Hawkes. Copyright © 1968 by Alex D. Hawkes. Reprinted by permission of Simon & Schuster, a Division of Gulf & Western Corporation. **St. Martin's Press** "Asparagus Sald," "Baking Powder Biscuits," "Oatmeal Snacks," from *The Book of Whole Grains*, by Marlene Anne Bumgarner. Copyright © 1976 by Marlene Anne Bumgarner. All rights reserved. **Ten Speed Press** "Minestrone," "White Rabbit Salad," "Tabouli," "Vegetable Stew," "High Protein-Low Calorie Dressing," from *The Moosewood Cookbook*, by Mollie Katzen. Copyright 1977. Reprinted by Ten Speed Press P.O. Box 7123, Berkeley, CA. 94707. $8.95 paper, $11.95 cloth. **Times Books** "Beef Goulash," "Broiled Fish" and "Ginger Cookies." Copyright © 1980 by Craig Claiborne. Reprinted by permission of Times Books, a division of Quadrangle/The New York Times Book Co., Inc. From *Craig Claiborne's Gourmet Diet*, by Craig Claiborne with Pierre Franey. Copyright © 1977 by Giuliano Bugialli. Reprinted by permission of Times Books, a division of Quadrangle/The New York Times Book Co., Inc. From *The Fine Art of Italian Cooking*, by Giuliano Bugialli. "Oven-Roasted Sweet Corn in the Husk." Copyright © 1977 by Jean Anderson. Reprinted by permission of Times Books, a division of Quadrangle/The New York Times Book Co., Inc. From *The Grass Roots Cookbook*, by Jean Anderson. **The Viking Press** "Chicken Broth," and "Pork Chops Baked with Orange," from *American Home Cooking*, by Nika Hazelton. Copyright © 1980 by Nika Hazelton. Reprinted by permission of Viking Penguin Inc.; "Paris Broil" and "Black Beans and Rice," from *Good Cheap Food*, by Miriam Ungerer. Copyright © 1973 by Miriam Ungerer. Reprinted by permission of Viking Penguin Inc.; "Haddock Chowder (Passamaquoddy Bay)," from *North Atlantic Seafood*, by Alan Davidson. Copyright © 1979 by Alan Davidson. Reprinted by permission of Viking Penguin Inc.; "French Cauliflower Pie," "Potato-Tomato Bake," "Figs in Wine," from *A Passion for Vegetables*, by Vera Gewanter. Copyright © 1980 by Vera Gewanter. Reprinted by permission of Viking Penguin Inc. **U.S. Department of Agriculture** "Oriental Beef," "Onion Sauce," and "Orange Smothee," from *Food, Home and Garden Bulletin 228,1979*," "Banana-Nut Bread," "Bean Salad," "Chicken Cacciatore," "Chili Bean Dip," "Corn Bread," "Gingerbread," and "Vegetable Chowder," from *Ideas for Better Eating*, Science and Education Administration, 1981.

Index

The Recipe Index begins on page 411.

A

Abalone, 140
Absorption, 31
  malabsorption, 372
Accidents
  weight and, 282
Achilles tendon, 336
  tendonitis, 337
Acids
  in cooking beans, 162
  digestion and, 10, 363, 364
Acidophilus milk, 154
Acne, diet and, 314, 354
Acupuncture, 282, 287
Additives, 199–201
  dye in Cheddar, 156
  dye in peanut spreads, 167
  dye in pistachios, 167
  dye in processed cheese, 157
  in infant's diet, 309
  in milk products, 154–55
  in sausages, 151
  in pork, 148
  in soy sauce, 163
Adipose tissue, 20
Adolescents, 314–17
  balanced diet for, 291
  calorie needs of, 12
  meal plan for, 302–3
  pregnancy and, 306, 316
Aerobic capacity, 326–27
Aerobic conditioning, 334–35
  in court and field sports, 346
Aerobics, 321, 334–51
Age
  calories and, 12
  exercise and, 324, 342, 351
  See also age groups, e.g., Adolescents; Elderly.
Aging process
  aerobics and, 334
  inflexibility and, 321
  See also Elderly.
Alcohol, 190–91
  as calories, 14
  in cooking, 218
  in reducing diets, 294
  gaining weight and, 301
  grains as source of, 168, 171
  pregnancy and, 306
  and water requirements, 50
Alcoholics, ketogenic diets and, 287
Alfalfa sprouts, 121, 164–65
Allergens, 369, 370
Allergies
  to eggs, 356
  of infants, 308, 309, 370
  to mangoes, 129
  to milk, 154
  to papayas, 131
  special diets and, 368
Alligator pears. *See* Avocados.
Allspice, 178
Almonds, 80–81, 166
American Academy of Pediatrics, 21

American Board of Nutrition, 356
American Celiac Society, 372
American Dietetic Association, 356
American Medical Association, 290
Amino acids, 10, 24–27, 285, 390–91
  essential, 25
  in liquid protein, 289
  in soybeans, 162–63
  vegetarian diets and, 354
  See also Proteins.
Amphetamines, 288
Anaerobics, 334
Analogs 25, 163
Anemia, 319, 355
Anger,
  digestion and, 11
  eating habits and, 300, 301
Anoretic drugs, 288
Anorexia nervosa, 314, 316–17, 388
Antibiotics, 38, 114, 355
Anxiety, 14, 300
Appetite, 283
  in children, 311
  in the elderly, 318–19
  exercise and, 321
  fasting diets and, 289
  gaining weight and, 301
  of infants, 308
  loss of, 284, 306, 354
  of people living alone, 304
  during pregnancy, 306
  running and, 337
  suppression of, 287
  of teenagers, 314
Apples, 64–65, 124
Aquaexercises, 344–45
Arthritis, exercise and, 324, 342, 351
Artichoke, 108
Arugula, 108
Asparagus, 84–85, 108
Atherosclerosis, 22, 356
Athlete's diet, 395–97
Atkins' Diet Revolution, Dr., 290
Aversions. *See* Food aversions.
Avocado, 66–67, 109

B

Baby. *See* Infant.
Back muscles, 325, 349
Back pain, 328, 330
Back problems, 342
Back strain, 329
Bacon, 60-61, 148
Badminton, 347, 348, 349
Baking soda, 377
  with beans, 164
Ballet, 331, 348
Bananas, 66-67, 125
Banting, William, 286
Barley, 168
  sprouts, 165
Barley flour, 174
  in breads, 270
Basal metabolism rate (BMR), 98–99

food choices and, 12
Basic Four Food Groups, 20, 96–107
Basil, 176, 178
Basketball, 346, 347
Bass, 136–39
Bay leaf, 178
Beach peas, 180
Beans, 82–83, 86-87, 109, 161-65
  flatulence and, 164
  See also Black-eyed peas; Flageolets; Green beans; Lentils; Soybeans.
Bean sprouts, 86–87, 164–65
Beef
  buying guide for, 142–43
  cuts of, 142–43
  fat content of, 285
  food chart, 60–63
  in sausages, 151
  variety meats of, 150–51
  See also Veal.
Beer, 190, 191, 395
Beets, 86–87, 109
Behavior modification, 293, 294, 296, 300–301
Bel Paese cheese, 155
Berman, Edith, 294
Berries, 125
Beverages, 182–91
  in brownbag lunches, 313
  for the elderly, 319
  food chart, 64–71, 84–85, 92
  gaining weight and, 301
  herbs and spices for, 179
  during pregnancy, 306
Bicycling, 323, 340–41, 348
Bile, 11
Biotin, 12, 36–37
  in foods, 37, 150, 153
Blackberries, 66–67
Bladder stones, 373
Bland diet, 355–56
Bland foods, meal planning and, 302
Blood pressure
  exercise and, 320, 322, 334, 351
  lowering of, 320, 333
  weight and, 282
  See also Hypertension.
Blood-sugar level, 14, 15, 16, 17
  fiber and, 18
Blueberries, 66–67, 126
Blue cheese, 52–53, 155
Bluefish, 60–61, 138
Body type, exercise and, 324
Body weight, calories and, 12
Bokchoy (pakchoi), 88–89, 110
Bones, 319, 337
  calcium and, 36–37,44, 307, 354
Bouquet garni, 176
Bowel movements, 365
  celiac disease and, 355, 372
Brains (food), 150
Brain (human), 13
Bran, 19, 171, 366
  bran flakes, 74–75
Brazil nuts, 82–83, 166
Breads, 72–73, 174

402

baking at home, 270–72
in brownbag lunches, 313
complex carbohydrates in, 15
for the elderly, 318, 319
flours and, 173–74
high fiber, 19
rolls, 80–81
white vs whole wheat, 72–73, 174
Breakfast
for children, 311–12
meal planning, 302–3, 304
Breast-feeding. *See* Pregnancy and breast-feeding diet.
Brick cheese, 155–56
Brie cheese, 156
Broccoli, 86–87, 110
Brody, Jane, 300–301
Brownbag lunches, 312–13
Brussels sprouts, 86–87, 110
Buckwheat, 168
Buckwheat flour, 74–75, 174
in breads, 270
Buffalofish, 136
Bulgur, 74–75, 171
Bulking agent, 288
Butter, 154–55
nutrition in, 52–53
shelf list, 304
Butterfish, 138
Buttermilk, 54–55, 154
for oral candidiasis, 355
Buying guide for foods, 108–79

C

Cabbage, 86–89, 110
Caciocavallo cheese, 156
Caffeine, 188–89
bland diet and, 355, 362, 364
in diet pills, 288
pregnancy and, 306
weight gain and, 301
Calciferol. *See* Vitamin D (calciferol).
Calcium, 44, 46
for adolescents, 33, 314, 315
bones and, 36–37, 44, 307, 354
children and, 33, 311, 371
elderly and, 319
food chart, 51–93
in foods, 44, 46, 108, 109, 110, 111, 112, 113, 115, 116, 117, 118, 120, 121, 122, 123, 126, 128, 129, 140, 154, 163, 166, 167, 170, 173, 174
phytic acid and, 174
during pregnancy, 33, 307
RDA, 33
Calisthenics, 328–31
aquaexercises, 344–45
Calorie expenditure
by body size, 299
by exercise, 323, 334, 346, 350
with illness, 299, 358
Caloric requirements, 12
of adolescents, 314–15
of adults, 298–99, 318
of children, 310, 311
of infants, 308
in pregnancy, 306–7

Calories, 12
in carbohydrates, 17, 286
deficit of, 282, 285
dieting and, 283–86, 288, 290
empty, 14, 15
energy and, 12, 283, 298
excess, 20, 285
in fats, 14, 17, 21, 286
in fiber, 18
in foods, 51–93, 154, 155, 164, 166, 168, 169, 316, 390
meal planning and, 302
in proteins, 12, 17, 24, 286
in sweeteners, 17
Calories Don't Count diet, 290
Camembert cheese, 52–53, 156
Cancer
diet and, 357, 365, 386–87,
high-fiber diet and, 365
laetrile and, 43
Candidiasis, 355
Candy, 82–85, 288, 372
Canoeing, 323, 325, 343, 349
Cantaloupes (muskmelons), 68–69, 130
Capon, 152
Caraway, 178
Carbohydrate loading, 396–97
Carbohydrates, 130–19
for adolescents, 315
in American diet, 10, 13, 14, 15
calories supplied by, 12
child's need of, 310
in balanced diet, 218, 284, 291, 278–79, 302
deficiency, 285
dieting and, 283–86, 292, 294
digestion of, 11
for the elderly, 318
energy supplied by, 13, 14, 15, 285
fiber in, 15, 17, 18, 285
food chart, 51–93
in milk, 154
Carbohydrates, complex, 15, 285
beans and flatulence, 164
diabetes and, 16
fiber and, 18
in foods, 161
meal planning and, 218, 278–79, 302
Cardiorespiratory system, 334
exercise and, 320, 321, 322, 323, 327, 338, 347
Cardiovascular disease, 21, 333
See also Blood pressure.
Cardiovascular fitness
exercise for, 349
Pritikin Program, 292
Carp, 136
Carrots, 13–14, 88–89, 110–11
as sweetener in recipes, 17
Cashews, 82–83, 166
Catfish, 136
Cattail, 180
Cauliflower, 88–89, 111
Celeriac, 111
Celery, 88–89, 112
Celiac disease, 355, 372
Cellulose, 19
elimination and, 12
Cereals (breakfast), 72–75, 172, 360

for adolescents, 314, 315
complex carbohydrates in, 15
for infants, 309
intolerance to, 372
during pregnancy, 307
shelf list, 304
Cereals and meals. *See* Grains.
Cheddar cheese, 52–53, 156
Cheeses, 155–59
cholesterol in, 23
nutrition in, 52–53
shelf list, 304
tofu as substitute for, 163
Cherries, 66–67, 126
Chervil, 176, 178
Chestnuts, 166
Chicken, 64–65, 152
Chicken broth, 355
Chicory, 113
Chick-peas, 161, 164
sprouts, 165
Children
body weight and, 12
eating habits and, 300, 310–13
eating sensibly and, 296, 310–13
exercise and, 312, 324, 351
meal planning for, 302–3
RDA, 32–33
Chinese cabbage, 110
Chives, 117, 176
Chloride, 45, 46
in foods, 45, 46, 138, 142, 153, 154
Chocolate allergy, 368–69
Cholesterol, 20–23
elderly and, 318–19
exercise and, 322
fat-controlled diet, 384–86
fatty acids and, 51
fiber and, 18
in foods, 140, 142, 153, 161, 163, 167
heart disease and, 288, 376
Pritikin Program, 292
Chyme, 10–11
Cigarette smoking
exercise and, 322
hypnosis and, 287
during pregnancy and breast-feeding, 306, 307
trying to gain weight and, 301
Cinnamon, 178
Cisco, 136
Claiborne, Craig, 49, 376
Clams, 60–61, 140
Cloves, 178
Cobalamin. *See* Vitamin B_{12} (cobalamin).
Coconuts, 82–83, 166
Cod, 138
Coenzymes, 31
Cofactors, 31
Coffee, 186–89, 301, 306
See also Caffeine.
Coffee whiteners, 154
Colby cheese, 156
Colds, diet for, 358
Cold remedies, PPA in, 288
Colitis, ulcerative, 362
Collard greens, 88–89, 112

403

Index

Competitive sports, 324, 336, 346
   court and field, 346
   personality type and, 324
   running, 336–37
Complementary combinations. *See* Protein.
Condensed milk, 154
Conley, Betsy, 316–17
Constipation, 18, 19
   in the elderly, 318, 319
   high-fiber diet and, 319, 363, 365
   during pregnancy, 306
Consumer Guide
   on Diet Workshop, Inc., 294
   on rating a diet, 291
Cookies, 76–77
Cooking, 212–17
   recipes, 218–77
Cooling down, 326, 327, 328, 338, 343, 350
Coordination, 321, 322, 338
Copper, 45–47
   in foods, 46, 47, 140, 150, 168, 173
Coriander, 178
Corn (grain), 168–69
   breakfast cereals, 74–75
Corn (vegetable), 88, 112–13
   complex carbohydrates in, 15
   high-fiber diet and, 365
Cornmeal, 76–77, 168–69
   in breads, 270
Cornstarch, 169
Cottage cheese, 52–53, 155, 156
Crab, 60–61, 140
Crackers, 76–77
Cramps
   allergic reactions and, 368
   during pregnancy, 307
   swimming and, 343
Cranberries, 66–67, 126
Crappie, 136
Crayfish, 140
Cream cheese, 52–53, 156
Creams
   buying guide, 154–55
   imitation, 54–55, 154
   nutritive value of, 52–55
Crustaceans, 140
Cucumbers, 88–89, 113
Cumin, 178
Currants, 125

D

Daikon radish, 119
Dairy products
   allergies to, 371
   fats in, 21
   for infants, 309
   food chart, 52–57
   See also Milk products.
Dance, 331, 349
Dandelion, 88–89, 180
Dates, 66–67, 126
Day lily, 180

Dehydration, 358
   lack of carbohydrates and, 14
Dental problems, 17
   special diets and, 361
Department of Agriculture, U.S.
   Basic Four Food Groups, 20, 96
   cheeses graded by, 155
   fruits graded by, 124
   poultry graded by, 152
   milk graded by, 154
   nutritive value of foods, 51
   nuts graded by, 166
   sausage graded by, 151
Depression
   eating habits and, 300
   in the elderly, 318–19
   exercise and, 320
Desserts
   in brownbag lunches, 313
   cholesterol in, 23
   eating out and, 305
   for the elderly, 318
   herbs and spices for, 179
   for infants, 309
   for reluctant milk drinkers, 302
Desserts, milk, 56–57, 155
Dextrose. *See* Glucose (dextrose).
Deutsch, Ronald M., 285
Diabetes, 16
   diet and, 356, 365, 374
   exercise and, 322
   fiber in diet and, 18
   sugar and, 354
   weight and, 282
Diarrhea
   as allergic reaction, 368, 372
   bland diet for, 362
   dehydration and, 358
   in the elderly, 318
   high-fiber diet and, 365
Diet candy and gum, 288
Dieting, 282–95
Diet pills, 283, 288, 294
Diets
   athlete's, 395–97
   balanced, 286, 290–95, 296, 302
   bland, 355, 362–64
   cancer and, 357, 365, 384–85
   drugstore diets, 288
   elimination, 368–70
   fad, 284, 374, 395
   fasting, 284, 286, 289–90
   liquid, 359–60
   low-carbohydrate, 14, 17, 286–89, 290
   reducing, 282–95
   sodium-controlled, 376–80
   soft, 361
   special, 354–94
   therapeutic, 354–94
   vegetarian, 390–94
   weight control, 282–94
Diet Workshop, Inc., 293, 294
Digestion, 10–12
   absorption and, 31
   bland diet and, 361, 362
   cholesterol and fat, 22
   evening meal and, 304
   fiber and, 18
   of infant, 308, 309

proteins and, 24–25
Digestive problems, 362
   acidophilus milk and, 154
   of the elderly, 318–19
   yogurt and, 155
Digitalis, 357
   as diet pill, 288
Dill, 176, 178
Disease, diet and, 354–89
Diuretics, 38
   as diet pill, 288
Diverticulitis, 18, 362, 364
Diverticulosis, 365
Dizziness, exercise and, 322, 327, 337
DNA (deoxyribonucleic acid), 25, 31
Doctor's Quick Weight Loss diet, 286, 290
Drug interactions
   elderly and, 319
   with foods, 38–39
   sulfa drugs and PABA, 43
Drugs, diet, 288
Drum, freshwater, 136
Dry milk, nonfat, 154
Duck, 152–53
Ductless glands. *See* Endocrine (ductless) glands.
Durum wheat, 171, 174

E

Eating habits, 296–319
   of children, 310, 311
   of the elderly, 318–19
   infants and, 308
   meal planning and, 302–3
   of person alone, 304
   reducing diets and changing one's, 283, 286, 288–89, 291, 292, 295
Eating out, 304, 305
Edam cheese, 156
Eggnog, 56–57, 359, 360
Eggplant, 113
Eggs, 58–59, 153
   allergy to, 369
   cholesterol in, 23
   for infant, 309
   during pregnancy, 307
   in frozen custard, 155
Elderly
   body weight and, 12
   cooking for one, 304
   eating sensibly and, 296, 297, 318–19
   exercise and, 320, 321, 324, 351
   meal planning for, 302–3
   swimming for, 342
   soft diet and, 361
Elimination, 12, 18, 285
Elimination diet, 368
Emulsifiers
   gum arabic in cream cheese, 156
   in processed cheese, 156
   in sweet cream, 154
Endive, 88–89, 113
Endocrine (ductless) glands, 31
   hormones of, 31
Endurance, 321, 338
Energy sources

calories, 12, 283, 298–99
carbohydrates, 13, 14, 15, 285
food and, 12
glucose as source of, 13, 14, 334, 396
proteins, 24
Enzymes
in cheese, 155
defined, 31
digestion and, 10, 11
proteins and, 24
Ergot, 171
Escarole, 113
Esophagus, 10
Ethylene gas, 123
Evaporated milk, 154
Exchange plans, 374, 377
Exercise, 320-51
dieting and, 293, 294, 301

F

Fad diets, 284, 374
Farina, 72–73, 171, 172
Farmer cheese, 156
Fast foods, 315, 316
Fasting diets, 284, 286, 289–90
Fatigue
from diet, 285
eating habits and, 300
exercise and, 321, 322, 337, 343
overexertion and, 337
swimming cramps and, 343
Fats, 10–12, 20–23
in adolescent diet, 315
aerobics burning off, 334
in American diet, 10, 13, 14, 21, 218
in animal protein, 14, 21, 185
in bland diet, 363
as body weight, 282
calories per gram, 12
in childrens' diet, 310
in diet of the elderly, 318–19
fat-controlled diets, 384–86
in foods, 51–93, 109, 136, 140, 144, 150,
  151, 152, 154–55, 161, 163, 168, 171,
  174
for gaining weight, 301
hydrogenated, 21, 167
ketogenic diets and, 286, 287
in low-carbohydrate diet, 288
meal planning and, 278–79
in nondairy creamer, 154
during pregnancy, 307
reducing amounts in diet, 21, 374
in yogurt, 155
See also Oils; Shortenings.
Fatty acids 10, 20, 21, 22, 51–93, 166, 167
in ketogenic diets, 287
monounsaturated, 20, 51
polyunsaturated, 20, 21, 22, 51
polyunsaturated, in foods, 166, 167
saturated, 20, 21, 22, 51-93, 163, 166
unsaturated, 20, 21, 51-93
Fava beans. See Beans, broad.
Favism, 161
Feces, 12
Fennel, 114, 178
Feta cheese, 156

Fever
calories and, 358
Fiber, 18–19
bread and, 174, 270
in carbohydrates, 15, 17, 285
elimination and, 12, 18
in foods, 17, 15, 18, 19, 108, 110, 116,
  124, 125, 161, 166, 168, 169, 170, 171
in soft diet, 362
Fiber diet, 136–39
Figs, 126–27
Filberts, 82–83, 166
Finnan haddie, 138
Fish
allergy to, 369
buying guide, 136–41
cholesterol in, 23
fillets defined, 136
food chart, 60–61
as protein, 390
shelf list, 304
Fitness trail, 338
Fixx, Jim, 337
Flageolets, 161
Flatulence
beans and, 164
bland diet and, 362
digestive system of the elderly and, 318
Flavorings
in peanut spreads, 167
in milk products, 154–55
Flexibility, 321, 322, 323, 328, 329, 333,
  336, 351
Flounder, 138
Flours, 80–81, 173–74
in recipes, 218
soy flour, 163, 270, 372
Fluoride, 45–47
in foods, 46, 47, 138, 140
for infant, 308
Folacin (folic acid), 36–37
in foods, 37, 39, 40, 150, 173
during pregnancy and breast-feeding,
  33, 307
RDA, 33
Fontina cheese, 156
Food allergies. See Allergies.
Food and Drug Administration, U.S.,
  199, 289
Food aversions, 368
Food avoidance, 356
Food diary, 297, 300, 368
Food phobias, children learning, 311
Freezing foods, 207, 209, 313
refreezing, avoidance of, 140, 207, 208,
  309, 313
Fried foods, bland diet and, 362
Frozen custard, 155
Fructose, 13, 16
Fruits
in bland diet, 362
buying guide, 124–35
complex carbohydrates in, 15
in diet, 218
food chart, 64–71
foods from the wild, 181
for the elderly, 318
for infant, 309

during pregnancy, 307
shelf list, 304

G

Galactose, 13
Gallbladder, 11
Garbanzos. See Chick-peas.
Garlic, 114, 117
Gastric stapling, 282, 287
Ginger, 114, 178
Gjetost cheese, 156
Glucose 13, 14, 16, 17, 20
diabetes and, 16
energy supplied by, 13
for fueling the muscles, 334
Gluten
in flours, 173–74, 270–71
intolerance to, 355
oats and, 169
rye and, 171, 174
soy flour and, 163
in wheat, 171
Glycogen, 13, 14, 20
Goat's milk, 154
Goose, 152-53
Gooseberries, 125
Goosetongue greens, 181
Gorgonzola cheese, 157, 361
Gouda cheese, 157
Grading of foods
fruits, 124
meats, 142, 144, 146
Graham flour, 174
Grains
for adolescents, 314
buying guide, 168–75
in diet, 218, 372
fiber in, 366
food chart, 72-81
during pregnancy and breast-feeding,
  307
protein combinations, 285
sprouts from, 164–65
whole, in bread, 270
Grapefruit, 66–67, 127
Grapes, 66–67, 128
Green beans, 86–87, 109
Greens. See specific greens.
Grits, 168
Groats, 170
Growth
of adolescents, 314
children and calories, 310, 311
Gruyere cheese, 157
Guavas, 128

H

Haddock, 60–61, 138
Hake, 138
Halibut, 138
Handicaps, exercise and, 324
Hazelnuts, 166
Headaches
allergic reactions and, 368–79
exercise and, 330, 350

405

Index

Health clubs, 333, 346
Heart
  aerobics and, 334
  dynamic fitness and, 321
  exercise and, 320, 321, 351
  See also Atherosclerosis; Blood pressure; Cardiovascular disease; Heart disease; Pulse rate.
Heart (meat), 150
Heartburn
  bland diet for, 362
  constipation and, 365
  during pregnancy, 306
Heart disease
  cholesterol and, 22
  dieting and, 291, 292
  exercise and, 322, 324
  low-carbohydrate diet and, 288,
  stress test, 322
  sugar and, 17
  overweight and, 282
Heart disease, coronary, 322, 365, 374
Heart rate. *See* Pulse rate.
Heiden, Eric, 340
Hemorrhoids, 18, 306, 365
  during pregnancy, 306
Herbs and spices
  in bland diet, 363
  buying guide, 176–79
  herbal remedies, 357
  shelf list, 304
  as substitute for salt, 49, 176, 178, 218
  substituting dried herbs for fresh, 176
Hiatus hernia, 365
High-fiber diet, 18, 365–67
Hominy, 72–73, 168
Homogenization of milk, 154
Honey, 84–85
Hormones, 22, 31, 288, 314
  digestion and, 10
  proteins and, 24
Horseradish, 114
Household chores as exercise, 350–51
Huckleberries, 125
Hunger
  defined, 283
  fiber and, 18
Hydrochloric acid, 10–11
Hydrogenated fats, 21, 167
Hypertension, 356, 374
Hypnosis, 282, 287
Hypoglycemia, 16

I

Ice cream, 56–57
Ice milk, 56–57, 155
Ices, 155
Illness
  basal metabolism rate (BMR) and, 299
  and diet, 354–57
Indigestion, 364
Infants
  allergies of, 308, 309, 370
  breast-feeding and, 307
  eating sensibly and, 308–9
  RDA, 32–33
  swimming and, 342
Injuries
  exercise and, 348, 349
  from jogging, 337
Inorganic defined, 31
Inositol, 43
Insomnia
  exercise and, 320, 321, 328, 350
  warm milk for, 301, 355
Insulin, 15, 16
Inulin, 115
Intestines, digestion and, 11–12
  bland diet for, 362–64
  high-fiber diet for, 365–67
  problems in elderly, 318–19
  surgical bypass for, 287
Iodine, 46, 47
  in foods, 46, 47, 138, 140
  during pregnancy and breast-feeding, 33, 307
  RDA, 33
  in salt, 47–48
Iron, 45–47
  for adolescents, 33, 314, 315
  for children, 33, 310, 311
  deficiency of, 46, 355
  for the elderly, 318, 319
  excess mineral supplement of, 44, 46
  fiber and, 18
  food chart, 51–93
  in foods, 46–47, 108, 109, 110, 111, 113, 115, 116, 118, 121, 126, 142, 150, 153, 161, 163, 166, 167, 169, 170, 171, 174
  for infant, 33, 308, 309
  phytic acid and, 174
  during pregnancy and breast-feeding, 33, 307
  RDA, 33
  soy flour interfering with absorption of, 163
Isokinetics, 332, 333
Isometrics, 321, 332–33

J

Jane Brody's Nutrition Book (Jane Brody), 300–301
Jarlsberg cheese, 158
Jaw wiring, 282, 287
Jerusalem artichokes, 115
Jogging. *See* Running and jogging.
Jolliffe, Dr. Norman, 291, 292, 295, 384
Juices, 184–85
  for adolescents, 315
  for infants, 309

K

Kale, 88–89, 115
Kasha, 168
Kayaking, 343
Ketones
  in ketogenic diets, 287
  See also Fatty acids.
Ketosis, 14
  fasting diet and, 289
  ketogenic diet and, 286–89
Kidneys (human), 12, 373
  ketogenic diet and, 286–89
Kidneys (meat), 150
Kiwi fruit, 128
Kohlrabi, 115
Kraus-Weber tests, 322, 329, 330

L

Labels, 192, 194–99
  of liquid protein, 289
  natural, 172
  sodium in food, 48
  special diets and, 371, 372
Lactation. *See* Pregnancy and breast-feeding diet.
Lactose, 13
  intolerance to, 13, 371
Laetrile (amygdalin), 43
Lamb, 146–47
  food chart, 62–63
  variety meats of, 150–51
Lamb's quarters, 181
Lard, 58–59
Laxatives
  as diet pill, 288
  elderly and, 319
  during pregnancy, 306
Lecithin, 20, 43
Leeks, 115
Legumes
  buying guide, 161–65
  in diet, 218, 369
  during pregnancy, 307
  protein in, 15
  protein combinations, 285, 390
  See also specific beans; peas; and peanuts.
Lemons, 68–69, 129
Lentils, 82–83, 162
  sprouts, 165
Lettuce, 88–89, 116
Liederkranz cheese, 158
Limburger cheese, 158
Limes, 68–69, 129
Lindauer, Lois Lynns, 294
Linn, Dr. Robert, 289
Linoleic acid, 20, 286
  in foods, 51–93
Liquid diets, 286, 289, 359–60
Liquid protein diets, 284, 289
Liquids. *See* Beverages.
Liver (human), 11
  cholesterol made in, 22
  glycogen and, 14
  ketogenic diets and, 287
  storage of fat and, 12
Liver (meat)
  buying guide, 150
  food chart, 62–63
  as iron source, 302, 355
Lobster, 140
Loganberries, 125
Longevity

exercise and, 351
weight and, 298
Lower back pain
    exercise and, 328, 330
    yoga and, 33l
Low-salt diets
    saltwater fish in, 138
    shellfish in, 140
Luncheon meat, 62–63, 151
Lunches
    brownbag lunches, 312–13
    for children, 312–13
Lunge, 349
Lungs
    cardioresperatory system, 334
    exercise and, 320, 321
Lysine, 26, 390

M

Macadamias, 166
Mackerel, 138
Macrominerals, 44
Macronutrients, defined, 31
Magnesium, 45, 46
    in foods, 45, 46, 115, 129, 142, 154, 167, 168, 173
    RDA, 33
Maltose, 13, 16
Manganese, 45–47
    in foods, 46, 47, 168, 173
Mangoes, 129
Manz, Esther, 293
Margarines
    in breads, 270
    as butter substitute, 218
    cholesterol in, 23
    gaining weight and, 301
    hydrogenated, 21
    nutritive value of, 58–59
    shelf list, 304
Marjoram, 176, 178
Mayer, Jean, 283
Meal planning, 278–79
    for adolescents, 315
    balanced, 302–4
    brownbag lunches, 312–13
    for children, 311–13
    for the elderly, 318–19
    food chart and, 51
    for infants, 309
    for one, 304
    trying to gain weight and, 301
Meals (grains), in breads, 270
Meals on Wheels, 318
Meat extracts
    in bland diets, 362
    ulcers and, 363
Meatless menu, 279
Meats
    cholesterol in, 23
    cutting down on fat intake, 21
    in diet, 218
    food chart, 60–65
    herbs and spices for, 178
    for infant, 309
    during pregnancy, 307
Meat tenderizer

cubed steaks, 144
    papain in, 131
Medical letter, on Dr. Atkins' Diet Revolution, 290
Melons, 130
Menstruation
    anorexia nervosa and, 317
    exercise and, 324
    iron and, 315
Menus, 278–79
    See also Meal planning.
Metabolism, defined, 31
Methylcellulose, 288
Micronutrients, 31
Milk and milk products, 154–55
    for adolescents, 314–15
    allergies to, 368, 368
    amino acid pattern of, 26
    buying guide, 154–55
    in child's diet, 311, 368
    cholesterol in, 23
    cutting down on fat intake, 21
    to encourage sleep, 301, 355
    for infants, 309
    for the elderly, 319
    food chart, 52–57
    lactase deficiency and, 13
    nutrients in, 15
    nutritive value of, 52-57
    for pregnancy and lactation, 306–7
    shelf list, 304
    soy milk, 154, 163
    sugars in, 13
Milk toast, 360
Milkweed, 181
Millet, 169
Minerals, 10, 44–49
    in carbohydrates, 15
    dieting and, 283, 286, 292
    for the elderly, 318
    food chart, 51–93
    pregnancy and, 307
    RDA, 33
    See also specific minerals.
Mint, 176, 178
Miso, 163
Mollusks, 140
Molybdenum, 45–47
    in foods, 46, 150, 168, 173
Monterey cheese, 158
Mormons, 357
Morning sickness, 306–7
Mozzarella cheese, 52–53, 158
Mucin, 11
Muenster cheese, 158
Mullet, 138
Mung bean sprouts, 86–87, 121, 164–65
Muscles, 325
    aquaexercises and, 344–45
    building strength of, 320, 321, 322, 332–33, 344
    fueling of, 334
    muscle-bound, 333
    neglected, 348, 349
    soreness from overexertion, 337
    strength tests for, 329
    warm-ups and, 327, 328, 337, 342
Mushrooms, 90–91, 116
Muskmelons, 130

Mussels, 140
Mustard greens, 90–91, 116

N

National Academy of Sciences, 21
National Jogging Association, 336
Nausea
    exercise and, 322, 327, 337
    during pregnancy, 306–7
Nectarines, 130
New England Journal of Medicine, 22
Niacin, 36–38
    for adolescents, 33, 315
    food chart, 51-93
    in foods, 37, 38, 109, 118, 138, 140, 142, 150, 161, 167, 168, 170, 171, 173, 174
    during pregnancy and breast-feeding, 33, 307
    RDA, 33
Nickle, 47
Nidetch, Jean, 294-95
Nitrogen, ketogenic diet and, 286
Nonvitamins, 43
Noodles, 175
Nucleic acids, 31
Nursing women. *See* Pregnancy and breast-feeding.
Nutmeg, 178
Nutrient density, defined, 15
Nutrients, essential, 10–12
Nuts
    buying guide, 166–67
    shelf list, 304
    soy nuts, 163

O

Oat flour, 174
Oats, 169–70
Oatmeal, 72–73, 170
    in breads, 270
Obesity
    in adolescents, 316
    fats and, 21
    See also Overweight; Weight control.
Octopus, 140
Oils
    in breads, 270
    cholesterol in, 23
    for cooking, 214
    fat-controlled diets, 384–86
    fats in, 21
    gaining weight and, 301
    nutritive value of, 58–59
    during pregnancy, 307
    soy oil, 163
    vegetable oil as substitute for olive oil, 218
Okra, 90–91, 117
Oleic acid, 51–93
Olympic records, 324
Onion, 90–91, 117
    See also Leeks; Shallots.
Oral candidiasis (thrush), 355

407

Index

Oranges, 68–69, 130–31
Oregano, 176–78
Organic, defined, 31
Organic fitness, 321
Osteoporosis, 319, 354
Overeaters Anonymous, 293
Overweight, 12, 282–95
   in childhood, 312
   costs of, 282
   exercise and, 320, 33422
   hormones and, 31
   as risk factor, 322
   See also Dieting.
Oxtails, 150–51
Oxygen, aerobic conditioning and, 334
Oysters, 60–61, 141

P

PABA (para-aminobenzoic acid), 43
Pain, exercise and, 320, 322, 327, 330, 331, 337
Pakchoi. *See* Bokchoy.
Pancreas, 11
Pangamic acid (pangamate), 43
Pantothenic acid, 12, 36–37, 40
   in foods, 37, 40, 138, 140, 150, 153, l73
Papaya, 68–69, 131
Para-aminobenzoic acid, 43
Parcours, 338
Parmesan cheese, 52-53, 158
Parsley, 90–91, 177
Parsnips, 90–91, 118
Pasta, 175
   complex carbohydrates in, 15
   for infant, 309
   macaroni, 78–79
   noodles, 78–79, 175
   semolina and, 171, 173
   shelf list, 304
Pasteurization
   of milk, 154
   of processed cheese, 157
Peaches, 68–69, 131
Peanut butter, 82–83, 167
Peanuts, 82–83, 166–67
   soy nuts compared to, 163
Pears, 68–71, 132
Peas (fresh), 90–91, 118
   beach peas, 180
   black-eyed peas, 86
Peas (dried), 82–83, 86–87, 161, 163, 164
   as substitute for mung beans, 162
   See also Chick-peas.
Pecans, 82–83, 167
Peppers, 90–91, 118
Peristalsis, 10, 11
Persimmons, 132
Personality, 324
Perspiration
   exercise and, 326, 336
   warm-up suits and, 321
pH, digestion and, 10
Phosphorus, 44–46
   calcium and, 315
   food chart, 51–93
   in foods, 45, 46, 108, 110, 111, 115, 118, 119, 125, 138, 140, 142, 152, 154, 161, 163, 166, 167, 168, 169, 170, 173
   RDA, 33, 307
Physical fitness, defined, 322
Phytic acid, 174
Pig's feet, 148
Pineapple, 70–71, 132
Pine nuts, 167
Pistachios, 167
Plantains, 125
Pizza, 80–81
Plums, 70–71, 132–33
Pomegranate, 133
Popcorn, 15, 80–81, 169
Porgy, 138
Pork, 148
   food chart, 62–65
   in sausages, 151
   variety meats of, 150–51
Portions
   for the elderly, 318
   dieting and, 287, 294
   eating out and, 305
   of fish, defined, 136
   in recipes, 218
   Weight Watchers International, Inc., and, 294
Port Salut cheese, 158
Posture
   eating sensibly and, 301
   exercise and, 328, 329
Potassium, 45, 46
   diuretics and, 38
   food chart, 51–93
   in foods, 38, 45, 46, 108, 109, 110, 111, 112, 113, 115, 117, 118, 119, 120, 121, 125, 126, 128, 129, 130, 142, 154, 161, 163, 166, 169, 170, 173
Potatoes, 90–91, 119
   for infant, 309
   during pregnancy, 307
Pot cheese, 156
Poultry
   buying guide, 152–53
   cholesterol in, 23
   in diet, 218
   food chart, 64–65
   hearts of, 150
   livers of, 150
PPA (phenylpropanolamine), 288
Pregnancy and breast-feeding diet, 306–7
   alcohol and, 16
   basal metabolism rate, 299
   caloric needs, 12
   exercise and, 306–7, 324
   ketosis, 287
   Prudent diet for, 291
   RDA, 32–33
Preservatives, added to foods, 163, 166, 167
Prickly pear cactus, 181
Pritikin, Nathan, 292
Pritikin Program, 284, 292
Processed cheese, 52–53, 157
   additives and, 199–20l
   in diet, 218
Progressive resistance, 332
Protein deficiency, 285, 290, 292
Protein, 24–29
   for adolescents, 32, 314, 315
   allergic reactions and, 369
   in American diet, 10, 13, 14
   animal proteins, 26, 285, 290
   in balanced diet, 218, 284, 292
   calories supplied by, 12, 14
   child's need of, 310
   complementary combinations, 26–27, 285
   complete, 26, 285
   conversion to fat, 24
   dieting and, 283–86, 292
   digestion of, 11
   for the elderly, 318, 319
   food chart, 51–93
   in foods, 109, ll8, 136, 140, 142, 152, 153, 154, 161, 162–63, 166, 167, 168, 169;, 170, 171, 173, 174, 285
   incomplete, 26, 285
   in ketogenic diets, 286
   liquid protein, 289
   meal planning and, 302
   in milk, 154, 390
   protein-sparing diet, 24, 284
   RDA, 32, 307
   in soybeans, 163
   vegetable protein, 15, 25, 285, 290
Protein supplements, 284, 289
Provolone cheese, 52–53, 158
Prudent diet, 291, 295
Prunes, 70–71, 132
Pulse rate (heart rate)
   aerobics and, 334
   exercise and, 322, 326–27
   field and court sports and, 346
   household work and, 350
   target area, 326, 327, 328, 337
Pumpernickel flour, 174
Pumpkin, 90–91, 119
Pumpkin seeds, 82–83, 167
Pyridoxine (vitamin B_6), 36–39
   in foods, 37, 39, 138, 140, 150, 168, 173
   RDA, 33

Q

Quince, 133

R

Raclette cheese, 159
Radishes, 92–93, 119
Rashes (allergic reaction), 368
Raspberries, 70–71, 134
Rechtschaffen, Dr. Joseph S., 351
Recipes, 218–77
Reduce and Stay Reduced (Jolliffe), 291, 292
Rennin, 155
Resistance training, 332–33

Retinol. *See* Vitamin A.
Rhubarb, 70–71, 134
Riboflavin (vitamin B$_2$), 36–38
  for adolescents, 33, 315
  food chart, 51–93
  in foods, 36–38, 109, 110, 140, 150, 154, 161, 166, 168, 170, 171, 173, 174
  during pregnancy and breast-feeding, 33, 307
  RDA, 33
Rice, 80–81, 170–71
  amino acid pattern of, 26–27
  brown rice, 170
  complex carbohydrates in, 15
  in recipes, 218
  white rice, 170
  wild rice, 170–71
Rice flour, 174
Rickets, 34, 37, 355
Ricotta cheese, 52–53, 159
RNA, 31
Roasts
  beef, 142–43
  lamb, 146–47
  pork, 148–49
  veal, 144–45
Rock Cornish game hen, 152
Romano cheese, 159
Root, Waverley, 170
Roquefort cheese, 159
Rosemary, 177, 178
Roughage. *See* Fiber.
Rowing, 323, 325, 334, 343
Running and jogging, 336–37
  reciprocal training for, 349
  training for, 326
  women and, 324
Rutabaga, 120
Ryan, Albert J., 337
Rye, 171
Rye flour, 174
  in breads, 270

S

Sage, 178
Salad dressings, 58–61
Salads
  foods from the wild, 180–81
  herbs and spices for, 179
Saliva, 10
Salmon, 60–61, 138
Salmonella, 152, 153
Salsify, 120
Salt, 48–49
  in breads, 270
  in butter, 155
  in buttermilk, 154
  in cooking beans, 162
  herbs and spices as substitute for, 49, 176, 178, 218
  in infant's diet, 309
  meal planning and, 302
  in peanut butter, 167
  during pregnancy, 307
  in recipes, 218
  reducing amounts in diet, 374, 376–80
Sandwiches, in brownbag lunches, 312–13

Sapsago cheese, 159
Satiety, defined, 283
Sauerkraut, 92–93
Sausages, 64–65, 151
Savory, 177, 178
Scallions, 117
Scallops, 60–61, 141
Scarsdale diet, 286
Sculling, 344
Scurvy, 36–37, 40–41, 355
Seafood
  in diet, 218
  See also Fish; Shellfish.
Seatrout, 138
Sea trout (brown trout), 137, 138
Seeds
  buying guide, 166–67
  sprouts from, 164–65
Selenium, 45–47
  in foods, 46, 138 152, 168, 173
Self-defense, 330, 331
Semolina, 171, 173
Sesame seeds, 167
Seventh-Day Adventists, 357, 366, 367
Shad, 60—61
Shallots, 120
Shelf list, 304
Shellfish, 140–41
  cholesterol in, 23
Sheraton, Mimi, 358
Sherbet, 56–57, 155
Shopping
  buying guide,
  children and, 312
  eating habits and, 301
  shelf list, 304
Shortenings
  in breads, 270
  cholesterol in, 23
  hydrogenated, 21
Shrimp, 60–61, 141
Silicon, 47
Skating, 323, 325, 348–49
Skiing, cross-country, 323, 325, 334, 341
Sleep
  evening meal and, 304
  milk and, 355
  trying to gain weight and, 301
Smelt, 136–37
Smoking
  bland diet and, 364
  See also Cigarette smoking.
Snacks
  boredom and, 350
  for children, 311
  eating habits and, 300, 301
  eating out and, 305
  fiber and, 19
  for gaining weight, 301
  for the elderly, 318–19
  high fiber, 366
  for infants, 309
  for teenagers, 314
  for ulcer patients, 363
Snap beans. *See* Green beans.
Snapper, 139
Sodium, 45, 46, 48–49
  in foods, 45, 46, 48-49, 111, 112, 138, 140, 142, 151, 153, 154, 155, 161, 163, 168, 173

  ketogenic diet and, 287
  lack of carbohydrates and, 14
  maximum for adolescents, 315
Sodium nitrate, 148, 151
Sodium nitrite, 148, 151
  in pork, 148
  in sausages, 151
Soft drinks, 185
  adolescents and, 314–15
  calcium and, 315
Sole, 139
  flounder sold as, 138
Sore throats, special diets for, 358, 361
Sorghum, 171
Soups
  herbs and spices for, 178
  shelf list, 304
Sour cream, 54–55, 154–55
  butter made with, 154
Soybeans, 25, 154, 372
  dried, 162–63, 164
  fresh, 109
  protein in, 390
  sprouts, 163, 164–65
Soy flakes, 163
Soy flour, 163, 174
Soy nuts, 163
Soy oil, 163
Soy sauce, 163
Soy sprouts, 163, 164–65
Spaghetti, 80–81
  See also Pasta.
Spaghetti squash, 121
Spareribs, 146, 148
Spas, 333
  dieting and, 293
Spices. *See* Herbs and spices.
Spinach, 92–93, 121
Sports
  personality and, 324
  body type and, 324
  coordination and, 321
Sprouts, 121, 164–65
  soybean, 163, 164–65
Squash (sport), 346, 348
Squash (vegetable), 92–93, 122
  See also specific squashes; Pumpkin.
Squash, spaghetti, 121
Squid, 141
Staples, shelf list, 202, 304
Starches, 13, 15
  in grains, 168, 173
Stare, Dr. Frederick, 290
Steaks
  beef, 142–43
  of fish, defined, 136
  veal, 144–45
Stillman's Quick Weight Loss diet, Dr., 286, 290
Stilton cheese, 159
Stomach, 10–11
Strawberries, 70–71, 134–35
Strength, 329, 338
Stress
  basal metabolism rate (BMR) and, 299
  exercise and, 320, 321, 330
Stress test, 322
String beans. *See* Green beans.

Index

Stroke, 22
Sucrose, 13, 16
Sugars, 16–17
  in American diet, 13, 15–17
  cereals and, 172
  in diet, 218, 374
  food chart, 84–85
  in grains, 168
  in high-fiber diets, 365
  meal planning and, 302
  in milk products, 154–55, 157
  reducing amounts in diet, 302
Sulfa drugs, PABA and, 43
Sulfur, 45, 46
  in foods, 45, 138, 142, 152, 153, 154
Sunflower seeds, 82–83, 167
Supplements, 32, 42
  fasting diets and, 286
Support groups, dieting and, 293–95
Surgery
  bland diet following, 358
  weight loss by, 282
Sweat. *See* Perspiration.
Sweetbreads, 151
Sweeteners, in bread, 270
Sweet potatoes, 92–93, 122
Sweets, 16–17
Swimming, 322, 342–43, 349
  aquaexercises, 344–45
  for back-pain sufferers, 330
  body types and, 324
  sprints as interval training, 326
Swiss chard, 122
Swiss Emmentaler cheese, 52–53, 159
Swordfish, 139
Synthetic
  natural vitamins and, 42
  vs inorganic, 31
Syrups, 84–85

T

T'ai chi ch'üan, 331, 349
Take Off Pounds Sensibly (TOPS), 293
Taller, Dr. Herman, 290
Tamari, 163
Tangelo, 135
Tangerine, 70–71, 135
Tarragon, 178
Tea, 187–88
  gaining weight and, 301
  pregnancy and, 306
Teenagers. *See* Adolescents.
Teeth, sweets and, 17
  See also Dental Problems.
Tennis, 347, 348, 349
  dynamic fitness and, 322
Tension
  eating habits and, 300
  exercise and, 321, 328, 330
  walking and, 334
  yoga exercises and, 331
Thawed foods. *See* Freezing foods.
Thiamin (vitamin B_1), 35–37
  for adolescents, 33, 315
  destroyed by baking soda, 164
  food chart, 51–93
  in foods, 36, 37, 110, 118, 138, 140, 148, 150, 161, 163, 166, 168, 170, 171, 173, 174
  during pregnancy and breast-feeding, 33, 307
  RDA, 33
Thrush (oral candidiasis), 355
Thyme, 177, 178
Thyroid hormones, for dieting, 288
Tilsiter cheese, 159
Tin, 47
Tocopherol. *See* Vitamin E.
Tofu, 163, 285
Tomatoes, 92–93, 123
  in bland diet, 362
Tongue (meat), 151
Tooth decay. *See* Dental problems.
TOPS (Take Off Pounds Sensibly), 293
Toxicity
  herbal remedies and, 357
  of laetrile, 43
  shellfish and polluted waters, 140
  vitamin chart, 36–37
Trace minerals, 44–49
Tripe, 151
Triticale, 171
Triticale flour, 174
Trout, 137
Tuna, 60–61, 139
Turkey, 64–65, 153
Turnips, 92, 123

U

Ugli fruit, 135
Ulcers
  diet and, 355
  milk and, 363
Underweight, among adolescents, 314–17

V

Vacations, 351
Vanadium, 47
Varicose veins
  constipation and, 365
  resistance training and, 333
Variety meats, 150–51
Veal, 144–45
  food chart, 64–65
  variety meats of, 150–51
  See also Beef.
Vegetables
  for adolescents, 314
  in bland diet, 362
  in brownbag lunches, 313
  buying guide, 108–23
  complex carbohydrates in, 15
  cooking, 319, 361
  in diet, 218
  fiber in, 366
  food chart, 86–93
  herbs and spices for, 179
  home grown, 114
  for infant, 309
  in gaining weight, 301
  during pregnancy, 307
  protein combination, 285
  shelf list, 304
Vegetarian diets, 354, 390–94
  for weight control, 284
Villi, 11
Violet, 181
Vitamin A (retinol), 20, 32–34, 36–37
  for adolescents, 32, 315
  children and, 32, 311
  during pregnancy and breast-feeding, 32, 307
  RDA, 32
  food chart, 51–93
  in foods, 34, 37, 108, 109, 110, 111, 112, 113, 114, 115, 116, 117, 119, 120, 121, 122, 123, 124, 126, 127, 128, 129, 130, 131, 132, 133, 135, 150, 153, 154, 163, 164, 168
Vitamin B complex
  in foods, 115, 117, 164, 173, 174
  See also specific B vitamins.
Vitamin B_1. *See* Thiamin (vitamin B_1).
Vitamin B_2. *See* Riboflavin (vitamin B_2).
Vitamin B_3. *See* Niacin.
Vitamin B_6. *See* Pyridoxine (vitamin B_6).
Vitamin B_{12} (cobalamin), 36–37, 40
  in foods, 37, 40, 140, 142, 150, 153, 154
  RDA, 33
Vitamin B_{15}. *See* Pangamic acid.
Vitamin B_{17}. *See* Laetrile (amydalin).
Vitamin C (ascorbic acid), 36–37, 40–41
  for adolescents, 32, 315
  for children, 33, 310
  food chart, 51–93
  in foods, 37, 41, 108, 109, 110, 111, 112, 115, 116, 117, 118, 119, 120, 121, 122, 123, 126, 127, 128, 129, 130, 131, 132, 135, 163, 164, 181
  during pregnancy and breast-feeding, 33, 307
  RDA, 33
Vitamin D (calciferol), 20, 34, 36–37
  for adolescents, 32, 315
  for children, 310
  cholesterol and, 22
  in foods, 37, 138, 150, 153, 154, 174
  for infant, 32, 308, 309
  during pregnancy and breast-feeding, 32, 307
  RDA, 32
Vitamin E (tocopherol), 20, 34–37
  in foods, 35, 37, 150, 163, 166, 171, 173, 174
  RDA, 32
Vitamin H. *See* Biotin.
Vitamin K, 20, 35–37
  in foods, 35, 37
  large intestine and, 12
Vitamins, 10, 30–43
  in carbohydrates, 15
  dieting and, 283, 286, 292
  for the elderly, 318
  fat soluble, 20, 32–35
  food chart, 51–93
  megadoses, 42–43, 356
  over-the-counter, 42–43

pregnancy and, 307
RDA, 32–33
in seed husks, 165
toxicity symptoms, 36–37
water soluble, 32–33, 35–41
See also specific vitamins.
Vomiting
allergic reactions and, 368
clear liquid diet for, 359
dehydration and, 358
ice cubes for, 359
during pregnancy, 306–7

W

Waffles, 80
Walking, 320, 334–35, 337, 338, 350
as aerobic conditioning, 334–35
weight loss and, 321
Walnuts, 82–83, 167
Warming up, 326, 327, 328, 337, 338, 343
Warm-up suits, nonporous, 321, 336
Water, 10, 12, 50
in cheese, 155
in cucumbers, 113
in foods, 51–93

elderly and, 319
fasting diet and, 289
fluoridated, 47
gaining weight and, 301
high-fiber diet and, 365
illness and, 306
during meals, 301
in milk, 154
Watercress, 123
Watermelon, 70–71, 130
Wax
on cheese, 155
on cucumbers, 113
on eggplant, 113
Wax beans, yellow, 86–87, 109
Weight, ideal, 296, 298–99
Weight control, 282–95
Weight lifting, 332, 349
Weston, Edward Payson, 335
Wheat, 171
breakfast cereal, 72–75
cracked wheat, 171
intolerance to gluten and, 355, 369
wheat sprouts, 165
whole-wheat grains, 171
See also Whole grain; Whole wheat.

Wheat flours, 80–81, 173
Wheat germ, 74–75, 171
Whitefish, 137
Whole grain
defined, 169
storage of, 168
Whole-wheat flour, 173
Wild foods, 180–81
Wild fox grapes, 181
Wine, l90–91, 218, 301, 364

Y

Yams, 122
Yeast, in breads, 270
Yoga, 331, 349
Yogurt, 56–57, 155

Z

Zen macrobiotic diet, 290
Zinc, 46, 47
fiber and, 18
in foods, 46, 47, 140, 150, 167, 173
RDA, 33

Recipe Index

Note: Numbers in **boldface** *refer to recipe sections.*

A

Acorn squash and cranberries, 255
Appetizers, **218–21**
bean salad as, 257
broiled tomato halves, 218–19
carrot, celery, and egg salad, 219
chili bean dip, 218
eggplant salad, 219
French cauliflower pie, 220
marinated chick-peas, 220
marinated leeks, 219–20
Mediterranean ratatouille as, 256
melon and ginger, 220
peanuts-go-lightly dip, 219
polenta cheese squares, 221
ricotta cheese soufflés, 220–21
roasted chick-peas as, 264
vegetarian nut patties as, 265
Apples
baked, 275
baked carrots and apples, 251
in Indian pudding, 276
in Louisiana sweet potato salad, 258
in rhubarb compote, 274
Artichokes, Jerusalem, 252–53
Asparagus salad, 257
Aspic, chicken and vegetables in, 233
Austrian curd cake, 277

B

Baking powder biscuits, whole-wheat, 268–69
Ballpark mustard, 380
Banana-nut bread, 269
Bananas
in fruit snowball, 274
as substitute in basic buttermilk bran muffins, 366
Barbecue
Indian barbecued chicken, 233
sauce, 247
See also Charcoal grilling.
Barley
casserole, 266–67
mushroom, egg, and barley casserole, 243–44
Bass
French fish soup, 225–26
wrapped fish, 228–29
Beans, **262–64**
bean salad, 257
Boston baked beans, 263
caldo Gallego (Portuguese stew), 244–45
chili bean dip, 218
in kasha pie, 241
pasta e fagioli (noodles and beans), 260–61
roast lamb and beans, 237–38
vegetable broths, 227
See also specific beans.
Bean sprout salad, 257
Beef, **235–37**
basic pot roast of beef, 235
beef goulash, 236–37
beef tacos, 236
beef with onions and tomatoes, 236
curry marinade for, 247
goulash soup, 227
ground, in black beans and rice, 262
ground, broiled hamburgers, 235
Oriental beef, 236
Paris broil, 235
peppered roast beef, 235
s'chee (Russian cabbage soup), 223–24
as substitute in crisp-fried turkey breast, 234
Beets
beets and greens, 248
beets with tuna, 258
Biscuits, whole-wheat baking powder, 268–69
Black beans
black beans and rice, 262
black bean soup, 225
Haitian black beans, 263

411

Recipe Index

Black-eyed peas
   black-eyed pea soup, 224
   hoppin' John (black-eyed peas and rice), 263
Blueberries, fruit with honey-lime dressing, 274
Bluefish
   bluefish with citrus juices, 229
   broiled fish, 230
Bombay-style sole, 228
Boston baked beans, 263
Boston lettuce
   lettuce and asparagus stew, 252
   peas and lettuce, 252
Bouillon, tomato, 221
Bran muffins, basic buttermilk, 366
Breadcrumbs, seasoned, 268
Breads, 267–72
   whole-wheat bread, 272
   yeast breads, 270–72
Broccoli
   broccoli dressing, 246
   broccoli harlequin, 248–49
   broccoli with eggs, 249
   linguine with broccoli, 261
   in mustard greens and onions, 252
   as substitute in bean sprout salad, 257
   as substitute in French cauliflower pie, 220
   as substitute in pureed celeriac, 250
Brook trout, cooked on a plate, 227
Broths
   chicken, 226
   vegetable, 227
Brussels sprouts
   Brussels sprouts with water chestnuts, 249
   onion sauce for, 246
Buckwheat groats, roasted (kasha)
   kasha and red peppers, 265
   in kasha pie, 241
   kasha stuffing, 265
Buckwheat groats, unroasted, kasha pie, 241
Bulgur
   bulgur wheat with yogurt, 266
   fruited bulgur, 266
   Italian soybean-grains casserole, 244
   tabouli (Middle Eastern salad), 259
Buttermilk
   basic buttermilk bran muffins, 366
   buttermilk gazpacho, 222
   buttermilk pancakes, 268
   high-protein, low-calorie dressing, 246
   tarragon-buttermilk dressing, 245
Butternut squash, in squash and onions, 255

C

Cabbage
   five-minute soup, 222
   green, as substitute in red cabbage, 250
   green cabbage and garlic, 250
   s'chee (Russian cabbage soup) 223–24
   as substitute in French cauliflower pie, 220
Cabbage, red, 250
   kidney beans with red cabbage and apples, 264
Cakes
   Austrian curd cake, 277
   fresh fruit cake, 275
Caldo Gallego (Portuguese stew), 244–45
Calves' liver. See Liver, calves'.
Cantaloupes
   fruit with honey-lime dressing, 274
   melon and ginger, 220
   melon cooler, 277
Carrots
   baked carrots and apples, 251
   bean sprout salad, 257
   carrot, celery, and egg salad, 219
   carrots with dill, 251
   casserole of spring garden vegetables, 242
   Israeli carrot salad, 257
   Italian carrot torte, 276
   marinated carrot relish, 379
   in potato salad Tzapanos, 258
   stir-fried watercress with carrots, 251
   as substitute in pureed celeriac, 250
Casseroles
   barley casserole, 266–67
   casserole of spring garden vegetables, 242
   green bean casserole, 250
   Italian soybean-grains casserole, 244
   mushroom, egg, and barley casserole, 243–44
   Spanish casserole, 244
   See also One-dish meals.
Cauliflower
   broccoli harlequin, 248–49
   French cauliflower pie, 220
   pueblo cauliflower, 249
   as variation in potato salad Tzapanos, 258
Celeriac, pureed, 250
Celery, in carrot, celery, and egg salad, 219
Cereal
   granola, 267
   scallion-cheese cereal, 267
Charcoal grilling
   barbecue sauce, 247
   broiled chicken breasts with lime juice, 232
   tandoori chicken (Indian barbecue chicken), 233
   lamb shish kebab, 238
Cheeses
   blue cheese, as substitute in pears with Gorgonzola, 273
   Cheddar in green bean casserole, 250
   Cheddar in polenta cheese squares, 221
   Gorgonzola, pears with, 273
   mozzarella in eggplant Parmesan, 243
   mozzarella in lasagna, 241
   mozzarella in pizza rustica, 240–41
   Parmesan in eggplant Parmesan, 243
   Parmesan in ricotta cheese soufflés, 220–21
   ricotta in lasagna, 241
   ricotta cheese soufflés, 220–21
   Swiss cheese in lasagna, 241
   See also Cottage cheese.
Chicken, 231–34
   barbecue sauce for, 247
   broiled chicken breasts with lime juice, 232
   chicken and vegetables in aspic, 233
   chicken broth, 226
   chicken cacciatore, 231
   chicken in a pot, 226–27
   chicken salad, 260
   chicken with citrus fruits, 232
   chicken with wine vinegar, 231
   country captain, 232–33
   curry marinade for, 247
   garbure (French vegetable soup with meat), 245
   high-protein, low-calorie dressing for, 246
   roast chicken, 233
   roast chicken with Canadian bacon and cottage cheese, 234
   Romanian chicken stew, 232
   Spanish casserole, 244
   stuffed chicken breasts, 231
   tandoori chicken, 233
   tarragon-buttermilk dressing, 245
Chick-peas
   bean salad, 257
   gratin of chick-peas with spinach, 264
   marinated chick-peas, 220
   in minestrone, 223
   roasted, 264
   in vegetable paella, 243
Chili bean dip, 218
Chowders
   haddock chowder, 225
   vegetable chowder, 222–23
   Yankee bean chowder, 224
Clams, baked, 230
Cod
   baked on a bed of aromatic vegetables, 228
   in tomato crown haddock, 229
   wrapped fish, 228–29
Colache (Mexican vegetable medley), 256
Collard greens
   assorted greens, 251
   mustard greens and onions, 252
Cookies
   ginger, 276
   oatmeal snacks, 276
Corn
   colache (Mexican vegetable medley), 256
   oven-roasted sweet corn in the husk, 249
Cornmeal
   cornbread, 268

corn pone, 268
polenta cheese squares, 221
Cottage cheese
   in Austrian curd cake, 277
   in high-protein, low-calorie dressing, 246
   in lasagna, 241
   in roast chicken with Canadian bacon and cottage cheese, 234
   in scallion-cheese cereal, 267
   in Swiss chard and cheese pie, 242
   in white rabbit salad, 257
Country captain, 232–33
Crab, as substitute in halibut salad with dill, 260
Cracked wheat, in tabouli, 259
Cranberries, acorn squash and, 255
Cream of wheat, in farina dumplings, 266
Croutons, 269
Cucumbers
   grated cucumber relish, 248
   as variation in potato salad Tzapanos, 258

D

Daikon radish, in rutabaga pancakes, 254
Desserts, **273–77**
   Austrian curd cake, 277
   baked apples, 275
   figs in wine, 275
   fresh fruit cake, 275
   fruit snowball, 274
   fruit with honey-lime dressing, 274
   gingerbread, 277
   ginger cookies, 276
   ginger pears, 273
   Indian pudding, 276
   Italian carrot torte, 276
   mixed fruits, 273
   oatmeal snacks, 276
   orange-pineapple cup, 274
   pears with Gorgonzola, 273
   poached fresh peaches with raspberry sauce, 273
   red plum compote, 275
   rhubarb compote, 274
   roast pineapple, 274
Dips
   broccoli dressing, 246
   chili bean dip, 218
   eggplant salad as, 219
   hummus as, 391
   peanuts-go-lightly dip, 219
   for tofu, 392
Dressings. *See* Salad dressings; Stuffings.
Drinks, **277**
   melon cooler, 277
   orange smoothee, 277
Dumplings, farina, 266

E

Eggnog, 359
Eggplant
   eggplant Parmesan, 243
   eggplant salad, 219
   Mediterranean ratatouille, 256
   peppers and eggplant, 253
Eggs
   broccoli with eggs, 249
   carrot, celery, and egg salad, 219
   eggnog, 359
   in French cauliflower pie, 220
   gratin of spinach and hard-boiled eggs, 242
   mushroom, egg, and barley casserole, 243-44
   ricotta cheese soufflés, 220–21
Escarole, as substitute in stir-fried watercress with carrots, 251

F

Farina dumplings, 266
Fennel salad, 258
Figs in wine, 275
Fish, **227–30**
   baked on a bed of aromatic vegetables, 228
   bluefish with citrus juices, 229
   Bombay-style sole, 228
   broiled fish, 230
   Florida Keys red snapper, 229
   French fish soup, 225–26
   mustard sauce for, 246
   Scandinavian dry-baked flounder, 227–28
   tomato crown haddock, 229
   trout cooked on a plate, 227
   vegetable sauce for, 247
   wrapped fish, 228–29
   See also specific fish.
Flank steak
   Oriental beef, 236
   Paris broil, 235
Florida Keys red snapper, 229
Flounder
   baked on bed of aromatic vegetables, 228
   broiled fish, 230
   in French fish soup, 225–26
   Scandinavian dry-baked flounder, 227–28
   as substitute in Bombay-style sole, 228
Fowl, chicken in a pot, 226–27
French cauliflower pie, 220
French vegetable soup with meat (garbure), 245
Fruits, **273–75**
   fresh fruit cake, 275
   fruited bulgur, 266
   fruit snowball, 274
   mixed fruit, 273
   See also specific fruits.

G

Gado gado (Indonesian salad), 259
Garbure (French vegetable soup with meat), 245
Gazpacho, buttermilk, 222
Gingerbread, 277
Ginger cookies, 276
Ginger pears, 273
Goulash, beef, 236–37
Goulash soup, 227
Grains
   granola, 267
   Italian soybean-grains casserole, 244
   See also specific grains.
Gratin of spinach and hard-boiled eggs, 242
Great Northern beans, in roast lamb and beans, 237–38
Green beans
   chili bean dip, 218
   green bean casserole, 250
   as variation in potato salad Tzapanos, 258
Green peppers, as substitute in bean sprout salad, 257
Greens
   assorted greens, 251
   as substitute in baked kale, 251–52
   as substitute in stir-fried watercress with carrots, 251
   See also specific greens.
Grey sole, whole fish baked on a bed of aromatic vegetables, 228

H

Haddock
   haddock chowder, 225
   tomato crown haddock, 229
Haitian black beans, 263
Halibut
   halibut salad with dill, 260
   in tomato crown haddock, 229
   wrapped fish, 228–29
Ham
   caldo Gallego (Portuguese stew), 244–45
   garbure (French vegetable soup with meat), 245
   ham steak baked in milk, 239
   in stuffed chicken breasts, 231
Hamburgers, broiled, 235
Honeydew melons
   fruit with honey-lime dressing, 274
   melon and ginger, 220
   as a variation in melon cooler, 277
Hoppin' John (black-eyed peas and rice), 263
Hummus, 391

Recipe Index

I

Indian barbecued chicken (tandoori chicken), 233
Indian kedgeree (rice and lentils), 262
Indian pudding, 276
Indonesian salad (gado gado), 259
Israeli carrot salad, 257
Italian carrot torte, 276
Italian soybean-grains casserole, 244

J

Jerusalem artichokes, braised, 252–53

K

Kale
  baked, 251–52
  cream of vegetable soup, 222
  as substitute in Swiss chard and cheese pie, 242
Kasha
  kasha and red peppers, 265
  kasha pie, 241
  kasha stuffing, 265
Kedgeree, Indian (rice and lentils), 262
Ketchup, tomato, 246
Kidney beans
  bean salad, 257
  chili bean dip, 218
  in kasha pie, 241
  kidney beans with red cabbage and apples, 264
  white, in Romanian chicken stew, 232

L

Lamb, 237–38
  lamb shish kebab, 238
  lemon lamb roast, 237
  shoulder lamb chops braised with onions and peppers, 238
  as substitute in beef with onions and tomatoes, 236
Lasagna, 241
Leeks, marinated, 219–20
Legumes, 260–64
  See also specific beans and peas.
Lentils
  Indian kedgeree (rice and lentils), 262
  liver with lentils and yogurt, 240
  pasta e fagioli (noodles and beans), 260–61
Lettuce, Boston
  lettuce and asparagus stew, 252
  peas and lettuce, 252
Lettuces
  cream of vegetable soup, 222
  five-minute soup, 222
Linguine with broccoli, 261
Liver, calves', 239–40
  liver with lentils and yogurt, 240
  sautéed liver with wheat germ, 239–40
Lobster, as substitute in halibut salad with dill, 260
Louisiana sweet potato salad, 258

M

Marinades
  curry marinade, 247
  lamb shish kebab, 238
  marinated chick-peas, 220
  marinated leeks, 219–20
  Paris broil, 235
Mayonnaise, 247
Meal planning, 278–79
Meatless protein dish, Italian soybean-grains casserole, 244
Meat loaf, onion sauce for, 246
Meats, 235–40
  broccoli dressing as dip for, 246
  vegetable sauce for, 247
  See also specific meats.
Mediterranean ratatouille, 256
Melons
  fruit with honey-lime dressing, 274
  melon and ginger, 220
  melon cooler, 277
Mexican vegetable medley (colache), 256
Middle Eastern salad (tabouli), 259
Milk toast, 360
Minestrone, 223
Muffins
  basic buttermilk bran muffins, 366
  oatmeal-banana, 269
Mung bean sprouts, bean sprout salad, 257
Mushroom, egg, and barley casserole, 243–44
Mussels, 230
Mustard, ballpark, 380
Mustard greens
  assorted greens, 251
  mustard greens and onions, 252
  as substitute in Swiss chard and cheese pie, 242
Mustard sauce, 246

N

Navy beans
  Boston baked beans, 263
  caldo Gallego (Portuguese stew), 244–45
  Yankee bean chowder, 224
Nectarines, fruit with honey-lime dressing, 274
Noodles and beans (pasta e fagioli), 260–61
Nuts
  in kasha pie, 241
  in lasagna, 241
  vegetarian nut patties, 265

O

Oats, rolled
  granola, 267
  oatmeal-banana muffins, 269
  oatmeal snacks, 276
  oatmeal pancakes, 267
One-dish meals, 240–45
  caldo Gallego (Portuguese stew), 244–45
  casserole of spring garden vegetables, 242
  eggplant Parmesan, 243
  garbure (French vegetable soup with meat), 245
  gratin of spinach and hard-boiled eggs, 242
  Indian kedgeree (rice and lentils), 262
  Italian soybean-grains casserole, 244
  mushroom, egg, and barley casserole, 243–44
  Spanish casserole, 244
  Swiss chard and cheese pie, 242
  vegetable paella, 243
Onions
  mustard greens and onions, 252
  onion and roasted tomato relish, 248
  roasted, 253
  sauce, 246
  squash and onions, 255
Oranges
  mixed fruit, 273
  orange-pineapple cup, 274
Orange smoothee, 277
Oriental beef, 236
Oysters, baked, 230

P

Paella, vegetable, 243
Pancakes,
  buttermilk pancakes, 268
  oatmeal pancakes, 267
  pancake mix, 267
  rutabaga pancakes, 254
Parsley
  parsley soup, 221
  as substitute in cream of vegetable soup, 222
Parsnips, as substitute in casserole of spring garden vegetables, 242
Pasta, 260–61
  pasta e fagioli (noodles and beans), 260–61
  pasta marinara, 261
  spaghetti alla matriciana, 260
Pastry, for pizza rustica, 240
Pea beans, in Yankee bean chowder, 224
Peaches
  in fresh fruit cake, 275
  fruit with honey-lime dressing, 274
  poached fresh peaches with raspberry sauce, 273
  spinach creamed with peaches, 254

Peanut butter, 167
Peanuts-go-lightly dip, 219
Pears
    ginger pears, 273
    pears with Gorgonzola, 273
    as substitute in spinach creamed with peaches, 254
Peas
    peas and lettuce, 252
    spring pea soup, 224
    vegetable paella, 243
Peas, split, in minestrone, 223
Peppers, pickled, 247–48
Peppers, green or yellow sweet, in peppers and eggplant, 253
Peppers, red, kasha and, 265
Pies
    French cauliflower pie, 220
    kasha pie, 241
    pizza rustica, 240–41
    Swiss chard and cheese pie, 242
Pineapples
    in fresh fruit cake, 275
    melon cooler, 277
    mixed fruit, 273
    orange-pineapple cup, 274
    roast pineapple, 274
Pinto beans, in Boston baked beans, 263
Pizza rustica, 240–41
Plums, in red plum compote, 275
Polenta cheese squares, 221
Pork, **238–39**
    curry marinade for, 247
    ham steak baked in milk, 239
    pork bits, 381
    pork chops baked with orange, 239
    pork chops with spinach, 239
    pork sausage patties, 238
Portuguese stew (caldo Gallego), 244–45
Potatoes
    caldo Gallego (Portuguese stew), 244–45
    cream of vegetable soup, 222
    haddock chowder, 225
    potato salad Tzapanos, 258
    potato-tomato bake, 253
    pureed celeriac, 250
    steamed new potatoes in broth, 253
    as substitute in French cauliflower pie, 220
    turnip-potato puree, 254
Potatoes, sweet
    Louisiana sweet potato salad, 258
    as substitute in turnip-potato puree, 254
Pot roast of beef, 235
Poultry, **231–34**
    mustard sauce for, 246
    See also Chicken; Turkey.
Prosciutto, as substitute in stuffed chicken breasts, 231
Pueblo cauliflower, 249

R

Radish, daikon, in rutabaga pancakes, 254
Ratatouille, Mediterranean, 256
Red cabbage, 250
    kidney beans with red cabbage and apples, 264
Red plum compote, 275
Red snapper. See Snapper.
Relishes, 248
    ballpark mustard, 380
    marinated carrot relish, 379
    salsa fria, 379
    whole tomato chutney, 379
Rhubarb compote, 274
Rice
    black beans and rice, 262
    "dirty," 261–62
    green, 262
    hoppin' John (black-eyed peas and rice), 263
    Indian kedgeree (rice and lentils), 262
    Italian soybean-grains casserole, 244
    rice salad vinaigrette, 259
    Spanish casserole, 244
    as substitute in tabouli (Middle Eastern salad), 259
    vegetable paella, 243
Romaine lettuce, in cream of vegetable soup, 222
Romanian chicken stew, 232
Russian cabbage soup (s'chee), 223–24
Rutabagas
    crisp rutabaga salad, 258
    rutabaga pancakes, 254
    as substitute in casserole of spring garden vegetables, 242

S

Salad dressings
    broccoli dressing, 246
    high-protein, low-calorie dressing, 246
    mayonnaise, 247
    simple vinaigrette, 245
    tarragon-buttermilk dressing, 245
Salads, **257–60**
    asparagus salad, 257
    bean salad, 257
    bean sprout salad, 257
    beets with tuna, 258
    carrot, celery, and egg salad, 219
    chicken salad, 260
    crisp rutabaga salad, 258
    eggplant salad, 219
    fennel salad, 258
    gado gado (Indonesian salad), 259
    grated cucumber relish, 248
    halibut salad with dill, 260
    Israeli carrot salad, 257
    Louisiana sweet potato salad, 258
    marinated chick-peas, 220
    marinated leeks as, 219–20
    potato salad Tzapanos, 258
    rice salad vinaigrette, 259
    tabouli (Middle Eastern salad), 259
    white rabbit salad, 257
Salsa fria, 379
Sauces and relishes, **245–48**
    barbecue sauce, 247
    broccoli dressing, 246
    cold vegetable sauce, 247
    curry marinade, 247
    grated cucumber relish, 248
    high-protein, low-calorie dressing, 246
    mayonnaise, 247
    mustard sauce, 246
    onion and roasted tomato relish, 248
    onion sauce, 246
    pickled peppers, 247–48
    simple vinaigrette, 245
    tarragon-buttermilk dressing, 245
    tomato ketchup, 246
Sausage
    pork sausage patties, 238
    roast turkey with sausage dressing, 234
Scallions
    scallion-cheese cereal, 267
    as substitute in marinated leeks, 219–20
Scandinavian dry-baked flounder, 227–28
S'chee (Russian cabbage soup), 223–24
Sea bass
    baked on a bed of aromatic vegetables, 228
    as substitute in Florida Keys red snapper, 229
Shellfish, **230**
    baked oysters or clams, 230
    mussels, 230
Shish kebab, lamb, 238
Shrimp, as substitute in halibut salad with dill, 260
Snacks
    chili bean dip, 218
    gingerbread, 277
    grated cucumber relish, 248
    oatmeal snacks, 276
    orange smoothee, 277
    peanut butter, 167
    pork bits, 381
    roasted chick-peas, 264
Snapper
    baked on a bed of aromatic vegetables, 228
    Florida Keys red snapper, 229
    in French fish soup, 225–26
Snow peas, as substitute in bean sprout salad, 257
Sole
    baked on a bed of aromatic vegetables, 228
    Bombay-style sole, 228
    as substitute in Scandinavian dry-baked flounder, 227–28
    tarragon-buttermilk dressing for, 245
Soufflés, ricotta cheese, 220–21

Recipe Index

Soups, 221–27
  black bean soup, 225
  black-eyed pea soup, 224
  buttermilk gazpacho, 222
  chicken broth, 226
  chicken in a pot, 226–27
  cream of vegetable soup, 222
  five-minute soup, 222
  French fish soup, 225–26
  garbure (French vegetable soup with meat), 245
  goulash soup, 227
  haddock chowder, 225
  melon cooler, 277
  minestrone, 223
  parsley soup, 221
  s'chee (Russian cabbage soup), 223–24
  spring pea soup, 224
  tomato bouillon, 221
  vegetable broths, 227
  vegetable chowder, 222–23
  Yankee bean chowder, 224
Soybeans
  Italian soybean-grains casserole, 244
  kasha pie, 241
Spaghetti
  pasta e fagioli (noodles and beans), 260–61
  pasta marinara, 261
  spaghetti alla matriciana, 260
Spanish casserole, 244
Spinach
  five-minute soup, 222
  gratin of chick-peas with spinach, 264
  gratin of spinach and hard-boiled eggs, 242
  spinach creamed with peaches, 254
  as substitute in baked kale, 251–52
  as substitute in cream of vegetable soup, 222
  as substitute in stir-fried watercress with carrots, 251
  as substitute in Swiss chard and cheese pie, 242
Squash, acorn, and cranberries, 255
Squash, butternut, and onions, 255
Squash, yellow summer, as substitute in grated zucchini, 255
Steak, flank
  Oriental beef, 236
  Paris broil, 235
Steak, sirloin, beef goulash, 236–37
Stews
  vegetable, 256
  See also specific meats.
Strawberries
  in fresh fruit cake, 275
  fruit snowball, 274
Stuffings
  bread stuffing, 269
  kasha stuffing, 265
  roast turkey with sausage dressing, 234
  stuffed chicken breasts, 231
Summer squash, yellow, as substitute in grated zucchini, 255

Sweet potatoes
  Louisiana sweet potato salad, 258
  as substitute in turnip-potato puree, 254
Swiss chard and cheese pie, 242

T

Tabouli (Middle Eastern salad), 259
Tacos, beef, 236
Tandoori chicken, 233
Tofu
  dip for, 392
Tomato bouillon, 221
Tomato ketchup, 246
Tomatoes
  baked cherry tomatoes, 255–56
  broiled tomato halves, 218–19
  onion and roasted tomato relish, 248
  pasta marinara, 261
  potato-tomato bake, 253
  in salsa fria, 379
  spaghetti alla matriciana, 260
  tomato crown haddock, 229
  whole tomato chutney, 379
Trout, cooked on a plate, 227
Tuna, beets with tuna, 258
Turkey
  barbecue sauce for, 247
  crisp-fried turkey breast, 234
  in garbure (French vegetable soup with meat), 245
  roast turkey with sausage stuffing, 234
Turnip greens
  assorted greens, 251
  as substitute in baked kale, 251–52
  as substitute in cream of vegetable soup, 222
  as substitute in mustard greens and onions, 252
  as substitute in Swiss chard and cheese pie, 242
Turnips, casserole of spring garden vegetables, 242
Turnips, white
  chili bean dip, 218
  in crisp rutabaga salad, 258
  crisp shredded turnips, 254
  in rutabaga pancakes, 254
  turnip-potato puree, 254
Turnips, yellow
  turnip-potato puree, 254
  crisp shredded turnips, 254

V

Veal
  as substitute in crisp-fried turkey breast, 234
  veal stew, 237
Vegetables, 248–56
  broccoli dressing as dip for, 246
  casserole of spring garden vegetables, 242

chicken and vegetables in aspic, 233
  chicken broth, 226
  colache (Mexican vegetable medley), 256
  cold vegetable sauce, 247
  cream of vegetable soup, 222
  dips for, 218, 219
  fish baked on bed of, 228
  gado gado (Indonesian salad), 259
  garbure (French vegetable soup with meat), 245
  marinated leeks, 219–20
  minestrone, 223
  rice salad vinaigrette, 259
  simple vinaigrette for, 245
  tabouli (Middle Eastern salad), 259
  in tomato bouillon, 221
  vegetable broths, 227
  vegetable chowder, 222–23
  vegetable paella, 243
  vegetable stew, 256
  See also specific vegetables.
Vegetarian nut patties, 265
Vinaigrette, simple, 245

W

Water chestnuts, Brussels sprouts with, 249
Watercress
  cream of vegetable soup, 222
  stir-fried watercress with carrots, 251
Watermelon, as variation in melon cooler, 277
Weakfish, broiled fish, 230
Wheat, cracked, in tabouli (Middle Eastern salad), 259
Wheat germ
  sautéed liver with wheat germ, 239–40
  as substitute in baked carrots and apples, 251
White beans
  caldo Gallego (Portuguese stew), 244–45
  garbure (French vegetable soup with meat), 245
  roast lamb and beans, 237–38
  white beans in olive oil, 263
White rabbit salad, 257
Whiting, backed on a bed of aromatic vegetables, 228
Whole-wheat
  baking powder biscuits, 268–69
  bread, 272

YZ

Yankee bean chowder, 224
Yogurt
  high-protein, low-calorie dressing, 246
  as substitute in orange smoothee, 277
Zucchini
  grated, 255
  Mediterranean ratatouille, 256
  zucchini and fresh dill, 255